Anterior Controllable Antedisplacement and Fusion

Anterior Controllable Antedisplacement and Fusion
Technique in Spinal Surgery

Edited by

Jiangang Shi

Chief Physician of the Department of Spine Surgery in Changzheng Hospital, and Chairman of Academic Association

ELSEVIER　　SCIENCE PRESS

Publisher: Sarah E. Barth
Acquisitions Editor: Humayra R. Khan
Editorial Project Manager: Matthew Mapes
Project Manager: Selvaraj Raviraj
Cover Designer: Greg Harris

3251 Riverport Lane
St. Louis, Missouri 63043

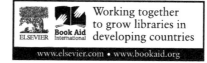

Working together to grow libraries in developing countries

www.elsevier.com • www.bookaid.org

Contents

Foreword

This book is a monograph compiled by the team of Prof. Shi Jiangang from Shanghai Changzheng Hospital based on their years of clinical experience on a new surgical strategy for ossification of the posterior longitudinal ligament (OPLL), making breakthrough reforms and innovations both in theory and technique. As a senior doctor with a practice dating back decades ago, I am honored to preface this monograph upon invitation. Taking this opportunity, I would like to touch upon OPLL-related academic topics.

OPLL was first recorded by British doctor Key in 1838, more than 180 years ago. Given the primitive status of medical development and inefficient communication, people knew little about OPLL and few doctors paid attention to the disease entity until the 1960s when a Japanese professional identified the abnormally ossified tissues of the posterior longitudinal ligament (PLL) on cadaver specimens and named it OPLL in 1964. It was described as a pathology of heterotopic ossification in the PLL, more commonly in East Asians with elusive pathogenesis. Cervical OPLL is also found in patients with diffuse idiopathic skeletal hyperostosis (DISH), a common condition in Europeans and Americans. With the advancement of imaging diagnostics in the past 30 years, the detection rate of OPLL has increased dramatically. Epidemiological surveys have shown that it affects 1.7%—3% of the general population. Indeed, OPLL has become a major disease in the spectrum of spinal pathologies.

The PLL's ossified tissues may be present for a long time with imaging findings but without spinal cord compression, called asymptomatic OPLL. Technically, cervical OPLL refers to conditions where the ossified tissues have caused signs and symptoms through the spinal cord and nerve root compression. This lesion is unique because it is located anteriorly in the spinal canal with marked contact with the spinal dural sac. Among the diverse surgical techniques described for OPLL, laminoplasty has been a constant dominant technique described by Japanese surgeons to initially avoid the shortcomings of total laminectomy. This technique achieves spinal cord decompression by expanding the spinal canal at the diseased segment and allowing the spinal cord to shift backward. However, it was gradually noted in clinical practice that the progression of ossification caused neural deterioration, and cervical kyphosis was a contraindication for laminoplasty. The direct removal of the ossified tissues through the anterior approach achieves definitive decompression, which is more conducive to the restoration of cervical curvature and the shape and volume of the spinal canal. The anterior approach provides significantly better results than the indirect decompression through the posterior approach but comes with more technical challenges and morbidities.

In the mid to late 1970s, the Department of Spine Surgery of Shanghai Changzheng Hospital, the authors' unit, developed rapidly and achieved brilliant results in basic and clinical research, setting it as one of the leading programs in spine surgery in China. Entering the 21st century, the program has focused on OPLL and accomplished outstanding achievements. In 2006, Prof. Chen Deyu's team designed and implemented the segmental decompression technique of the OPLL with increased surgical efficacy and significantly reduced complications, and laid the foundations for the innovative techniques that follow.

In 2016, Prof. Shi Jiangang's team developed and carried out the anterior controllable antedisplacement fusion (ACAF) technique, a controllable technique that expands the spinal canal with reduced complications typically seen in anterior procedures and aligned with the advantages of minimally invasive surgery. Based on the anatomical features of the cervical spine, this technique anteriorly displaces the vertebrae and the OPLL as a whole while maintaining the natural location of the spinal cord of the involved segments, thus expanding the spinal canal and relieving the compression. As a landmark breakthrough innovation, this technique represents brand-new ideas about OPLL treatment.

This monograph, compiled by Prof. Shi Jiangang, focuses on the basics and procedures of the innovative ACAF technique based on the biological, pathological, and anatomical profiles of OPLL. With a unique theme and distinctive features, it is an invaluable surgical monograph that addresses a specific disease of the cervical spine, featuring a well-structured fundamental and technical explanation with exhaustive technical pearls. My endorsement goes to this work from Prof. Shi Jiangang and his team not because he is my protege but, indeed, it provides invaluable guidance for clinical practice. My definition for an excellent professional is one who keeps pondering over his field of interest, the everyday work, and the variability among cases, which is the only way a surgeon can make progress in each patient whom he provides care.

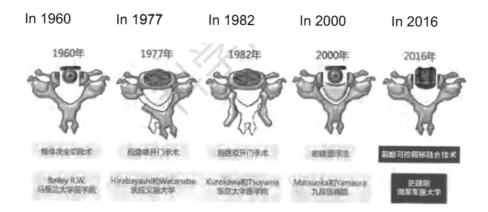

| In 1960 | In 1977 | In 1982 | In 2000 | In 2016 |

Sub-total Corpectomy
Posterior Single-door Laminoplasty
Posterior Double-door Laminoplasty
Anterior Floating Method
Anterior Controllable Antedisplacement and Fusion

Bailey R.W.
University of Maryland School of Medicine

Hirabayashi and Watanabe
Keio University

Kurokawa and Tsuyama
Graduate School of Medicine, The University of Tokyo

Matsuoka and Yamaura
Kudanzaka Hospital

Shi Jiangang
Shanghai Changzheng Hospital

As an excellent monograph that summarizes the experience gained from practice and scientific analysis, this work from Professor Shi Jiangang will become a classic one.

March 2019

Preface

—— A Brief Overview of the ACAF Technique

I was overwhelmed by excitement when I began with this introduction.

An ancient Chinese quote has it that "It has taken me ten years to sharpen a sword, and now I'm going to test its edge." It has been 16 years since we first had the idea of the anterior controllable antedisplacement fusion (ACAF) technique, which was later promoted nationwide and even worldwide. Looking back on the past 16 years, I would like to introduce its chronological development as the start of this monograph.

The ACAF technique is the fruit of the decades of cervical spine practice of the Department of Orthopedics of Shanghai Changzheng Hospital. It is a new surgical technique for severe cervical ossification of the posterior longitudinal ligament (OPLL) that my team and I described for the first time in international literature based on the fundamentals of in situ spinal cord decompression.

In October 2003, my colleagues and I planned surgery on a patient with severe OPLL, a professor from Fudan University. Since an anterior approach was particularly risky when the stenosis involved over 65% of the canal, we performed a posterior laminectomy for better surgical safety. After the operation, the patient had significantly improved muscle strength of the lower limbs but persistent and worsen numbness of the arms. The imaging studies revealed adequate decompression and marked posterior shift of the spinal cord. The patient's anguish of "increased arm numbness" triggered our team's dedication to seeking causes and solutions.

By November 2005, anterior cervical decompression surgery typically included the Cloward technique, the Smith-Robinson technique, and subtotal corpectomy and decompression, with the latter providing more extensive and thorough decompression than the former two techniques. However, with the increased number of segments involved in decompression and fusion, the bone graft fusion rate declines, and the cervical spine becomes destabilized due to the absence of a significant part of the vertebra. As such, Prof. Yuan Wen described an innovative extended decompression technique with subtotal corpectomy that preserves the posterior wall of the vertebra in November 2005. Featuring sufficient decompression through safe and straightforward operation, this technique boasts improved bone graft fusion rate and cervical spine stability and recognizes the importance of the spinal canal integrity. It also provided the clinical basis for the overall antedisplacement of the vertebral-OPLL complex (VOC) and spinal canal reconstruction and turned into the principles of the ACAF technique.

In April 2009, in view of severe complications in patients with severe OPLL undergoing anterior surgery, hemilaminectomy was adopted as a risk-reduction strategy in Shanghai Changzheng Hospital under the guidance of Prof. Jia Lianshun. This technique was effective in most patients, but some of them still had numbness in the arms and fingers and imaging evidence of compressed spinal cord and nerve roots. In performing the hemilaminectomy, we realized that removing only half of the lamina achieved decompression without risks of aggravating radiculopathy because the lamina that remained prevents the posterior shift of the spinal cord. This procedure was a significant step forward because it provided us a practical basis for in situ spinal cord decompression. In the same year, Prof. Chen Deyu summarized years of experience in the surgical treatment of patients with cervical OPLL and described the approach through the "safe interval" in the hope of reducing the risk of the ossification resection procedure, in particular, the incidence of cerebrospinal fluid (CSF) leakage. However, it was not easy to identify this safe interval during the operation, leaving CSF leakage as a constant risk for spine surgeons. The attempts made in this period served as an essential clinical basis for the concept of "vertebral-OPLL-dura complex."

In July 2012, with the long-term follow-up of a large number of patients undergoing the conventional anterior or posterior surgery, we found that excessive anteroposterior or lateral displacement or rotation of the spinal cord caused nerve root traction injuries and unfavorable clinical prognosis. Such observation provided evidence for the development of the concept of in situ spinal cord decompression.

In November 2012, to further demonstrate the logic and feasibility of ACAF, we started a two-year anatomic study at the Second Military Medical University and the Teaching and Research Section of Anatomy of Fudan University.

In January 2015, we completed specimen studies and published the first edition of Anatomical Illustration of Spinal Surgery, which demonstrated that the cervical nerve roots were anchored by the surrounding ligaments at the neural exit foramina. Therefore, the excessive drift of the spinal cord would inevitably lead to nerve root traction injuries. Follow-up anatomical studies have validated our understanding that only by restoring the malpositioned spinal cord to its original natural state can a better clinical effect be achieved, a state only achievable through anterior surgeries.

In February 2016, we reviewed the imaging data of a large number of patients with OPLL who had undergone anterior surgery and concluded that the vertebra, OPLL, and the dura at the lesion became an adhered complex. It is the destruction of this complex in conventional techniques that lead to CSF leakage. Enlightened by this clinical fact, we wondered if we can achieve thorough decompression of the spinal cord and nerve roots through the antedisplacement of the entire complex without resecting it. By then, based on the pathological characteristics of OPLL, the concept of "OPLL complex" had become increasingly evident. My team and I then began to design the model and conduct anatomical experiments. Dr. Sun Jingchuan and colleagues conducted multiple experiments on human models and modified the surgical procedure step by step, paving the way for the clinical application of the ACAF technique.

In a national conference I attended as a moderator in May 2016, I presided over a session of reports on Surgical Exposure of the Vertebral Artery. The interaction with the speakers reaffirmed our understanding of the anatomical structure and profiles of the vertebral arteries and provided evidence for our technique of "bilateral groove development" on the vertebrae, an essential step of the ACAF technique. Returning from that meeting, I immediately convened the team to refine the proposed procedure, conducted a biomechanical study on the experimental models that we developed, and went through ethical evaluation.

In July 2016, the ACAF technique was successfully performed on a patient with severe OPLL and visual impairment. The fingers' tactile sensation is the second pair of eyes for people with compromised vision, and this patient had been despondent with his digital numbness, whose resolution rest upon decompression of multiple nerve roots. At the preoperative discussion meeting, my team had divided opinions on which approach to take, the anterior or the posterior. To make it work in the complex surgery involving multiple segments, I decided to take this challenge. With meticulous planning and preparation, we performed the ACAF technique for the patient. The operation lasted for more than six hours. At two o'clock in the morning, when the patient awoke from anesthesia and told us that his fingers did not feel numb anymore, our team cheered the ACAF technique's success. Within that month, we successfully carried out the procedure on a second complex case, a dependent patient with 90% cervical canal stenosis wheeled in on admission. During the operation, I developed grooves on both sides of the vertebrae to thoroughly decompress the pairs of nerve roots of each segment and displaced the complex forward in a controllable manner. Being "controllable" ensures the steady process of the entire decompression, a prerequisite for successful decompression from an anterior approach regardless of the size and dimension of the OPLL. The patient recovered well after the operation and walked out of the hospital upon discharge in no need of assistance.

In August 2017, the ACAF technique was reported internationally for the first time.

In October 2017, to continuously improve the ACAF technique and verify the difference in stability between it and the conventional surgical techniques, we cooperated with the team of Academician Zhong Shizhen from the Institute of Clinical Anatomy of Southern Medical University in the comparative biomechanical studies among multiple surgical techniques. The results reaffirmed us that the ACAF technique had comparable stability to the conventional anterior cervical discectomy and fusion (ACDF) technique and significantly better stability than the anterior cervical corpectomy decompression and fusion (ACCF) technique. We validated the safety of the ACAF technique in terms of the risk of vertebral artery injuries and investigated the limit of the disease where the ACAF technique is applicable, providing guidelines to its use in the wide-based and extreme lateral OPLL. After studying the spinal cord and nerve roots of post-ACAF fresh specimens, we found that the ACAF technique left a larger decompression width than conventional surgical techniques, which resulted in relieved neural exit foramina and compression-free roots and courses of multiple groups of nerve on both sides. This finding lent support to the application of the ACAF technique in cervical spinal stenosis and revision surgeries.

In December 2017, the first national course on the ACAF technique was held.

In November 2018, a focused discussion on the ACAF technique was held at the 13th Annual Congress of the Chinese Orthopaedic Association. By then, the ACAF technique had been reported six times by peers around the world at international academic conferences.

By October 2019, the ACAF technique had been widely carried out in China. This surgical technique achieves four breakthroughs in anterior surgery for severe OPLL: ① Conventionally, anterior surgery is contraindicated when the lesion involves more than three segments, but ACAF can manage up to six segments. ② OPLL above C2 is no longer a contraindication for anterior surgical decompression. ③ The indication of the anterior procedure has been expanded to include spinal canal stenosis up to 80%. ④ It minimizes the incidence of complications, such as CSF leakage.

The ACAF technique has been applied to the surgical treatment of cervical spinal stenosis and cervical revision surgeries. We also applied this novel surgical idea to the ossification of the thoracic posterior longitudinal ligament and the ossification of the ligamentum flavum (OLF). When adapted to the thoracic spine, the technique becomes antedisplacement for the thoracic OPLL and posterior displacement of OLF. These new techniques have achieved good efficacy and provide new solutions to severe ossification of the thoracic ligaments.

That is our journey, starting with the professor with OPLL from Fudan University in 2003 and marked with the description of the ACAF basic principles, the "basics of in situ spinal cord decompression," the "concept of vertebral-OPLL complex," and the implementation of ACAF technique. With more than 10 years of persistence, we have fed the concept-practice-concept loop with relentless practicing, thinking, and studying. Now, this technique has been valued by expert spine surgeons in many countries and regions with growing influence and popularity. "Success and achievements cannot be made without talents." Facing a high incidence of OPLL in, we hope that more and more spine surgeons can understand and address this disease and that this book can guide more spine surgeons to apply the ACAF technique. Let's work together for the benefit of more OPLL patients.

I would like to take this opportunity to extend my sincere thanks to Shanghai Changzheng Hospital, where I work. The resources here have inspired me to develop profound thinking from my practice so that I am able to apply and improve my thoughts in the clinical practice. My gratitude also goes to Prof. Jia Lianshun, my mentor, as well as Academician Qiu Guixing, Academician Zhang Yingze, Academician Tian Wei, Academician Zhong Shizhen, Prof. Yuan Wen, Prof. Xiao Jianru, Prof. Chen Deyu, Prof. Ni Bin, Prof. Ye Xiaojian, Prof. Xu Rongming, Prof. Qiu Yong, Prof. Lv Guohua, and other experts and professors for their guidance, encouragement, and support. Finally, I would like to thank my team members for their long-standing hard work, perseverance, and dedication. This technique has been available for only around 10 years. Though achieving extraordinary clinical efficacy for the moment, it still needs to be validated with a large number of cases and improved with modified basics. I hope that the spine experts across China will work together to enrich and advance this technique in clinical practice.

Just like a newborn baby who needs care and love, this new technique requires many of us to practice and verify in order to become more and more established.

When a child comes of age, the gratitude towards parenting prevails. Similarly, when a new technique has manifested benefits on a larger population, the dedication of the care providers prevails. Gathering the wisdom and experience of all experts, we will advance health to a new level in China.

October 19, 2019
Shanghai

Introduction

With the change of lifestyles and pace, patients' expectations for quality life are growing, posing new challenges to the surgical treatment of cervical spine diseases. Particularly, due to great difficulty in treatment and high risk of surgery, serious diseases such as ossification of the posterior longitudinal ligament (OPLL) and cervical spondylotic myelopathy (CSM) with multisegment spinal stenosis put tremendous pressure on spine surgeons and heavy burdens on patients.

Based on the years of experience in the treatment of OPLL, the authors of this book have described a new technique of anterior controllable antedisplacement and fusion (ACAF) through repeated attempts, innovative ideas, and investigations. The ACAF technique provides a new surgical method for the compression between the vertebra and the spinal cord. Effective in treating a series of posterior compressions such as OPLL and multisegment spinal stenosis, it has been carried out in many spine centers. This textbook provides a comprehensive description of the ACAF technique with principle, procedure, indications, and case series and explains the surgical steps and pearls. We have compiled this textbook in the hope of communicating profoundly with peers and promoting the ACAF technique to benefit more patients with spine diseases.

The book is composed of four chapters. Chapter 1 introduces the concept and surgical principles of the ACAF technique and provides a historical review of cervical spine surgery. Chapter 2 focuses on the indication of the ACAF technique in CSM and OPLL by analyzing the characteristics of the diseases and reviewing previous surgical techniques. Chapter 3 focuses on the procedure of the ACAF technique and explains in detail how to complete a standard ACAF operation with proper surgical steps, techniques, key skills, instruments, and devices. Chapter 4 includes a large number of ACAF cases with an individualized discussion of case profile and surgical details as a supplement to the first three chapters.

This book objectively and exhaustively records the detailed process of the ACAF technique from design to application, for the reference of spine surgeons and rehabilitation physicians at all levels.

Principles of the anterior controllable antedisplacement and fusion technique

Section 1: A brief history of cervical spine surgery

Cervical spine surgery is a time-honored and constantly evolving surgical treatment that involves sophisticated anatomical relationships and neurological relevance and thus requires surgeons to operate meticulously. However, this subject has never been devoid of courageous and intelligent pioneers who have kept exploring and trying. The earliest spinal treatment was described in Edwin Smith Papyrus from ancient Egypt [1] where one of the scenes depicts resting, immobilization, and wound binding for patients with cervical spine fractures. In ancient Greece, anatomy developed rapidly. Hippocrates invented manual reduction with rope traction and splinting for patients with spinal fractures. During the same period, doctors made various surgical attempts, including laminectomy. In ancient Rome, Galen became the first person who removed bone fragments from the spine. In the 7th century AD, the Greek Paulus became the first scholar who proposed the idea of reconstructing the spine through surgery built upon the summary of achievements of ancient Greek medicine. Later, as Europe entered the Dark Ages, spinal medicine there almost stagnated. It was not until the Renaissance that research in spine practice revived. Interestingly, although based on mostly isolated and rough case reports, these ancient explorations represent early forms of the concepts of modern spinal surgery, including spinal realignment, compressor removal, and segmental stabilization [2].

The 19th century, the critical hundred-year initial development of modern surgery, saw bacteriology founded by Louis Pasteur, the aseptic practice of surgery initiated by Joseph Lister, the introduction of ether as an anesthetic by Crawford Long, and X-ray discovered by Wilhelm Röntgen. Driven by these great inventions and discoveries, the development of cervical spine surgery accelerated. Chipault, a French doctor, described his idea of anterior cervical surgery in his book about neurosurgery in 1895, which did not develop into a relatively mature surgical technique until more than 50 years later [3].

The 20th century saw surgeons trying out surgical interventions on the cervical spine with their deepened understanding of the local structure and pathologies. Walton and Paul, when performing a posterior cervical exploration in 1905, found the

Anterior Controllable Antedisplacement and Fusion. https://doi.org/10.1016/B978-0-323-88049-7.00001-8

jagged anterior contour of the spinal cord due to the compression of an epidural mass at the intervertebral level of indeterminate nature, being an intervertebral disc or a tumor, despite pathological analysis. In 1914, Sudeck described the structured method of interpreting anteroposterior (AP) spine radiographs in an article. In 1911, Fred Albee, an American doctor, described the first posterior spinal fusion surgery in a case where tuberculosis-related spinal deformity was corrected by interspinous fusion with an autologous tibial graft [4]. In 1925, Davis took the first standard X-ray of the spine. In the same year, Charles Elsberg reported the first case of posterior cervical discectomy following laminectomy but mistook the resected disc as a chondroma [5]. In 1934, American doctor Mixter reported posterior surgical resection of intervertebral discs as a treatment of disc herniation, pioneering surgical treatment of spinal degeneration. In 1943, American surgeon Ralph Cloward reported the first posterior lumbar interbody fusion with good results, from which he later expanded this technique to the cervical spine.

The year 1955 became a watershed because, due to technical and other constraints, cervical intervertebral disc surgery had always been performed via the posterior approach, and the feasibility of an anterior approach was rarely explored prior to that year. In 1955, Smith and Robinson pioneered the removal of the prolapsed intervertebral disc from the front of the cervical spine, followed by intervertebral bone grafting and fusion. In 1958, being experienced in trephination and lumbar fusion, Cloward reported the cervical decompression and fusion technique via an anterior approach, which he believed had a broader scope of indications than the posterior surgery and became widely accepted in the field of spinal surgery [6].

After nearly a 100 years of development, anterior surgery gradually integrates and modifies various techniques, including decompression, fusion, and instrumentation, and evolved into the anterior cervical decompression and fusion surgery primarily used today. Anterior surgery enables direct decompression by removal of the exact intervertebral discs, osteophytes, and ossifications that compress the cervical spinal cord. For patients with reduced cervical lordosis or even kyphosis, the anterior surgery restores intervertebral height and curvature through interbody bone grafting. This helps restore the stress distribution of the cervical spine and retension the ligamentum flavum, which prevents the hypertrophic tissue from flopping into the spinal canal and impinging on the spinal cord and nerve roots. In addition, as the anterior spinal artery provides 75%−80% of the blood supply to the ventral spinal cord, one of the critical advantages of the anterior surgery is the protection of the blood supply of the spinal cord through the decompression from its ventral side. The innovation of the anterior cervical approach has been further boosted by the more profound and specific researches on the anatomical structure of the cervical spine, as well as the increased accessibility of advanced technologies such as lumination systems and spinal surgery instrumentations. These advancements have helped surgeons to operate with higher accuracy and reduced risk to the vital tissues and organs around the cervical spine.

In Asia, due to objective factors such as socioeconomy and industrialization, the development of cervical spine surgery has been deeply influenced by that in Europe and the United States while carrying its traits. In Europe and America, the first posterior cervical discectomy was carried out as early as 1925. In contrast, anterior cervical surgery was hardly accepted until the 1950s due to technical barriers. Therefore, posterior procedures for cervical spine diseases dominated the first half of the 20th century in Europe and America, from which it spread to Asia as mature and widely applied procedures. On the other hand, with the spectrum of cervical spondylosis distinct from that in the European and American populations, the Asian population has different expectations for cervical spine surgery, which triggers the divergence of surgical method innovation.

Take the ossification of the posterior longitudinal ligament (OPLL) as an example, which predilects the Asian population. It is difficult to resect the ossification that spans multiple segments with the anterior approach, which often leaves residual ossification and the risk of dural and neural injuries from the resection maneuvers.

These constraints, though, promoted the development of posterior surgeries, such as laminectomy and laminoplasty [7].

For cervical degenerative diseases, the posterior surgeries aim to expand the volume of the posterior spinal canal, so that the spinal cord can drift backward to achieve indirect decompression.

As one of the first posterior surgical strategies, laminectomy made surgeons realize that the resection of lamina seriously compromised the load-bearing function of the posterior column of cervical spine, which lead to a high incidence of complications of cervical instability such as kyphosis and anterior subluxation. With technological development, the modified laminoplasty became widely carried out in the 1970s in that it restored spinal canal stability to a certain extent by expanding the spinal canal while retaining most of the posterior structures.

Spinal instrumentation came on stage thanks to the advancing biomechanics and material science. In the 1960s, the titanium alloy initially used in the aerospace field was turned into a material for the spinal instrumentation systems, a type of internal fixation. The typical internal fixation with screws and plates was used as early as 1886 by Schede and Hansmann on the extremities. That for the spine, however, was not available until 1953 by Holdsworth and Hardy, who instrumented a patient with a thoracolumbar fracture with plates and screws. After the first anterior cervical plate introduced in 1964, a variety of plates became available, including Arbeitsgemeinschaft für Osteosynthesefragen (AO) plate, Caspar plate, Spinetech plate, Orion plate, and Zephier plate. In the 1980s, Caspar applied the anterior cervical plate fixation technique in the routine cervical surgery to reduce graft-related complications and enhance the stability of the cervical spine during flexion, extension, lateral flexion, and axial rotation. In 1986, the first AO locking plate was applied in cervical instrumentation by Morshcer, where the screw head generated a tight fit and created a robust and more reliable construct with the plate, screw, vertebra, and bone graft [8].

After the birth of the anterior cervical decompression and fusion technique in 1955, surgeons struggled with the limited availability of autogenous bones. Initially, they tried to use other materials as alternatives to the autologous bone, which yielded

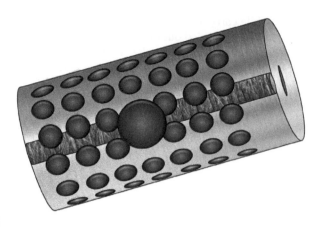

FIGURE 1-1-1

Bagby bone basket.

a suboptimal fusion effect. Ultimately, the idea of a "cage" filled with autogenous bone fragments was brought into play as the American doctor George Bagby tried it out on horses suffering from cervical spondylosis in 1988. The eponymous "Bagby Bone Basket" features a fenestrated and hollow cylinder of stainless steel used when being filled with bone fragments (Fig. 1-1-1). By the 1990s, this cage-based technique was gradually applied to the treatment of human cervical spondylosis with a safe, stable, and long-lasting effect.

Since then, this field has embraced a series of cage designs of various materials (including titanium, stainless steel, cobalt-chromium alloy, and polyether ether ketone) and shapes.

Historically, the cages were classified by design into threaded and square cages. Based on the Cloward technique, the threaded cage, as an early version of the design, was represented by the BAK-cage introduced in 1994, a porous titanium alloy cylindrical cage with high stiffness that enables expeditious fusion (Fig. 1-1-2). However, its use and investigation over time revealed the shortcomings: it resulted in stress concentration on the endplate, loss of the intervertebral height, and cage subsidence. The square cage, in a similar idea as the horseshoe bone graft in the Smith—Robinson method, was primarily designed with rough upper and lower surfaces for enhanced anchorage in the intervertebral space. It was later modified with curved upper and lower surfaces to match the endplate contour.

Moving into the 21st century, in order to restore the natural curvature of the cervical spine, the square cage was further modified into a wedge shape, with the higher side facing the front. At the same time, the trapezoid cage that supplements the arc of the endplate was developed to increase the stability of the cervical spine during lateral flexion, forward flexion, and axial rotation.

Progress was also made in surgical visualization. In 1967, the Swiss neurosurgeon Yasargil introduced the microscopic technique in discectomy, which evolved into microscopic discectomy. In the United States, orthopedic surgeon Kambin

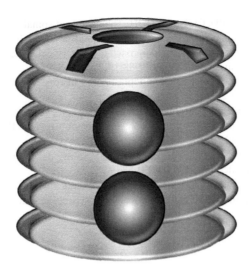

FIGURE 1-1-2

BAK-cage.

took the lead in using arthroscopy for discectomy via a posterolateral approach in 1992, which constituted arthroscopic microdiscectomy [9]. Five years later, neurosurgeon Foley established microendoscopic discectomy with a tubular retraction system and endoscope, used in spinal surgery for the first time. In particular, this tubular system provides working accesses of various calibers and accepts both endoscopes and surgical microscopes, whose versatility has been widely recognized by spine surgeons [10].

Advances in technology have brought about ongoing renovations in cervical spine procedures, from fusion immobilization to functional reconstruction for anterior procedures, and from laminectomy to laminoplasty for the posterior ones. Meanwhile, many highly specific hybrid and combined procedures have been in use to tailor to specific clinical needs since a century ago, demonstrating the outstanding creativity and expertise of spine surgeons.

References

[1] Goodrich TJ. History of spine surgery in the ancient and medieval worlds. Neurosurgical Focus 2004;16(1):1–13.

[2] Knoeller SM, Seifried C. Historical perspective: history of spinal surgery. Spine 2000; 25(21).

[3] Keller T, Holland MC. Some notable American spine surgeons of the 19th century. Spine 1997;22(12):1413–7.

[4] Albee FH. Bone surgery with machine tools. Scientific American 1936;154(4):178–81.

[5] Castro ID, Santos DPD, Christoph DDH. The history of spinal surgery for disc disease: an illustrated timeline. Arquivos de Neuro-Psiquiatria 2005;63(3a):701—6.

[6] Cloward RB. The anterior surgical approach to the cervical spine: the Cloward procedure: past, present, and future. Spine 1988;13(7):823—7.

[7] Kurokawa R, Kim P. Cervical laminoplasty: the history and the future. Neurologia Medico-Chirurgica 2015;55(7):529—39.

[8] Elizabeth C, Matthew HP, Mobbs RJ, et al. The design evolution of interbody cages in anterior cervical discectomy and fusion: a systematic review. BMC Musculoskeletal Disorders 2015;16(1):99.

[9] Kambin P, Cohen LF. Arthroscopic microdiscectomy versus nucleotomy techniques. Clinics in Sports Medicine 1993;12(3):587—98.

[10] Fengzeng J, Tie F. Introduction to the development history of western neurospine surgery. Chinese Journal of Neurosurgical Disease Research 2015;14(5):385.

Section 2: Origin and development of the ACAF technique

Founding basis of the ACAF technique

Thanks to the advances in imaging and material science, the anterior and posterior cervical spine surgical procedures have developed rapidly, with increasingly mature surgical techniques and device applications. In the treatment of cervical spondylosis, spinal stenosis, OPLL, and other degenerative cervical spine diseases, anterior surgical techniques represented by anterior cervical discectomy and fusion (ACDF) and anterior cervical corpectomy and fusion (ACCF), and posterior surgical techniques represented by laminoplasty have been widely applied clinically with good results. The anterior and posterior approaches are entirely different in the surgical concept. After the 1950s, against the background of technological progress, the pioneers of the anterior approach used imaging technology to locate the compressed levels, lighting equipment to improve the safety of surgery, instrumentation to ensure the stability of the cervical spine, and the retraction systems to ensure full exposure. With all these advancements, they achieved the direct removal of the compressors from anterior approaches. Nowadays, the anterior approach has become the most widely used cervical spine surgery due to its advantages of small surgical access trauma and reliable curative effect. Practitioners of the posterior approach have made enormous surgical attempts during a prolonged period, which can even date back to the ancient Greek period. It was applied in the treatment of spinal trauma and other diseases very early with its safe and straightforward procedure of spinal cord exposure that allows surgeons to directly remove the posterior compressors such as a broken lamina or bone fragments. It is also very advantageous in restoring the dislocated zygapophyseal joint. For the anterior source of compressions, the posterior approach expands the spinal canal and allows the spinal cord to shift backward and dodge the compressor. Driven by the development of modern science, the posterior approach has also been greatly improved, especially since the emergence of laminoplasty and the lateral mass screw technique. Fairly speaking, the anterior approach is a sprouting technique thanks to the advancement of science and technology, whereas the posterior approach represents a time-honored and constantly improving one.

However, objectively, both surgical procedures have their own inherent downsides. Let's take OPLL as an example. In using the anterior approach to treat extensive (e.g., involving more than three segments), thick (e.g., ossification of more than 50% of the spinal canal diameter), and deep lesions (e.g., osteophytes at the back of the vertebra), surgeons must balance adequate decompression with safety, fusion, and stability. The disadvantages of the posterior approach are as follows. First, it does not allow a direct relief of the compression on the front of the spinal cord. Second, it is not as good as the anterior approach in realigning the cervical spine [13]. In addition, the backward drift of the spinal cord causes problems that have long plagued surgeons and patients such as nerve root palsy, deterioration of cervical spine curvature, and ossification progression [1]. Therefore, in summary, there is still room for improvement in outcome satisfaction among the existing cervical spine surgeries. From the perspective of disciplinary development, the barriers in using the classic surgical procedures are the reference for improvement, and our analysis of these barriers can guide the innovation of cervical spine surgery. Now we are going to discuss the common difficulties in cervical spine surgery based on our clinical work.

Limitations of the anterior approach
High surgical risk
The anterior approach is developed by the distraction of the tracheoesophageal sheath and carotid sheath, which course longitudinally, to expose the vertebra and intervertebral disc. This approach has been made significantly safer with the advancement of technology and equipment. However, because the damage of the abovementioned vital structures may lead to adverse events such as hematoma-induced compression, esophageal perforation, and fatal bleeding, the anterior approach still carries considerable risks. At the same time, anterior decompression via the intervertebral space is achieved sometimes via the potential space between the posterior wall of the vertebra and the dural sac. Due to the small space and limited vision, the surgeon must operate carefully to avoid spinal cord injury. Especially for patients with OPLL, the ossification is resected while instruments such as rongeur repeatedly access the spinal canal. Such frequent disturbance to the spinal cord may cause neurologic deterioration. When the ossification and the dura are adhered, the removal maneuver is even more difficult and dangerous, which increases the risk of dural tear.

Implant-related complications
Since anterior decompression requires the removal of the source of compression, the intervertebral disc or vertebra from the front, and the anterior and middle column of the spine are the mainstay of biomechanical stability, and the biomechanical stability of the cervical spine is significantly compromised during the anterior decompression. Instrumentation for anterior reconstruction is distinct from the pedicle screw system used in the posterior approach. Implant- and instrumentation-related complications are inherent to ACDF and ACCF, in particular the latter one. Nevertheless, the use of instrumentation provides a better decompression effect. Implant-related complications include implant displacement and dislodgement, in particular the breakage, subsidence, and bone nonunion encountered in the ACCF technique. In the ACCF technique, space initially occupied by the vertebra is primarily maintained

by the titanium mesh. The titanium mesh provides support almost alone, unlike the construct used in the ACDF technique where the vertebra is preserved, and the cage provides extra support. This role of the titanium mesh requires a better fit with the vertebra. According to the literature, an ideal titanium mesh is one that fits the curvature of the endplate with a smooth surface that avoids damage to the endplate, in a suitable diameter to reduce stress concentration and withstands the distraction manipulation on the vertebrae. Therefore, the application of the titanium mesh is less convenient and reliable than that of a cage.

When treating multisegment cervical lesions through ACCF with long cylindrical titanium mesh, the risk of complications is far from negligible, such as titanium mesh subsidence and screw loosening. In the multisegment ACCF technique, since only four screws can be used to fix the longer plate on the cephalad and caudal vertebrae adjacent to the decompression levels, the overall purchase of the construct is weak, and the bone—screw interface in the vertebra is prone to micromotion, which will eventually lead to screw loosening and pull out [2,3]. In addition, as the result of the intervertebral fusion depends on the creeping substitution initiating from the bone—implant interface, the distance it takes to complete this process is markedly longer in cylindrical titanium mesh. Thus, there is a risk of osteonecrosis and fusion failure.

In order to address the complications related to the cylindrical titanium mesh, some surgeons combine ACDF and ACCF, namely, the hybrid decompression and fixation (HDF) technique to avert the risk of long-segment vertebral resection and cylindrical titanium mesh. Good results have been reported with HDF. The "skip" corpectomy was described by Dalbayrak in 2010 [4] in the treatment of cervical spondylotic myelopathy (CSM) and OPLL in more than three segments, where the C4 or C5 vertebra is skep during corpectomy. This preserved vertebra separates the extended cavity from the corpectomy and serves as a "bridge pier" or intermediate point of fixation. As such, two shorter titanium meshes are used instead of a long cylindrical one. They are inserted to the endplates of the preserved vertebra on the cephalad and caudal side, respectively, and constitute a "nunchaku" construct. This technique bears enhanced hardware stability and fusion rate with better screw purchase from the additional pair of screw and shorter meshes that reduces the distance needed for the creeping substitution of bone fusion. However, these two modified procedures also have their limitations, that is, insufficient decompression in the segment where the vertebra is preserved, and a limited role in continuous-type OPLL with spinal stenosis. These downsides stem from the unresolved contradiction between complete decompression and structure preservation in anterior surgeries. The bony structure that compresses on the spinal cord is located at the posterior wall of the vertebra. In order to reveal and remove it, the anterior part of the vertebra must first be cut to provide access, resulting in the sacrifice of "innocent" noncompressing structures.

Limitations of the posterior surgery

Incapable of direct decompression

The inability to achieve direct decompression is one of the main disadvantages of posterior surgery. In posterior surgeries, decompression is achieved by allowing the spinal cord to shift posteriorly and away from the ventral compressor, a behavior similar to a bowstring. The extent of decompression gained depends entirely on how much the cord has shifted dorsally. As the protruding intervertebral discs, osteophytes, and ossifications are still left in their original positions, once the compression advances and the spinal cord shifts forward, the spinal cord compression will recur. For example, characterized as a gradually evolving disease entity, OPLL can continue to develop after posterior surgery and neutralize the decompression effect. This is especially relevant in the case of hill-shaped ossification. To overcome these constraints, Japanese surgeons introduced the "K-line" concept in 2008 to assess the severity of OPLL [5] and recommended against the posterior procedure for patients with K-line negative disease because the insufficient dorsal shift of the spinal cord is highly probable.

Worsen neurological dysfunction

The posterior surgery exerts a significant impact on the natural structure of the cervical spine. In a laminectomy, due to the destruction of the load-bearing and tension-resistant structure of the posterior column and the sacrifice of muscle attachments, the load-bearing axis gradually shifts to the anterior column, resulting in continuous contraction of the posterior muscles and increased stress of the vertebra and intervertebral disc. In the long term, the vertebra and the intervertebral disc tend to be deformed under constant stress, and the posterior counter-tension muscles gradually become fatigued, which causes cervical kyphosis. The progressing kyphosis forces the spinal cord to bend forward and lean against the posterior margin of the vertebra and result in recurrent cord compression (Fig. 1-2-1) [6]. The literature shows that cervical lordosis less than 10° or the presence of focal kyphosis will significantly offset the effect of posterior decompression [7,8]. In addition, the backward shift and rotation of the spinal cord following posterior surgery can lead to nerve root tethering, which in turn causes nerve root palsy and counteracts symptom improvement (Fig. 1-2-2).

To address the worsened cervical curvature and maintain neurological improvement, laminoplasty and laminectomy combined with lateral mass (pedicle) screw fixation have been attempted from "dynamic" and "static" perspectives.

Laminoplasty respects the importance of the posterior cervical muscles in maintaining spinal stability. By preserving the lamina, laminoplasty minimizes the sacrifice of the muscle attachment area and the elevation of the ligament structure, thus preserving the cervical range of motion. Some surgeons further modified these techniques and described C3 laminectomy combined with laminoplasty, laminoplasty sparing the C7 spinous process, and selective laminoplasty, aiming to protect the posterior cervical muscles better. In terms of the results, laminectomy has been

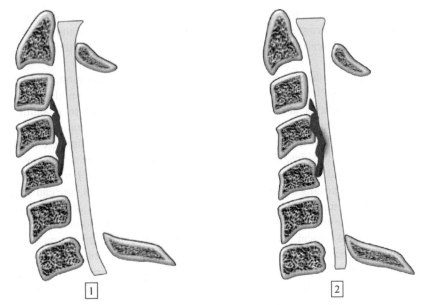

FIGURE 1-2-1

The effect of cervical curvature on decompression through the posterior approach.
(1) The cervical lordosis is present, and the spinal cord drifts back sufficiently.
(2) The cervical lordosis straightened, and the spinal cord moves forward and is compressed again.

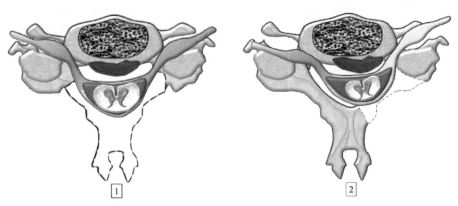

FIGURE 1-2-2

Schematic diagram of nerve root tethering due to posterior shifted or rotated spinal cord.
(1) Nerve roots tethered by the backward drifted spinal cord.
(2) Nerve roots tethered by the rotated spinal cord.

better, but laminoplasty still carries the adverse effect of reduced cervical range of motion and kyphosis progression. Prolonged immobilization, the spontaneous fusion of facet joints, and scarring of the posterior neck tissue may be the underlying causes.

Laminectomy combined with lateral mass (pedicle) screw fixation, through its strong "three-column" fixation, effectively avoids cervical segmental instability. The sustained benefit is also expectable as the cervical curvature is buttressed with a prebent titanium plate. However, this operation is more complicated, and caution should be taken in the screw placement process to avoid damage to blood vessels and nerves. Besides, this technique exerts greater damage to the posterior cervical muscles and impact on the cervical range of motion than laminoplasty.

Based on summarizing the shortcomings of traditional surgeries, one can see that the various postoperative complications are the composite result of many factors, some of which may still be unknown. Therefore, the attempts to solve the compression or tethering of a focal part in isolation may not achieve concrete improvement of the surgical procedure. However, if a surgical procedure intends to minimize its impact on the cervical spine structure and cervical spinal cord and restore the structure to how it is physiologically as much as possible, such modified technique could generate fewer adverse results.

On this basis, the author's team developed the concept of in situ decompression of the spinal cord as another arrow in the quiver [9]. With the principle of in situ decompression to the spinal cord, reflecting the features of groove development in ACCF, laminoplasty, and other techniques, the author's team developed the anterior controllable antedisplacement fusion (ACAF) technique for OPLL and cervical spondylosis with compression dorsal to the vertebra [10,14]. This procedure immobilizes and moves the anterior wall of the spinal canal to expand the spinal canal while directly eliminating the compressor anterior to the spinal cord. It achieves the composite result of decompression, spinal canal reconstruction, and restoration of the shape and position of the spinal cord.

The concept of spinal cord in situ decompression

The concept of in situ decompression of the spinal cord has been derived from the two fundamental principles of decompression and stabilization in spinal surgery, with the key lying in "in situ." "In situ decompression" aims to correct the malposition of the spinal cord caused by the disease, restore the natural shape and spatial position of the spinal cord, and prevent it from being in another pathological state. To fulfill this concept, spinal surgery needs to achieve adequate decompression in a quantifiable and controllable manner and optimize the compression-free environment for the spinal cord. As such, the decompressed spinal cord is in an ample buffer space with neuroprotective content free of abnormal curvature, drift, or rotation. The spinal cord in its natural state bears the following two advantages, which are also the fundamentals of the concept of in situ decompression [9,10−12].

Advantages of the in situ spinal cord

Consistency with evolutionary anatomy

During the evolution of primates from crawling on all fours to walking upright on both feet, the spine has changed gradually from being in "C" shape with only one curve to the "S" shape made up of sacral kyphosis, lumbar lordosis, thoracic kyphosis, and cervical lordosis. This change has occurred to maintain gait stability in the upright posture and reflected the coordination and compensation of each segment of the spine. This ergonomic posture maintains the balance needed for the centered gravity line of the human body while enabling head-up and horizontal gaze with the least effort. It represents a status where the vertebrae, intervertebral discs, and facet joints are under the minimal tensile and compressive loads. Inhabiting in the spinal canal, the spinal cord adapts its shape to that of the canal during evolution [13]. The spinal cord grows within the spinal canal but at speed slower than that of the spine, making it shorter than the spinal column and creating a difference between the segments of the spinal cord and the vertebral level. Therefore, after branching from the spinal cord, the 31 pairs of spinal nerves travel for a certain distance in the spinal canal before they reach the corresponding intervertebral foramen where they leave the spinal canal to form the peripheral nervous system. According to the different functions of the segments, certain levels of the spinal cord have undergone adaptive changes in volume, such as the cervical enlargement and lumbar enlargement. Therefore, the natural shape of the human spinal nerve and its spatial relationship with the spine represent the result of the prolonged evolution process. With structural and functional harmony, it is such a delicate component that it adequately and efficiently transmits sensory and motor signals.

Consistency with the mechanics of anatomy

The spinal cord is wrapped by three layers of connective tissue: pia mater, arachnoid, and dura mater. The pia mater adheres to the surface of the spinal cord. Its triangular lateral extension based medially and pointing outward on both sides, known as the denticulate (or dentate) ligament, anchors the dura mater. The dentate ligament is distributed along the entire length of the spinal cord and is often located between the upper and lower nerve roots. Anchoring the spinal cord to the dura mater, it plays a role in restricting spinal cord rotation and the rostral–caudal movement but does not hinder its ventral–dorsal mobility [14]. There is also a connection between the dura mater and the spinal canal. The spinal dura mater joins the cranial dura at the edge of the foramen magnum and the filum terminale caudally and is secured to the sacrum and coccyx. On the ventral and dorsal side of the dura mater, the Hoffman ligament and the posterior epidural ligaments connect the dural sac with the ligament lining the inner surface of the spinal canal. These connection structures are crucial not only for the physiological position of the spinal cord but also for the protection of the spinal cord against pathological conditions. For example, Wadhwani described that in the case of intervertebral disc herniation, if without Hoffman ligament that pulls the dural sac anteriorly, the nerve root is bound to be stretched and cause pain no matter how minimally the canal is occupied by the disc material [15].

The natural position of the spinal cord in the spinal canal is maintained by the nerve roots and ligaments of each segment. Nerve roots, bundles of efferent motor and afferent sensory nerve fibers, branch off the spinal cord and exit through the intervertebral foramen, where they maintain tension due to the constrain of the surrounding ligaments and blood vessels. In bending posture, the spinal cord, nerve roots, and denticulate ligaments are under physiological tension [16]. The tension of the nerve root and denticulate ligament on the nerve root can be broken down into two components. The axial component of the force intends to balance gravity and the traction from nerve roots and denticulate ligament of other segments, which alleviates the tethering on the spinal cord. The transverse component, in contrast, featuring a balanced summation of each vector, keeps the spinal cord centered in the spinal canal surrounded by enough buffer space to minimize collision and shock [17]. Therefore, as a whole, the nerve roots and ligaments along all the segments provide axial support for the spinal cord against gravity and axial traction while maintaining traction on the transverse plane that results in a centered position and rotational constraint.

However, the connecting structures such as nerve roots and ligaments also complicate the vector profile of the spinal cord. According to the Saint Venant's principle in material mechanics, the stress measured at any point on an axially loaded cross-section is uniform, given that the measured location is far enough away from the point of load application. The resultant load moment is related only to the force and its moment arm. In other words, a new load forces a change in the stressed state only in the regions close to the applied load. However, this principle is poorly applicable in the spinal cord, anchored by the nerve roots and surrounding ligaments. A load exerted on any specific area causes changes in the spinal cord tension extensively across this knitted structure. For example, in patients with tethered cord syndrome, the direct tethering of the filum terminale results in extensive neural dysfunction of the saddle area and lower extremities due to the concurrent traction of the denticulate ligament [18]. Therefore, a surgery planned to address the abnormal stress states of the spinal cord shall aim to reconstitute its typical load distribution profile. Specifically, this can be achieved by restoring the natural position of the spinal cord in the spinal canal and the relative spatial relationship between the nerve roots, ligaments, and the spinal cord.

Overview of abnormal profile of the spinal cord

Physiologically, the spinal cord is centered in the spinal canal with an oval cross-section equally distributed on the left and right. In the sagittal plane, it forms a smooth curve along the curvature of the spine [19]. Under the influence of factors such as degeneration, deformity, and iatrogenic intervention, the spinal cord may undergo not only morphological changes, such as depression and bending [20,21], but also spatial position changes such as drift and rotation. In spite of a dearth of systematic research on the physiological and pathological significance of the spinal cord in abnormal profiles, its potential relation with neurological symptoms has attracted increasing attention.

The posterior drift of spinal cord

In diseases such as CSM, OPLL, and cervical spinal stenosis, the posterior decompression via posterior cervical approaches allows the spinal cord to drift backward and clear off the ventral compression. During this posterior cord drift, the tethering effect of the nerve roots constitutes important pathogenesis of nerve root palsy [22,23]. Studies have shown that the backward drift of the spinal cord is restricted by anatomical elements where the maximum distance of the drift is between 6.0 and 6.5 mm [24]. This indicates the traction force in front of the spinal cord.

Clinical observation also reveals spatial and temporal relations between the backward drift of the spinal cord and nerve root tethering. Hyakumachi found that the backward drift distance of the spinal cord of patients with C5 neuropathy was significantly greater than that of patients who were free from the disease [25]. Takashi Shiozaki found that in the early stage (24 hours) after laminoplasty, the dural sac expanded rapidly and resulted in a significant drift of the spinal cord, in particular at the C5 nerve root. Two weeks later, the spinal cord moved forward slightly, which alleviated the excessive drift seen immediately after surgery [26]. The concurrence of the excessive dorsal drift of the spinal cord and C5 radiculopathy accounts for the frequent timing (within one week after surgery) of onset of C5 neuropathy and the self-limiting nature of the disease. In addition, Dai Liyang found that the duration of radiculopathy was negatively correlated with the recovery rate of the spinal cord function measured by Japanese Orthopaedic Association (JOA) score. To be specific, patients with sustained radiculopathy experienced suboptimal cord recovery. This shows that the dorsal drift of the spinal cord may cause not only nerve root palsy but also spinal cord injury.

When the cervical spine becomes straightened or even kyphotic, the spinal cord tends to move forward and rest against the vertebra. Logically, if the cervical spine resumes lordosis through surgery, the spinal cord will drift back to its natural position. This is one of the theoretical foundations for anterior and posterior combined surgery for patients with cervical kyphosis. However, problems such as excessive interspace distraction, use of cage too high for the interspace, and excessively prebent posterior rod may cause excessive lordosis of the cervical spine and backward drift of the spinal cord. Minoda and Kim, among others, found that the attempt to provide adequate room for posterior spinal cord drift by restoring the cervical spine to an overly lordotic position via ACDF would increase the incidence of C5 neuropathy [27].

Some surgeons also tried to reduce the traction of nerve roots by controlling the degree of the backward drift of the spinal cord in order to strike a balance between definitive decompression and excessive backward drift. Yoichiro Hatta compared the effects of selective versus extensive laminoplasty and found that they achieved comparable neurological recovery because the former retained the posterior arch of the vertebra, constrained the posterior drift of the spinal cord, and caused fewer C5 neuropathy [28]. It can be argued that the concept of selective laminoplasty is to achieve better neurological recovery by trying to restrict the shift of the spinal cord.

Spinal cord rotation

In spinal orthopedics, the derotation maneuver for deformity correction can cause spinal cord tethering and blood supply impairment, leading to spinal cord injury [29]. Qiu Yong found through animal studies that rotating the spinal column twisted and pulled the tracts within the spinal cord, leading to changes in somatosensory-evoked potentials and in pathological examinations such as hemorrhage, demyelination, and glial cell infiltration. Chen Deyu found in in vitro studies on the cervical spinal cord that the rotation of the cervical spine drove the spinal cord to twist and produced abnormal shear forces at the level where the twist was most severe. Elastic mechanics analysis shows that the rotation of the compressed spinal cord increases the stress at the compression site and aggravates spinal cord damage.

Spinal cord rotation resulting from local compressors, such as intervertebral discs and ossification, also exerts secondary damage to nerve roots. Postoperative C5 radiculopathy in OPLL patients is highly related to spinal cord rotation. In OPLL, the causes of spinal cord rotation can be classified into two categories. ① Preexisting rotation prior to surgery: because of asymmetric or eccentric ossification, the left and right sides of the spinal cord suffer from different degrees of compression. On the side with more severe compression, the spinal cord deforms and shifts more markedly, resulting in spinal cord rotation. ② Postoperative rotation: after surgical decompression, the potential energy accumulated in the spinal cord before the operation is transformed into the kinetic energy of the cord derotation. In addition, in single-door laminoplasty, because the lamina is removed only on one side, the spinal cord is unevenly decompressed on both sides. The laminectomy side sees a more posterior shift of the spinal cord so that the spinal cord tends to rotate (Fig. 1-2-3). This phenomenon has been evidenced by studies comparing

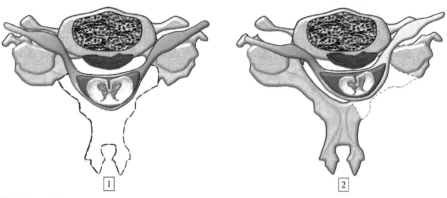

FIGURE 1-2-3

Spinal cord rotation caused by single-door laminoplasty for OPLL.
(1) Asymmetric compression from OPLL.
(2) Asymmetric decompression after single-door surgery.

posterior single-door and double-door laminoplasty. Shuichi Kaneyama found that the incidence of C5 neuropathy was higher in patients undergoing single-door surgery than in those undergoing double-door surgery, and multivariate analysis revealed single-door surgery is a significant risk factor for C5 neuropathy [30]. He believes that the spinal cord can drift along the midline after double-door surgery, thereby avoiding spinal cord rotation. In contrast, single-door surgery tends to induce spinal cord rotation. It is worth noting that the symptoms of nerve root palsy after single-door surgery can appear on the door side, or the hinge side, or even on both sides. The author believes that after the lamina is cut, the compressor will generate a torque on the spinal cord that drives it to rotate. As a reaction, the tethered nerve roots on both sides generate a pair of moments to counteract the rotational torque. Therefore, the nerve roots on both sides are subject to traction injury during spinal cord rotation [31,32].

A number of studies have found a strong correlation between the spinal cord rotation angle on the preoperative magnetic resonance imaging (MRI) axial image and the incidence of postoperative C5 neuropathy, regardless of anterior or posterior surgery. Arunit J.S. pointed out in the study that the larger the preoperative spinal cord rotation angle, the higher the incidence of postoperative nerve root traction [17,33]. Spinal cord rotation is categorized into mild ($0° \sim 5°$), moderate ($6° \sim 10°$), and severe ($\geq 11°$), and moderate or above rotation is regarded as a predictor of the onset of C5 neuropathy [34,35]. It is worth noting that patients with C5 neuropathy may have a rotated spinal cord before the operation but do not show symptoms. Instead, they complain of weakness of elevation and shoulder pain only after surgical decompression. In this regard, the author argues that, first, spinal cord rotation is a chronic process as a response to compression where nerve roots gradually tolerate the mechanically stable traction. Second, after surgical decompression, as the elastic potential energy accumulated in the rotated cord is quickly transformed into the kinetic energy for cord rotation, the nerve roots undergo rapid changes in the magnitude and direction of the traction force and sustain neuropathy of C5.

The anterior shift of the spinal cord

As mentioned above, the excessive backward shift of the spinal cord is closely related to nerve root palsy. Similarly, excessive forward displacement of the spinal cord also compromises the nerve root. Takase found in the study that the anterior shift of the spinal cord after ACCF induces C5 neuropathy. As the central part of the compressing vertebra is removed during ACCF, which serves as a natural barrier of cord motion, the spinal cord drifts significantly forward unimpededly. Such anterior shift is more evident in patients undergoing multilevel corpectomy [36,37]. As a result, the nerve root easily impinges on the posterior edge of the resected bone (Fig. 1-2-4). Also, nerve tethering occurs in a fashion similar to that in the posterior shift of the spinal cord. Meanwhile, when removing the central part of the vertebra in the ACCF, as the access of the instrument is constrained by the structures on both sides, the surgeons tend to remove less bone laterally as they proceed. This leaves a "funnel-like" cavity with a big opening and a small bottom (Fig. 1-2-5),

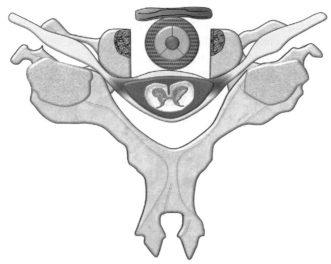

FIGURE 1-2-4

Nerve root compression following the anterior shift of the spinal cord.

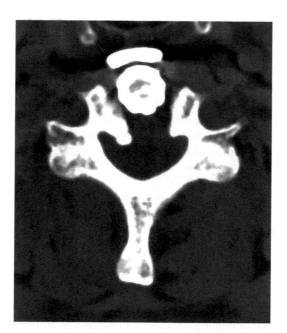

FIGURE 1-2-5

The "funnel-shaped" cavity developed in ACCF.

predisposes the nerve root to compression at its exit canal, and aggravates the nerve root compression. Ikenaga conducted a quantitative analysis of the associations mentioned above and concluded that after anterior surgery, the greater the dural sac expands, the higher the incidence of C5 radiculopathy [38].

Saunders reported a "restrictive decompression technique" that narrows the distance between the grooves in the ACCF technique from 20 to 15 mm to prevent excessive advancement of the spinal cord, which resulted in reduced incidence of postoperative C5 neuropathy. Odate also put forward a similar argument that reducing the width of the anterior decompression to less than 15 mm and developing symmetrical grooves help reduce the incidence of C5 neuropathy [39]. However, these modifications inevitably diminish the effect of decompression surgery [39,40].

Pathogenesis of the abnormality of spinal cord profile

The way to decompress the spine is to isolate the compressive sources and the spinal cord. Intraoperatively, the surgeons use direct visualization and imaging to determine whether the pressure-induced material and the dura mater are separated via evidence of resumed cerebrospinal fluid (CSF) zone and distension of the indented spinal cord. However, in clinical practice, surgeons gradually realized that even in the absence of evidence of compression, some patients still had symptoms around the spine and the innervation area. For example, axial pain related to the excessive distraction of the intervertebral space [41,42], C5 nerve root disease associated with the excessive posterior drift of the spinal cord, tethered cord syndrome, and lumbosacral bowstring diseases [43,44]. These symptoms or diseases can be improved after alleviating or eliminating the abnormal tension status of the spinal cord, shown in a myriad of investigations. For example, the proper distraction of the intervertebral space and the use of cages of appropriate height during ACDF help reduce the incidence of axial symptoms [45]. Patients with tethered cord syndrome obtain significant improvement in symptoms after spinal shortening surgery distributed evenly across multiple segments [46]. The incidence of axial pain and nerve root palsy is significantly reduced in OPLL patients after controlled decompression with the ACAF technique. To conclude, despite the fact that relatively few basic and biomechanical studies have been directed to the abnormal profile of the spinal cord, spine surgeons have corrected the abnormal cord profile in practice and traced its pathogenic mechanism from a clinical perspective. Based on the literature and the author's research work, the pathological mechanism of the abnormality in the spinal cord profile is detailed in the following three aspects.

Nerve root traction

Nerve root palsy is a common complication after cervical anterior and posterior decompression, with C5 nerve root being the most common victim. C5 neuropathy manifests as dyskinesia, sensory changes, and pain in the C5 innervation area first reported in a case of posterior cervical decompression by Scoville in 1961 [47]. In the past 20 years, various assumptions and validations on the cause of C5 neuropathy have been put forward, among which "the theory of tethered nerve roots" is one of the primary explanations. The theory attributes C5 nerve root disease to traction caused by the spinal cord drift, the mechanism by which posterior surgeries, such as laminectomy and laminoplasty, work. As the spinal cord drifts dorsally and avoids the ventral compressor, the nerve roots of the same level, still immobilized to the elements around the intervertebral foramen, become stretched. Moreover, the frequent involvement of C5 has been ascribed to the anatomical delineation that the C5 nerve root travels a short distance in the spinal canal after branching off the spinal cord at the most lordotic vertebral segment. Similarly, the ventral advancement of the spinal cord can also lead to C5 radiculopathy [40,57].

Although studies have analyzed the relation of C5 radiculopathy and neuronal injury of the anterior horn of the spinal cord, this alone does not account for the general picture of C5 symptomatology. When investigating the etiology of C5 nerve root disease, Hajime Takase and colleagues failed to conclude any difference in postoperative cord injury, shown as hyperintensity signals in spinal cord MRI, between the diseased and the control groups [36]. Subsequently, he quantitatively analyzed the correlation between the distance of the posterior drift of the spinal cord and C5 nerve root disease and concluded that the increase of the drift distance is associated with a higher risk of the C5 radiculopathy. He also recognized that the onset of C5 radiculopathy was a few days after surgery, rather than immediately after surgery. This delayed onset indicates that it takes time to develop symptoms from the nerve root being stretched. It is a period when the continuous mechanical traction gradually aggravates the local mechanical and metabolic insults, and finally causes symptoms.

There are two prerequisites for developing an evident anterior or posterior drift of the spinal cord in the spinal canal: ① the pressure difference between the front and back of the spinal cord due to bone removal of the spinal canal and ② the bony resection spanning multiple vertebral segments. Meeting these criteria, the spinal cord of sufficient length moves forward or backward under a sufficient bending moment and pulls the nerve roots. This process of pathogenesis is consistent with the finding of previous studies that C5 radiculopathy is particularly likely to occur in multisegment decompression surgery [48].

In addition to ventral and dorsal drift, the rotation of the spinal cord also causes asymmetrical traction of nerve roots. Spinal cord rotation can work synergistically with ventral or dorsal drift, increasing the risk of C5 nerve root disease [35,49]. Kaneyama described the single-door laminoplasty for irregular-shaped OPLL as a technique of "asymmetric decompression for asymmetric lesion" [30]. Irregular-shaped ossification generates compression unevenly across the spinal cord, putting it in an "impending state of malposition" before surgery that predisposes the cord to rotation or shift. Therefore, the compression of the ossification and unilateral decompression procedure synergistically drive the spinal cord to drift dorsally or laterally, or twist, and ultimately aggravate the traction of the nerve roots.

Stress-induced spinal cord changes

With a mechanical profile similar to a long rod, the spinal cord reflexes the Poisson effect, a law of material mechanics, to some extent. This law has it that a compression load causes an object to become shorter in the direction of the compressive load and wider laterally and vice versa [50]. Cadaveric studies have confirmed that the cervical spinal cord is elongated in the forward flexion position and shortened in the extension position. Correspondingly, the cross-sectional area becomes smaller in an extended spinal cord in a forward flexed cervical spine but larger in a shortened spinal cord in an extended cervical spine [50]. Biomechanically, when a tensile load is applied to the spinal cord, the load—deformation behavior of the spinal cord is represented in a curve with two distinct stages. In the initial stage, a smaller tensile force produces a considerable deformation, whereas, in the second stage, a larger force only produces a smaller deformation (Fig. 1-2-6). This phenomenon is determined by the inherent pliability of the spinal cord in response to flexion and extension.

In physiological flexion and extension, the cervical spinal cord adapts to the spinal canal environment by inherent pliability similar to an accordion. It is readily ductile in the initial stage of the tensile load. However, its pliability and ductility feature works only within 70%—75% of the maximum extension and flexion of the spinal column. Once the accordion-like mechanism is run out, the spinal cord directly bears the subsequent tensile force and sustains exponential load (Fig. 1-2-7).

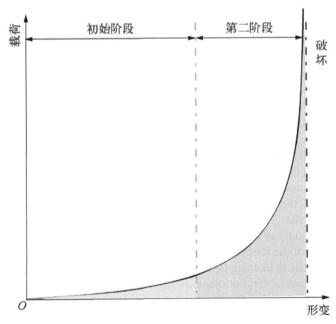

FIGURE 1-2-6

Load—deformation curve of the spinal cord. Initial stage, second stage, damage, load, and deformation.

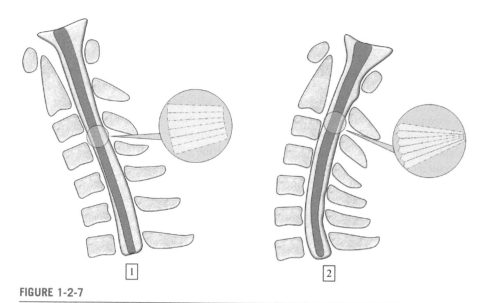

FIGURE 1-2-7

The relationship between cervical spine dynamics and spinal cord morphology.
(1) Pulled spinal cord in the flexed cervical spine.
(2) Pushed spinal cord in the extended cervical spine.

This mechanism explains the symptomatology of Hirayama disease. In this condition, the spinal cord is already tense in the neutral cervical position since the cervical column and the spinal cord have grown in unequal speed. Therefore, when sustaining tensile force, driven by the nature of traveling in the shortest path, the cervical spinal cord is left with no option but to lean forward against the posterior wall of the vertebra. This eventually causes dynamic anterior cord compression [51]. Therefore, restoring the curvature of the spinal cord is conducive to protecting the pliability of the spinal cord and allowing it to resist the abnormal load.

A compressed spinal cord responds to stress in a more complicated manner. In addition to the local contact pressure from the compressor, the spinal cord is subject to longitudinal tensile loads centered on the compression point. Besides, under the fulcrum effect of the compressor, the spinal cord sustains a bending load on the opposite side of the compressor (Fig. 1-2-8). At the same time, the spinal cord, with a cross-sectional area already reduced due to compression, is further pinched under the impact of the tensile load. Since the tensile stress on the spinal cord is proportional to the tensile load applied and inversely proportional to the cross-sectional area, the spinal cord of smaller diameter suffers higher stress per unit on the cross-sectional area. As such, if left not corrected by surgery, the spinal cord in pathological curvature will deteriorate under the synergistic effect of multiple stress forms.

Fukushima found that patients whose spinal cord cross-sectional area is still less than 45 mm^2 have poor neurological recovery [52]. Kameyama and colleagues proved that the cross-sectional area of the spinal cord of the healthy Japanese

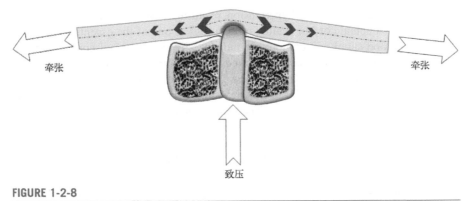

牵张   牵张

致压

FIGURE 1-2-8

The effect of compressing objects on the stress status of spinal cord. Tensile load and impingement.

population is between 51 and 59 mm^2. When the cross-sectional area of the spinal cord is reduced to 1/3 of the average value, the gray matter will be damaged [19]. This finding indicates that the resumption of the cross-sectional area of the spinal cord is associated with the recovery of neural function, and a procedure that simply removes the compressors without restoring the cross-sectional area of the spinal cord may provide little benefit. However, there are also reports that some patients with spinal cord cross-sectional area less than 40 mm^2 remain neurologically normal. Therefore, it is not enough to evaluate the status of the spinal cord by analyzing the individual geometric parameters in isolation, such as the cross-sectional area of the spinal.

The stress on any point in the spinal cord is the collection of all the stress components in the cross-section of that point. A tensile load of a particular magnitude affects the spinal cord differently in various areas. Those with a large cross-sectional area are subject to less stress, and vice versa. Therefore, to a certain extent, the restoration of the cross-sectional area of the spinal cord is conducive to the restoration of the stress status of the spinal cord, which is a precondition to guard against mechanical and metabolic disorders of neurons and nerve fibers. However, in addition to the longitudinal pull, the spinal cord is subject to various forms of stress, such as pushing, deflection, shear, and even torsion due to the constraint of the spinal canal, nerve roots, and ligaments. As such, the spinal cord of each segment is distinct in its stress profile, and segments of the same cross-sectional size may display completely different stress patterns. Therefore, to reestablish the stress profile of the spinal cord, it is necessary to restore such morphological indicators as spinal cord position, curvature, and cross-sectional area.

Blood supply disorder of the spinal cord

The spinal cord is a soft tissue with densely distributed blood vessels. Changes in its curvature and position can distort and narrow its blood vessels, or constrict the blood vessels through intramedullary hypertension, resulting in ischemic lesions of the spinal cord [53]. A spinal cord in healthy morphology is one of the essential prerequisites for its blood supply. In compressor-induced changes in spinal cord curvature, abnormal pressure and shear stress are often present at the level of the compression [50]. At this compressed site, the intramedullary blood vessels parallel to the stress buckle while those perpendicular to the stress stretch [50], resulting in the disrupted circulation of the blood supply area. The small blood vessels in the spinal cord are particularly vulnerable to traction and local hypertension, and prone to occlusion and spasm, resulting in spinal cord ischemia (Fig. 1-2-9) [29].

Shimizu found that spinal kyphosis leads to kyphotic change and flattening of the spinal cord, which resulted in compression of blood vessels and diminished blood supply on the ventral part of the spinal cord and suboptimal recovery of neurological function [54]. The impaired blood supply in the conus medullaris constitutes one of the causes of tethered cord syndrome. The excessive longitudinal stretch generates significant pull of the spinal cord along its axis, leading to ischemia and hypoxia of the neural element and neural deficit of the saddle area. Through animal studies, Yamada and colleagues observed that longitudinal traction of the filum terminale

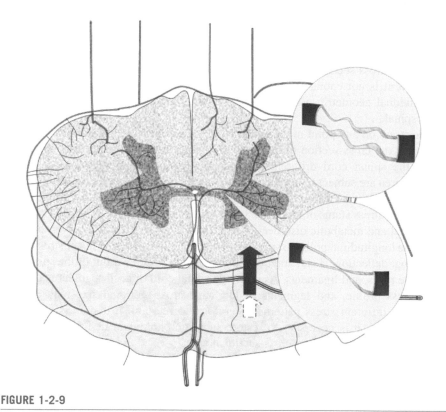

FIGURE 1-2-9

The effect of shear load on the spinal cord blood vessels.

leads to the deformation and thinning of the feeding vessels, neuronal hypoxia, significant reduction of mitochondria quantity toward the end of the spinal cord, which reflects mechanical and metabolic injuries to the spinal cord [55].

Blood vessels are narrowed by the perpendicular load while twisted by the parallel load.

Objectives of the in situ decompression of the spinal cord

According to the theory of in situ decompression of the spinal cord, the objectives of spinal surgery include removing spinal cord compression, restoring spinal cord position and shape, and resuming the immediate environment of the spinal cord. As the core task of spinal surgery is to support and restore spinal nerve function, the author believes that spinal surgery should focus on the overarching role of the spinal cord in the treatment process. The three objectives described above have been focused on the spinal cord and intended to reestablish its natural status. The solution for these goals addresses the discord among the spinal cord and the compressors, the intracanal environment, and the various parts of the cord itself. Each of the three goals serves specific purposes: the removal of compression aims to solve the cause of the disease, the restoration of the position and shape of the spinal cord aims to optimize its stress profile, and the resumption of its immediate environment aims to ensure long-term benefit of the treatment. The ACAF technique has been developed from the existing surgical experience for the three objectives above.

Removing spinal cord compression

The widely used cervical spine surgeries, such as ACDF, ACCF, and single-door laminoplasty, are characterized by the composition of spinal canal decompression, cervical fusion, and instrumentation. However, in history, these three categories of techniques did not emerge simultaneously. The spinal canal decompression was the first to be acknowledged and applied, which reflects that to relieve spinal cord compression has always been our burning need: whether it is trauma, degeneration, tumor, or immune disease, compression of the spinal cord is the leading cause of symptoms and disability.

The development of the ACAF technique was driven by a desire to achieve safe, direct, and thorough decompression for OPLL, a typical compressive cervical spine disease involving multiple compression mechanisms. According to studies and the author's observations, OPLL is associated with four primary compression mechanisms: ① the static compression by the ossification protruding into the spinal canal, ② the dynamic compression present in the localized and segmental types of ossification, ③ the imminent compression state of the stenosed spinal canal that is precipitated by intervertebral disc degeneration and minor trauma at any time, and ④ progressive and repeated compression by the advancing ossification. As such, a well-performed decompression is one that removes the ossification, relieves spinal stenosis, and guards against the impact of a progressing ossification. Attaining this goal is not likely with either traditional anterior or posterior surgery alone.

Jia Lianshun of Shanghai Changzheng Hospital held that the most effective decompression was one that removes the compressor directly. In other words, wherever the compression is, the compressor should be removed right there on the spot. Since the compressor in OPLL comes from the posterior longitudinal ligament (PLL) ventral to the spinal cord, only anterior procedure can achieve direct and complete decompression and eliminate the risk of ossification progression. Therefore, generations of spine surgeons have kept seeking ways to remove ossification directly from the anterior approach. Historically, the ACDF and the ACCF techniques have been the mainstay anterior surgeries for localized and continuous OPLL, respectively. However, because the ossification is deep within the surgical wound and often adhered to the dura, it is difficult and risky to remove it directly and it often leaves residual lesion.

Therefore, methods that move the OPLL anteriorly rather than resecting it have been described, for example, the floating method of isolating the OPLL from the bony perimeter and let it float on the pulsating dura, the modified floating method of thinning the ossified tissue and leaving the intractable parts as "islands" on the dura, and the suture-assisted floating of the thinned and freed ossification. This category of techniques marks the shift of mindset from "prioritized resection" to anterior displacement of OPLL and encourages other novel techniques. Based on the previous experience and the close anatomical connection between the ossification and the vertebra, the ACAF decompression technique was described. It is the first time that surgeons anteriorize the ossification and the vertebra as a whole. Such anterior displacement not only moves the compressor away from the spinal canal and spinal cord and into the intervertebral space but also integrates it as the new anterior wall of the spinal canal and a part of the anterior cervical column. After that, even if the ossification progresses, it does not generate compression on the spinal cord in the spinal canal. Multisegment cervical spondylosis and spinal stenosis have similar pathology as continuous and mixed OPLL, with compression posterior to the vertebrae across multiple segments. From years of clinical practice, we have delivered the decompression benefit of the ACAF technique in these disease entities as well.

Restoring the position and shape of the spinal cord

The normal cervical spine maintains a lordotic arc, which shapes and locates the spinal cord [56]. It has been shown in myriads of studies that restoring the physiological curvature of the cervical spine through surgery reestablishes the mechanical status of the vertebrae, intervertebral discs, ligaments, and muscles, thereby reducing long-term degeneration and neurological complications. The literature on the relationship between the physiological curvature of the cervical spine and the efficacy of cervical spine surgery is reviewed here. Uchida K. believed that correcting cervical spine curvature via anterior approaches significantly improves the patient's neurological recovery. Lau D identified cervical curvature was an important parameter for surgical benefits from the neurological evaluation of patients who had received posterior surgery for multilevel spondylosis. Buell T. J. and colleagues ascribed poor surgical or neurological outcome to the straightened or even kyphotic cervical spine, which subjects the spinal cord to increased longitudinal tensile load and intramedullary pressure and poorer arterial blood supply. After investigating the cervical curvature and symptom improvement in 127 patients who had received surgery for OPLL, Liu et al. concluded that the anterior procedures bear better lordosis and clinical recovery than the posterior ones. Based on the evidence, systems such as Caspar lamina spreader, customized titanium mesh, and lateral mass screw and rod system for posterior approaches have been increasingly used [12,57−60]. To the spinal cord, the restoration of the curvature of the cervical spine and the shape of the spinal canal resumes the suitable space for the spinal cord, a prerequisite for its natural position and shape.

Modified techniques keep emerging thanks to generations of surgeons who strive to improve outcomes and resolve the abnormal profile of the spinal cord and avoid unintended stress. A case in point is the aforementioned selective laminectomy [28] and restrictive anterior decompression [40] aiming to reduce excessive spinal cord drift. To take another example, the spine-shortening osteotomy for tethered cord syndrome has partially reducted the spinal cord by realigning the spinal column and the cord. However, the tips to avoid malpositioning the spinal cord while achieving adequate decompression and to control the position and shape of the spinal cord for optimal recovery are elusive in conventional techniques. Typically, the position and shape of the spinal cord are indirectly restored through the correction of cervical curvature via interspace spreading and the use of cages of appropriate height in anterior surgeries or via precontoured rods in posterior techniques. Such curvature improvement is general rather than specific on each segment, however, leaving it incapable of controlling the position of the spinal cord. In terms of spinal cord position control, the ACAF technique has unique advantages. The anterior wall of the spinal canal is mobilized and migrated forward in the ACAF technique as the surgeon tightens the vertebra screw so that the distance of ventral displacement of each level is under the surgeon's control. This technique is conducive to the precise adjustment of the spinal alignment and the AP diameter of the spinal canal, and better control of the position and curvature of the spinal cord. What is more, a precise in situ decompression is guaranteed as the surgeon can observe the degree of vertebral advancement through the C-arm X-ray machine and make necessary changes at any time.

Reconstituting the immediate environment of the spinal cord

The CSF in the dural sac, the liquid environment which the spinal cord relies on for its physiological activities, plays a vital role in maintaining buffer, protection, nutrition, transmission, and appropriate pressure.

The application of MRI has enabled physicians to appreciate the CSF in the spinal canal noninvasively with unprecedented clarity. Subsequently, the space available for the cord (SAC) and the ratio of spinal cord/CSF column area, among others, have been introduced to assess the room of the dural sac. With these parameters, the imaging evaluation has been narrowed down to the spinal cord and its immediate environment for subsistence. Doctors can determine the effect of surgical

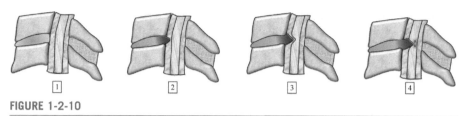

FIGURE 1-2-10

Schematic diagram of Kang's grading: Panel 1, grade 0; Panel 2, grade 1; Panel 3, grade 2; Panel 4, grade 3.

decompression from signs of separation between the pressure-inducing component and the spinal cord, resumed width of the CSF column, and the resumed volume of the spinal cord indented previously. Kang, a Korean surgeon, proposed Kang's grading system of cervical canal stenosis based on CSF obliteration and the signs of compressive myelopathy. It comes with four grades: 0, 1, 2, and 3. Grade 0 refers to the absence of spinal canal stenosis; grade 1, the obliteration of the arbitrary subarachnoid space of more than 50%; grade 2, spinal cord deformity; and grade 3, spinal cord signal changes (Fig. 1-2-10). The higher the grade, the more severe the neurologic deficit.

Wu Desheng reviewed and analyzed CSM patients undergoing the ACCF technique and found that patients with a larger cross-sectional area of the spinal cord or spinal canal and a wider spinal cord or CSF column before surgery attained more significant benefit from the surgery. He noted that the ACCF technique optimizes the volume and shape of the spinal canal to which the spinal cord adapts.

With the further application and development of MRI comes doctors' endeavor in describing the dynamics of CSF in the spinal canal and its function. In 1997, Greitz reported his MRI and radionuclide imaging study on the CSF circulation and noted that after produced from the ventricular choroid plexus, the CSF enters the subarachnoid space through the midbrain aqueduct and the median and lateral apertures of the fourth ventricle. Driven by the arterial pulsation of the brain and spinal cord, CSF gradually distributes in the subarachnoid space and returns to the blood through the venous system of the brain and spinal cord. Enzermann clarified the relationship between CSF dynamics and the cardiac cycle and the dynamics of CSF in the spinal canal in two phases: during cardiac systole, the cerebral tissue and intracranial vasculature expand and compress the ventricles, which forces CSF craniocaudad; alternatively, during diastole, CSF flows caudocranially. Phase-contrast magnetic resonance (PC-MR), spinning off from MRI technology, measures changes of fluid dynamics in the human body and computes the speed and direction of fluid movement. In recent years, it has been increasingly applied to assess CSF circulation and spinal cord movement in patients with cervical spine diseases. With this technology, surgeons have looked to associate the effect of surgical decompression with CSF movement.

Yoshizawa [61] revealed in the study that spinal stenosis interrupted the steady and rapid flow of CSF and generated focal turbulence and stasis, which then blocked the nutrient supply and waste removal of the spinal cord and caused spinal cord cell edema and even death. Watable investigated CSM patients and elaborated on the correlation between spinal myopathy symptoms, spinal canal cross-sectional area, and CSF flow rate. The more severe the symptoms, the smaller the cross-sectional area, and the slower the flow rate. Through the PC-MR technology, Yun observed that in patients with Kang's Grade 0 and 1 spinal stenosis, the CSF flow was present on the ventral and dorsal sides of the spinal cord. It was present on only one side in patients of Kang's Grade 2 and absent in those with Kang's Grade 3 spinal stenosis (Fig. 1-2-11). The study of Tominaga [62] demonstrated in patients with extensive OPLL that the CSF flow rate was significantly increased after laminoplasty, and the magnitude of increase was positively correlated with the neurological recovery rate. This finding indicates that the CSF flow channel is cleared by decompression. However, for patients with short OPLL undergoing the ACDF and ACCF, their neurological function recovered well after surgery, but not the CSF flow rate. He then suggested that compared to the anterior approach that only addresses segmental compression, multiple-segment posterior surgeries achieve "overall" decompression of the cervical spinal cord and resume the patency of the CSF channel. In their retrospective study, the author's team also noted that OPLL patients with better neurological recovery after surgery were associated with more significant increases in the area of the spinal cord, CSF, and spinal canal on axial MRI images.

At present, despite divided opinions on the best surgical procedures that resume CSF circulation, many studies have established that compressors such as intervertebral discs, osteophytes, and ossification impinge the dural sac and disrupt CSF circulation. Meanwhile, since the recovery of CSF circulation is related to the recovery of spinal cord function, CSF can serve as one of the indicators for surgical decompression. In brief, the CSF circulatory disturbance affects the spinal cord in three

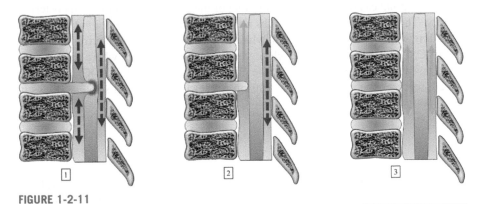

FIGURE 1-2-11

Abnormal flow of cerebrospinal fluid.
(1) Absent CSF flow on the ventral and dorsal side in a severely impinged spinal cord.
(2) CSF flow present on the ventral side only in an impinged dura mater.
(3) CSF flow unobstructed in the absence of cord compression.

aspects: ① squeezed by the compressor, CSF diverts away at the compressed level in the dural sac cavity and provides less buffer or protection to the spinal cord; ② the aberrant CSF flow generates varying intensity of pressure on the surface of the spinal cord and causes spinal cord injury; ③ CSF circulatory disorders cause biochemical changes and affect spinal cord metabolism. Therefore, restoration of the natural CSF circulation and distribution through surgery is of great significance to protecting spinal cord function.

In spinal stenosis, OPLL, and other diseases, anterior and posterior surgeries achieve a certain extent of decompression by modifying the "bony environment" (i.e., expanding the narrowed spinal canal) where the spinal cord is. However, for the "liquid environment" (CSF in the dural sac), in the absence of purposeful intervention, surgeons have to rely on the spontaneous expansion of the spinal cord after decompression. Composed of connective tissue, the dural sac may adhere to the pressure origins such as intervertebral disc, ossified tissue, and osteophytes, and thin out under the sustained compression. In this case, the dural sac becomes vulnerable to injury during surgery and results in CSF leakage. Therefore, instead of seeking to restore the natural state of the "liquid environment," surgeons pursue techniques to minimize surgical maneuver to the dural sac and avoid CSF leakage.

The ACAF technique, guided by the theory of in situ decompression to the spinal cord, reestablishes the CSF environment in a unique manner, which is explained here with the example of multisegment OPLL. First of all, the ACAF technique averts direct removal of the ossified tissue as the surgeon does not have to dissect the potential plane between the ossification and the dural sac. This significantly reduces the iatrogenic irritation to the CSF environment. Second, the ACAF technique achieves spinal cord decompression and the reconstruction of the anterior wall of the spinal canal wall through vertebrae-ossification complex (VOC) antedisplacement. This advancement not only clears the compression ventral to the spinal cord but also expands the spinal canal, a result similar to that of the combined anterior and posterior surgery. Therefore, the ACAF provides not a segmental decompression but overall unloading of the cervical spinal cord, which is conducive to the concurrent resumption of CSF channel patency in each segment. Finally, for cases where the ossified tissue has adhered to the dura mater, the dural sac, as a part of the VOC, is antedisplaced, representing a purposeful expansion of the collapsed dural sac that allows it to reposition in the spinal canal.

References

[1] Chen Y, Chen D, Wang X, et al. C5 palsy after laminectomy and posterior cervical fixation for ossification of posterior longitudinal ligament. Journal of Spinal Disorders & Techniques 2007;20(7):533−5.

[2] Matsuda R, Goda K, Nakase H, et al. Case of hydrocephalus after cervical laminoplasty for cervical ossification of the posterior longitudinal ligament. Brain and nerve=Shinkei Kenkyū no Shinpo 2009;61(1):89−92.

[3] Das K, Couldwell WT, Sava G, et al. Use of cylindrical titanium mesh and locking plates in anterior cervical fusion. Journal of Neurosurgery 2001;94(1):174−8.

[4] Dalbayrak S, Yilmaz M, Naderi S. "Skip" corpectomy in the treatment of multilevel cervical spondylotic myelopathy and ossified posterior longitudinal ligament. Journal of Neurosurgery: Spine 2010;12(1):33−8.

[5] Fujiyoshi T, Yamazaki M, Kawabe J, et al. A new concept for making decisions regarding the surgical approach for cervical ossification of the posterior longitudinal ligament. Spine 2008;33(26):e990−3.

[6] Andaluz N, Zuccarello M, Kuntz C. Long-term follow-up of cervical radiographic sagittal spinal alignment after 1-and 2-level cervical corpectomy for the treatment of spondylosis of the subaxial cervical spine causing radiculomyelopathy or myelopathy: a retrospective study. Journal of Neurosurgery: Spine 2012;16(1):2−7.

[7] Beatty RA, Odate S, Shikata J, et al. Extremely wide and asymmetric anterior decompression causes postoperative C5 palsy. Spine 2014;39(7):632.

[8] Xiaowei L, Deyu C, Xinwei W, et al. The effect of K-line on the curative effect of two kinds of posterior cervical surgery in patients with cervical ossification of the posterior longitudinal ligament. Chinese Journal of Spinal Cord 2013;23(1):6−10.

[9] Haisong Y, Jingchuan S, Jiangang S, et al. In-situ decompression to spinal cord during anterior controllable antedisplacement fusion treating degenerative kyphosis with stenosis: surgical outcomes and analysis of C5 nerve palsy based on 49 patients. World Neurosurgery 2018:115.

[10] Haisong Y, Jingchuan S, Jiangang S, et al. Anterior controllable antedisplacement fusion as a choice for 28 patients of cervical ossification of the posterior longitudinal ligament with dura ossification: the risk of cerebrospinal fluid leakage compared with anterior cervical corpectomy and fusion. European Spine Journal 2019;28(2):370−9.

[11] Haisong Y, Jingchuan S, Jiangang S, et al. Anterior controllable antedisplacement fusion (ACAF) for severe cervical ossification of the posterior longitudinal ligament: comparison with anterior cervical corpectomy with fusion (ACCF). World Neurosurgery 2018;115:e428−36.

[12] Jingchuan S, Jiangang S, Ximing X, et al. Anterior controllable antidisplacement and fusion surgery for the treatment of multilevel severe ossification of the posterior longitudinal ligament with myelopathy: preliminary clinical results of a novel technique. European Spine Journal 2018;27(6):1469−78.

[13] Harrison DE, Cailliet R, Harrison DD, et al. A review of biomechanics of the central nervous system—part I: spinal canal deformations resulting from changes in posture. Journal of Manipulative and Physiological Therapeutics 1999;22(4):227−34.

[14] Hogan Q, Toth J. Anatomy of soft tissues of the spinal canal. Regional Anesthesia and Pain Medicine 1999;24(4):303−10.

[15] Wadhwani S, Loughenbury P, Soames R. The anterior dural (Hofmann) ligaments. Spine 2004;29(6):623−7.

[16] Harrison DE, Cailliet R, Harrison DD, et al. A review of biomechanics of the central nervous system—part II: spinal cord strains from postural loads. Journal of Manipulative and Physiological Therapeutics 1999;22(5):322−32.

[17] Chugh AJS, Weinberg DS, Alonso F, et al. Comparing the effectiveness of sagittal Balance, foraminal stenosis, and preoperative cord rotation in predicting postoperative C5 Palsy. Clinical Spine Surgery 2017;30(9):e1256−61.

[18] Yamada S, Lonser RR. Adult tethered cord syndrome. Clinical Spine Surgery 2000;13(4):319−23.

[19] Kameyama T, Hashizume Y, Sobue G. Morphologic features of the normal human cadaveric spinal cord. Spine 1996;21(11):1285–90.

[20] Jones CF, Cripton PA, Kwon BK. Gross morphological changes of the spinal cord immediately after surgical decompression in a large animal model of traumatic spinal cord injury. Spine 2012;37(15):E890–9.

[21] Chu WCW, Man GCW, Lam WWM, et al. Morphological and functional electrophysiological evidence of relative spinal cord tethering in adolescent idiopathic scoliosis. Spine 2008;33(6):673–80.

[22] Kawaguchi Y, Kanamori M, Ishihara H, et al. Minimum 10-year followup after en bloc cervical laminoplasty. Clinical Orthopaedics and Related Research 2003;411:129–39.

[23] Denaro V, Longo UG, Berton A, et al. Favourable outcome of posterior decompression and stabilization in lordosis for cervical spondylotic myelopathy: the spinal cord "back shift" concept. European Spine Journal 2015;24(Suppl. 7):826–31.

[24] Lee JY, Sharan A, Baron EM, et al. Quantitative prediction of spinal cord drift after cervical laminectomy and arthrodesis. Spine 2006;31(16):1795–8.

[25] Seichi A, Takeshita K, Kawaguchi H, et al. Postoperative expansion of intramedullary high-intensity areas on T2-weighted magnetic resonance imaging after cervical laminoplasty. Spine 2004;29(13):1478–82.

[26] Shiozaki T, Otsuka H, Nakata Y, et al. Spinal cord shift on magnetic resonance imaging at 24 hours after cervical laminoplasty. Spine 2009;34(3):274–9.

[27] Kim S, Lee SH, Kim ES, et al. Clinical and radiographic analysis of C5 palsy after anterior cervical decompression and fusion for cervical degenerative disease. Journal of Spinal Disorders & Techniques 2014;27(8):436–41.

[28] Hatta Y, Shiraishi T, Hase H, et al. Is posterior spinal cord shifting by extensive posterior decompression clinically significant for multisegmental cervical spondylotic myelopathy? Spine 2005;30(21):2414–9.

[29] Yong Q, Qiqi L, Weiguo L, et al. Experimental study on spinal cord conduction dysfunction caused by rotation and stretching of the spine. Chinese Journal of Orthopedics 2004;24(12):751–6.

[30] Kaneyama S, Sumi M, Kanatani T, et al. Prospective study and multivariate analysis of the incidence of C5 palsy after cervical laminoplasty. Spine 2010;35(26):e1553–8.

[31] Sakaura H, Hosono N, Mukai Y, et al. C5 palsy after decompression surgery for cervical myelopathy: review of the literature. Spine 2003;28(21):2447–51.

[32] Tianwei S, Hang Z, Shouliang LU, et al. Clinical analysis of C5 nerve root palsy in hinge side and different angles in lamina open-door after expansion of open-door cervical laminoplasty. Chinese Journal of Reparative and Constructive Surgery 2011; 25(11).

[33] Imagama S, Matsuyama Y, Yukawa Y, et al. C5 palsy after cervical laminoplasty: a multicentre study. Journal of Bone & Joint Surgery British Volume 2010;92(3):393–400.

[34] Chugh AJ, Gebhart JJ, Eubanks JD. Predicting postoperative C5 palsy using preoperative spinal cord rotation. Orthopedics 2015;38(9):e830.

[35] Eskander MS, Balsis SM, Chris B, et al. The association between preoperative spinal cord rotation and postoperative C5 nerve palsy. JBJS 2012;94(17):1605–9.

[36] Takase H, Murata H, Sato M, et al. Delayed C5 palsy after anterior cervical decompression surgery: preoperative foraminal stenosis and postoperative spinal cord shift increase the risk of palsy. World Neurosurgery 2018;120:e1107–19.

[37] Yang L, Min Q, Huajiang C, et al. Comparative analysis of complications of different reconstructive techniques following anterior decompression for multilevel cervical spondylotic myelopathy. European Spine Journal 2012;21(12):2428–35.

[38] Ikenaga M, Shikata J, Tanaka C. Radiculopathy of C5 after anterior decompression for cervical myelopathy. Journal of Neurosurgery Spine 2005;3(3):210–7.

[39] Odate S, Shikata J, Yamamura S, et al. Extremely wide and asymmetric anterior decompression causes postoperative C5 palsy: an analysis of 32 patients with postoperative C5 palsy after anterior cervical decompression and fusion. Spine 2013;38(25):2184–9.

[40] Saunders RL. On the pathogenesis of the radiculopathy complicating multilevel corpectomy. Neurosurgery 1995;37(3):408–13.

[41] Jia L, Yongqian L, Fanlong K, et al. Adjacent segment degeneration after single-level anterior cervical decompression and fusion: disc space distraction and its impact on clinical outcomes. Journal of Clinical Neuroscience 2015;22(3):566–9.

[42] Tingsheng L, Chunshan L, Beiping OY, et al. Effects of C5/6 intervertebral space distraction height on pressure on the adjacent intervertebral disks and articular processes and cervical vertebrae range of motion. Medical Science Monitor International Medical Journal of Experimental & Clinical Research 2018;24:2533–40.

[43] Jiangang S, Ximing X, Jingchuan S, et al. Diagnosis and treatment analysis of 30 cases of lumbosacral bowstring disease. Chinese Journal of Medicine 2017;97(11):852–6.

[44] Qingjie K, Ximing X, Jingchuan S, et al. Correlation analysis of spinal nerve hypertension and intervertebral disc degeneration. Chinese Journal of Medicine 2017;97(43). 3416–20.

[45] Jiayue B, Xin Z, Di Z, et al. Impact of over distraction on occurrence of axial symptom after anterior cervical discectomy and fusion. International Journal of Clinical and Experimental Medicine 2015;8(10):19746–56.

[46] Haibo W, Ximing X, Jingchuan S, et al. Analysis of bladder function in the treatment of tethered cord syndrome with uniform spinal cord shortening and axial decompression. Chinese Journal of Spinal Cord 2018;28(05):440–6.

[47] Scoville WB. Cervical spondylosis treated by bilateral facetectomy and laminectomy. Journal of Neurosurgery 1961;18(4):423–8.

[48] Odate S, Shikata J, Kimura H, et al. Hybrid decompression and fixation technique versus plated 3-vertebra corpectomy for 4-segment cervical myelopathy: analysis of 81 cases with a minimum 2-year follow-up. Clinical Spine Surgery 2016;29(6):226–33.

[49] Shuichi K, Masatoshi S, Koichi K, et al. Prospective comparative study of the incidence of postoperative segmental motor paralysis between open-door and double-door laminoplasty. Spine Journal Meeting Abstracts 2008:7.

[50] Panjabi M, White A. Biomechanics of nonacute cervical spinal cord trauma. Spine 1988;13(7):838–42.

[51] Yu F, Xinglong P, Jun Z, et al. Morphological changes of the lower cervical spinal cord under neutral and fully flexed position by MRI in Chinese patients with Hirayama's disease. Amyotrophic Lateral Sclerosis 2008;9(3):156–62.

[52] Fukushima T, Ikata T, Taoka Y, et al. Magnetic resonance imaging study on spinal cord plasticity in patients with cervical compression myelopathy. Spine 1991;16(10): s534–8.

[53] Collins WF. A review and update of experiment and clinical studies of spinal cord injury. Paraplegia 1983;21(4):204–19.

[54] Shimizu K, Nakamura M, Nishikawa Y, et al. Spinal kyphosis causes demyelination and neuronal loss in the spinal cord: a new model of kyphotic deformity using juvenile Japanese small game fowls. Spine 2005;30(21):2388–92.

[55] Yamada S, Won DJ, Pezeshkpour G, et al. Pathophysiology of tethered cord syndrome and similar complex disorders. Neurosurgical Focus 2007;23(2):1–10.

[56] Goto S, Kita T. Long-term follow-up evaluation of surgery for ossification of the posterior longitudinal ligament. Spine 1995;20(20):2247–56.

[57] Rui W, Fei Y, Haibo P, et al. Individual designed titanium mesh used in bone graft fusion and internal fixation to restore cervical curvature. Chinese Journal of Tissue Engineering Research 2014;67(4):281–4.

[58] Herman JM, Sonntag VK. Cervical corpectomy and plate fixation for postlaminectomy kyphosis. Journal of Neurosurgery 1994;80(6):963–70.

[59] AI-Shamy G, Cherian J, Mata JA, et al. Computed tomography morphometric analysis for lateral mass screw placement in the pediatric subaxial cervical spine. Journal of Neurosurgery: Spine 2012;17(5):390–6.

[60] Takemitsu M, Cheung KM, Wong YW, et al. C5 nerve root palsy after cervical laminoplasty and posterior fusion with instrumentation. Journal of Spinal Disorders & Techniques 2008;17(4):267–72.

[61] Yoshizawa H. Presidential address: pathomechanism of myelopathy and radiculopathy from the viewpoint of blood flow and cerebrospinal fluid flow including a short historical review. Spine 2002;27(12):1255–63.

[62] Tominaga T, Watabe N, Takahashi T, et al. Quantitative assessment of surgical decompression of the cervical spine with cine phase contrast magnetic resonance imaging. Neurosurgery 2002;50(4):791–5.

Section 3: Surgical options and indications of the ACAF technique

In 1911, Hibbs and Albee reported the spinal fusion decompression technique to treat spinal tuberculosis. Since then, the fusion-decompression idea has guided the surgical treatment of traumatic and nontraumatic spinal diseases. Especially in the cervical spine, whether it is caused by infection, fracture, congenital and developmental deformity, or degenerative disease, a space-occupying entity in the spinal canal that compresses the spinal cord will lead to motor, sensory, reflex, and sphincter dysfunction and skin dystrophy that correspond to the disease high up in the spine, which seriously affects the ability of work and daily activities in patients. Achieving evident decompression of the spinal cord should be a key element in designing the spine surgical procedures. In this section, we are going to discuss the characteristics of various spinal cord compression diseases to which the ACAF technique is applicable and the selection of surgical procedures.

Ossification of the posterior longitudinal ligament
Overview

The PLL travels longitudinally along the anterior wall of the spinal canal, from C2 to the sacral canal. Its fibers extend to the bilateral intervertebral foramen and the capsule of the uncinate process, as known as the Luschka joints. OPLL is caused by the heterotopic bone formation in the PLL and the gradual OPLL. As this ossified structure compresses the spinal cord and nerve roots, it then produces neurological symptoms such as paresthesia of the hands, feet, and trunk, motor paralysis, and bladder and bowel dysfunction. This disease is mostly chronic, progressive, and difficult to treat.

In 1838, Key became the first person to point out that the ossification of spinal ligaments could lead to spinal cord injury and paralysis. In 1960, based on an autopsy, Tsukimoto attributed spinal movement restriction and nerve damage to OPLL, which drew significant attention at that time and lead to the term of "calcification of posterior longitudinal ligament." This disease was later renamed as "ossification of the posterior longitudinal ligament" as pathological evidence from Terayama in 1964 revealed ossified components in the diseased ligament tissue of patients with calcification of PLL.

Epidemiological-wise, the incidence of OPLL is high in Asia and low in Europe and the United States. It affects people over the age of 40 years more often, with a male-to-female ratio of 2:1 to 3:1. According to surveys of many Japanese hospitals, the incidence of OPLL in adult outpatient is 1.5%−2.4%. Its incidence varies from 0.4% to 3% in other Asian countries and stands at around 0.1% in North America and Germany, according to the study of Yamauchi and Izawa.

The primary complaints of patients with incipient OPLL are neck discomfort and symmetrical numbness of the upper extremities, in particular the hands. As the disease progresses, typical symptoms of OPLL include sensorimotor dysfunction of the upper and lower extremities, tendon hyperreflexia, positive pathological signs, and bladder dysfunction. Usually, tetraplegia develops around the same time as sphincter dysfunction.

The cause of OPLL is not yet clear, but genetic factors and metabolic disorders have been proved to have played an important role in the pathogenesis of OPLL. Genetic studies have revealed the familial clustering in OPLL. Terayama found that the incidence of OPLL was 24% among the second-degree relatives of OPLL patients. A twin study involving eight pairs of identical twins and two pairs of fraternal twins conducted by the OPLL Research Society of Japan showed that both twins in six pairs of identical twins developed the disease. In comparison, only one of the twins in the remaining four pairs did so. This study suggested that genetic factors play an essential role in the pathogenesis of OPLL. A human leukocyte antigen haplotype analysis on siblings for OPLL found that individuals who shared two identical haplotypes with the proband had a much higher incidence than those with only one identical haplotype, and those who did not share the same haplotype with the proband did not develop OPLL at all. Nonparametric linkage analysis indicated that the collagen $\alpha 2$ (XI) gene might be a potential key gene in the pathogenesis of OPLL. In addition, abnormal metabolism of glucose, vitamin A, and vitamin D is also related to the onset of OPLL.

OPLL of the cervical spine is a complex and continuous process from early hyperplasia, punctate calcification, and chondrogenesis to complete ossification (Fig. 1-3-1). At first, chondrogenic and fibroblast-like spindle cells with mesenchymal characteristics in the PLL keep proliferating under the effect of various growth factors, causing fibrous and nonfibrous tissue proliferation. Infiltrated by the vascular tissue, the PLL gradually degenerates with chondroid traits. Finally, osteogenesis develops within the chondroid tissue in the degenerated PLL, and the ossified PLL is gradually substituted with mature lamellar bone. With the continuous growth of ligament ossification, the spinal canal further narrows, and the patients' symptoms worsen as the spinal cord is increasing compressed. However, not all cervical OPLL causes cervical spondylosis, and the ossified lesion can remain static for a long time in some patients without progression.

Diagnosis

In observing the dural ossification (DO) among OPLL patients, Mizuno classified DO into three types: isolated, double-layered, and en bloc. In the en bloc DO, the ossified dura mater is wholly integrated with the ossified PLL.

Patients with OPLL present similar to CSM, but their disease progresses significantly faster than common cervical degenerative diseases.

X-ray examination, the mainstay of diagnosis and classification of OPLL, has been applied in a large number of epidemiological investigations and analyses

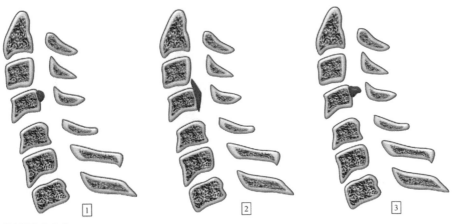

FIGURE 1-3-1

Growth direction of ossification of posterior longitudinal ligament.
(1) Original posterior longitudinal ligament ossification.
(2) Longitudinal growth of the ossification.
(3) Horizontal growth of the ossification.

carried out by Japanese physicians. OPLL presents as an abnormally dense mass along the posterior margin of the vertebra. According to the shape of the ossification, OPLL can be roughly classified into the following four types: ① continuous type where the ossification, in the shape of a band or a cord, spans multiple segments; ② segmented type where the ossification is confined to the space behind the vertebra without crossing the disc space; ③ mixed type where the disease manifests the combined elements of continuous and segmented types; and ④ circumscribed or localized type where the ossification is contiguous with the intervertebral disc and forms a mound-shaped protrusion (Fig. 1-3-2). Compared with Japanese investigators, those in Europe preferred computed tomography (CT) to diagnose and investigate OPLL. In 1992, Epstein studied the cervical CT data of Caucasian patients and found the punctate calcification on hypertrophic PLL and related this finding with the development process of OPLL. With advantages in showing the shape and location of ossification, the shape of the spinal canal, and the spinal cord compression in different planes, CT and MRI can be used to identify incipient and minimal ossification lesions and plan the surgery.

In Caucasian patients in European and American countries, OPLL is regarded as a subtype of diffuse idiopathic skeletal hyperostosis (DISH). As put forward by Resnick, DISH was a common disease that caused axial and nonaxial bone hyperplasia in Caucasians over 50 years of age that featured the calcification and ossification of the ligaments along with the vertebrae. About 50% of DISH patients also have OPLL. Therefore, OPLL can be distinguished from DISH as the patients are assessed for ossification of other parts of the body.

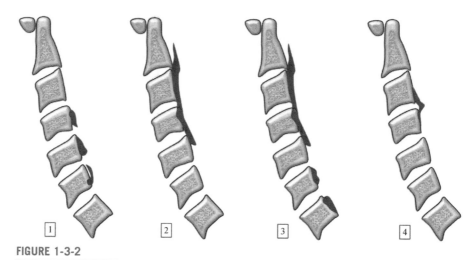

FIGURE 1-3-2

OPLL classification.
(1) Segmented type.
(2) Continuous type.
(3) Mixed type.
(4) Localized (circumscribed) type.

Imaging studies are an indispensable means to diagnose OPLL and characterize its morphology and relationship with the spinal cord. The primary feature of OPLL on the X-ray image is the abnormally dense strip shadow on the posterior margin of the vertebrae (Fig. 1-3-3). On a noncontrast CT scan, the disease manifests itself as a hyperdense ossification mass at the posterior margin of the vertebrae protruding into the spinal canal, with stenosed and narrowed spinal canal. On axial CT images, the degree of spinal stenosis is measured by the ratio of the reduction of the spinal canal. The three-dimensional CT reconstruction can be used to provide a complete understanding of the magnitude of the OPLL (Fig. 1-3-4). On the T1-weighted and T2-weighted images of MRI, the OPLL often presents as hypointense masses that protrude into the spinal canal, accompanied by diminished extradural fat and compressed dural sac. On the axial image at the affected levels, a hypointense mass on the posterior margin of the vertebra indents the spinal canal and compresses the spinal cord and nerve roots (Fig. 1-3-5).

Surgical treatment

Surgical intervention can change the natural history of spinal ligament ossification and prevent spinal cord deterioration. The reasonable selection of the timing and type of surgery is critical to ensure the surgical efficacy in OPLL patients.

Because some patients are free of neurological symptoms and signs for a long time, not all patients with OPLL require surgery. It has been a consensus that

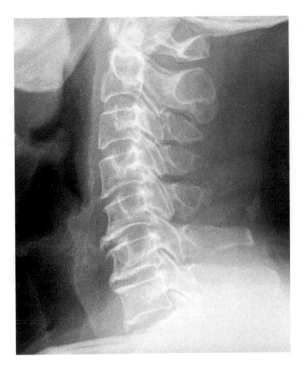

FIGURE 1-3-3

OPLL X-ray image.

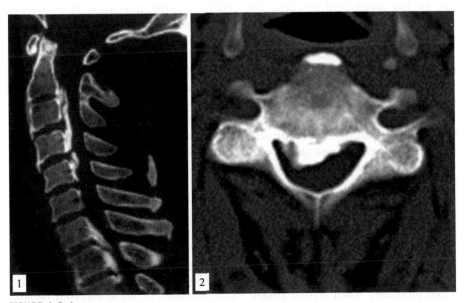

FIGURE 1-3-4

OPLL CT images.
(1) Sagittal view.
(2) Transverse view.

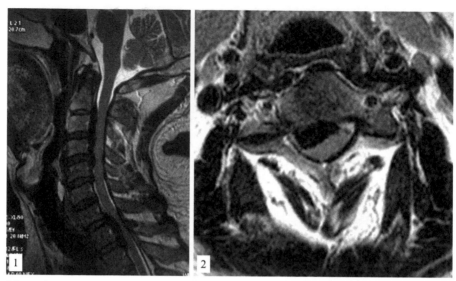

FIGURE 1-3-5

OPLL MRI images.
(1) Sagittal view.
(2) Transverse view.

surgical intervention before the occurrence of irreversible pathological changes in the spinal cord changes the disease's natural history, helps prevent further deterioration of the spinal cord function, and obtains a better prognosis. In a 14-year follow-up study of patients with cervical myelopathy caused by OPLL undergoing laminectomy, Kato et al. found that young patients and those with a higher score of JOA had a good prognosis and recommended early surgical decompression for patients with cervical OPLL and myelopathy. Spinal ligament ossification progresses slowly, and it takes a long time from the onset of symptoms to the severity that patients need surgery. According to a report from the Ministry of Health, Labour and Welfare of Japan in 1984, 54.8% of the patients with mild myelopathy OPLL had no change in the quality of daily life after more than five years of conservative treatment, 26.7% had improved quality of life, and only 18.5% had worsening symptoms which required surgical treatment. When studying the quality of life of elderly OPLL patients [1], Matsunaga et al. found that OPLL patients with no or only mild myelopathy (Nurick grade 1 to 2) could obtain a satisfactory quality of life for the long term through conservative treatment. In patients with moderate myelopathy (Nurick grade 3 to 4), surgical treatment was much more effective than conservative treatment. Furthermore, patients with severe myelopathy (Nurick grade 5) consistently ended up with poor quality of life regardless of the type of treatment. Therefore, they suggested that surgery be provided before Nurick becomes grade 5 and preferably when Nurick grades 3 to 4. Meanwhile, some surgeons believe that asymptomatic OPLL can be observed continuously for 6 to 12 months or even years, and surgery can be postponed until the patient develops symptoms of spinal cord compression with CT or MRI evidence of severe nerve compression, intramedullary signal hyperintensity in T2-weighted MRI, or a change in somatosensory-evoked potential. The surgery principles are to resolve the compression of the OPLL on the spinal cord and nerve roots and provide a favorable biological and biomechanical environment for the recovery of nerves and spinal cord.

Conventional anterior surgeries

The conventional anterior surgeries are ACDF and ACCF techniques. Their indications include segmental OPLL of C3 to C7, severe spinal canal stenosis, especially spinal canal stenosis greater than 60%. The conventional anterior surgeries are advantageous in that they are performed with facilitating patient positions, techniques easy to learn, high fusion rate with bone grafting, restoration of the physiological curvature of the cervical spine, and thorough decompression. The anterior surgeries have been shown superior to the posterior ones in OPLL patients with more severe stenosis in the outcomes of spinal canal volume expansion, symptom relief, and JOA score [2]. Since the compressing object of OPLL is in front of the spinal cord, the anterior surgery can directly remove the compressing object, which constitutes the most effective way of decompression.

However, the anterior surgeries bear unique challenges: ① Difficulty in exposure: In OPLL of unusual shapes, such as a wide-based or paracentral lesion, it is difficult to fully expose the ossification through the prepared intervertebral space or grooves from corpectomy. Also, they leave limited space for instrument maneuvers. What is worse, the bleeding from ossification removal further blurs the vision in the narrow operating wound. The combined effect of the above factors can result in oblique bone cuts and residual ossification (Fig. 1-3-6). For ossifications extending proximally (e.g., those involving C2) or distally to the thoracic spine, anterior access becomes more inhibiting [3]. ② Resection risk: Since the ossification is often attached or even adhered to the dura mater, while the ossification is resected in a piecemeal fashion, the dura mater may flutter. In return, the ossification sways and fails the removal maneuvers, causing secondary spinal cord injury and tear of the adhered dura [4]. ③ Difficulty in reconstruction: during ossification resection, many vertebral structures in the anterior column irrelevant to the compression are resected as well, which significantly changes the force distribution pattern of the anterior and posterior spinal columns. Moreover, for long-segment ossification, the surgeon needs to reconstruct with structural bone or long titanium meshes, which increases the risk of nonunion and dislodgement of grafts [5]. The anterior approach mainly includes the following types.

ACDF technique

This procedure is suitable for circumscribed OPLL at the intervertebral space that does not affect the posterior wall of the vertebra. The procedure involves removing the intervertebral disc and the attached ossification followed by intervertebral fusion and instrumentation with screw and plate.

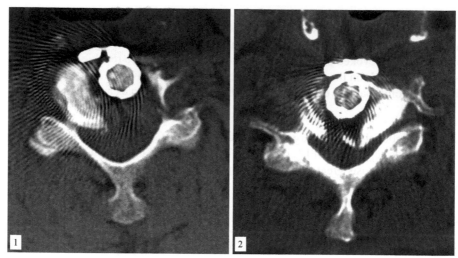

FIGURE 1-3-6

CT images displaying ACCF technique and the groove developed.
(1) Oblique groove.
(2) Ossification residue.

ACCF technique

Studies have shown that patients with spinal stenosis greater than 60% undergoing anterior surgery obtained better results than those undergoing posterior surgery, though they had a similar complication rate [6]. Besides, the anterior procedure has many advantages. First, there is straight-forward patient positioning, less bleeding due to intermuscular approaches, shorter surgical duration, and surgeon-friendly features. With the direction of approach consistent with cord compression, the anterior approach achieves the most effective direct decompression. It also provides partial and appropriate correction for the spinal curvature and stabilization with bone graft fusion, which is especially suitable for patients with cervical kyphosis. The most frequent complications include hyponatremia, throat irritation, lung infection, and CSF leakage. Injuries to the recurrent laryngeal nerve, trachea, esophagus, spinal cord, and nerve roots, and loosening and dislodgement of instrumentation can also occur from time to time [7].

OPLL can encroach on the dura mater, resulting in adhesion and even ossification of the dura mater. This explains the residual ossification and tearing of the dura mater in the ACCF surgery. As such, Yamaura issued the first report of the anterior floating surgery that does not directly remove the ossification [8]. Rather than completely removing the ossified lesion, this technique leaves the ossification and achieves decompression by allowing the lesion and the ossified dura to drift forward slowly under the CSF shove. In this procedure, a corpectomy is performed for ossification exposure, followed by OPLL dissection from the front and sides. This procedure allows the OPLL to move forward into the groove to achieve decompression.

Indeed, the ossification floats ventrally, which is an uncontrollable process [9]. Literature shows that it takes an average of two weeks to achieve a radiologically measurable drift. This process may fail in some patients as the ossification drifts back again and or does not adequately drift forward due to the barrier of the residual vertebra. Therefore, decompression achieved through this procedure is unpredictable in speed and efficacy [10]. Chen Deyu described a modified technique in which the ossifications were first thinned as much as possible. As such, the floating can be achieved with a minimum ossification on the dura mater [11]. However, these two methods are technically demanding and bear the risks associated with long-segment implants.

Based on the summary of the conventional anterior surgeries that resects the ossification, Chen Xiongsheng described the "en bloc ossification resection" to address spinal cord irritancy of repeated instrument entries into the spinal canal [12]. In this procedure, a subtotal corpectomy of the responsible vertebra is performed first, which preserves the posterior wall of the vertebra. Then the posterior wall of the vertebra is dissected with a burr to generate a complex of the posterior wall and the ossification. Finally, the complex is clamped out as a whole to achieve the decompression. The technique was deemed innovative as it advocates the "principle of minimal spinal cord irritancy" and remove the ossification en bloc instead of in a piecemeal fashion. As such, it helps reduce bleeding and prevent iatrogenic spinal cord injury. However, this procedure achieves a limited number of resected levels, a constraint shared by the conventional ACCF technique, and carries a significant risk of spinal dural injury during the bone resection.

Posterior surgeries

Indications of posterior surgeries include ① K-line-positive OPLL of three or more segments; ② OPLL involving C1 or C2 or extending to the thoracic spine; ③ concomitant dorsal compression of the spinal cord; ④ developmental spinal stenosis that constitutes significant risk and challenge in anterior approach decompression; and ⑤ patients with acute onset spinal cord injury requiring extensive decompression [13]. Posterior surgeries are advantageous as they provide adequate decompression in a safe and straight-forward manner. The rationale behind the indication mentioned above is threefold. First, the thick and extensively fused continuous OPLL causes minimal instability or disc herniation. Second, there is a high risk of nonfusion and dislodgement of long-segment intervertebral implants. Finally, OPLL that extends to the upper cervical spine or thoracic spine can hardly be decompressed adequately through the anterior approach, let alone the meager access constrained by anatomy.

Lamina decompression, fusion, and instrumentation

This conventional technique has been described above. With the use of pedicle screw providing good purchase, this technique stabilizes the spine and corrects the cervical curvature, factors that protect against kyphosis after laminoplasty in the longer term. However, because OPLL often exists with severe spinal stenosis, the instruments' repeated entries into the spinal canal can easily injure the spinal cord. Meanwhile, as the spinal canal is vented posteriorly and the dura mater exposed to the adjacent structures, dural adhesion and scar may develop, leading to spinal stenosis. Thus, this technique has fallen out of favor.

Laminoplasty

The aforementioned "Z"-shaped, single-door, and double-door laminoplasty are applicable to OPLL treatment. They all achieve decompression by enlarging the posterior part of the spinal canal (Fig. 1-3-7). In view of the frequent coexistence of spinal stenosis in OPLL, laminoplasty has the following three advantages: ① Less intrusion in the spinal canal. The only step that involves the spinal canal is groove development. The groove is cut on the posterolateral ring of the spinal canal in an outside-in fashion with significant freedom of maneuver and minimal disturbance to the spinal cord. ② The posterior wall of the spinal canal is mostly preserved. With the hinge healed, the lamina continues to be the posterior barrier to the spinal cord to guard against the compression from scars. Therefore, it provides patients with better postoperative mobility than anterior surgeries. ③ The technique is relatively easy to master, and it can be successfully applied in elderly patients with multiple-segment OPLL or multiple underlying diseases. With shorter operation duration, it provides a good option for patients with suboptimal physical fitness.

Despite the above advantages, posterior surgeries also bear many complications inevitably. Based on a large number of retrospective studies, researches have concluded the primary complications of posterior surgeries as postoperative cervical axial pain, C5 nerve palsy, and recurrent cord compression secondary to ossification progression. Cervical axial pain is tied to the destruction of the posterior spinal

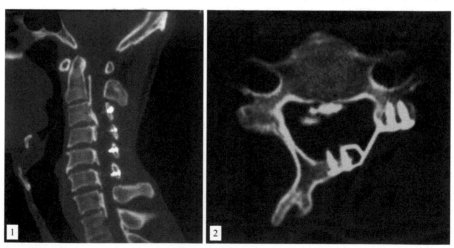

FIGURE 1-3-7

CT images after single-door laminoplasty for OPLL.
(1) Sagittal view.
(2) Transverse view.

structure due to such procedures as muscle elevation, the use of electrocautery for hemostasis, and the destruction of articular processes. Ischemia–reperfusion injury of the nerve root artery primarily accounts for C5 palsy. The overcorrection of cervical kyphosis and nerve root tethering caused by the posterior shift of the spinal cord also causes C5 palsy.

Matsunaga et al. followed up 450 patients for 10 years [1] and found that after any kind of posterior decompression surgery, the ossification continued to develop. Transversely, 42% of the disease developed while 86% developed longitudinally. The progressing ossification diminishes the long-term efficacy of posterior-only procedures. For better long-term effects, the anterior surgeries are increasingly preferred. Put it another way, patients with longer life expectancy are recommended against the posterior-only surgeries.

Combined anterior and posterior surgery

Indications of the combined anterior and posterior surgery have been concluded as: ① spinal canal stenosis of 50% or higher caused by anterior spinal cord compression with concomitant developmental or degenerative cervical spinal canal stenosis; ② severe cord compression from ventral bony indentation at multiple segments (with spinal canal stenosis much higher than 50% or even above 75%) despite the absence of developmental or degenerative component; ③ "pincer-type" impingement on the spinal cord and spinal canal stenosis above 50% at one, two, or more levels caused by anterior bony indentation.

Although the combined anterior and posterior approach has composite advantages, it also carries a higher incidence of surgical complications related to each of the anterior and posterior approaches. It increases the treatment cost and the financial burden of patients as well. Therefore, more caution should be taken when considering the combined anterior and posterior approach. Indeed, with the advent of the ACAF technique, the combined anterior and posterior approach is indicated for a fewer number of cases. The ACAF technique can be applied to most cases where the ossification was previously thought to be too severe, with a reduced possibility of complications.

ACAF technique

For OPLL patients, the indications of the ACAF technique include ① ossification posterior to vertebra unresectable through the intervertebral space; ② ossification involving one to four vertebra segments (or even up to six segments if custom-made long plates are available); ③ ossification involving C2 or T1 levels; and ④ prominent localized ossification unlikely to benefit from a posterior decompression. In particular, for severe OPLL of more than three vertebrae, or at least 5 mm thick, or with spinal canal stenosis above 60%, direct resection is noticeably difficult and risky, and the choice of surgical treatment has remained a topic of controversy [3]. For these patients, the ACAF technique has obvious advantages.

The ACAF technique provides a new direct decompression option for some "massive" OPLL used to be in a dilemma between the posterior and the combined AP approach.

First of all, the ACAF technique prepares for decompression by dissecting VOC from its surrounding structure. Therefore, it applies to cases where ACCF is not an option, such as cases with problematic exposure due to the wide-based or paracentral disease. Another example is OPLL extending beyond the pedicles, where direct resection of the lateral parts is almost impossible. In such a case, the ACAF technique simply involves a modified groove position without the complicated exposure process and converts it to a much straight-forward operation.

Second, the ACAF technique averts the removal of the ossification behind the vertebra, effectively reducing the risks of epidural hematoma, dural injury, and spinal cord injury. Therefore, the surgery is less affected by unfavorable factors such as bulky lesions and severe spinal canal stenosis. Finally, the significant parts of the vertebra and ossification preserved in the ACAF technique serve as the basis for reconstructing the anterior spinal column and the anterior wall of the spinal canal. Thus, the ACAF technique is a safer option in treating multilevel OPLL independent of the risk of nonfusion and massive hardware-associated complications.

Another common challenge for the conventional anterior and posterior approaches is ossifications involving the C2 or the thoracic spine. However, in the ACAF technique, this is readily addressed with a recess, like a bird nest, developed in the posteroinferior rim of the C2 or the posterosuperior rim of the T1 vertebra in an undercut fashion through the disc space. When the VOC is moved forward, the ossification at the C2 and T1 segments also moves and rests into the "bird nest" to achieve decompression. In this sense, ACAF provides a new idea for OPLL treatment [14].

Cervical spondylotic myelopathy
Overview

Cervical spondylosis refers to a group of clinical diseases caused by vertebra degeneration, intervertebral disc, facet joints, and ligaments. The most common cause of degeneration is aging, followed by sustained occupational injuries (such as axial loading), genetic susceptibility, smoking, and Down syndrome. CSM is the most severe type of cervical spondylosis that manifests with spinal cord compression and is the most common cause of nontraumatic upper motor neuron paralysis.

The process of cervical spine degeneration generally begins with the loss of disc integrity. With the progress of intervertebral disc degeneration, the water content of the nucleus pulposus gradually decreases, and the disc may even collapse. Subsequently, the inner fiber ring buckles inward while the outer one protrudes outward. This process, called intervertebral disc herniation, results in intervertebral space narrowing and an impaired cushion effect of the disc. In an autopsy study, Christe described the pathological process of intervertebral disc herniation as central cystic degeneration, annulus fibrosus layer malalignment, and progressing radial fissures. These changes eventually increase the stress on adjacent vertebral endplates [15].

Without the disc's cushioning effect, the endplates sustain loads directly as a motion unit, which results in hyperostosis in the subcortical bone and osteophytes formed on the ventral side of the spinal canal. From a biomechanical perspective, osteophyte formation results from the compensation that stabilizes the spine during segmental motion by increasing the contact area between the vertebrae. On the other hand, osteophytes encroach the spinal canal and compress the spinal cord and nerve roots. Osteophytes can also form at the uncovertebral and facet joints, causing ventral stenosis of the intervertebral foramen. On the posterior side of the spinal canal, the ligamentum flavum in reduced tension buckles due to the loss of the disc height, protruding into the spinal canal. The combined effect of these pathological changes is circumferential stenosis of the spinal canal that leads to CSM (Fig. 1-3-8).

Arnold found a high correlation between the sagittal diameter of the spinal canal and the occurrence of myelopathy in an autopsy study [16]. At the C3 to C7 segments, the sagittal diameter of the spinal canal is typically 17−18 mm, while that

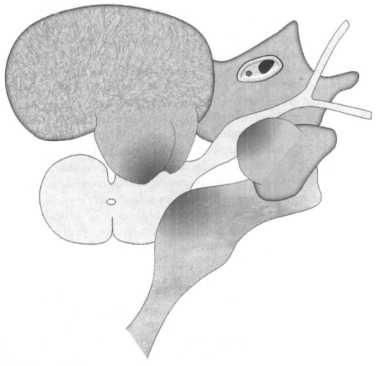

FIGURE 1-3-8

Spinal nerve compression caused by degeneration of intervertebral discs, facet joints, and ligaments.

of the spinal cord approximately 10 mm. Therefore, there is a 7—8 mm long anterior and posterior space to the spinal cord to cushion the mild stenosis caused by degeneration. The sagittal diameter of the spinal canal less than 12 mm has been found in multivariate analysis to be one of the risk factors for CSM onset. For example, patients with congenital spinal stenosis are less tolerant of degenerative stenosis than the general population and are vulnerable to CSM.

In addition to the above static mechanical stressors, dynamic factors can also induce CSM. Dynamic factors such as flexion and extension can exacerbate the existing spinal nerve root compression, especially in patients with cervical spondylosis, OPLL, or congenital spinal stenosis. During cervical flexion, the spinal cord is stretched and pulled to the ventral side, getting closer to the osteophytes protruding into the spinal canal. When the neck extends, the ligamentum flavum buckles and protrudes into the spinal canal, increasing the risk of the "pincer-type" impingement from concomitant anterior and posterior stressors on the spinal cord. Using a computer model to simulate the mechanical properties of the gray and white matter of the spinal cord, Ichihara measured the intramedullary pressure of the spinal cord under dynamic conditions. The results showed that in patients with severe spinal stenosis, the shear force generated by repeated hyperextension of the cervical spine on the front and back of the spinal cord was comparable to that in acute spinal cord trauma.

Although CSM's main pathogenesis is the compression of the nerve tissue under both static and dynamic factors, more and more evidence now shows that spinal cord ischemia is also an essential disease contributor. Many studies have shown that CSM histopathological changes are similar to those observed in spinal cord ischemia. Studies have also confirmed that oligodendrocytes are very sensitive to ischemic changes and can lead to early demyelination of the corticospinal tract. Also, patients with various severity of spinal cord compression have been identified with pathological changes in the lateral corticospinal tract similar to spinal cord ischemia. The pattern of spinal cord ischemia depends on the types of blood vessels involved. At the damaged segments, the common direct causes of ischemia are decreased blood flow of the venous plexus of the pia mater, venous congestion, and compression of large blood vessels (such as the anterior spinal artery).

As CSM causes a heterogeneous spectrum of signs, it is difficult to detect the symptoms during the early stage. Since natural history varies vastly among the population, the prognosis is often unpredictable. Clark and Robinson reported the natural history study of CSM involving 120 patients in 1956 for the first time. Studies have shown that CSM can cause slowly progressing nerve damage and acute symptom aggravation. In untreated patients, the symptoms are rarely entirely relieved, and neural damage hardly recovers. Most patients will live with varying degrees of permanent disability. Lees and Turner reported in a 10-year follow-up study that due to the insidious onset and slow progress, patients with CSM had consistent symptoms long before symptom aggravation that prompted health-seeking behavior. Symon and Lavendar indicated that CSM was anything but a "benign" disease because even after surgery, 67% of the patients still experienced continuous neurological deterioration. Sadasivian shared the same view in his study that CSM's natural history was characterized by progressive deterioration. A study also found that patients with CSM had an average delay of 6.3 years from onset to diagnosis, during which the patients' ambulation deteriorated on average by two grades, measured with Nurick score.

In addition to neurogenic neck pain, CSM patients often complain of nonspecific stiffness and numbness, pain, and muscle weakness in the neck and the innervated area associated with the disease level. The most typical symptoms of CSM are gait disturbance and weakness and stiffness of the lower limbs. Patients may also experience decreased hand dexterity and paresthesia, manifested as clumsy movements in buttoning, zippering, and writing. Sphincter and detrusor dysfunction are rare, but some patients report symptoms of urgency, frequent urination, and constipation.

The crux of physical examination is to identify and locate the abnormalities of upper motor neurons, including deep reflexes, ankle-knee clonus, muscle spasm, Babinski sign, and Hoffman sign. The pathological reflex originates from the loss of upper motor neurons' inhibitory function and is often associated with spinal cord disease.

Gait disturbance is an initial symptom in some CSM patients. At first, patients may feel imbalance when walking or discordant steps when taking turns or complain of the inability to walk long distances. As the disease progresses, patients may experience stiffness or cramps while walking. During the examination, the typical findings include a wide-based stance and hesitant step initiation. With deteriorating motor coordination, the patient may have to maintain balance by toe walking or heel landing.

In terms of the upper extremities' motion, CSM patients often manifest weakness of the triceps and intrinsic hand muscles. In severe cases, muscle atrophy may occur. The positive finger escape sign indicates diminished strength of the intrinsic hand muscle where the small finger spontaneously abducts as the patient holds fingers extended and adducted. The 10-second grip and release test is another way to examine the intrinsic hand muscles. Patients struggling to make a fist and release 20 times 10 seconds indicates impaired signaling along the spinal cord and spinal cord compression. In the lower extremities, the proximal muscles are more affected than the distal ones, and muscle weakness is more common in the iliopsoas and quadriceps femoris muscles.

CSM involves a broad spectrum of paresthesia. It typically starts at the fingertips, being nondermatomal and confined to the hands. Impaired sense of vibration and proprioception of the extremities associated with the dorsal tract's injury is also one of the early signs of myelopathy. A positive Lhermitte sign indicates injury to the spinal cord's dorsal funiculus, where extreme cervical flexion leads to shock-like sensations that radiate down the spine and into the extremities. In contrast, the sensory disturbances caused by spinothalamic tract injury are characterized by asymmetry.

CSM patients, especially those with spinal stenosis who sustain a hyperextension injury, can also present with the acute central cord syndrome, which manifests as weakness in the upper extremity weakness and less severe weakness of the lower extremity extremities, sensory disturbances below the level of injury, and myelopathies, such as spasms and urinary retention.

Among the many scales introduced to assess CSM are the Nurick score mentioned above, which focuses on patients' walking function. The most widely used scale is the JOA score that integrates the movement, sensation, and bladder function. Its modified version or mJOA, described by Benzel, has been adopted to a more considerable extent.

Diagnosis

MRI is the most crucial imaging study for diagnosing CSM. Compared with X-ray and CT, MRI delineates the pattern of the spinal cord and the CSF zone, and reflects the extent of the disease through signal intensities, thereby assisting physicians in the differential diagnosis and assessment of the disease. Therefore, all cervical spondylosis patients with myelopathy signs should undergo MRI for proper diagnosis (Fig. 1-3-9).

CT has advantages in displaying delicate bony structures and is used in conjunction with MRI for diagnosis and surgical planning. X-ray images provide a global view of the shape of the cervical spine. Specifically, lateral X-ray images show intervertebral stenosis, endplate osteophytes, spinal canal stenosis, and cervical alignment; posteroanterior X-ray images demonstrate uncovertebral hyperplasia and scoliosis (Fig. 1-3-10); dynamic radiographs reveal the changes of the range of segmental motion (Fig. 1-3-11); and the oblique images depict the size of the intervertebral foramen (Fig. 1-3-12).

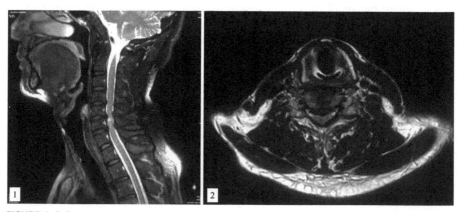

FIGURE 1-3-9

MRI images of cervical spondylosis.
(1) Sagittal view.
(2) Axial view of the C5/6 intervertebral space.

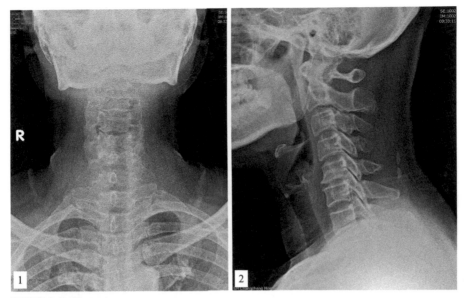

FIGURE 1-3-10

X-ray images of cervical spondylosis.
(1) Lateral view.
(2) Posteroanterior view.

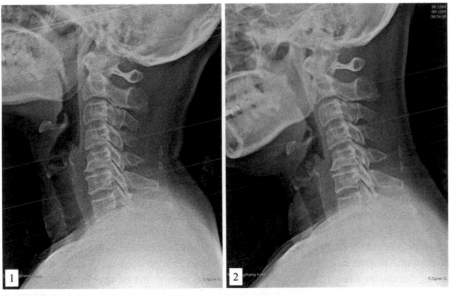

FIGURE 1-3-11

X-ray images of cervical spondylosis.
(1) Hyperextension.
(2) Hyperflexion

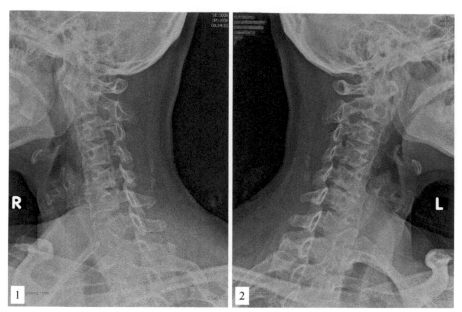

FIGURE 1-3-12

X-ray images of cervical spondylosis.
(1) Right oblique view.
(2) Left oblique view.

CSM should be distinguished from various diseases, and the key to the correct diagnosis is the precise understanding of all the causes of myelopathy.

The infectious causes of myelopathy include abscesses (bacterial, fungal, and tuberculosis), human immunodeficiency virus infection, West Nile virus infection, tropical spastic paralysis, and neurosyphilis. Vascular causes include infarction, hematoma, and vascular malformations. The causes of noninfectious inflammation and demyelinating include multiple sclerosis, acute disseminated encephalomyelitis, transverse myelitis, and optic neuromyelitis. Rheumatic diseases related to immunological injury to the spinal cord are, for example, systemic lupus erythematosus, Sjogren's syndrome, sarcoidosis, and rheumatoid arthritis. In addition, syringomyelia is easily confused with CSM, and imaging studies hold the key to the correct diagnosis.

When no structural abnormalities are evident in imaging results, nutritional and metabolic diseases should be considered. Vitamin B12 deficiency can lead to subacute degeneration of the posterior and lateral corticospinal tracts. The deficiency of copper, vitamin E, and folic acid can also lead to myelopathy. Glioma, meningiomas, neurofibromas, and metastases can cause symptoms of myelopathy through compression and invasion. When the tumor involves the vertebra (such as prostate cancer bone metastasis and multiple myeloma), patients can experience severe pain, bone destruction, and spinal instability, triggering spinal cord compression.

Paraneoplastic syndromes may have myelopathy manifestations, often accompanied by elevated levels of biomarkers. In patients receiving radiotherapy, the parts of the spinal cord exposed to radiation may develop myelopathy. Motor neuron diseases such as ALS can also interfere with the diagnosis of CSM.

Surgical treatment

Nonsurgical treatment is primarily indicated for patients with mild myelopathy (mild hyperreflexia without dysfunction) or patients unfit for surgery. It also applies to individuals with only MRI signs of spinal cord compression but not frank symptoms. Nonsurgical treatment includes the following methods: isometric exercises, collar and cervical braces that reduce nerve irritancy and relieve of cord symptoms; physical therapy that strengthens neck muscles, unloads the cervical spine, and slows down cervical degeneration; nonsteroidal antiinflammatory drugs and other drugs that provide analgesia by inhibiting periarticular inflammation in the early stage of the disease; and neuromodulation drugs (gabapentin or pregabalin) and tricyclic drugs (amitriptyline or nortriptyline) for persistent neck pain and upper limb pain. It should be noted that epidural administration of steroids and neck traction provides mainly symptom relief and helps little with myelopathy's improvement. In addition, patients need to adopt a better lifestyle and daily habits, avoid activities that may aggravate the condition, and, in particular, prevent falls and trauma that may precipitate cervical hyperextension.

For CSM patients, the primary purpose of surgical treatment is to relieve the spinal cord's compression and restore blood supply, and secondly, to stabilize the motion segments to avoid dynamic injuries and deformities, thereby avoiding continued nerve deterioration. Before surgery, surgeons conduct a comprehensive assessment of the patient's symptoms, the severity of nerve damage, and imaging findings to determine whether they need surgery. Surgery is usually recommended for patients with rapidly deteriorating neurological function in a short time or with significantly affected quality of life (e.g., walking, bladder and bowel function, and hand functions). Patients with mild symptoms but severe imaging evidence of compression are also counseled to surgical treatment in case of disease progression. The selection of surgical technique hinges on the location of compression, the involved segments, the vertebral alignment, and the presence of instability. Surgical techniques are classified into two types: anterior and posterior surgeries.

Conventional anterior surgeries

The indications of the anterior surgeries in CSM include: ① cervical intervertebral disc herniation (extrusion) compressing spinal nerves; ② hyperostosis at the posterior wall of the vertebra, resulting in compression; and ③ destabilized cervical spine due to intervertebral instability. The anterior surgery's primary rationale is discectomy or corpectomy of one or multiple segments, followed by bone grafting and fusion. The overarching value of the anterior surgery lies in that it removes the anterior compressors, which cause compression on the ventral spinal cord, and realigns the cervical vertebrae.

Given the various anterior techniques, the selection of a specific one is based on compression.

ACDF technique

This technique applies to compressions mostly confined to the intervertebral space with minimal intervertebral height loss. In this procedure, the surgeon first removes the degenerated nucleus pulposus, and then the osteophytes on the upper and lower rims of the posterior wall of the vertebra through the intervertebral space. After intervertebral decompression, endplate preparation and bone grafting are performed with proper screw and plate instrumentation. Beneficial to restoring the intervertebral height and the physiological curvature of the cervical spine, ACDF represents the option of choice with predictable results and few complications for patients with myelopathy with isolated intervertebral impingers [17]. However, for multisegment lesions, ACDF is less favored due to limited exposure space and scope of decompression. Technically straight-forward though, ACDF requires careful patient selection, and patients with complex diseases are counseled with other surgical methods.

ACCF technique

This technique is recommended for patients with multisegment spinal cord compression and evident compressors behind the vertebra. In this procedure, the surgeon inserts the distractor screws into the upper and lower vertebrae adjacent to those to be removed to facilitate the subsequent vertebra resection. The intervertebral discs on both ends of the vertebrae to be removed are cleared with care taken to retain the bony endplates to prevent the mesh subsidence into the vertebra. After that, along the medial edge of the longus cervicalis, the anterior cortical and cancellous bone of the responsible vertebra are removed until the posterior wall of the vertebra is accessible. The posterior wall of the vertebra is separated from the PLL with an elevator, the cortical bone at the posterior margin of the vertebra removed, the responsible vertebra resected in a piecemeal fashion, the PLL exposed, and the decompression extended to the surrounding areas. The PLL is resected as thoroughly as possible to decompress the spinal cord fully. Finally, a long bone graft or titanium mesh is implanted for fusion, and screws and plate placed for instrumentation.

The ACCF technique provides a broader space for maneuvers, better visualization, and a better decompression than the ACDF technique. It is an essential anterior cervical treatment for multisegment anterior spinal cord compression. Compared to the posterior surgeries, the ACCF technique directly removes the compressors and has more advantages in maintaining the physiological lordosis of the cervical spine [18]. However, since most vertebrae have been removed, the patient is prone to significant surgical insult and complications such as hematoma at the surgical site and dural tear [19]. It has significantly changed the load distribution of the cervical spine and created challenges for reconstructing the load-bearing element of the cervical spine. On the one hand, the application of the anterior plate and the titanium mesh has provided support to the fusion segment and restored and maintained the cervical spine's curvature. On the other hand, such a construct carries the risk of complications such as mesh subsidence, graft dislodgement, and nonfusion [20]. Especially in the multisegment ACCF technique, the plate and mesh spanning a long-distance become malleable and may destabilize under longitudinal loads, quickly causing fusion failure [20]. Therefore, compression in more than three segments is recommended against ACCF technique to prevent complications such as fusion failure of the implant.

Posterior surgeries

The posterior surgeries constitute another group of essential strategies for spinal stenosis and multilevel spinal cord compression. For most patients with cervical spondylosis, because the intervertebral discs and osteophytes on the posterior wall of the vertebra are the main compressors, the anterior approach is often used for direct decompression, especially for patients with poor cervical curvature, where posterior surgeries are not recommended [18]. However, posterior surgeries are still good options in cases with preserved cervical curvature and with concomitant articular process hyperplasia, impingers dorsal to the spinal cord, such as hypertrophic ligamentum flavum, compression involving more than three segments, dismal prospect for a successful fusion, and cases where an anterior surgery is too risky.

Easy to learn and practice, laminectomy used to be a standard posterior approach for cervical spondylosis and was widely used. However, it has been fallen out of favor as the severe complications gradually surfaced, such as cervical kyphosis, segmental instability, and advanced neurological deterioration. In the 1980s, Japanese surgeons sought to treat cervical spondylosis with laminoplasty, which preserved cervical motions while preventing destabilization. Laminoplasty and laminectomy share the objective of enlarging the spinal canal and facilitating the posterior shift of the spinal cord. However, laminoplasty has the edge over laminectomy in cervical stability as bone stock and muscular insertion are preserved. What is more, it has the edge over anterior surgeries in maintain cervical motion [21]. Nevertheless, cervical kyphosis is a contraindication of any posterior surgeries. If decompression in the posterior surgery is achieved with the spinal cord shifted dorsally and away from the ventral indentation, a process guided by cervical lordosis and the pressure difference between the cord's back and front. This mechanism does not work in a kyphotic cervical spine. The major posterior surgeries are described as follows.

Hemilaminectomy decompression technique

This procedure applies to patients with mild spinal stenosis and unilateral symptoms. In this procedure, the surgeon first removes the lateral part of the lamina to be resected from the interlaminar space. Then the surgeon removes the lamina of the responsible segments proximal and distal and dissects and mobilizes the ligamentum flavum until he reaches the dural sac. As such, decompression is completed. Finally, bone grafts are placed between the resected lamina. In laminectomy for more than five segments, lateral mass screws and rods are placed for segmental stability. This procedure has a small impact on the stability of the vertebral segments.

Total laminectomy decompression technique

This procedure is indicated for patients with severe spinal stenosis. The decompression is performed similarly to that of hemilaminectomy except that both sides of the laminae are removed to expose the entire posterior dura mater for bilateral decompression. Since the entire lamina is removed, this highly destabilizing technique makes the patient prone to postoperative cervical kyphosis. Therefore, it is often supplemented with the interlaminar grafting with iliac bone, or the "H-shaped" interspinous bone grafting, and lateral mass screw placement (Fig. 1-3-13).

Laminoplasty

This indication of this procedure is similar to that of laminectomy, namely patients with more than three segments involved and spinal stenosis. It includes single-door and double-door surgery. In the single-door surgery, the surgeon first removes the lamina's posterior cortex on one side and the cut through the lamina on the other side. The lamina is then flipped open from the cut-through side with the contralateral side as the hinge and stabilized, lengthening the lamina to achieve decompression. With a straightforward technique and predictable outcome, single-door surgery is widely applied in clinical practice. In the double door surgery, the surgeon first

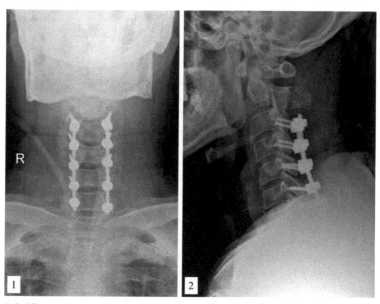

FIGURE 1-3-13

X-ray images of laminectomy with concomitant screw and rod instrumentation.
(1) Posteroanterior view.
(2) Lateral view.

removes the posterior cortex on the lamina on both sides. Then the surgeon splits the spinous process along the midline, flips them laterally, and fixes them. The volume expansion obtained via this procedure is more significant and symmetrical, thus better in decompression. However, it is more challenging and less adopted than single-door surgery [22].

Compared with the anterior surgeries, the posterior ones are easier to adopt and safer as they avert disruption to the anterior structures such as the carotid sheath, trachea, and esophagus. However, the posterior surgeries achieve only indirect decompression and do not eliminate the herniated discs and osteophytes located ventrally. Also, the changes in the morphology of the cervical spine and spinal cord from posterior surgeries have left patients vulnerable to complications such as deformities, axial pain, and nerve root paralysis. As such, it is not the first choice for multisegmental CSM [22].

Combined anterior and posterior surgery

The combined anterior and posterior approach is preserved for patients with severe cervical kyphosis and multisegment cord compression. Posterior instrumentation enhances the stability of the anterior structure and provides a reliable decompression environment for the anterior approach, whereas the anterior procedure aims to restore cervical spine alignment and achieve spinal cord decompression. For example, in a two- to three-segment corpectomy, the posterior procedure is performed first for screw and rod instrumentation to prevent translation and torsion of the spine, reduce implant-related complications, and increase fusion rate. As new techniques are emerging, this procedure has fallen out of favor.

ACAF technique

The ACAF technique is primarily indicated for multisegment cervical spondylosis with spinal stenosis, osteophytes behind the vertebra, and poor cervical curvature. It has unique roles in treating various congenital, developmental, and degenerative cervical spinal stenosis with an AP diameter of the spinal canal less than 12 mm or a Pavlov ratio less than 0.75 [23]. It achieves neural decompression posterior to the vertebrae via displacing the vertebrae forward. The ACAF technique is distinct from the ACCF technique in that it retains and moves the vertebrae forward, thus resolving the conflict between decompression and reconstruction [24]. By preserving the most parts of vertebrae and osteophytes and utilizing them as the concrete basis for spinal canal reconstruction, the ACAF technique effectively avoids the risk of cervical spine instability and mesh subsidence after multisegment corpectomy. Thus, it achieves a significantly higher fusion rate than the ACCF technique. For spinal stenosis treatment, the ACAF technique incorporates the concept of spinal canal expansion characterized in posterior surgeries. Reconstructing the spinal canal anterior wall with the vertebra—ossification complex, the ACAF technique has been proven to surpass the ACCF technique in spinal canal expansion. In managing suboptimal cervical curvature, the ACAF technique achieves partial resection of the anterior vertebra and VOC advancement tailored to the thickness of the ossification of that level. As such, the vertebral alignment is fine-tuned to restore the cervical spine and spinal canal closer to their natural pattern. It is especially helpful for long-segment lesions [24]. Moreover, the ACAF technique is less technically demanding and less morbid than the ACCF technique. For patients with severe and complex cervical spondylosis, the ACAF technique can substitute the conventional combined anterior and posterior surgery with good surgical results and significantly less morbidity.

Complications of ACAF
Cerebrospinal fluid leakage

Cerebrospinal fluid leakage (CSFL), or CSF egressing via a tear in the dura, a major complication to anterior cervical surgery, results from mechanical injury of the dura with surgical tools, in particular during adhesiolysis. In addition, spinal canal stenosis and cervical OPLL, among other conditions, thin out the dura and predispose the host to CSFL. Compared with patients without OPLL, those with OPLL have been found with 13.7-fold risk of dural tear in anterior cervical surgery [1]. If left unnoticed or unaddressed, CSFL may cause intracranial hypotension, increased risk of infection, delayed wound healing, local cysts, or even extensive subcutaneous CSF collections that may compromise ingestion or respiration (Figs. 1-3-14 and 1-3-15). Principal management includes control of the leak (with pressure dressing, lumbar drain, or dural repair), preventing infection, and promoting wound heal. ACCF has been associated with dural tear as the dura may be involved in the surgical tool during adhesiolysis between the dura and PLL. Especially when the dural is ossified, resection may result in a large dural defect and cause the CSFL to persist. Anterior cervical approach provides limited room for surgery, which calls for better options to prevent and repair dural tear.

In contrast to conventional procedures, ACAF significantly reduces the risk of dural tear due to minimal instrument contact with the dura and obviates adhesiolysis between the dura and the PLL. CSFL among patients with cervical OPLL has been reported as 4.6%−32% [2] after ACCF but 3.5%−5.9% after ACAF. Caution should be exercised in ACAF though in cases with DO or ossification attached to the dura. DO can be specifically identified with double-layer sign in preoperative CT, where the hyperdense ossified ligament is separated by a hypodense and nonossified central component (Fig. 1-3-16). A study comparing ACAF and ACCF in cervical OPLL with this double-layer sign showed CSFL in both groups, but the ACAF group had a markedly lower incidence than the ACCF group (3.5% and 22.6%) [3]. CSFL in ACAF has been ascribed to excessive antedisplacement of the levels where the ossification has been adhered to the dura. What is more, continuous and long-spanning OPLL generates extra risk as extra maneuver is involved when the surgeons decide to sever the OPLL at certain intervertebral levels. Therefore,

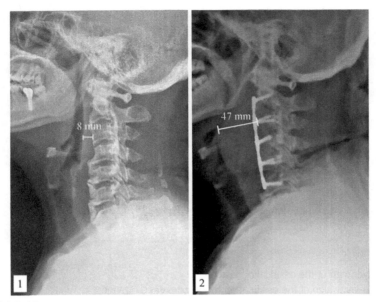

FIGURE 1-3-14

X-ray images of subcutaneous CSF collection
(1) Preoperative cervical lateral X-ray shows soft tissue anterior to C3 measuring 8 mm.
(2) Postoperative cervical lateral X-ray shows extensive subcutaneous fluid collection due to CSFL, resulting in swollen soft tissue anterior to C3 of 47 mm.

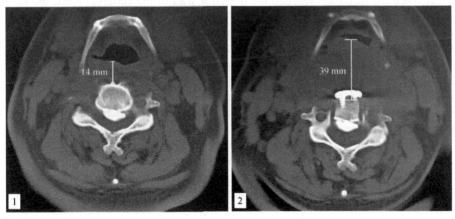

FIGURE 1-3-15

CT images of subcutaneous fluid collection due to CSFL.
(1) Preoperative cervical axial CT image shows the anterior wall of C3 vertebral body is 14 mm posterior to the posterior wall of trachea.
(2) Post-ACAF cervical axial CT image shows extensive subcutaneous fluid collection due to CSFL and C3 vertebral body 39 mm from the trachea.

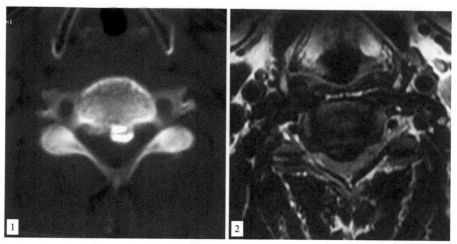

FIGURE 1-3-16

Double-layer sign of the ossification lesion.
(1) Double-layer sign of the ossification lesion on axial CT image.
(2) Double-layer sign of the ossification lesion on axial MRI image.

antedisplacement of all the levels should be consistent and moderate to avoid undue tension to the dura in patients with double-layer OPLL in preoperative CT scan.

For levels with wide-based OPLL, the gutters are developed lateral to the base of the OPLL to avoid leaving residual ossification at the bottom of the gutter. Otherwise, when the gutter has reached the posterior wall of the vertebral body, the surgeon will still need to separate the OPLL from the dura. When performed all within the narrow gutter, this step is particularly challenging for ossification resection and high risk for CSFL. When CSFL is identified during ACAF, the tear can be sealed with autologous fascia or synthetic material, which is fixed by the vertebral bodies. Small tear or minimal leak may go unnoticed during surgery, but it may develop into a major leak after surgery upon position changes, increased motion, or increased tension on the dura. Thus, a prompt repair is always warranted whenever CSFL is suspected during surgery.

In case of small dural tear with adequate surgical repair and drainage of less than 200 mL/day and decreasing within 48 hours, pillowless sleeping, keeping supine, and delayed ambulation help prevent intracranial hypotension syndrome. Supportive care includes monitoring drainage volume, fluid replenishment, keeping electrolytes, and albumin in balance, and using high-grade antibiotics (such as third-generation cephalosporins). To maintain interstitial pressure and reduce leak, the wound is pressure-dressed with sandbag or elastic bandage while allowing normal swallowing and breathing. In contrast, in case of larger tear with suboptimal surgical repair and drainage of more than 200 mL/day after 48 hours, the lumbar drainage is maintained. Subarachnoid drainage facilitates dural and wound healing as it directs CSF flow to the drainage and prevents it from infiltrating the wound area. Also, in patients with subcutaneous CSF collection, lumbar drainage unloads interstitium and resolves dysphagia and dyspnea. When physical exam and imaging studies performed upon dyspnea reveal subcutaneous CSF collection around the wound, an ultrasound-guided CSF drainage provides immediate symptom relief.

Dysphagia

Dysphagia constitutes a major complication of anterior cervical surgery, characterized by discomfort in the throat or when swallowing or foreign body sensation around the back of the throat within 3 days after surgery. It is usually self-limited and rarely last more than two months. The condition has been associated with mass effect of the titanium plate, swollen tissue anterior to the spine, injury to the superior laryngeal nerve, among others [4]. Riley's study on 454 cases of anterior cervical surgeries registered incidences of 19.8%, 33.3%, and 39.1% three months later in surgeries involving single, double, and three or more levels [5]. This correlation between the morbidity and the number of surgical levels has been also observed in our practice. Studies have yield inconsistent results on the potential impact of plate profile and width on dysphagia. Lee recommended narrow and low-profile plate as a prevention [6], whereas Chin disproved association between plate profile and dysphagia when the plate measured between 3 and 7 mm thick [7]. Data from China revealed 6% of dysphagia incidence after ACCF [8], whereas early ACAF procedure resulted in 6.7% of dysphagia. In addition, post-ACAF dysphagia may also be related to the plate's compression and tension over the fascia and excessive intervertebral distraction.

The prevertebral fascia is closely related to anterior structures of the neck. The prevertebral fascia comes with two layers. Its thinner deep layer encircles the vertebral body and overlies the bilateral longus colli and scalene muscles, whereas its tougher superficial layer extends laterally, surrounds the common carotid artery and internal jugular vein, and becomes the carotid sheath. Fibrous connections are present between the prevertebral fascia and the tracheoesophageal sheath, and the visceral sheath is able to move between the deep and superficial layers of the prevertebral fascia in relation to the spine. Hence, the traction on the prevertebral fascia is transmitted via fibrous tissue to the esophagus, causing irritation (Fig. 1-3-17). In ACAF, usually a multilevel procedure, the proximal and distal ends of the surgical field are exposed to a lesser extent to reduce surgical trauma. Therefore, surgeons should be on guard during instrumentation and avoid trapping the prevertebral fascia beneath the plate at both ends of the construct. It is also important to use a nerve hook or elevator to ensure the prevertebral fascia lies over the plate before closure. Another measure to prevent dysphagia is to achieve a gentle distraction of the proximal and distal intervertebral spaces with vertebral body screws (see Chapter 2, Section 5) instead of Caspar pins, which are prone to overdistraction. In conventional anterior cervical surgeries, Caspar pins are used to distract the intervertebral space to 2—3 mm for decompression of the neural exit foramina. However, in the ACAF technique, usually on three or more levels, higher risk of dysphagia is present

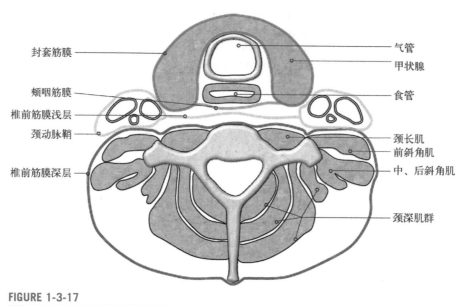

封套筋膜
颊咽筋膜
椎前筋膜浅层
颈动脉鞘
椎前筋膜深层

气管
甲状腺
食管
颈长肌
前斜角肌
中、后斜角肌
颈深肌群

FIGURE 1-3-17

Anatomy of prevertebral fascia and the surrounding structures.

as multiple distractions result in significant increase of the entire cervical spine and axial shear force between the prevertebral fascia and tracheoesophageal sheath. Therefore, to avoid overdistraction in ACAF procedure, our team generally uses small cage and vertebral body screws to distract the proximal and distal intervertebral space of the construct and reproduces the natural intervertebral height.

Other preventive measures include protecting the superior laryngeal nerve from direct insult by intermuscular dissection, intermittent relaxation of the retractors over the tracheoesophageal sheath, and iced saline irrigation. It also helps to prescribe trachea push exercise before surgery to relax soft tissue. It is administered two days before surgery, twice daily, and for 30 minutes each session (refer to Chapter 2, Section 1).

Complications of fusion

Reliable instrumentation and definitive fusion are necessary as anterior cervical surgery of any type will compromise stability. Patients who need multilevel decompression in anterior surgery are especially prone to a failed fusion. ACCF involves additional risk of poor stability and failed fusion since much of the vertebral body is removed and the fusion depends on only two interfaces (in the single-mesh situation) between the titanium mesh and vertebral bodies. For better post-ACCF cervical stability, Dalbayrak et al. described a skip ACCF technique, where the middle level is preserved in a three-level ACCF procedure, so that stress is better distributed with the preserved vertebral body. This technique has been proved helpful in reducing instrumentation failure [9]. In contrast, ACAF shares more similarities with ACDF when it comes to fusion due to the increased contact areas between cages (or bone grafts) and vertebral bodies. Also, the stress between the instrumentation and bone is better distributed by the multiple screws and cages in the reconstructed anterior cervical column. However, ACAF bears two concerns for suboptimal fusion. First, partial anterior corpectomy is required in ACAF, but when performed excessively, it reduces the area available for bone grafting. Second, the releases between vertebral bodies may compromise blood supplies to the surrounding structure.

To ensure bone grafting and fusion, the authors have adopted the following techniques to retain adequate grafting surface and blood supplies to the vertebral bodies. ① Ensure at least 12 mm of AP length of the residual vertebral body after partial corpectomy. This 12 mm has been based on the common size of cervical cages used among Chinese patients. This will provide adequate size above and below the cages for maximized fusion. Also, as most vertebral body screw systems start with 10–12 mm for screw length, residual vertebral bodies of this size or above help ensure screw purchase and overall stability of the construct. Given that the cervical vertebral bodies measure about 18 mm in AP length among Chinese patients, vertebral body resection should be performed within 6 mm in depth. At levels with ossification of more than 6 mm thick, the plate should be prebent with increased curvature to accommodate increased antedisplacement of this level. ② Graft the bilateral gutters of the prepared vertebral bodies. After antedisplacement, strips of autologous or allogenous bone grafts are placed along the gutters on both sides to increase the area for fusion. ③ Preserve the unossified PLL at the bottom of the gutters. This preserves the vasculature between the PLL and the vertebral bodies and promotes fusion. (See Chapter 2, Section 2).

In another study performed by the authors to characterize the fusion after ACAF, patients with cervical OPLL who had received ACAF of three or more levels received radiological assessment at the third, sixth, and twelfth months. The two arms showed comparative fusion at the third and twelfth months. At the sixth month, 24.75% of patients reached Eck grade I fusion (fused with trabeculae across the endplate) [10]; by the 12th month, 100% patients reached Eck grade I. In another study of patients with cervical OPLL receiving long-span ACAF (4.5 levels on average), follow-up of six to twelve months revealed 6.7% cage settling, and all patients were free from pseudoarthrosis, cervical kyphosis, screw loosening or pullout, or hardware breakage [3,11]. In a previous biomechanical study, the authors simulated three-level ACAF and ACCF on human cadavers and analyzed postoperative cervical stability by documenting neck motion of flexion, extension, side bend, and axial rotation. They concluded that neck stability experienced a more rapid decline after repetitive load in the ACCF specimen than in the ACAF model, though both specimens demonstrated comparable overall stability. This conclusion was reproduced in the comparison between ACDF and ACCF. This suggests similar biomechanical profiles between ACAF and ACDF. Both procedures provide reliable immediate and long-term cervical stability whereas ACCF is less favorable in load to failure.

With all these data available, ACAF provides favorable fusion outcome, though longer-term studies are warranted.

Nerve injuries

Spinal cord injury represents the most severe complication of spinal surgery, which may even cause paralysis [12,13]. Although the advancing surgical technology has reduced spinal cord injuries from malpositioned cage or mesh and poor screw entry points or trajectories, spinal cord safety in cervical surgeries should always be emphasized. In anterior cervical surgeries where ossification and protruded disc materials are to be removed, surgical instruments work near the dura and frequently reach deep to remove lesion and address compression. Therefore, iatrogenic cord injuries from instruments are particularly relevant and unsalvageable. Therefore, adequate exposure, good control of instruments, and thorough hemostasis are prerequisites for cord safety. The key concept in ACAF is the vertebra−OPLL complex, where the OPLL and the ventral vertebra are treated as one piece. In the ACAF procedure, direct decompression is achieved by release and antedisplacement of the vertebral body, leaving alone the ossification−dura interface. Therefore, ACAF obviates the iatrogenic insult to the dura and spinal cord from surgical tools. ACAF minimizes inadvertent cord injury during surgery as it does not aim for lesion removal. In addition, surgical maneuvers are directed lateral to the spinal cord around the uncovertebral joints, staying away from the cord and its blood vessels along the anterior median fissure. Since its adoption, ACAF has registered zero spinal cord injury [3]. C5 nerve palsy received the most attention among various nerve injuries. This condition is characterized by decreased power of the deltoid and/or biceps brachii without myelopathy deterioration after cervical surgery, and 50% patients also report concomitant pain or numbness of the C5 region. With etiology yet to be clarified, C5 palsy is also found in cases that do not experience noticeable nerve injury during surgery. Tethering effect has been frequently assumed as a cause of C5 palsy. Based on "in situ decompression," ACAF reduced the key generator of C5 palsy—spinal cord displacement. In the ACAF technique, the vertebra−OPLL complex serves as the new anterior wall of the spinal canal and a barrier to the dura and spinal cord so that they do not displace anteriorly, as seen where defect is left anterior to the neural elements. Therefore, ACAF provides adequate decompression and prevents tethering effect and C5 palsy. Its incidence has been reported as 2.4% after ACAF procedure in contrast to the 3.2%−28.6% after ACCF [14−16]. Nevertheless, caution is still warranted to respect the natural position of the spinal cord and prevent nerve tethering. To avoid shift of excessive antedisplacement of the spinal cord, surgeons prevent asymmetrical or excessive antedisplacement of the bony structure. To this end, gutters are developed along the vertical plane to facilitate the symmetrical and ventral elevation of the vertebra−OPLL complex. The extent of antedisplacement should be based on the thickness of the ossification and the cervical curvature [17]. In some patients who developed C5 palsy after ACAF, the dura and/or the spinal cord did not resume its normal shape and position yet

(Figs. 1-3-18 and 1-3-19). This was attributed to the asymmetrical recovery of spinal canal after ACAF. Also, when the reconstructed spinal canal encourages excessive flow of the thecal sac and the CSF ventral to the spinal cord, the cord may shift, pulling on the C5 nerve roots and causing palsy. Therefore, the antedisplacement should be adequate to restore the normal AP dimension of the spinal canal. In other words, the antedisplacement should allow the ossification to just clear off the spinal canal.

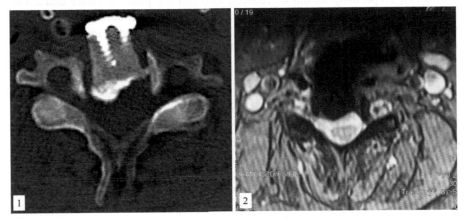

FIGURE 1-3-18

The thecal sac distended to the left ventral side after ACAF.
(1) CT axial image.
(2) MRI axial image.

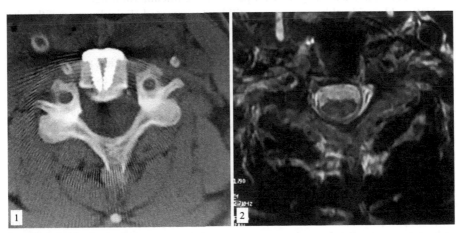

FIGURE 1-3-19

ACAF with excessive antedisplacement.
(1) CT axial image.
(2) MRI axial image.

Theoretically, this perfect antedisplacement can be achieved when the extent of anterior corpectomy is consistent with the ossification thickness. However, the plate curvature also drives antedisplacement of the vertebral bodies. With a more curved plate, the distance for the vertebral body to elevate is longer, so that the vertebral body ends up being antedisplaced further than the planned distance. This results in excessive enlargement of the AP dimension of the spinal canal. Therefore, in cases with reduced cervical lordosis where a prebent plate is planned, the extent of anterior corpectomy should be reduced to offset the plate curvature and avoid excessive antedisplacement. To measure the correct extent of anterior corpectomy, the prebent plate can serve as a template and nerve hook used to measure the distance between the plate and the vertebral body.

Hemorrhage and hematoma

Injury to the internal vertebral venous plexus and partial resection of vertebral bodies are the principal causes of intraoperative hemorrhage and postoperative hematoma of anterior cervical surgeries. The anterior internal vertebral venous plexus travels posterior to the PLL and is closely related to the dura. In the presence of compression, such as with ossification, the venous drainage within the spinal canal is blocked, causing distention of the thin-walled veins. In such case, the veins are at increased risk of injury from surgical steps and inadequate hemostasis. Thicker veins around the uncovertebral joints (Luschka joints) and nerve roots constitute particular risk of hemorrhage beyond the efficacy of tamponade. Cancellous bone bleeding is another important source in ACAF where partial corpectomy is performed, in particular in multilevel decompression. Heavy bleeding and insufficient drainage will cause hematoma manifesting as local pain and significant swelling.

Noticeable epidural hematoma can still be documented clinically even with subtle intraoperative hemorrhage and thorough hemostasis. Case review identified hypertension, diabetes mellitus, and other underlying diseases as risks for coagulopathies due to increased blood velocity, endothelial injuries, and disturbance of vasoactive substances. Therefore, hematoma develops as soon as bleeding occurs before blood is drained with vacuum during surgery, and persistent wound bleeding aggravates hematoma and compresses the spinal cord. To address this issue, the authors have resorted to D-dimer test before surgery. Plasma levels of D-dimer, the primary degradation product of cross-linked fibrin, are elevated with increased risk of a blood clot and increased fibrinolysis. With the action of thrombin, cross-linked fibrin gets rid of peptide A and peptide B and forms fibrin I and fibrin II. Fibrin degradation from activated plasmin produces D-dimer. Patients requiring a second surgery to clear hematoma have been found with D-dimer level several dozen folds higher than usual in previous studies. In addition to the risk of wound infection, the danger of hematoma also lies in cord compression and dyspnea within 24 hours after surgery. Thus, as soon as hematoma is suspected, a prompt action should be taken to clear the suture materials and the hematoma and address hemorrhage while maintaining unobstructed respiration.

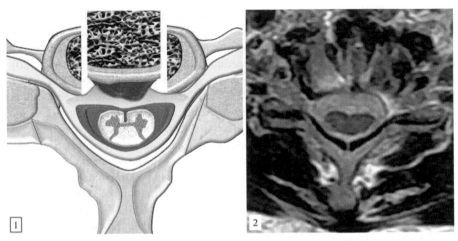

FIGURE 1-3-20

Illustration and imaging result of the "tenting effect."
(1) Illustration of the "tenting effect" after ACAF.
(2) Imaging results of "tenting effect" after ACAF.

The authors have adopted the following practices to prevent internal vertebral venous plexus injury and reduce hemorrhage from vertebral bodies during ACAF procedures. First, the antedisplacement of vertebra—OPLL complex removes the compression over internal vertebral venous plexus. The venous drainage becomes patent again so the undistended vein is less vulnerable to injuries. Second, the antedisplaced vertebra—OPLL complex serves as the new anterior wall of the spinal canal, leaving little room for hematoma to develop. Therefore, even when mild hemorrhage occurs anterior to the spinal cord, it is unlikely to aggravate into hematoma and compress the cord. Third, when the dura become attached to the ossified PLL, as antedisplacement occurs, the dura is moved ventrally and acts like a tent with proper tension. This "tenting effect" further obliterates the room for hematoma development. These are the three features of ACAF that guard against hematoma and cord compression (Fig. 1-3-20). For the bone bed hemorrhage from anterior vertebral body resection and bilateral gutter development, using harmonic scalpel or high-speed burr as the cutting tool helps reduce hemorrhage, in addition to applying bone wax. Also, during surgery, hemostasis can be provided by tamponade over the venous plexus dorsal to the vertebral bodies with the vertebra—OPLL complex and materials such as bone wax and gelatin sponge via the gutters. Earlier data showed ACAF resulted in 328 mL of average blood loss without causing cord compression or dyspnea [18].

Vertebral artery injury

A rare complication with severe consequence after cervical surgeries, vertebral artery injury may lead to vertebral artery occlusion, arteriovenous fistula, pseudoaneurysm, massive hemorrhage, cardiac arrest, neurological sequela, and even death. It occurs in 0.3%−0.5% of cases of anterior cervical surgeries [19]. The most common mechanism of vertebral artery injury features excessive lateralization of surgical tools, violating the medial wall of the transverse foramen [20]. Since ACAF has been associated with wider span of decompression than ACCF (17.9 ± 1.0 mm vs. 15.1 ± 0.8 mm), ACAF may bear higher risk of vertebral artery injuries from surgical tools than ACCF procedure. However, the authors have not experienced any vertebral artery injury since the adoption of ACAF.

The uncinate processes have been used to guide anterior corpectomies. Similarly, uncinate process serves as the principal marker in ACAF, where the gutters are centered over the anterior slope of uncinate processes, also known as the transition from the anterior rim of the uncinate process to the anterior edge of vertebral bodies. This helps avoid directing the gutters medially or laterally, and thus prevents vertebral artery injuries or narrow decompression span. The authors measured the distance between the gutters and vertebral arteries in ACAF using CT imaging and cadavers. The distance was represented as the distance between the anterior slop of uncinate process and the medial wall of the transverse foramen, and the distance between the gutter wall and the medial wall of the transverse foramen. Such measurement showed that the distance between the gutter wall and the medial wall of the transverse foramen was consistently more than 2 mm and was slightly longer than that between the anterior slop of uncinate process and the medial wall of the transverse foramen across C3 to C6. In other words, even though the gutter location is subject to the size of bone cutting tools (such as burr diameter or rongeur width), the actual gutter wall was lateral to the anterior slope of the uncinate process, and a safety gap of at least 2 mm was consistently present between the gutter wall and the medial wall of the transverse foramen. Therefore, gutter development does not violate the medial wall of the transverse foramen or the vertebral artery as long as the cutting tool is directed vertically and along the parasagittal plane.

However, maintaining adequate width of the decompression can still bear risk of artery injury in cases of aberrant vertebral arteries infringing the medial wall of transverse foramen. Conventional anatomic landmarks no longer work in such situation, so preoperative mapping of vertebral artery course with CT and MRI is imperative, where tortuosity warrants further investigation. Digital subtraction angiography is the gold standard for proving vertebral artery aberration while CTA and magnetic resonance angiography provide essential noninvasive means (Fig. 1-3-21).

Insufficient antedisplacement

The release and antedisplacement of vertebra−OPLL complex hold the key to the ACAF procedure which features instrumentation and fusion of the antedisplaced bony structure. Vertebral body release is the prerequisite for antedisplacement and the latter facilitates neural decompression. To achieve safe antedisplacement, the authors use plate and screws as the anchorage and driver for vertebral body

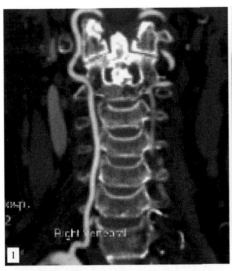 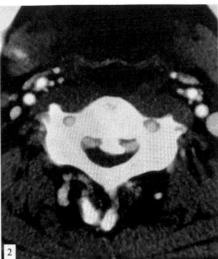

FIGURE 1-3-21

Vertebral artery images.
(1) CTA images of vertebral artery.
(2) CT Images of vertebral artery.

antedisplacement. Compared to freehand antedisplacement that may cause inadvertent vertebral body movement, using plate and screws as the pull ensure antedisplacement as expected and neural safety. Even so, a small number of cases still experience challenging and suboptimal antedisplacement, resulting in gaps between the plate and vertebral bodies. This gap is also shown in postoperative CT and lateral X-ray images. As a result, spinal canal is not restored to the natural size, leaving residual compression (Fig. 1-3-22).

Among cases of insufficient antedisplacement, the most common cause is oblique gutters mentioned earlier. This manifests in postoperative axial CT images as parallel but oblique gutters on both sides. Oblique gutters result in residual ossification on the ipsilateral side and blocked antedisplacement on the contralateral side. During antedisplacement, the eave-shaped or trapezoid wall on the contralateral side blocks and rubs against the vertebra—OPLL complex, causing insufficient antedisplacement.

The antedisplacement is not possible without thorough release of the vertebra—OPLL complex from the surrounding bony structures. During the procedure, sometimes, deeper gutter may constitute challenges to visualization, making it difficult to determine if the gutter resection is complete. For antedisplacement, if the screws are tightened before the complete isolation of the vertebra—OPLL complex, this may result in screw loosening and incomplete ventral displacement of the vertebral body. Screw trajectory may also determine the readiness of antedisplacement. Two screws, one on each side, are used for each vertebral body to provide desirable

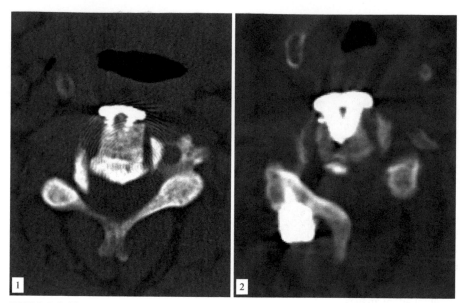

FIGURE 1-3-22

Post-ACAF CT images of insufficient antedisplacement.

(1) The gap is present between vertebral bodies and the plate. Subject to rotational vector, the posterior edge of the vertebra—OPLL complex runs into the gutter wall, blocking antedisplacement.

(2) The gap is present between vertebral bodies and the plate. During instrumentation, the overly convergent screws came into contact at the screw tips and blocked screw insertion. As a result, the extent antedisplacement was less than desired.

screw purchase and plate fixation. If the two screws are overly convergent, their tips may come into contact and stop the inserting process. When the screw and plate construct is not fixed with the vertebral body, the antedisplacement process stops prematurely.

The ring apophysis along the anterior and posterior edge of vertebral bodies may also block the antedisplacement process. In typical cervical intervertebral space, there is anterior ring apophysis of the lower endplate of the cephalad vertebra and the posterior ring apophysis of the upper endplate of the caudad vertebra. This ring apophysis is more prominent in the upper than the lower cervical spine. During antedisplacement in ACAF, the anterior or posterior ring apophysis may collide with cages and stop the antedisplacement process. Specifically, the anterior ring apophysis may block the cage insertion whereas the posterior ring apophysis may ventralize the cage placement. This results in suboptimal antedisplacement and anterior case placement, if not anterior cage protrusion. In vertebral bodies associated with insufficient antedisplacement, 70% are with anterior and posterior ring apophysis. Thus, intervertebral preparation should involve adequate resection of the anterior and posterior ring apophysis to ensure the endplates are parallel, eliminating friction or blockade during antedisplacement. In addition, intraoperative 3D CT images from O-arm radiography help determine if ring apophysis is thoroughly removed (see Chapter 2, Section 5) [25].

Residual ossification

The thorough decompression from ACAF is not possible without the complete release of the vertebra—OPLL complex. If the lateral ossification is not removed during vertebra—OPLL complex preparation, the bony residual in the spinal canal will offset the benefit of decompression and may affect patient outcome [17] (Fig. 1-3-23). A study of 115 patients undergoing ACAF for cervical OPLL revealed 8.7% incidence of residual ossification. It occurs more frequently, at 71.4%, to wide-based ossification beyond the anterior slop of the uncinate process [17].

The location and trajectory of the gutters determine if all the ossification bulk is entirely included in the vertebra—OPLL complex. The gutters should be placed lateral to the edge of the ossification and directed vertically without mediolateral angulation. Correctly placed gutters are based on preoperative accurate measurement of the ossification and precise surgical procedure. The gutters should always be placed lateral to the edge of the ossification. Once the gutter is placed, the proper

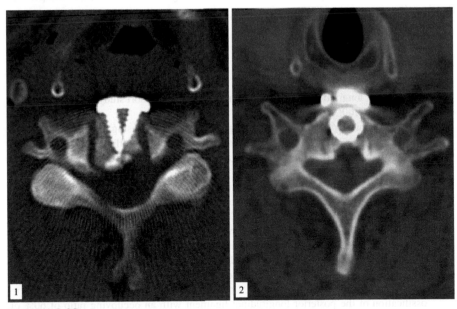

FIGURE 1-3-23

CT images of residual ossification.
(1) Residual ossification after ACAF.
(2) Residual ossification after ACCF.

trajectory of the gutter is essential to surgical success. The failure to develop the gutter along the parasagittal plane accounts for violation of the ossification or residual compression. During the ACAF procedure, standing on one side of the patients, surgeons remain mindful of developing oblique gutters along their visual projection. The failure to maintain visualization and surgical tools perpendicular to the floor will leave residual ossification on the ipsilateral side.

What is more, surgeons should keep an eye on the depth of the gutters. Once the posterior wall of the vertebral body is isolated, the cutting process is finished. Otherwise, further cutting into the PLL may leave out residual ossification. When developing the gutter on each side of the vertebral body, surgeons constantly ensure the correct trajectory and depth of the gutter with a nerve hook palpating the posterior wall of vertebral bodies to stop the cutting process as soon as the posterior wall is reached. Otherwise, they will end up cutting into the ossified PLL. To remove the last 1 mm or 2 mm of the posterior wall of the vertebral body in the gutter, a rongeur is used to access and remove the bottom of the gutter from intervertebral space. When the gutter is through, a nerve hook is used to palpate the bottom of the gutter and determine if all the ossification has been attached to the released vertebral body. Ossification present at the bottom of the gutter or lateral to the gutter suggests the gutter is not lateral enough. In such case, one should be expanding the gutter laterally rather than attempting to cut into the ossification at the gutter bottom. Otherwise, it will leave bony residuals lateral to the gutter bottom (see Chapter 2, Section 4).

References

[1] Matsunaga S, Sakou T, Taketomi E, et al. Clinical course of patients with ossification of the posterior longitudinal ligament: a minimum 10-year cohort study. Journal of Neurosurgery 2004;100(3):245–8.

[2] Yoshii T, Hirai T, Yamada T, et al. Intraoperative evaluation using mobile computed tomography in anterior cervical decompression with floating method for massive ossification of the posterior longitudinal ligament. Journal of Orthopaedic Surgery and Research 2017;12(1):12.

[3] Boody BS, Lendner M, Vaccaro AR. Ossification of the posterior longitudinal ligament in the cervical spine: a review. International Orthopaedics 2019;43(4):797–805.

[4] Pham MH, Attenello FJ, Lucas J, et al. Conservative management of ossification of the posterior longitudinal ligament. A review. Neurosurgical Focus 2011;30(3):e2.

[5] Mizuno J, Nakagawa H. Outcome analysis of anterior decompressive surgery and fusion for cervical ossification of the posterior longitudinal ligament: report of 107 cases and review of the literature. Neurosurgical Focus 2001;10(4):1–7.

[6] Fujimori T, Iwasaki M, Okuda S, et al. Long-term results of cervical myelopathy due to ossification of the posterior longitudinal ligament with an occupying ratio of 60% or more. Spine 2014;39(1):58–67.

[7] Iwasaki M, Okuda SY, Miyauchi A, et al. Surgical strategy for cervical myelopathy due to ossification of the posterior longitudinal ligament: part 2: advantages of anterior decompression and fusion over laminoplasty. Spine 2007;32(6):654–60.

[8] Yamaura I, Kurosa Y, Matuoka T, et al. Anterior floating method for cervical myelopathy caused by ossification of the posterior longitudinal ligament. Clinical Orthopaedics and Related Research 1999;359(359):27−34.

[9] Matsuoka T, Yamaura I, Kurosa Y, et al. Long-term results of the anterior floating method for cervical myelopathy caused by ossification of the posterior longitudinal ligament. Spine 2001;26(3):241−8.

[10] Yamaura I. Anterior decompression for cervical myelopathy caused by ossification of the posterior longitudinal ligament—anterior floating method of OPLL. Nihon Seikeigeka Gakkai Zasshi 1996;70(5):296.

[11] Haisong Y, Xuanhua L, Xinwei W, et al. A new method to determine whether ossified posterior longitudinal ligament can be resected completely and safely: spinal canal "Rule of Nine" on axial computed tomography. European Spine Journal 2015;24(8):1673−80.

[12] Xiongsheng C, Yin Z, Shengyuan Z, et al. Anterior en bloc resection of ossification in the treatment of cervical ossification of the posterior longitudinal ligament. Chinese Journal of Orthopedics 2018;38(24):1480−92.

[13] Shaobo W, Qinlin C, Gengding D, et al. Observation on the long-term curative effect of single-door cervical laminoplasty. Chinese Journal of Orthopedics 1999;19(9):519−21. e428−e436.

[14] Jingchuan S, Kaiqiang S, Shunmin W, et al. "Shelter technique" in the treatment of ossification of the posterior longitudinal ligament involving the C2 segment. World Neurosurgery 2019;125:e456−64.

[15] Christe A,L, Ubli R, Guzman R, et al. Degeneration of the cervical disc: histology compared with radiography and magnetic resonance imaging. Neuroradiology 2005;47(10):721−9.

[16] JR JGA. The clinical manifestations of spondylochondrosis (spondylosis) of the cervical spine. Annals of Surgery 1955;141(6):872−89.

[17] Papadopoulos EC, Huang RC, Girardi FP, et al. Three-level anterior cervical discectomy and fusion with plate fixation: radiographic and clinical results. Spine (Phila Pa 1976) 2006;31(8):897−902.

[18] Xuzhou L, Shaoxiong M, Hui Z, et al. Anterior corpectomy versus posterior laminoplasty for multilevel cervical myelopathy: a systematic review and meta-analysis. European Spine Journal 2014;23(2):362−72.

[19] Fouyas IP, Statham PF, Sandercock PA. Cochrane review on the role of surgery in cervical spondylotic radiculomyelopathy. Spine 2002;27(7):736−47.

[20] Yifu S, Le L, Jianhui Z, et al. Comparison between anterior approaches and posterior approaches for the treatment of multilevel cervical spondylotic myelopathy: a meta-analysis. Clinical Neurology and Neurosurgery 2015;134:28−36.

[21] Liping X, Hong S, Zhenhuan L, et al. Anterior cervical discectomy and fusion versus posterior laminoplasty for multilevel cervical myelopathy: a meta-analysis. International Journal of Surgery (London, England) 2017;48:247−53.

[22] Long Z, Jia C, Can C, et al. Anterior versus posterior approach for the therapy of multilevel cervical spondylotic myelopathy: a meta-analysis and systematic review. Archives of Orthopaedic and Tranmatic Surgery 2019;139(6):735−42.

[23] Yake, M., Rongxin, S., Shunmin, W., et al. Surgical skills and clinical analysis of anterior cervical vertebral compression complex forward fusion in the treatment of multilevel cervical spondylotic myelopathy. Chinese Journal of Bone and Joint Surgery 2018;11(10):13−7.

[24] Haisong Y, Yong Y, Jiangang S, et al. Anterior controllable antedisplacement fusion as a choice for degenerative cervical kyphosis with stenosis: preliminary clinical and radiologic results. World Neurosurg 2018;118:e562—9.

[25] Jiaquan L, Kai C, Sheng H, et al. Comparison of anterior approach versus posterior approach for the treatment of multilevel cervical spondylotic myelopathy. European Spine Journal 2015;24(8):1621—30.

Procedures of the anterior controllable antedisplacement fusion technique

Section 1: Preoperative preparation

Special technologies and equipment

Anterior controllable antedisplacement fusion (ACAF) technique can be successfully carried out with the techniques and equipment typically used in anterior cervical corpectomy and fusion (ACCF) surgery. Since adequate preparation can effectively reduce the risk and difficulty of surgery, the following assistive techniques and equipment are recommended: intraoperative electrophysiological monitoring, autologous blood transfusion technique, ultrasound bone knife and burr, carbon fiber operating table, O-arm X-ray machine, etc.

Ultrasound bone knife and burr

Ultrasound bone knife is generally used with a multipronged blade or a 2.5–3 mm ball or rasp tip.

Frequently used burrs tips are 2.5–3 mm spherical or teardrop tips.

One of the advantages of the ultrasound bone knife is that it generates less damage to the soft tissue.

The blade of the ultrasound bone knife should not stay in the same location for more than two seconds to avoid overheating.

Burrs running at low speeds tend to slip and damage soft tissues.

Care should be taken to prevent a spinning burr from entrapping the surrounding soft tissue.

When using an ultrasonic bone knife, gauze soaked with normal saline is applied to local soft tissue to protect against burns from the device's handle where heat is produced (Fig. 2.1.1, Table 2.1.1).

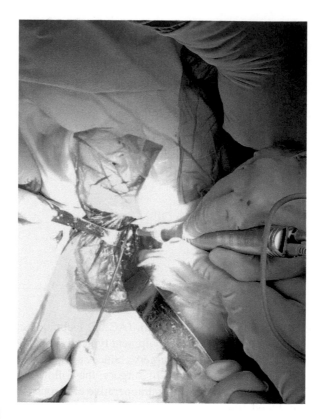

FIGURE 2.1.1

Surgeons create bilateral troughs using ultrasonic bone knife.
A large piece of gauze soaked with normal saline is placed under the ultrasonic bone knife
to avoid burns on the soft tissue as the device handle and cutter give off heat.

Table 2.1.1 Comparison of the advantages of the ultrasonic bone knife and
burr for bilateral osteotomies trough of the vertebral bodies.

Ultrasound bone knife	Burr
The blade is friendly to soft tissues	Efficient cutting
The blade does not entrap soft tissues	Widespread and easily accessible
Variable blade angles	
Good visualization with little debris	

Electrophysiological monitoring

Since most of the steps are performed outside the spinal canal, the ACAF technique
has a little impact on the neural elements, and the intraoperative electrophysiological
monitoring is less indispensable than in the ACCF technique. However, the

intraoperative electrophysiological monitoring technique is still recommended for higher surgical safety.

Autologous blood transfusion technique can reduce the demand for allogeneic blood transfusion. It is necessary for long-segment ACAF surgeries.

O-arm X-ray machine

The carbon fiber operating table is used in conjunction with the O-arm X-ray machine (Fig. 2.1.2) to confirm whether bilateral troughs are wide enough for the ossification of the posterior longitudinal ligament (OPLL), whether there are barriers for the antedisplacement, and to evaluate the effect of hoisting of the vertebra-ossification complex (VOC).

The O-arm machine can provide accurate information on the troughs' position and the effect of antedisplacement, which is extremely important for patients with long-segmental, wide-base, and severe OPLL. However, its downsides are extra time and radiation exposure. Therefore, it is not routinely used in less challenging ACAF cases in our practice (the evaluation of the surgical challenge of the ACAF technique will be discussed in detail in Section 7 of this chapter).

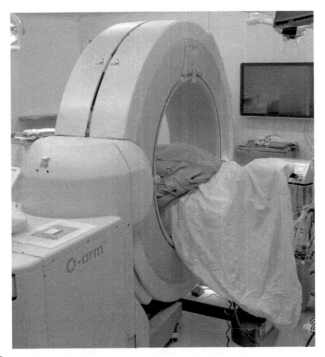

FIGURE 2.1.2

Intraoperative O-arm X-ray machine used with carbon fiber operating table.

Preparation of the approach

The ACAF technique is performed via an anterior cervical approach, and the feasibility of the approach needs to be thoroughly evaluated and prepared before surgery. The feasibility is usually based on the patient's neck length, mandible height, and the position of the sternal angle identified from physical examination and the cervical X-ray images of anterolateral, hyperextension, and flexion views.

Where a longitudinal incision may be used, the surgeon counsels the patient on the cosmetic and functional impact of the scar tissue.

Before surgery, patients perform exercises to isolate the trachea and esophagus to reduce the tension encountered during intraoperative exposure.

The tracheal isolation exercise usually starts two days before surgery and lasts for 30 minutes each time.

It intends to reduce the strength required in mobilizing the trachea and esophagus during the operation, and the likelihood of discomfort in swallowing after the operation.

The exercise can be conducted by the patient independently or with the assistance of others.

With slightly flexed fingers except for the thumb of the left hand, the patient palpates the right edge of the laryngeal prominence and pushes dorsally. Upon feeling the laryngeal prominence shifts to the left, the patient continues to push until the finger pulps are entirely on the prominence and gradually pushes the trachea toward the left (Fig. 2.1.3).

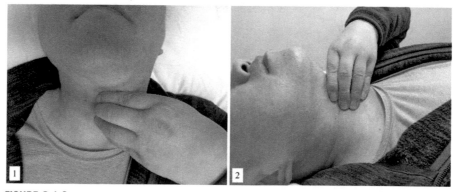

FIGURE 2.1.3

Self-administered tracheal isolation exercise in the supine position.
(1) Front view: the patient pushes the trachea and esophagus to the left with his left hand;
(2) Lateral view: with adducted fingers, the patient pushes deep posteriorly besides the laryngeal prominence before pushing it to the left. The four fingers can be placed caudally or cephalad according to the surgical exposure required for the segments to be treated.

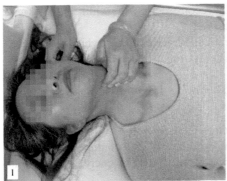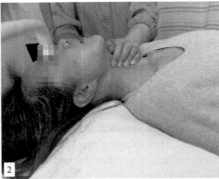

FIGURE 2.1.4

Assisted tracheal isolation training with the help of others.

(1) Front view: standing on the patient's left side, the helper pushes the patient's trachea and esophagus with his or her left hand to the left until the fingers reach beyond the midline;

(2) Lateral view: with adducted fingers, the helper pushes deep posteriorly besides the patient's laryngeal prominence before pushing it to the left. The four fingers can be placed caudally or cephalad according to the surgical exposure required for the segments to be treated.

When a helper is available, the patient lies in a supine position with a small pillow placed under the neck. Seated on the patient's left side, the helper provides the pushes with his or her left hand in the method described above (Fig. 2.1.4).

Patients commonly experience local soreness and choke during the exercise. However, exercise should be stopped if the patient has symptoms such as vomiting, dizziness, and blurred vision.

Preparation for decompression

Adequate decompression in the ACAF technique hinges on a detailed imaging measurements before surgery.

(1) Curvature and mobility of the patient's cervical spine and required amount of plate contour are measured from anterolateral, hyperextension, and flexion X-ray images.

(2) Cervical magnetic resonance imaging (MRI) is used to identify the segments of the compression, the segments for decompression, and, more importantly, the spinal cord's position that indicates the risk of spinal cord injury during decompression.

By identifying the cord compression on the sagittal MRI images, the surgeon can plan for thickness of anterior resected vertebral bodies (VBs).

The hoisting distance of the VOC is equal to the thickness of the OPLL in principle, depending on the resection of the anterior portion of VBs, is carefully measured on the axial computed tomography (CT) or MRI scans.

(3) Based on the three-dimensional (3D) CT reconstruction, the width and thickness of the OPLL at each segment are measured.

The OPLL's width and position are identified on the axial CT, which can be used as a basis for the distance between bilateral troughs when the VOC is isolated from the spine.

(4) CT angiography (CTA) can be used to delineate the course and variance of the vertebral arteries.

CTA of the vertebral arteries can be performed to identify any vertebral arteries' anomaly. This imaging modality is justifiable in the ACAF technique, where a primary concern is whether the vertebral artery turns medially and encroaches the bone (Fig. 2.1.5).

Preparation for reconstruction

Reconstruction is usually achieved with an anterior cervical plate and intervertebral cages in the ACAF technique as it generally does not involve vertebral body resection. Sometimes, to limit the number of the fusion segments, a small portion of vertebral bodies may be removed. Therefore, the anterior cervical titanium mesh should be made available. To facilitate fusion in the construct as troughs have been developed in the vertebral bodies, morselized bone or bone chips strip are made available to fill the bone bed.

Titanium plate

There are no specific criteria for the plate used in the ACAF technique. Any typical titanium plates 16 mm wide and around 2 mm thick will work.

Anterior cervical titanium plates of various specifications are made available to meet any need during surgery.

Screws

Screws ranging from 12 to 18 mm long are made available. The differences among self-tapping screws, self-drilling screws, nonrestrictive screws, semirestrictive screws, etc., will be described in detail in Section 4 of this chapter.

Intervertebral fusion and bone grafting

The cages appropriate for ACAF measure up to 14 mm wide (coronal dimension) and 12 mm long (sagittal dimension). Cages wider than this range may affect troughs on both sides, whereas those too long may block the antedisplacement process (see Section 4 of this chapter for details).

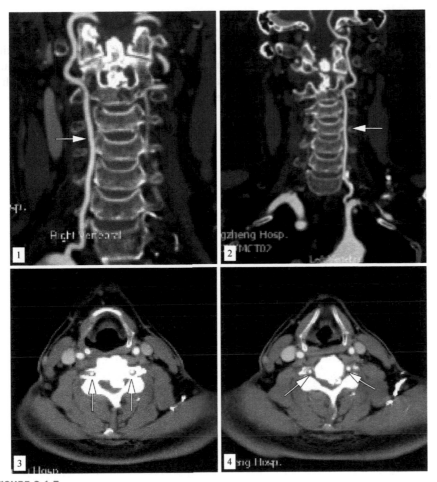

FIGURE 2.1.5

CTA of the vertebral arteries and contrast-enhanced cervical CT images.
(1, 2) CTA of the vertebral arteries demonstrating the courses of the arteries (arrow),
helpful for preoperative assessment;
(3, 4) Axial images of contrast-enhanced CT demonstrating hyperdense vertebral arteries
(arrows) in the transverse foramina. Vertebral artery anomaly is identified based on their
courses and relationship with the surrounding bone at each level.

    Bones resected from the anterior wall of the vertebral body are usually filled into
the intervertebral cage, and the fusion of the troughs on both sides needs to be
grafted.

    The commonly used bone grafting material is allogeneic or artificial bone, pref-
erably presented as long strips or pliable threads.

Salvage plan preparation

The conversion to a posterior surgery is the salvage plan for ACAF, which needs skin preparation on the neck and occiput area and surgical plaster table. Although the author's team has not had any conversion to a posterior surgery where ACAF fails, the preparation for a salvage plan is recommended in challenging cases.

Section 2: Surgical technique

Anesthesia and patient positioning

General anesthesia is usually adopted. Given the access affected by the mandible, transnasal intubation is used when the surgery involves C3 or above, whereas the transoral system can be used for surgeries below the C3 vertebral level.

The challenge of the transoral intubation is that the mouth is kept open by the endotracheal tube and the bite block, causing the mandible to block the upper cervical spine.

Transnasal intubation is usually required in cases where C3/4 intervertebral space preparation is expected.

If any difficulty is encountered during transnasal intubation, transoral intubation can be adopted with a bandage-based soft bite block instead of a plastic one to reduce the mandible's impact on surgical fields (Fig. 2.2.1).

The patient is placed in a supine position. A pillow and a roll are used to make the neck for a slightly extended position. Neck hyperextension should be avoided in case of increased tension on the trachea affecting intraoperative exposure (Fig. 2.2.2).

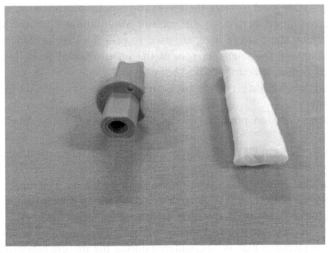

FIGURE 2.2.1

Hard (left) and soft bite block (right).

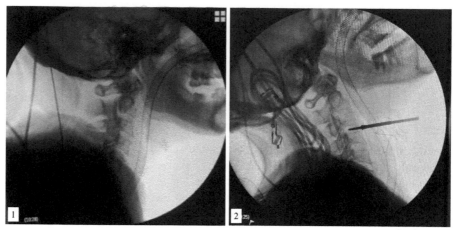

FIGURE 2.2.2

Access to C2 affected by the extent of neck extension.

(1) When the neck is insufficiently extended, the exposure of C2 is affected by the lower jaw;

(2) When the neck is in hyperextension, the trachea and esophagus are stretched, affecting the exposure.

Exposure

The selection of transverse versus longitudinal incisions is determined according to the number of surgical segments and patient's neck situation. The Smith–Peterson approach is typically used to expose the anterior spinal column. After exposure, vertebral screws are used to mark the level. The bipolar electrocoagulation is used to coagulate the blood vessels on the anterior longitudinal ligament initially. An electrotome and a sharp nerve hook are used to peel the longus colli muscle from subperiosteal toward the lateral margin of the uncovertebral joint. Hemostasis is then achieved with an electrotome and bone wax.

A longitudinal incision is recommended when the surgery involves three or more vertebral bodies.

A transverse incision provides access to four intervertebral levels in ACDF technique.

However, considering that ACAF requires more structure exposure and surgical fields, a longitudinal one is recommended if the ACAF involves three or more levels.

For longus colli elevation, an exposure is deemed adequate if it reaches the uncovertebral joints on both sides. The annular epiphysis along the upper and lower rims of the vertebral body is removed with a triple joint rongeur.

The nourishing blood vessels of the longus colli exit from the vertebral body on both sides, and bleeding may be encountered during the muscle elevation. In such a case, bone wax should be used instead of bipolar coagulation for hemostasis of the transected nourishing vessels on the bone surface.

Discectomy of the involved levels vertebral

The target disc spaces and the osteophytes along the anterior rims of the vertebral bodies are removed with a triple joint rongeur. The intervertebral disc is cleared with a pointed-tip scalpel, a curette, and a pituitary in this right order. The osteophytes on the posterior edges of the intervertebral space are removed with a laminectomy rongeur, exposing the posterior longitudinal ligament (PLL). The intervertebral spaces within the complex to be antedisplaced are prepared just to expose the PLL. In the intervertebral space adjacent to the upper and lower instrumented vertebrae, a weak point on the PLL is palpated with a nerve stripper, broken through, elevated, and extended to dissect the PLL with a pointed scalpel. The PLL at the intervertebral space is removed with a curette and a laminectomy rongeur to expose the dura mater (Fig. 2.2.3).

The intervertebral space should be prepared to the distance between the troughs, or decompression width, on the vertebral body, which is typically 18—20 mm for men and 16—18 mm for women.

When preparing the intervertebral space, the lateral margins of the preparation are defined first. The hypertrophic uncovertebral joints on both sides usually require resection with a laminectomy rongeur.

After removing the intervertebral disc and cartilage endplates, the dish-shaped endplates are prepared and flattened with a Kerrison rongeur. The preparation also involves the anular epiphysis on the anterior and posterior borders for the caudal

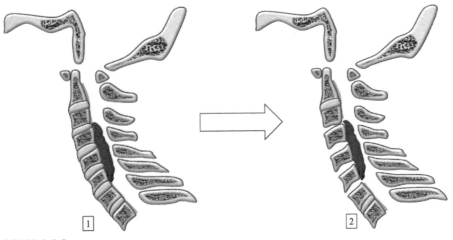

FIGURE 2.2.3

Illustration of intervertebral space preparation in the ACAF technique.
(1) OPLL extending from C4 to C6 vertebral level;
(2) The C3/4, C4/5, C5/6, C6/7 intervertebral discs are removed, the endplates prepared to be parallel to each other, and the PLL resected at C3/4 and C6/7. The rest of the PLL remains intact.

endplate and those posterior to the uncinate processes on both sides for cephalad endplate.

According to our experience, the PLL of each segment can be left intact as they rarely affect the anterior displacement of the vertebral body. The PLL dissection becomes necessary when there is imagery evidence of soft-tissue compression that protrudes from the PLL.

Space preparation of high quality is the basis for the successful ACAF procedure.

Resection of the anterior vertebral bodies of the VOC

The vertebral body's anterior part is resected with a triple joint rongeur by a depth consistent with the thickness of the ossification at each segment. The autogenous bone fragments generated are reserved for subsequent bone grafting. During the procedure, a prebent anterior cervical plate can be temporarily placed to evaluate if the space between the plate and remaining vertebral body is enough for the hoisting of the OPLL. Alternatively, this can be measured off the 3D reformatted images taken by a C-arm or O-arm X-ray machine. The titanium plate is taken off from the field. The vertebral bodies can be further removed with a burr or an ultrasonic osteotome if indicated by the measurement (Fig. 2.2.4).

The thickness of the bone removed from the front of the vertebral body is theoretically the same as that of the ossification at the back of the vertebral body.

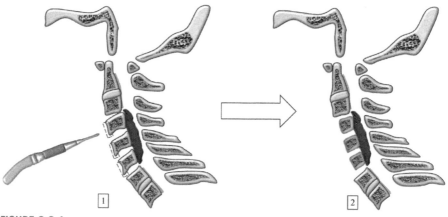

FIGURE 2.2.4

Illustration of removing the anterior part of the vertebral bodies in the ACAF technique.
(1) The amount of bone removed from the anterior part of the vertebral bodies, where the depth of removal is dependent on the thickness of the OPLL at each segment;
(2) A triple joint rongeur and a high-speed burr are used to remove the bone of the anterior part of the vertebral bodies.

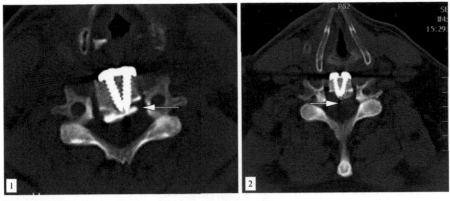

FIGURE 2.2.5

CT finding of the vertebral body screw penetrating the posterior wall.
(1) The vertebral body screws penetrating the vertebral body but not the ossification;
(2) The vertebral body screws passing through the posterior wall and the ossification and ending up in the spinal canal (arrow). ↑.

Excessive removal of the anterior part of the vertebral body will result in the insufficient anteroposterior diameter of the remaining vertebral body, resulting in a decrease in the purchase of the screws in the vertebral bodies during antedisplacement, screw penetrating the posterior wall of the vertebral body, and reduced area of intervertebral fusion (Fig. 2.2.5).

Important data: The average anteroposterior diameter of the vertebral body of East Asians is 18 mm for men and 16 mm for women. The commonly used screws are at least 12 mm long and cages 10 mm long in anteroposterior dimension.

If a bulky OPLL measures over 6 mm thick, the anterior resection depth is no longer consistent with the OPLL. To gain extra distance of advancement, the plate is properly contoured.

During the anterior resection, the surgeon gets to feel the hardness of the vertebral bone, which will guide the decision on the proper advancement strategy in later steps.

When placing the plate, the surgeon inserts the screws on the caudal vertebrae first to confirm whether the plate's length and contour are appropriate. Repeat plate contouring should be avoided.

Installation of the intervertebral cages and anterior cervical plate vertebral

The size of each intervertebral space is measured with trials. The cages filled with the autologous bone are placed in each intervertebral space. Note that the cages must be of appropriate height. A prebent plate of appropriate length is placed on

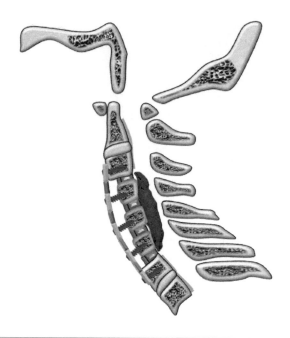

FIGURE 2.2.6

Illustration of the installation of the plate and the intervertebral cage in the ACAF technique.

The plate and screws must be put in place before the vertebral bodies are entirely isolated to ensure the stability of the vertebral bodies and the safety of the nerves during the dissection and advancement operations.

the anterior margin of the vertebral bodies. Screw tunnels are prepared with drill bits and tap before screws are inserted (Fig. 2.2.6). The screw heads are made contact with the plate, and no antedisplacement attempt is made at this time.

The cage's height is deemed appropriate when it can be inserted with ease instead of being impacted into the gap.

If even the smallest cage does not fit into the intervertebral space, the intervertebral space is checked to see if the surfaces are smooth, and the endplates on both sides are entirely parallel.

Small intervertebral space where even the 4 mm high cage has difficulty in ease insertion creates challenges for antedisplacement. When the intervertebral space is less than 2 mm, a fusion option is to place the morselized bone grafts without using a cage (Fig. 2.2.7).

The plate and screws are placed before thorough isolation to stabilize the vertebral bodies to be displaced and avoid cord injury during the bone cutting and vertebral body dissection.

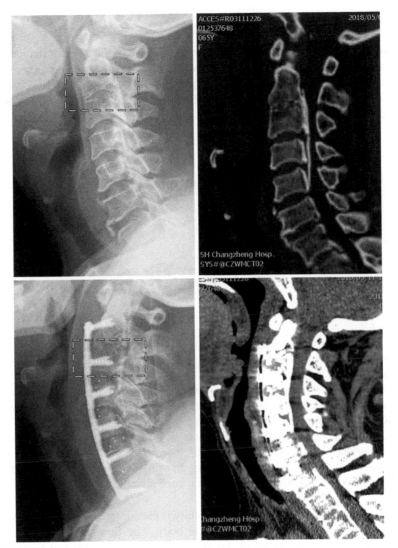

FIGURE 2.2.7

A case where the narrow intervertebral space is packed with morselized bone grafts.
In a case with narrow C2/3 intervertebral space (dashed frame) where a cage does not fit
in, fusion is provided by the packed morselized bone.

Screws are placed parallel to each other, perpendicular to the plate, and in line
with the antedisplacement force applied later. Care should be taken to avoid directing the screws toward the midline.

Bilateral osteotomies of the VOC trough vertebral

Bilateral osteotomies were performed through the base of the anterior uncinate process (anterior junction of the uncinate process base and the superior surface of the vertebra) using a high-speed drill. Subsequently, the posterior vertebral wall was removed using a Kerrison bone punch when the posterior cortex of the VBs was exposed (Fig. 2.2.8).

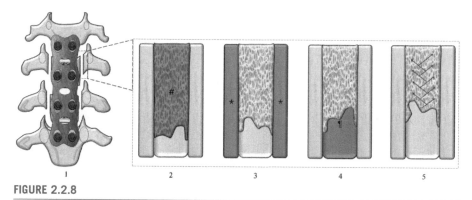

FIGURE 2.2.8

Illustration of bilateral osteotomies of the VOC in ACAF technique.
(1) After the plate and cages are in place, troughs are created on the vertebral bodies on both sides lateral to the ossification;
(2−5) To dissect the posterior cortex at the bottom of the trough, the potential space between the PLL and the vertebral body is separated with a nerve probe, and a Kerrison bone punch is used to remove the bone in a zigzag pattern. # indicates the bone at the bottom of the trough (the orange part in panel 2); *, the bone wall through which the trough is developed (the orange part in panel 3); the symbol, the PLL revealed after the bone at the trough bottom is removed (the magenta part); and the red arrow, the pattern of the bone resection maneuvers with a Kerrison bone punch.

There are two situations where the difficulty is encountered during the dissection between the posterior wall of the vertebral body. The first situation is when the OPLL spans beyond the border of the troughs transversely. This can be managed by thinning the ossification with an ultrasonic bone knife before taking it out with a 1 mm Kerrison bone punch. The other situation is that the decompression width between troughs is so broad that the trough reaches the base of the pedicle. This can be addressed by bypassing the pedicle from the inside. The proper strategy can be developed on preoperative imaging results and intraoperative assessment of the difficulty. Intraoperative CT offers some help as well.

We recommend that troughs are developed 1 mm lateral to the edge of the ossification, producing an 18−20 mm distance between the troughs.

When developing the troughs, the cutting instrument is directed vertically and downwards without deviation. Otherwise, the surgeon may lose the sense of the anatomical boundaries and lead to problems such as residual ossification and penetration into the pedicle or the transverse foramen (Fig. 2.2.9).

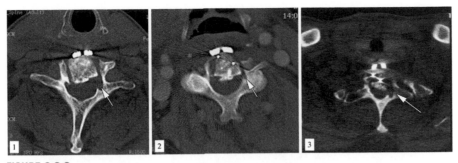

FIGURE 2.2.9

Deviation from the spinal canal due to oblique troughs.
The postoperative axial CT images demonstrating the consequence of oblique troughs,
and lateral mass and lamina (arrow) damaged by the cutter during operation.

When using high-speed burrs and ultrasonic osteotomes for trough development, the cutter size of 2.5—3 mm is appropriate. Ball or teardrop bits are preferred for burrs, and ball or rasp-shaped cutter for ultrasonic osteotome.

Troughs are developed 2.5—3 mm apart. A narrower decompression width limits the field of view whereas a wider one leaves too little bone in the residual vertebral body.

During trough development, when the burr reaches the end, or the posterior cortex, a nerve hook is used through the disc space to separate and palpate the potential plane between the PLL and the posterior wall of the vertebral body.

The probing with a nerve hook serves several purposes. First, it reveals the volume of bone left after resection. Second, it helps validate the trajectory of rongeur when cutting the bone. Third, and most importantly, it reveals whether there is ossification at the bottom of the trough. This step is particularly necessary when preoperative imaging studies suggest a wide-based lesion at a specific level. If ossification is identified where the trough will be developed, the trough is expanded laterally to ensure the dissected complex includes all the ossifications.

The remaining posterior wall of the vertebral body is removed with a 1—2 mm rongeur in a piecemeal fashion and zigzag pattern (Fig. 2.2.8).

Surgeons comfortable using burrs can complete the trough with the burr, though with increased risk. This may also leave residual ossification lateral to the trough in cases with wide ossifications.

A fitted plate may block the instrument when the surgeon tries to develop a trough on the opposite side. Therefore, the trough on the opposite side is developed before plate and screw placement. The trough on the surgeon's side can also be marked first to facilitate subsequent operations.

As soon as the trough is completed, a weak "pop" sound may be heard, which suggests the completion of the trough.

Hemostasis for the lateral wall of the trough is achieved with gelatin paste. Bone wax should be avoided in case of nonfusion of bone troughs. Bleeding of the PLL at

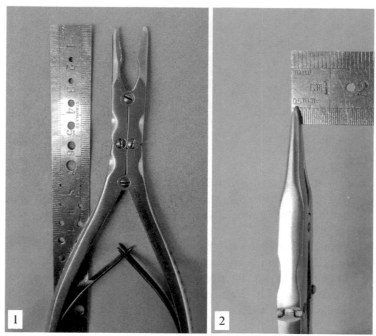

FIGURE 2.2.10

A small rongeur.
(1) Cutter length: 15 mm;
(2) Cutter width: 3 mm.

the bottom of the trough is stopped with bipolar electrocoagulation or absorbable gelatin sponge.

A special type of small rongeur can be used to complete the troughs more efficiently. The jaw of the small rongeur is 3 mm wide and 15 mm long (Fig. 2.2.10). With this small-profile design, it enters the intervertebral space with ease and develops the troughs efficiently, starting with the edges of the vertebral bodies defining the disc space. The troughs are developed as follows: first, a notch is cut with the small rongeur on the upper and lower rims of the vertebral body free of the adjacent disc materials. Bone resection is carried out as the jaw of the rongeur engages the notches. Thereafter, the two notches above and below serve as the starting points where bone resection is carried forward with a small rongeur until a thin layer of the posterior cortex is reached. As the surgeons become proficient, they complete this step in a shorter time. The final step of trough completion is performed with a burr carefully (Fig. 2.2.11).

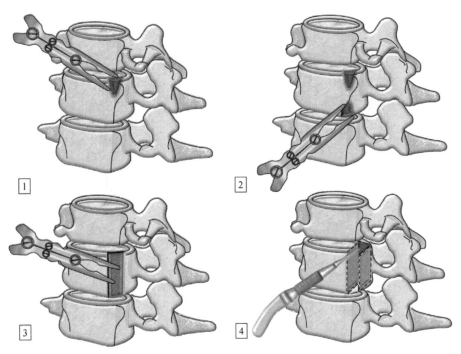

FIGURE 2.2.11

Illustration of trough developed with the small rongeur.

(1) A notch is created on the upper rim of the vertebrae to be antedisplaced and free of the adjacent disc materials;

(2) Another notch is created on the lower rim of the same vertebrae;

(3) With the two notches as the starting points, the central part of the trough is developed;

(4) The trough is completed on the posterior cortex of the vertebral body with a burr.

Hoisting (controllable antedisplacement) of the VOC

After the procedures mentioned above are completed, a neural probe is used to identify any bony connection between the VOC and the spine. An O-arm or G-arm can also be used for intraoperative CT 3D reconstruction to rule out any bony structure that may block the antedisplacement process. Multiple screwdrivers are used to simultaneously tighten the screws on the vertebral bodies that need to be advanced. During this step, surgeons can visualize the advancing vertebral bodies. If there is no perceivable advancement, the surgeon stops the advancement maneuver to check whether the VOC is still connected to the surrounding bony structures (Figs. 2.2.12 and 2.2.13).

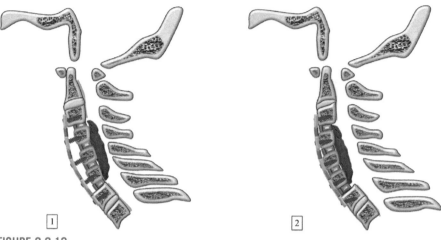

FIGURE 2.2.12

Illustration of VOC in ACAF technique.

(1) Plate and cages placed on the cervical spine. The plate and screws provide temporary stabilization, and the advancement process should not start until the VOC is entirely isolate;

(2) After the VOC is isolated completely, screws on the vertebral bodies of the advancement levels are gradually tightened. With the screw purchased in the bone, the vertebral bodies are advanced in a controllable and safe manner until they contact with the plate.

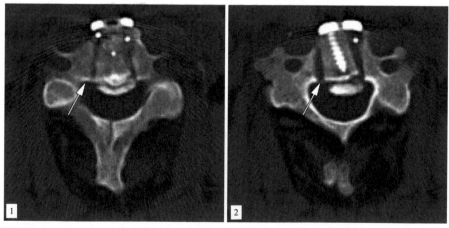

FIGURE 2.2.13

A case of the incompletely hoisted vertebrae vertebral in ACAF surgery.
The two panels indicate insufficient advancement due to incomplete isolation (arrow) of the complex.

The process of hoisting the VOC generally requires screws on one side only. Although the use of bilateral screws can increase their pullout strength in the bone, they may result in constraint or screw pull-out as all the screws may not be aligned with the direction of advancement.

Screws inserted on one side provide smaller but adequate purchases in the bone as long as the bony complex is entirely isolated.

In addition to incomplete dissection and bony barrier, excessive friction between an oversized cage and the endplates is another common cause of insufficient advancement.

To diminish the excessive friction, the screws at both ends of the plate are backed out, or cervical traction is applied before advancement maneuvers.

If resistance is felt during advancement, the surgeon should immediately stop tightening the vertebral screw. Otherwise, the screw tunnels may be damaged, and the advancement plan will fail.

The mechanism of compression screws can be used to distract the intervertebral space before antedisplacement. As the advancement finishes, the disc space is reduced as the screws are fitted from a new entry point and direction.

During vertebral body advancement, hemorrhage may occur from the spinal canal veins through the bone trough. Hemostasis can be obtained with absorbable gelatin sponge or gauze packed in the troughs.

Bone grafting, hemostasis, wound closure, and postoperative immobilization

After bone grafts are packed in the troughs on both sides, the bleeding stopped, wound lavaged, and one or two drainage tubes placed; the surgical wound is closed layer by layer. The head, neck, and chest braces are used for three months postoperatively to facilitate early isolation and bone fusion.

The bone graft materials in the form of granulates, chips, or threads work perfectly.

To facilitate bone grafting in the troughs, the graft materials can be placed before the plate is fitted on the bone. If so, grafts presented in threads are preferred to reduce resistance during antedisplacement.

Active bleeding in the wound should be carefully stopped using bipolar coagulation.

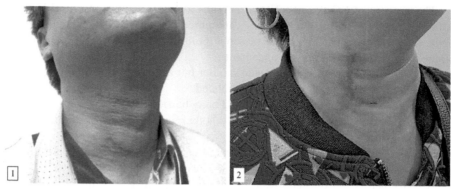

FIGURE 2.2.14

Comparison of the scars from transverse and longitudinal incisions.
(1) Transverse incision is less obvious and cosmetically suitable;
(2) Longitudinal incision is less cosmetically suitable.

After wound lavage with normal saline, gauze is packed in the operation field and kept there for one minute. The gauze is removed and the surgeon assesses for any bleeder. If the gauze is frankly soaked with blood, the surgeon must look for the bleeder and stop it.

The incision is sutured layer by layer. For transverse incisions, intradermal sutures are routinely used. Intradermal suturing is adopted for transverse incisions. For the longitudinal ones, the two sides of the wound are reapproximated with the dermatoglyph realigned and stitched with small needle and sutures with small intervals (Fig. 2.2.14).

Patients undergoing short-segment ACAF surgery wear the Philadelphia collar for three months. Those undergoing long-segment surgery are recommended to wear the head, neck, and chest brace for three months and reassessed for a full weight bear by X-ray (Fig. 2.2.15).

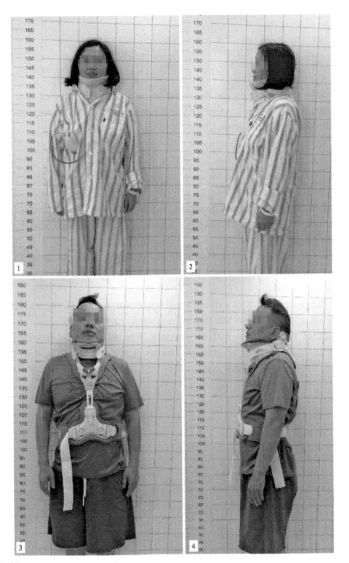

FIGURE 2.2.15

Comparison of patients wearing the Philadelphia collar and the head, vneck, and chest brace.

(1, 2) Philadelphia collar, smaller and comfortable to wear, indicated for short-segment operation where immobilizing is less demanding;

(3, 4) The head, neck, and chest brace, providing all-directional constraints in forward flexion, extension, rotation, and lateral flexion. With robust immobilization but less comfort, it is recommended for long-segment surgeries or compromised spinal stability.

Section 3: Exposure

The ACAF technique exposes the cervical spine from the anterior and reaches the vertebral bodies through space between the trachea-esophagus sheath and the carotid sheath (Smith–Robinson approach).

Preoperative planning

Good surgical exposure depends on adequate preoperative planning. Before surgery, the patient's neck condition should be thoroughly evaluated based on physical appearance and imaging results.

Dynamic X-ray images of the cervical spine can be used to assess the range of motion of the patient's cervical spine and the difficulty of exposing each segment with the neck extended.

Knowing the patient's history of cervical spine surgery is of great significance for the decisions on approach and the use of a gastric tube.

Cervical MRI is analyzed before surgery where any space-occupying lesion should come to the surgeons' attention. The team should identify the nature of the mass and how it affects surgical access (Fig. 2.3.1).

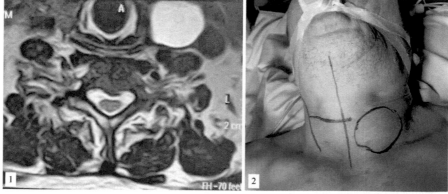

FIGURE 2.3.1

A cystic mass in the thyroid identified on preoperative MRI studies.

Patient positioning

The patient is placed in the supine position on a soft pillow under the shoulders and a saddle pillow under the neck so that the neck is slightly extended. Bean bags are used on both sides of the head for immobilization (Fig. 2.3.2). Neck hyperextension should be avoided in case of aggravating the preexisting hyperextension injury and tensioning the trachea and esophagus.

Patients with severe OPLL placed in the surgical position before being anesthetized to determine if the position deteriorates symptoms and how far the neck can be safely extended.

There should be no gap between the saddle pillow and the neck. A gap can be eliminated with a rolled towel to make the saddle pillow provide robust support and immobilization for the cervical spine.

After the patient is properly positioned, check for any potential glitch that may change the position. Extra immobilization can be provided with adhesive tapes.

The surgeon checks the tension of the patient's trachea-esophagus sheath by pushing them to the left and right. If they are too tense, the team adjusts the patient's position to reduce the neck extension.

For exposure of the vertebral bodies of the C6 and below, if the preoperative lateral X-ray image shows overlapping shoulders and C6, the patient's shoulders

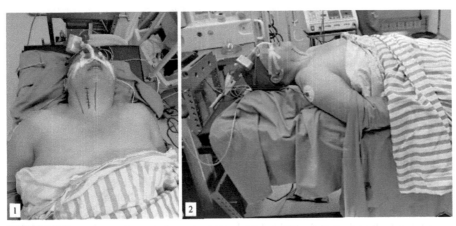

FIGURE 2.3.2

Patient positioning.
(1) Front view: Care should be taken to ensure the patient's head and neck are placed centered, and the midline of the neck and the medial edge of the sternocleidomastoid muscle is marked;
(2) Lateral view: The position is checked to see how extended the patient's neck is and any gap between the neck and the pillow. Ensure the patient is adequately immobilized to prevent any change in the position during surgery. The head holder's position is checked to ensure it does not block the field of intraoperative fluoroscopy.

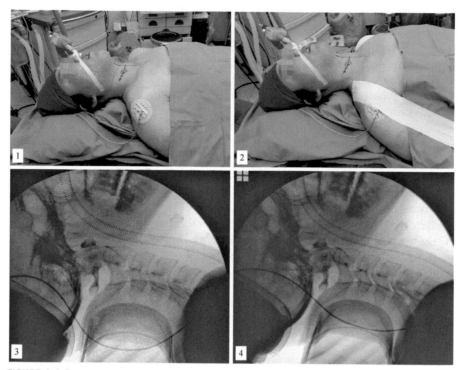

FIGURE 2.3.3

Patient positions and their lateral image. The cervicothoracic region is exposed better when the shoulders are pulled distally and fixed with adhesive tapes.
(1, 3) C6 overlapped with the shoulders on lateral X-ray when the shoulders are not pulled distally.
(2, 4) C6 well shown on lateral X-ray after the shoulders are pulled distally and fixed with adhesive tapes.

are pulled distally and fixed with adhesive tape after he or she has been anesthetized (Fig. 2.3.3).

Patients with ankylosing spondylitis often present with thoracic hyperkyphosis. Therefore, before anesthesia occurs, the patient is asked to lie supine on the operating table to be adequately padded and supported in their natural posture. If this is done when anesthetized, patients are prone to fractures (Fig. 2.3.4).

Incision

In the ACAF technique, a longitudinal incision is usually used when the surgery involves many segments and a transverse incision for shorter segments. Either long or short transverse incision works well. The transverse incision starts at or just lateral to

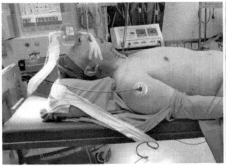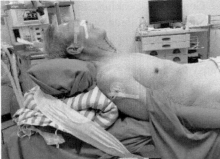

FIGURE 2.3.4

The positioning of patients with ankylosing spondylitis.
(1, 2) These are two patients with ankylosing spondylitis. The patient on the right panel with thoracolumbar hyperkyphosis is well supported with pads under the head, neck, and shoulders. Tapes are used to eliminate motions within the stack of positioning pads.

the midline of the neck, course laterally along the dermatoglyph, and ends around the inner edge of the sternocleidomastoid muscle or just beyond it. The longitudinal incision is located medial to the midpoint between the midline of the neck and the inner edge of the sternocleidomastoid muscle (Fig. 2.3.5).

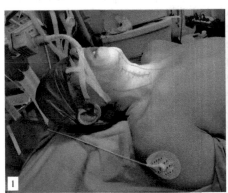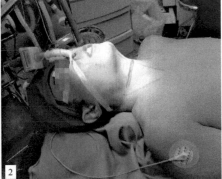

FIGURE 2.3.5

Photo of patients marked with incisions.
(1) Longitudinal incision: It is medial to the midpoint between the midline and the sternocleidomastoid muscle, reducing skin tension during retraction. Multiple short horizontal lines are drawn along the incision to facilitate skin realignment during skin closure;
(2) Transverse incision: It is made over the midpoint of the surgical vertebral segments along the dermatoglyph between midline and sternocleidomastoid muscle. It can be extended toward and beyond the midline if the need arises.

Generally speaking, the threshold for using a longitudinal incision is the advancement of three or more vertebral bodies, which is anything but an unbreakable rule. For example, in patients with thin subcutaneous fat tissue and lower shoulder positions, surgery on three vertebral bodies may be well managed with a transverse incision.

Whether transverse or longitudinal, incisions should be closer to the midline to reduce skin tension during the operation.

The right recurrent laryngeal nerve is anatomically unfavorable and vulnerable to iatrogenic damage, a risk for a right-sided anterior approach. But it comes just handy for surgeons with right-handed dominance. After surgery, patients seldom choke when drinking or develop hoarseness.

Incisions extended laterally do not help with the surgical approach where tasks are dominantly around the midline. When the need arises for a longer incision in a tight wound, it is extended medially and even beyond the midline.

Whether longitudinal or transverse, an incision provides maximum exposure from C2 to T1–T3 depending on the patient's condition.

The proximal-distal placement of incision

The proper placement of the incision along the cervical axis is essential for surgical exposure. A properly placed incision represents surgeon expertise and facilitates a successful and time-saving operation. Conversely, a poorly placed incision may complicate the procedure. In the ACAF technique, the incision is placed at a proper level along the cervical axis based on the diseased segments and cervical curvature.

The cervical segments are roughly represented by palpable anatomical landmarks: the lower edge of the mandible represents C2 vertebral body to C2/3 intervertebral space; hyoid bone, C3 vertebral body to C3/4 intervertebral space; thyroid cartilage, C4 vertebral body to C4/5 intervertebral space; and cricoid cartilage, C5/6 intervertebral space (Fig. 2.3.6).

These correspondences may vary among individuals, and preoperative imaging results provide relevant information.

When using a transverse incision, it is placed along the center of the surgical segments.

If a compromise is to be made, a proximal transverse incision is preferred to a distal one as the latter provides a more challenging exposure.

From the aesthetic point of view, the transverse incision generally chooses the naturally formed dermatoglyph that is close to the surgical segment as the surgical incision. A longitudinal incision should cover the most caudal and cephalad levels of the surgical segments.

Dissection of deep and superficial fascia

After the skin and subcutaneous adipose tissue are cut and bleeders coagulated, the platysma is exposed and bluntly dissected from the subcutaneous adipose tissue

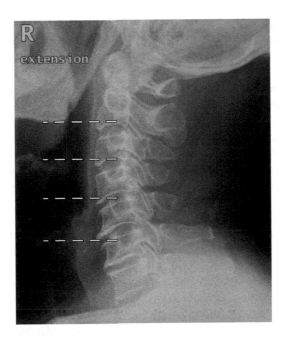

FIGURE 2.3.6

Relations between physical landmarks and cervical segments.
The relations are defined on preoperative hyperextension X-ray images, which is more representative of the intraoperative position. The relations are presented with dashed lines. From top to bottom, they are: the lower edge of the mandible (inferior surface of C2 vertebral body), hyoid bone (inferior surface of C3 vertebral body), thyroid cartilage (C4/5 intervertebral space), and cricoid cartilage (superior surface of C6 vertebral body).

along the span of the desired cervical segments. The pulsating carotid artery is palpated with fingers. Around 1 cm medial to the carotid artery, the platysma and the fibroareolar fascia below it are held and elevated with pick-ups and cut open with a bovie. The meningeal scissors go beneath the fibroareolar fascia and opened to bluntly dissect the space caudally and cephalad before the platysma and the fibroareolar fascia are split longitudinally with a bovie. The fibroareolar fascia is retracted to reveal the subhyoid muscles such as the omohyoid muscle. The intermuscular fascia is elevated with forceps and bluntly opened with meningeal scissors. With the index finger entering through the space between the tracheoesophageal sheath and carotid sheath, the vertebral bodies are palpated from anterior to posterior and dissected off soft tissues caudally and cephalad. An S retractor and a thyroid retractor are placed into the wound along the index finger to retract the tracheoesophageal sheath and carotid sheath, respectively.

When the platysma is to be opened, the communication between the jugular veins is seen crossing from lateroproximal to mediodistal. The platysma is often split lateral to this communication. If the communicating vein is unavoided, it can be ligated and cut off.

The platysma and fibroareolar fascia are incised longitudinally to reach all the desired segments.

The dense fibroareolar fascia deserves more attention during dissection. Under-dissected, it generates significant tension and restricts exposure of the vertebral bodies.

To avoid tension over the retractors held by the first assistant from the omohyoid muscle, when displacing the vertebral bodies of C5 and below, the spine is accessed from the medial side of the omohyoid muscle. When lifting C4 and the vertebral bodies above it, the surgeon should choose to enter from the outside of the omohyoid muscle.

In the long-segment surgeries, the omohyoid muscle can be cut off, suture-tagged at each end, and anastomosed after surgery. Alternatively, the vertebral bodies are accessed proximal and distal to the omohyoid muscles, respectively, for muscle preservation.

When palpating the vertebral body, the index finger starts by confirming the pulsation of the carotid artery laterally to ensure the finger is right between the trachea-esophageal sheath and the carotid sheath.

With retractors placed, sometimes there are neurovascular bundles beneath the deep fascia between the tracheoesophageal sheath and the carotid sheath. If they do not affect the exposure, they are pulled to one side with the retractor.

Upon excessive tension, the deep fascia is carefully and bluntly dissected with meningeal scissors to avoid damaging the arteries and nerves around it.

Exposing and locating the vertebral bodies and the intervertebral discs

As access is provided by the S retractor and the thyroid retractor that pull apart the trachea-esophageal sheath and carotid sheath, the wound is observed for any vascular bundle or esophagus. If present, they are mobilized to one side with a ball-tipped small periosteum detacher. The prevertebral fascia is elevated and held by forceps with serrated tip and bluntly opened with meningeal scissors to expose the vertebral bodies and the intervertebral discs. After locating the surgical segments through fluoroscopy, a periosteum detacher and a bovie are used to peel the longus colli laterally.

Any blood vessel on the vertebral body or medial to the longus colli is ligated with a bipolar coagulator.

The desired segments are located with Caspar pins in the intervertebral space lest screws on the vertebral bodies compromise bony structure and the displacement maneuvers (Fig. 2.3.7).

Before fluoroscopy, a gauze is placed between the locating pin and the trachea-esophageal sheath to protect the latter structures. After the fluoroscopy, the gauze is assessed for blood impregnation followed by hemostasis.

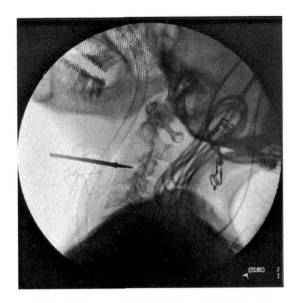

FIGURE 2.3.7

The desired segments located with Caspar pin with intraoperative C-arm X-ray fluoroscopy. When locating the cervical levels in the ACAF technique, the Caspar pin is placed in the intervertebral space whenever possible to preserve the vertebral body.

The longus collis should be peeled to both sides until the joints of the uncinate vertebrae.

The longus colli is always peeled subperiosteally in case injuring the sympathetic trunk on its surface, which leads to Horner syndrome. Bleeding from the nutrient vessels going through the vertebral cortex during muscle elevation is stopped with bone wax.

Illustration of the decision-making incisions in the ACAF technique with cases

Case 1

- Diagnosis—Cervical OPLL (segmental type, from C5 to C6).
- Surgical plan—ACAF technique with advancement of C5 and C6 segments.
- Incision—Anterior transverse incision. In this case, the C5 and C6 vertebral bodies, only two segments, were planned to be advanced, around the middle of the neck length. Therefore, the transverse incision was used to provide adequate exposure with a cosmetically suitable scar (Fig. 2.3.8).

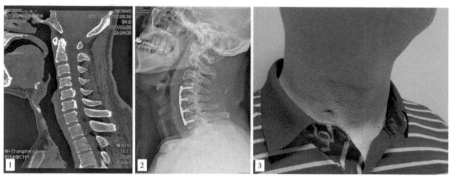

FIGURE 2.3.8

(1) Preoperative midline sagittal CT image;
(2) Postoperative lateral X-ray image;
(3) Physical appearance of the neck three months after the operation.

Case 2

- Diagnosis—Cervical OPLL (segmental type, from C2 to C6 vertebral bodies).
- Surgical plan—An ACAF technique with advancement of C3 to C6 segments.
- Incision—Anterior longitudinal incision. In this case, the ossification involved many segments. The antedisplacement from C3 to C6 vertebral bodies was planned, which was almost the entire cervical spine. The surgery posed significant challenge to surgical exposure, and the longitudinal incision was used with relative ease (Fig. 2.3.9).

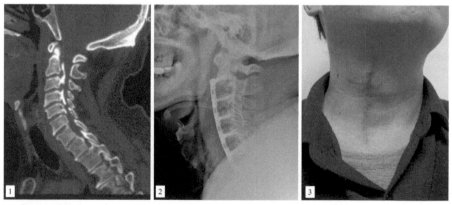

FIGURE 2.3.9

(1) Preoperative midline sagittal CT image;
(2) Postoperative lateral X-ray image;
(3) Physical appearance of the neck 12 months after the operation demonstrating scar contracture.

Case 3

- Diagnosis—Cervical OPLL (segmental type, from C3 vertebral body to C5/6 intervertebral space).
- Surgical plan—An ACAF technique with antedisplacement of C3 and C4 segments.
- Incision—Anterior transverse incision. This case features a short-segment disease in the proximal cervical spine. A transverse incision was used for cosmesis where care was exercised to achieve good dissection of the deep fascia (Fig. 2.3.10).

Case 4

- Diagnosis—Cervical OPLL (circumscribed type, behind C5 and C6 vertebral bodies, with myelopathy at the C3/4 intervertebral space level).
- Surgical plan—An ACAF technique with antedisplacement of C4 to C6 segments.
- Incision—Anterior transverse incision. Three vertebral bodies were to be ventrally displaced, representing a relatively long span. But a good exposure is expectable given that the desired levels are around the middle of the neck axis. To reduce scar contracture, a transverse incision was used (Fig. 2.3.11).

Case 5

- Diagnosis—Cervical OPLL (mixed type, at C2 to C3 and C5 to T3 vertebral bodies).
- Surgical plan—An ACAF procedure with antedisplacement of C5 and C6 segments, and an ACDF procedure for C3/4 decompression.

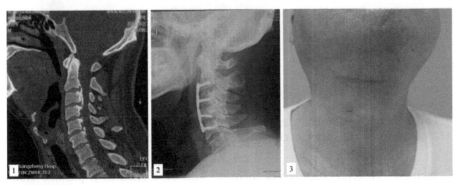

FIGURE 2.3.10

(1) Preoperative midsagittal CT image;
(2) Postoperative lateral X-ray image;
(3) Physical appearance of the neck three months after the operation.

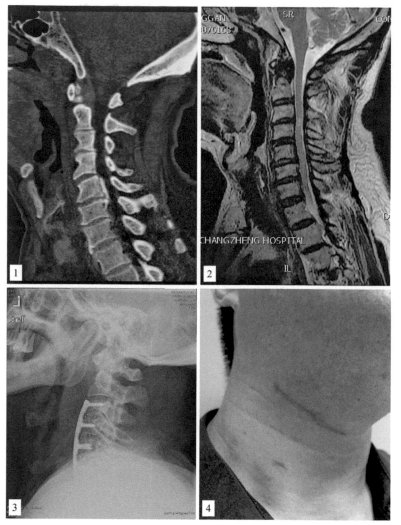

FIGURE 2.3.11

(1) Preoperative midsagittal CT image;
(2) Preoperative midsagittal MRI;
(3) Postoperative lateral X-ray image;
(4) Physical appearance of the neck three months after the operation.

- Incision—Anterior longitudinal incision. This case features a planned ante-displacement of C5 and C6 vertebral bodies, representing a short-segment procedure around the middle of the cervical axis that usually favors transverse incision. However, given a nodule (56 × 34 mm in size) in the left thyroid lobe, the tension from the trachea, and esophagus would be so significant that it might

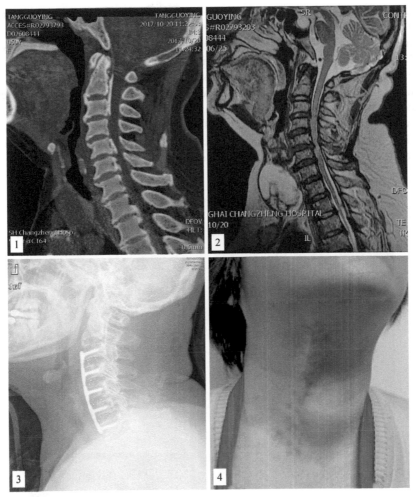

FIGURE 2.3.12

(1) Preoperative midsagittal CT image;

(2) Preoperative midsagittal MRI image;

(3) Postoperative lateral X-ray image;

(4) The appearance of the neck three months after operation with little scar contracture.

compromise exposure in a transverse incision. Therefore, a longitudinal incision was used instead to provide ease for exposure and extended caudally during surgery to diminish tension on the skin (Fig. 2.3.12).

Case 6

- Diagnosis—Cervical OPLL (mixed type, at C2/3 to C4/5 and C7 to T1/2 segments).

- Surgical plan—An ACAF procedure with advancement of C3 to C4, and C6 to T1 segments.
- Incision—Anterior dual transverse incisions. The levels to be antedisplaced were C3 to C4 and C6 to T1 segments, skipping a level in between. It was difficult to expose through a single transverse incision. If a longitudinal incision is used, it needs to be extended from the mandible to the clavicle, resulting in severe scar contracture. Since C5 was spared from the procedure, two transverse incisions were used to expose the proximal and distal segments separately. Specifically, a right transverse incision was used to expose the proximal C3 and C4 while the left transverse incision was used for the distal C6 to T1 (Fig. 2.3.13).

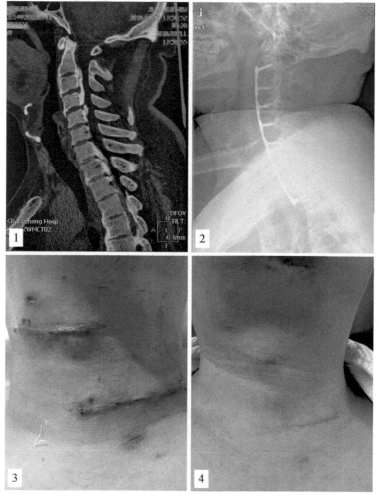

FIGURE 2.3.13

(1) Preoperative midsagittal CT image;

(2) Postoperative lateral X-ray image;

(3) The appearance of the neck one year after the operation with inconspicuous scars.

Case 7

- Diagnosis—Cervical OPLL (mixed type, at C2 to T1).
- Surgical plan—An ACAF procedure for C3 to C5 advancement and an ACDF for C6/7 intervertebral space decompression.
- Incision—Anterior dual transverse incisions. This case features the spinal cord consistently compressed from C2 to T1 segments due to a continuous ossification of C2 to C4 and a segmental one distally. The surgical plan was to antedisplace the C3 to C5 segments and decompress the C6/7 intervertebral space, involving five consecutive segments. Similar to Case 6, with C6 spared from the advancement, two transverse incisions were used for exposure. The upper one was for C2 to C5 and the lower one, C5 to C7 segments (Fig. 2.3.14).

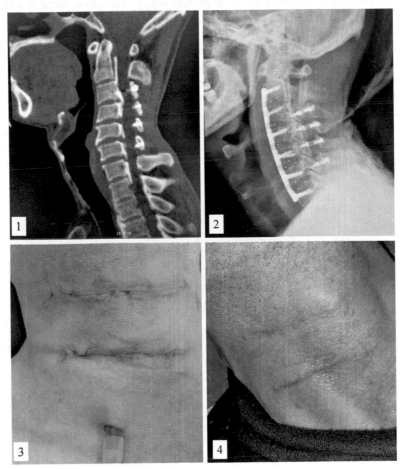

FIGURE 2.3.14

(1) Preoperative midsagittal CT image;
(2) Postoperative position X-ray image;
(3) The appearance of the neck three days after the operation, with normal appearance of skin flaps between incisions suggesting uncompromised blood supply;
(4) The appearance of the neck three months after the operation.

Section 4: Bilateral osteotomies

The ACAF technique hinges on two key steps, namely, the isolation and advancement of VOC. The crux of isolation, or dissection of the VOC from the surrounding bone, is to develop longitudinal bone cuts on both sides of the vertebral body. ACAF adopts a similar surgical exposure to ACDF, which is distinct from that in the ACCF where the spinal canal is exposed to evaluate the trough boundaries on both sides (Fig. 2.4.1). To incorporate the OPLL in the VOC, the bone cuts on both sides of the VOC should be wide enough. However, if the bone cuts are too wide apart, it increases the risk of vertebral artery or pedicle injury. Therefore, there is a proper range for the trough position (Fig. 2.4.2), and to determine the proper position of the troughs is a critical step in the ACAF technique.

Laminoplasty (LAM) also involves the proper placement of troughs on the bone across multiple segments. According to anatomical studies, the troughs are recommended to be placed at the junction between the lamina and the lateral mass, often identified with a change of the surface angle and a nutrient artery. If the trough is too medial, leaving a large proportion of the residual lamina on that side, it exerts little effect on decompression and expansion and posterior shift of the spinal cord. Rather, it may even cause nerve entrapment, aggravated upper limb symptoms, and lead to incomplete paraplegia in severe cases. On the contrary, if the trough is too lateral, it

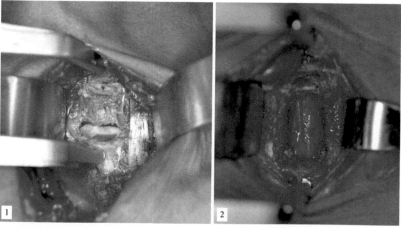

FIGURE 2.4.1

Human cadavers demonstrating the surgical fields of the ACDF and the ACCF techniques.
(1) The surgical field of the ACDF technique;
(2) The surgical field of the ACCF technique.

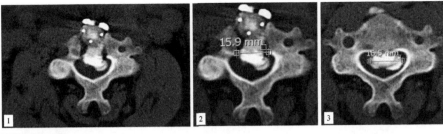

FIGURE 2.4.2

Failed antedisplacement of the VOC due to narrow decompression width or the distance between the two bone cuts.
(1) Insufficiently advanced ossification;
(2) The troughs 15.9 mm apart on postoperative images;
(3) The ossification measuring 16.5 mm before the operation.

can easily damage the articular processes and nerve roots and cause difficulty in opening the spinal canal (Fig. 2.4.3).

The ACAF technique is similar to LAM in that both involve developing troughs on both sides, and that the ossification, the spinal cord, the pedicle, and the nerve roots are not directly exposed. As anatomical evidence recommends the junction of the lamina and lateral mass as the landmark for the troughs in LAM, where do we locate the troughs in the ACAF technique? Is the uncinate process a reliable anatomical landmark? How does this landmark guide trough development (Fig. 2.4.4)? Are troughs developed off the uncinate processes incorporate a large part of the ossifications? Is this process blocked by the pedicles? Does it carry the risk of vertebral artery injury? To answer these questions, we need to review the anatomy of the trough sites in the ACAF technique.

A 100 vertebral bodies of C3 to C7 levels in 20 OPLL patients were measured for the following six coronal dimensions: the base distance of the uncinate process, the transverse foramen to the uncinate process, the pedicle to the uncinate process, the distance from posterior to anterior uncinate process, width of the VOC, and maximal width of OPLL (Fig. 2.4.5).

Through this series of measurements, the author's team found that the maximal width of OPLL is 13.2 mm on average and the mean width of the VOC in the ACAF cases is 16.8 mm on average. Because the VOC is wider than the maximum width of the OPLL, the troughs are adequately wide apart to incorporate the entire ossification.

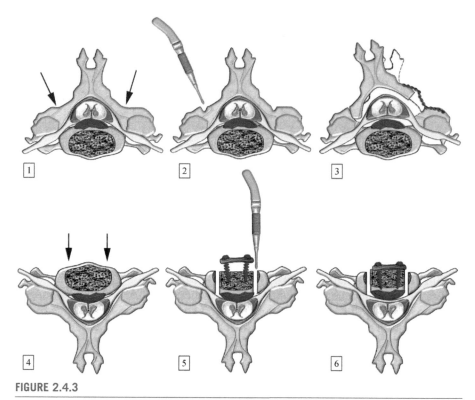

FIGURE 2.4.3

Illustration of the troughs developed in the ACAF and the LAM techniques. Width of the VOC of each case is the average value obtained from the most caudal level, most cranial level, and the middle level of OPLL.

(1–3) Trough position and decompression mechanism in LAM;

(4–6) Trough position and decompression mechanism in ACAF;

(1) Troughs (arrows) planned at junction of the lamina and the lateral mass on both sides in LAM technique;

(2) Troughs (arrows) developed at the junction of the lamina and the lateral mass on both sides with a burr;

(3) The lamina disconnected via the trough on one side and the spinal canal opened toward the opposite side, decompressing the spinal cord by allowing it to shift backward;

(4) Troughs (arrows) planned along the uncinate processes in ACAF technique;

(5) After plate installation, the vertebral body is cut along the uncinate processes with a burr;

(6) After VOC advancement, direct decompression of the spinal cord is achieved.

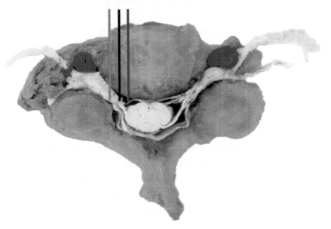

FIGURE 2.4.4

Top-down view of C5. The desired positions of the troughs are indicated in three colors. Red: through the posterior base of the uncinate process; black: through the anterior base of the uncinate process; and blue: through the medial wall of the pedicle.

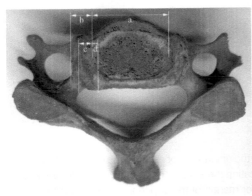 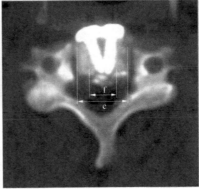

FIGURE 2.4.5

Illustration of cervical spine parameters.

(1) (Base distance of the uncinate process) Distance between the bilateral anterior the uncinate process base (anterior junction of the uncinate process base and the superior surface of the vertebrae).

(2) (Transverse foramen to the uncinate process) shortest distance between the sagittal plane across the anterior uncinate process base and the sagittal plane across the ipsilateral transverse foramen. The result is positive when the transverse foramen is lateral to the uncinate process, and the result is negative when the transverse foramen is medial to the uncinate process.

(3) (Pedicle to the uncinate process) shortest distance between the sagittal plane across the anterior uncinate process base and the sagittal plane across the ipsilateral pedicle. The result is positive when the pedicle lateral to the uncinate process, and the result is negative when the pedicle medial to the uncinate process.

(4) (Posterior to anterior uncinate process) Distance between the sagittal plane across the anterior uncinate process base and the sagittal plane across the ipsilateral posterior uncinate process base. The result is positive when the posterior uncinate process is lateral to the anterior uncinate process, and the result is negative when the posterior uncinate process is medial to the anterior uncinate process.

(5) (Maximal width of OPLL) Maximal width of OPLL.

(6) (Width of the VOC) Width of the VOC is the distance between the medial borders of bilateral osteotomies.

Anatomical study of the trough position
Trough developed at the anterior base of the uncinate process

During the bone cutting process, the pedicle, vertebral arteries, and other lateral structures are beyond direct visualization. Therefore, an easily identifiable and reliable landmark is needed to ensure the surgery is performed safely and effectively [1]. At constant locations and subject to little change in imaging studies, the easily identifiable anterior base of the uncinate process on both sides serves as the landmark for parasagittal bone cuts on the vertebral bodies in the ACAF technique (Fig. 2.4.6).

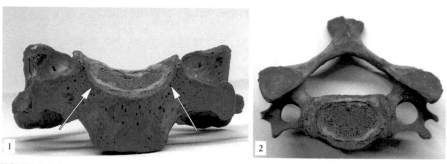

FIGURE 2.4.6

Anatomical location of the anterior base of the uncinate processes of the cervical spine.
(1) Front view of a cervical vertebrae, indicating the anterior base of the uncinate process (arrow) at the junction between the anterior margin of the superior endplate and the uncinate process;
(2) Top-down view of a cervical vertebrae.

The tip of the uncinate process is used as a surgical landmark for anterior cervical decompression by some surgeons. However, in cervical spine degeneration, it is difficult to locate the tip of the uncinate process due to hyperplastic osteophytes.

In the technique described here, the anterior base of the uncinate process is used as a landmark because it is less affected by degeneration or hyperostosis (Fig. 2.4.8).

The maximum width of OPLL averages 13.2 mm in the general population, 13.2 mm in men and 13.1 mm in women.

In the ACAF cases, the width of VOC averaged 16.8 mm in the composite cohort, 17.0 mm in men and 16.3 mm in women.

The distance between the planes of the anterior bases of the uncinate processes increases from C3 to C7 (Fig. 2.4.7), to a larger extent in men than in women.

In women, the average distance increases from 13.2 mm on C3 to 20.8 mm on C7.

In men, it increases from 16.0 mm on C3 to 24.5 mm on C7.

According to Lu's report, in West Asian, this parameter increases from 19.2 mm on C3 to 24.6 mm on C7 [2]. The difference between the author's team and that of Lu may represent genetic variance between East and West Asia.

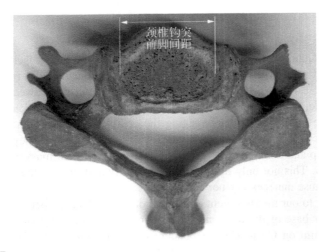

FIGURE 2.4.7

The base distance of the uncinate process.

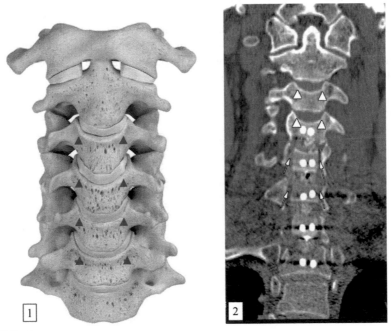

FIGURE 2.4.8

Anterior base of the uncinate process, the anatomical landmark for trough development.
(1) Front view of the cervical spine model, with the anterior base of the uncinate process marked (solid triangles);
(2) Coronal CT image of the patient after the ACAF procedure, with the anterior bases of the uncinate processes (solid triangles) and the troughs (arrows). The troughs and the anterior bases of the uncinate processes of the same side are aligned.

The relationship between the anterior base of the uncinate process and the pedicle

In the ACAF technique, when the bone cut on the vertebral body reaches the spinal canal, the cutting instrument may engage the ossification medially or the pedicle laterally (Fig. 2.4.9). Without understanding the relationship between the trough and the pedicle, it is challenging to assess if the cutting instrument keeps engaging bony structures. With the cutter engaging the pedicle, if the surgeon mistakes the pedicle as the vertebral body and continues with the cutting tool, they may end up going too deep and damaging the pedicle and even the lateral mass, which locates far posteriorly. This not only increases the difficulty and time of the operation but it may also cause unnecessary nerve damage.

According to our measurement of clinical data, the distance between the planes of the anterior base of the uncinate process and the medial edge of the pedicle is constantly 3 mm on C3 to C5 independent of the patient's sex. This distance is 1.8 mm on C6 and 0 mm on C7 (Fig. 2.4.10).

It measures about 3 mm at C3 through C5 in both men and women with little variance.

The coronal distance between the medial wall of the pedicle and the anterior base of the uncinate process at C6 averages 1.6 mm in men and 2.0 mm in women and measures significantly shorter than the vertebrae above C6.

At the C7 level, this distance is −0.2 mm in men and 0.2 mm in women.

Troughs developed off the anterior base of the uncinate process are clear of the pedicle all the way from C3 down to C6.

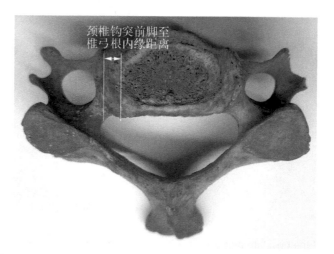

FIGURE 2.4.9

Distance between the anterior base of the uncinate process and the medial boundary of the pedicle.

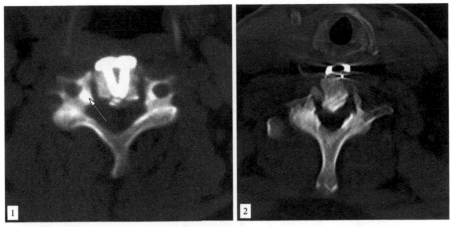

FIGURE 2.4.10

Comparison of C4 and C7 vertebral bodies with troughs developed off the anterior base of the uncinate process.

(1) Axial CT image of the C4 after ACAF in an OPLL patient. At C4, the uncinate process is 3 mm medial to the plane of the pedicle, enabling a safe zone (arrow) between the pedicle and the bone cut based off the anterior base of the uncinate process;

(2) Axial CT image after ACAF in an OPLL patient at the C7, where the minimal coronal distance between the uncinate process and the pedicle is 0.6 mm. As such, the cutter aiming for the anterior base of the uncinate process ended up in the pedicle.

The C7 vertebral body is cut 1 mm medial to the anterior base of the uncinate process for pedicle clearance independent of the patient's sex (Fig. 2.4.11).

The relationship between the anterior base of the uncinate process and the transverse foramen.

Vertebral artery injury constitutes a fatal complication in anterior cervical surgeries. As the troughs on the vertebral bodies in the ACAF technique are significantly wider apart than those in the ACCF technique, does the bone cut pose a risk to the vertebral artery? The coronal distance between the plane across the tip of the uncinate process and the transverse foramen of the same side has been reported at 3 mm on C2 to C4 and 1.5 mm on C5 to C7, and the coronal distance between the lateral wall of the uncinate process and the vertebral artery varies from 1.7 to 1.8 mm. Therefore, developing the trough off the uncinate process's tip poses a significant risk to the vertebral artery (Fig. 2.4.12). In contrast, the anterior base of the uncinate process, used by the author's team as a landmark in the ACAF technique, is about 3 mm medial to the plane of the uncinate process tip.

Through measurement, the author's team identified a safe zone of at least 5 mm wide between the planes of the anterior base of the uncinate process and the medial wall of the transverse foramen (Fig. 2.4.13).

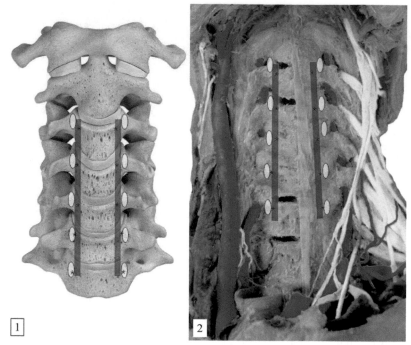

FIGURE 2.4.11

The relationship between the pedicles and the anterior bases of the uncinate processes, used as landmarks for trough development.
(1) Front view of the cervical spine model marked with the anterior base of the uncinate process (asterisks), the pedicles (ovals), and the desired bone cuts (red lines);
(2) The front view of a human cadaver specimen marked with the anterior bases of the uncinate processes (asterisks), the pedicles (ovals), and the desired bone cuts (red lines). Note that the right part of the anterior longitudinal ligament, the right side of the intervertebral discs, and the osteophytes laterally of the C2/3, C3/4, C6/7, and C7/T1 have been removed.

This safe zone measures 5.9 mm at the C7 level and 7.2 mm at the C3 among men.

It measures 5.1 mm at the C7 level and 6.4 mm at the C3 among women.

In general, the distance between the anterior base of the uncinate process and the transverse foramen varies between 4.6 and 7.2 mm.

The width of this safe zone remains constant across all cervical levels.

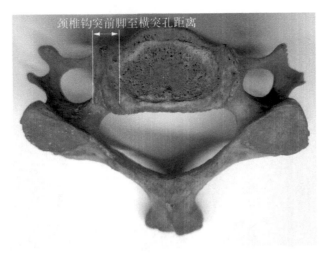

FIGURE 2.4.12

Distance between the planes of the anterior base of the uncinate process and the transverse foramen.

The relationship between the anterior and the posterior base of the uncinate processes

The posterior base of the uncinate process is always medial to the anterior base (Fig. 2.4.14). The distance between the parasagittal planes across the anterior and the posterior bases of an uncinate process tends to increase from C3 to C7. The osteophytes around the posterior part of the uncinate process can compress the spinal cord, nerve roots, and vertebral arteries and cause symptoms. To treat these diseases, foraminal decompression and osteophyte removal are usually necessary. The vertebral body cut at the anterior base of the uncinate process usually achieves 4.6 mm of decompression anterior to the spinal canal within the intervertebral space. Therefore, the ACAF technique provides satisfactory results for radiculopathy as well.

The coronal distance between the planes of the anterior and the posterior bases of an uncinate process increases from C3 to C7.

In men, it increases from −3.9 mm at C4 to −5.7 mm at C7 level.

In women, it increases from −3.7 mm at C3 to −5.6 mm at C7 level.

Summary of trough placement

An average desired placement of trough has been reached from imaging investigation.

For males, the longitudinal troughs are developed with bone cuts in the vertebral bodies at the anterior base of the uncinate process at the C3 to C6 and 1 mm medial to the anterior base at C7.

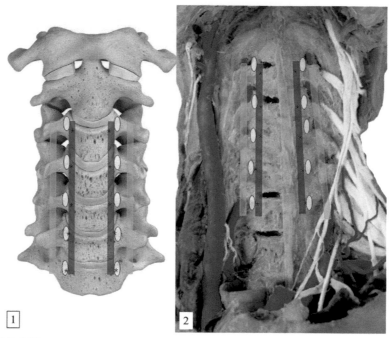

FIGURE 2.4.13

Relationship between the desired troughs off the anterior base of the uncinate process and the vertebral arteries.

(1) Front view of the cervical spine model marked with the anterior base of the uncinate process (asterisks), the pedicles (blue lines), and the desired bone cuts (red lines);

(2) The front view of a human cadaver specimen marked with the anterior bases of the uncinate processes (asterisks), the pedicles (blue lines), and the desired bone cuts (red lines). The right anterior longitudinal ligament has been resected; C2/3, C3/4, C6/7, C7/T1 intervertebral space, right osteophytes, and intervertebral discs have been removed.

For women, the longitudinal troughs are developed with bone cuts in the vertebral bodies 1.5 mm, 1 mm, and 0.5 mm lateral to the anterior base of the uncinate process at C3, C4, and C5, respectively, and 1 mm medial to the anterior base at C7.

The vertebral body troughs developed with this rule are clear of the pedicles laterally and with a 5 mm safe zone from the vertebral arteries.

Trough developed in this way provides sufficient decompression of the spinal cord and nerve roots.

A customized surgical plan is based on measurements from the preoperative CT images for each patient.

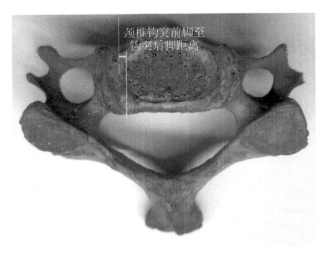

颈椎钩突前脚至
钩突后脚距离

FIGURE 2.4.14

The coronal distance between the planes of the anterior base and the posterior base of an uncinate process.

The sequence of the procedure in relation to plate placement

The ACAF technique has been broken down into steps in a previous section. Since the VOC is temporarily stabilized with instrumentation before adequate isolation to ensure a controllable advancement procedure, the plate and cages are placed before completing the troughs on both sides of the vertebral bodies, as recommended in the previous section. However, this recommendation is based on a perfect scenario rarely seen in the actual practice. In the anterior approach, the trachea and esophagus are pulled to the surgeon's opposite side to the extent that the longus colli of that side is seen in the wound. The excessive pull to these structures risks injuries to the trachea, esophagus, and vagus nerve. Softer than the tracheoesophageal sheath, the carotid sheath on the surgeon's side is prone to excessive retraction, causing carotid sinus syndrome, even cardiac arrest.

The typical exposure in the ACAF technique is shown in Fig. 2.4.15. The vertebral bodies are cut via an interval between retracted structures, with the tracheoesophageal retractor on the surgeon's opposite side and the thyroid retractor on the surgeon's side. Performing surgery via this plane developed through retraction is difficult. If the plate is placed before trough development, it becomes an unavoidable barrier in the small wound, compromising visualization and tool entries and complicating the bone cut procedure. Therefore, in the actual practice, the plate and cages are not placed before trough development on both sides of the vertebral bodies.

Indeed, during the actual practice, the trough on the surgeon's opposite side is developed first, followed by plate and cage placement. The trough of the surgeon's

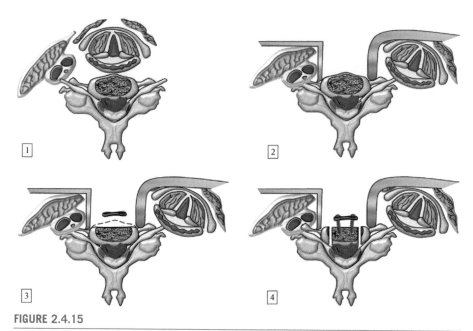

FIGURE 2.4.15

Illustration of the standard steps of exposure in ACAF technique.
(1) Before surgery;
(2) The carotid artery sheath and tracheoesophageal sheath retracted to each side;
(3) An anterior part of the vertebral body is resected and a plate placed;
(4) Screws placed in the vertebral bodies before they are cut on both sides.

side is then cut. Steps performed in this sequence ensure the VOC's stability during isolation without compromising surgical exposure and access of instruments. To enhance the exposure for trough development on the surgeon's side, the plate can be placed 1−2 mm off the midline toward the other side (Fig. 2.4.16).

The trough on the surgeon's opposite side is developed before placing a plate and cages in case of being blocked by the plate. However, in cases with a short distance between the bilateral uncinate processes, the trough on the opposite side can be covered by the plate, interfering with the surgeon's assessment on the decompression width or the distance between the troughs on both sides. To address this challenge, the procedure has been further modified so that in addition to the trough on the opposite, the desired location for the trough on the surgeon's side is etched with the bone cutter with care not to dissect the cortex at the bottom of the trough. In this way, the surgical exposure and space for trough development are obtained while ensuring the stability of bony structures before VOC isolation. After the plate and cages are placed, even if exposure and access are limited, the surgeon can feel comfortable finishing the trough on his or her side with a rongeur (Fig. 2.4.17).

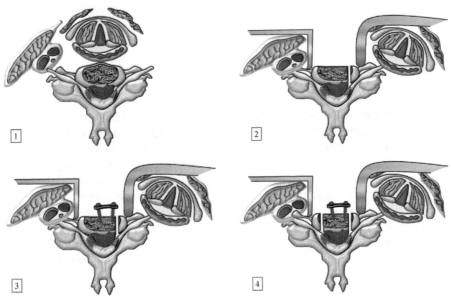

FIGURE 2.4.16

Illustration of modified steps of exposure in ACAF technique.

(1) Before surgery;

(2) A trough developed on the surgeon's opposite side;

(3) Plate and screws placed on the vertebral bodies;

(4) Trough on the surgeon's side developed.

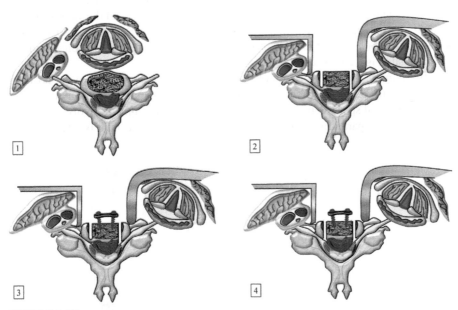

FIGURE 2.4.17

Illustration of another modified series of steps for exposure.

(1) Before surgery;

(2) A complete trough on the surgeon's opposite side and a half trough on the surgeon's side;

(3) Plate and screws placed;

(4) Completed trough on the surgeon's side.

Barriers of bone resection deep in the trough and strategies

To remove the bone toward the bottom of the trough, the surgeon proceeds with a rongeur while palpating the trough's location and depth with a nerve hook, as recommended by the authors. If the power platform (burr or ultrasonic osteotome) is used from initiating to finishing the trough, the surgeon may lose sight of the trough's position and depth and leave residual ossification. Also, burrs and the ultrasonic osteotome can cause thermal and mechanical damage to nerves.

If the power platform is used to cut bone, the surgeon also palpates the trough's bottom intermittently with a nerve hook via the intervertebral space to get a sense of how deep the trough is (Fig. 2.4.18). Before clearing the last 2 mm-thick bone toward the bottom, a rongeur is used instead to manually clear out the bone in a piecemeal fashion via the intervertebral space.

Specifically, the bone toward the bottom is removed with a 2 mm rongeur engaged from the caudal (with a right-dominant surgeon standing on the right side of the patient) or cephalad (with a right-dominant surgeon standing on the left side of the patient) disc space. If the surgeon prefers to engage the bone from the caudal disc space, they start from the most caudal level and work toward the cephalad direction (Fig. 2.4.19).

Preferably, the rongeur engages the bone via the space between the vertebral body and the PLL to spare the latter from damage. In OPLL, the ossification within the spinal canal pushes the spinal cord and dural sac caudally, and the venous plexus on both sides in the canal is often distended and tortuous. Sparing the PLL at the bottom of the bone trough avoids bleeding from the ruptured venous plexus in the spinal canal (Figs. 2.4.20 and 2.4.21).

After completing the grooving of the first vertebral body, the grooving position can be referenced and adjusted in the grooving of the second vertebral body. Since the intervertebral space between a vertebra and its distal segment involves preliminary endplate preparation without posterior ossification resection, it is often difficult

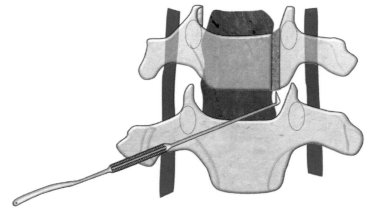

FIGURE 2.4.18

The posterior wall of the vertebral body palpated with a nerve hook.

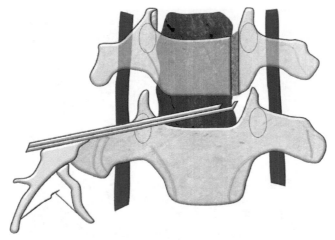

FIGURE 2.4.19

The bone toward the bottom of the trough removed with a rongeur engaged from the intervertebral space.

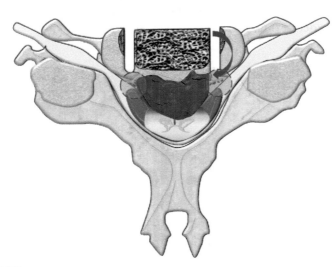

FIGURE 2.4.20

Illustration of bone removal at the bottom of the trough.
The PLL indicated with the green line, and bone is resected with rongeur engaged along the trajectory indicated with the red arrow. As such, the venous plexus behind the PLL is protected from surgical insult.

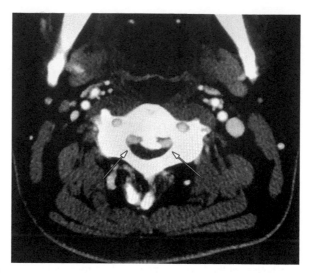

FIGURE 2.4.21

The venous plexus in the spinal canal shown on contrast-enhanced CT.
The venous plexus (arrow) with enhancement similar to that of the vertebral arteries.

to remove the bone at the bottom of the distal vertebral body from the intervertebral space. In the face of this constraint, the surgeon can extend the trough of the first vertebral body cephalad before approaching the bone at the bottom of the trough in the distal vertebral (Fig. 2.4.22).

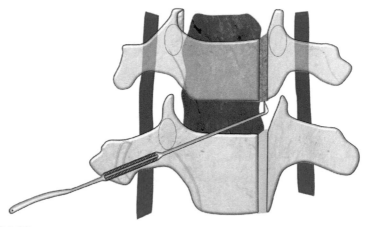

FIGURE 2.4.22

The trough on the distal vertebral body is completed, exposing the PLL (shown by the gray band). The surgeon then starts removing the bone at the bottom of the upper vertebral body.

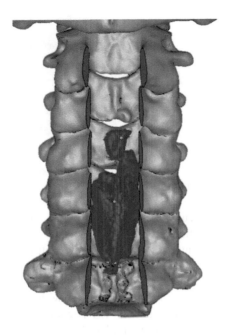

FIGURE 2.4.23

The coronal view of the three-dimensional reconstruction of the PLL of the cervical spine.

The ossification (red) of irregular. Caution should be taken during surgery to frequently palpating the edge of the OPLL when developing the troughs on the vertebral bodies.

If resistance is encountered when removing the bone from the trough bottom, the surgeon checks for any bony barrier with a nerve hook between the trough bottom and the PLL (Figs. 2.4.23 and 2.4.24). Care should be exercised to clear the bone at the trough bottom layer by layer instead of poking deep with the rongeur or power

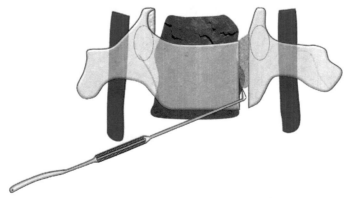

FIGURE 2.4.24

The interval between bone at the bottom of the trough and the posterior longitudinal ligament palpated with a nerve hook.

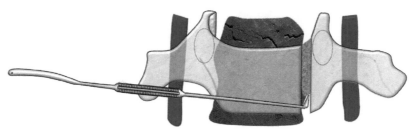

FIGURE 2.4.25

If the bony barrier is at the lower two-thirds of the vertebral body, the interval is explored with the nerve hook directed laterally.

tool lest complications occur, such as nerve injury, cerebrospinal fluid (CSF) leakage, or residual ossification.

The bony resistant encountered toward the trough bottom is assessed for possible nature according to its location. The bony resistance around the inferior two-thirds of the vertebral body is usually OPLL. The trough is then assessed to see if it is too medial, and the bony resistance here is compared with the OPLL at the broader width on preoperative CT scans. If an OPLL is confirmed, the surgeon explores laterally with a nerve hook and can often identify a gap (Fig. 2.4.25).

Upon palpating this gap, the bony barrier is bypassed as the surgeon expands the trough laterally with the 2 mm rongeur (Fig. 2.4.26). If the difficulty persists during the attempt to bypass the ossification, a nerve elevator is used again to explore, and the 1 mm rongeur is used instead.

The bony barrier around the upper one-third of the vertebral body is usually the pedicle. The surgeon explores medially for the gap, which is often present (Fig. 2.4.27).

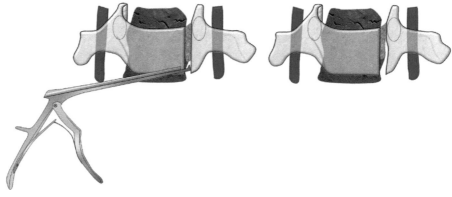

FIGURE 2.4.26

The trough is expanded laterally with a rongeur to bypass the bony barrier.

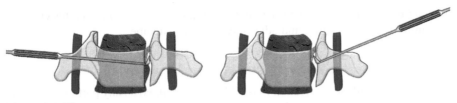

FIGURE 2.4.27

The bony barrier located at the upper third of the vertebral body is usually the pedicle, and the interval is explored with the nerve hook directed medially.

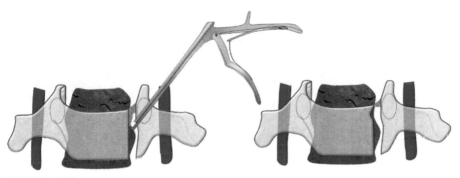

FIGURE 2.4.28

The trough is expanded medially with a rongeur, bypassing the bony resistance. Arrows indicate the residual ossification and dashed lines, VOC.

Upon reaching the interval, the nerve hook is substituted with a 2 mm rongeur to expand the trough laterally and bypass the bony barrier (Fig. 2.4.28). If it is still difficult to bypass the ossification, the nerve hook is used again for palpation, and the 1 mm rongeur is used for bone removal.

After the trough is completed, the nerve hook is used to palpate laterally along the bottom edge of the trough to identify any residual compressor or ossification. If present, it is removed with a rongeur.

Overview of residual ossification

As a key part of the ACAF technique composed of the PLL ossification and the vertebral body in front of it, the VOC is isolated, advanced, and stabilized as a whole for anterior direct decompression without ossification removal. All these procedures that follow are impossible without the en bloc isolation of the VOC.

The process of isolating a VOC en bloc is by no means easy. When a wide-based OPLL is treated with the ACCF technique, it is often difficult to remove the entire ossification, which poses challenges to the decompression and causes persistent cord impingement. Unexpectedly, to isolate the VOC in the ACAF technique is a challenging step. Failure to incorporate the lateral parts of the OPLL in the VOC results in residual ossification and adversely surgical outcome.

Definition of postoperative residual ossification mass

Postoperative residual ossification mass (PROM) is defined as any part of the OPLL left out by the VOC in the spinal canal observed in the postoperative axial CT images [3] (Fig. 2.4.29).

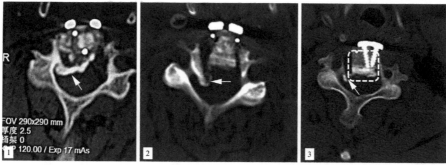

FIGURE 2.4.29

Transverse CT image of residual ossification.

Definition of wide-based OPLL

The spinal canal is divided into three parts with two sagittal planes through the anterior bases of the uncinate processes. An OPLL on the posterior wall of the vertebral body is deemed wide-based if it extends to the lateral zones. Otherwise, it is a narrow-based OPLL (Fig. 2.4.30).

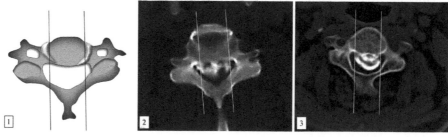

FIGURE 2.4.30

Illustration and imaging presentation of wide-based and narrow-based OPLL.
(1) Illustration of the axial view of the cervical vertebral body, divided into three parts by the two parasagittal lines through the anterior bases of the uncinate processes;
(2) A wide-based OPLL where the OPLL on the posterior wall of the vertebral body extends to the right lateral zone;
(3) A narrow-based OPLL where OPLL is not present in the lateral zones, despite being bulky.

Clinical data of residual ossification after ACAF

A review of 75 OPLL patients treated with the ACAF technique, including 6 (8%) with a wide-based OPLL, concluded a 4% (three cases) incidence of PROM with CT evidence (Fig. 2.4.31).

Further analysis of PROM incidence and imaging findings among wide-based OPLL cases identified all the patients developing PROM as those with wide-based diseases at baseline. Therefore, the incidence of residual ossification in patients with wide-based OPLL is as high as 50%. It is worth noting that all three patients with residual ossification on the right side of the VOC.

Further analysis of the six patients with wide-based OPLL showed that patients without residual ossification had good neurological recovery supported by

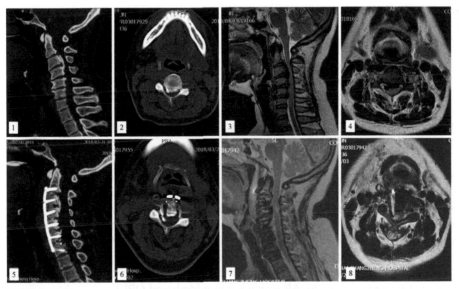

FIGURE 2.4.31

Imaging studies demonstrating postoperative residual ossification.
(1) Preoperative sagittal CT;
(2) Preoperative transverse CT at C4 where the ossification is wide-based on the right side;
(3) Preoperative sagittal MRI;
(4) Preoperative transverse MRI;
(5) Postoperative sagittal CT;
(6) Postoperative transverse CT demonstrating residual ossification on the right side posterior to the C4 vertebral body;
(7) Postoperative sagittal MRI at C4 demonstrating signal changes in the spinal cord;
(8) Postoperative transverse MRI at C4 vertebral body demonstrating the signal intensity of CSF present in the right trough, residual ossification compresses the spinal cord, and spinal cord signal changes.

significantly improved Japanese Orthopaedic Association (JOA) score. However, those with residual ossification did not reach neurological recovery as expected.

Among the patients without residual ossification, four (5.6%) developed CSF leakage, all of whom healed spontaneously within one week without special treatment. However, two (66.7%) with residual ossification developed CSF leakage, and both patients underwent lumbar puncture and drainage on the second day after surgery. The drainage lasted for two weeks until the leakage was brought under control and patients recovered. Two (2.7%) developed a transient neurological decline in patients without residual ossification, manifested as decreased strength of the right C5 innervating muscles. They recovered within three days. Among the patients with PROM, two developed weakness of the right biceps and deltoid muscles, which recovered gradually with proper rehabilitation training and the use of diuretics and steroids.

Strategies to avoid residual ossification

When using the conventional ACCF technique, OPLL is classified into open-based and close-based types according to the ossification morphology on CT scans. An open-based disease does not reach the pedicle on either side. In contrast, the closed-based OPLL joins the pedicle, making it is difficult to expand the bone cut laterally. Therefore, a closed-based OPLL is a contraindication for the ACCF technique.

The ACAF technique dissects and advances the VOC to obtain direct decompression without frequent instrument entries in the spinal canal that may cause spinal cord injury. An anatomical study conducted to evaluate the safety and decompression width between troughs on both sides of the vertebral body showed that when the base of an OPLL is wider than the distance between the bilateral uncinate processes, it may cause difficulties in trough development in the ACAF technique. A review of three patients with residual ossification after ACAF suggested a 50% incidence of residual ossification in wide-based OPLL. This result draws particular attention to applying the ACAF technique in wide-based OPLL.

Preoperative measurement of anatomical parameters

Preoperative planning is crucial in the ACAF technique. As the difficulty of the ACAF technique lies in the isolation of the VOC from the surrounding structures, the longitudinal span of the OPLL is measured beforehand to identify the desired levels of the VOC for antedisplacement. The OPLL is measured at every level for thickness (anteroposterior dimension) and width (coronal dimension) to guide the amount of bone resected from the anterior part of the vertebral bodies, the desired distance of antedisplacement, and the decompression width. The distance between the intended trough position and the intervertebral foramen is measured as well to avoid damage to the vertebral arteries laterally during the bone cut.

In managing wide-based OPLL, attention is paid to its position in the sagittal plane. If the ossification is found paracentral or beyond the typical location of the trough, it is measured at greater detail at the intervertebral, vertebral body, and pedicle levels (Fig. 2.4.32). Since OPLL is usually wider at intervertebral levels than vertebral body levels, it is more likely to extend beyond the desired trough at the intervertebral levels. Such details are documented before surgery to guide the surgeon to bypass the ossification at those levels. If a wide-based OPLL extends to the pedicle, its relation with the pedicle's medial wall is defined to guide the dissection medial to the pedicle's medial wall.

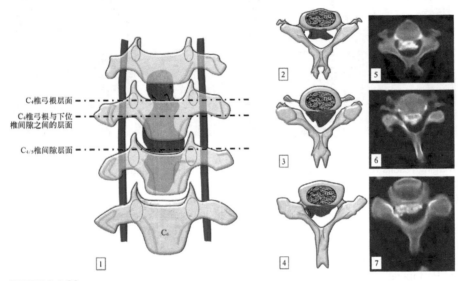

FIGURE 2.4.32

The shape and position of the OPLL at each level are defined.
(1) Illustration of the coronal view of the cervical OPLL dorsal to the posterior wall of the vertebral bodies of C3 to C5;
(2, 5) Illustration of the OPLL at C4 pedicle level;
(3, 6) Illustration of the OPLL at a level between the C4 pedicles and the caudal disc;
(4, 7) Illustration of the OPLL at C4/5 intervertebral level.

Avoid oblique troughs

Bone cut on the vertebral body toward the correct direction is the key to avoiding oblique bone troughs, insufficient antedisplacement, and residual ossification. A common cause of this mistake is when the surgeon uses a head-mount magnifier, which may trick the surgeon away from the vertical axis perpendicular to the floor. The surgeon may end up developing an oblique trough as they tend to tilt the cutter tool to their opposite side when developing the trough on their side. This may leave residual ossification on the same side (Figs. 2.4.33 and 2.4.34). Therefore, care should be taken to ensure that troughs are developed with the cutting tool perpendicular to the floor. Alternatively, the surgical table can be tilted 10−25° toward the surgeon to compensate for their natural line of sight. When a surgical microscope is

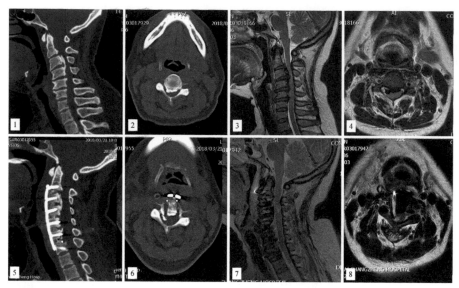

FIGURE 2.4.33

Imaging results revealing residual ossification due to oblique troughs on the vertebral bodies.

(1) Preoperative sagittal CT;

(2) Preoperative transverse CT at C4 where the ossification is wide-based on the right side;

(3) Preoperative sagittal MRI;

(4) Preoperative transverse MRI;

(5) Postoperative sagittal CT;

(6) Postoperative transverse CT at C4 where troughs are deviated toward the left, resulting in residual ossification on the right side;

(7) Postoperative sagittal MRI;

(8) Postoperative transverse MRI at the C4 vertebral body level with signal changes in the spinal cord due to compression of the residual ossification.

used, its field of view is maintained perpendicular to the surgical field to help avoid developing oblique troughs (Fig. 2.4.35).

Limit trough depth after discectomy, the nerve hook is used to palpate the plane between the posterior wall of the vertebral body and the PLL via the disc space to define the pedicle's location and the edge of the ossification to locate the trough. During the bone cut on the vertebral body, its posterior wall is frequently palpated with a nerve hook via the disc space to keep track of the trough's direction and depth and prevent the cutting tool from proceeding beyond the posterior cortex into the ossification. When the trough is palpated to be close to the posterior cortex, a rongeur of 1 mm or 2 mm is used to complete the resection. Engaging the posterior cortex from the disc space, the rongeur removes the posterior cortex in a

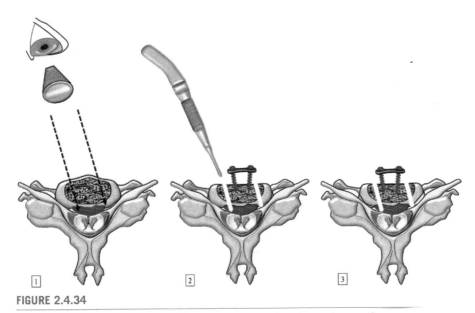

FIGURE 2.4.34

Illustration of oblique troughs as the surgeon uses a head-mount magnifier.

(1) The line of sight when the surgeon with a head-mount magnifier stands on the patient'
right side;

(2) Trough deviated toward the left when the surgeon cuts bone along their natural line of
sight;

(3) In OPLL wide-based on the right side, troughs deviated toward the left result in residual
ossification on the right side.

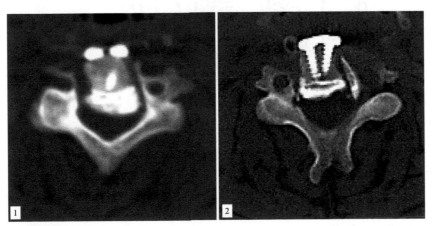

FIGURE 2.4.35

Axial CT views of cases ending up with oblique troughs.

(1) Oblique troughs;

(2) Insufficiently advanced vertebral body due to blockage of the trough's lateral wall.

piecemeal fashion. Then the nerve hook is used to palpate the edges of the trough bottom to determine whether the OPLL is entirely incorporated in the VOC (Fig. 2.4.36). If ossification is identified at or lateral to the trough, it indicates that the trough is not lateral enough. To avoid residual ossification, the surgeon expands the troughs laterally instead of proceeding with the bony resection at the trough's bottom.

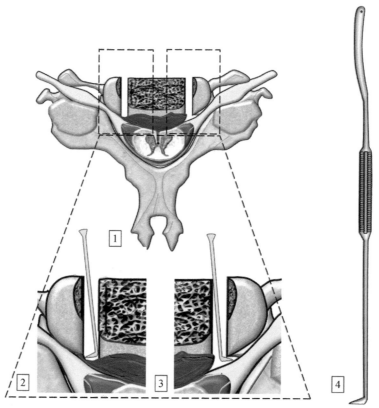

FIGURE 2.4.36

After removing the posterior wall of the vertebral body in the trough, use a nerve hook to palpate the bottom of the trough to check for any residual ossification.

(1) Illustration of the axial view of the cervical spine, marked with the OPLL (red) and the troughs on both sides of the vertebral body (dashed frame);

(2, 3) Larger view of each frame;

(2) Palpating the bottom of the right trough, the nerve hook finds residual ossification at the bottom of the trough and on its lateral edge. The trough is expanded laterally instead of removing the ossification;

(3) Palpating the bottom of the left trough, the nerve hook finds no ossification at the bottom of the trough and on its lateral edge, indicating that the ossification has been included in the VOC.

Intraoperative CT

Providing surgeons with images, intraoperative CT study is constructive for validating sufficient decompression in the technically demanding cases operated through anterior. In particular, CT taken during VOC advancement reveals oblique troughs or residual ossification so that surgeons can manage them properly. Among the three patients with residual ossification mentioned earlier in this chapter, intraoperative CT was used in none of them. In contrast, neither of the two cases with wide-based OPLL where intraoperative CT had been used developed residual ossification (Fig. 2.4.37).

Although rare in the ACAF technique, residual ossification may lead to a suboptimal recovery of neural function. Residual ossification can be avoided by obtaining accurate anatomical measuring anatomical before surgery, cutting the vertebral body along the anterior base of the uncinate process along the parasagittal direction, and using intraoperative CT.

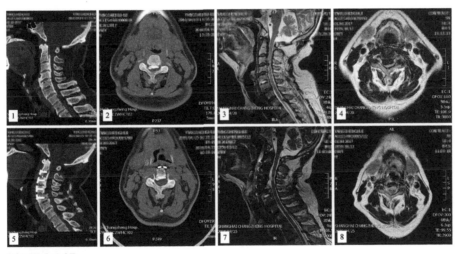

FIGURE 2.4.37

Images of a case of wide-based OPLL free of residual ossification after the operation.
(1) Preoperative sagittal CT;
(2) Preoperative transverse CT at C4 where the ossification is wide-based on the right;
(3) Preoperative sagittal MRI;
(4) Preoperative transverse MRI;
(5) Postoperative sagittal CT;
(6) Postoperative transverse CT showing parasagittal troughs and residual ossification;
(7) Postoperative sagittal MRI showing resumed cerebrospinal fluid zone;
(8) Postoperative transverse MRI at C4 where the spinal cord is fully decompressed.

References

[1] Haisong Y, Jingchuan S, Jiangang S, et al. Anterior controllable antedisplacement fusion (ACAF) for severe cervical ossification of the posterior longitudinal ligament: comparison with anterior cervical corpectomy with fusion (ACCF). World Neurosurgery 2018; 115:e428−36.

[2] Lu J, Ebraheim NA, Georgiadis GM, et al. Anatomic considerations of the vertebral artery. Journal of Spinal Disorders 1988;11(3):233−6.

[3] Jingchuan S, Ximing X, Yuan W, et al. How to avoid postoperative remaining ossification mass in anterior controllable antedisplacement and fusion surgery. World Neurosurgery X 2019;3:100034.

Section 5: Hoisting technique

The ACAF technique features the isolation, antedisplacement, and fusion of the vertebral bodies or VOC from the cervical spine through an anterior approach. Isolation and antedisplacement are key steps in this process. Nerve decompression hinges upon antedisplacement, and adequate isolation is the prerequisite for antedisplacement isolation (Fig. 2.5.1).

The core of the hoisting technique is to facilitate the stable and controllable antedisplacement of VOC with stabilization devices. The plate and screws provide stability and driving force for the VOC antedisplacement and stabilize the cervical spine after the hoisting process. As the plate and screw placement has been introduced in a previous session, this section will discuss the specific techniques of the screws for antedisplacement.

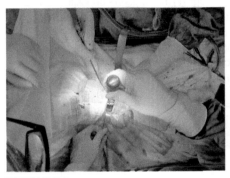 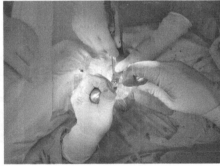

FIGURE 2.5.1

The antedisplacement process. Multiple screwdrivers are used to tighten the screws simultaneously to hoist the VOC to the ventral side.

Sequence of screw tightening for hoisting
Hoisting with bilateral screws

After the contralateral osteotomy was performed, the surgeon places a plate of appropriate length and contour between the troughs and fixes it with two screws on the cephalad and caudal vertebrae, respectively. Before inserting screws in vertebral bodies between the cephalad and caudal levels, a depth gauge is used to determine if the gap between the plate and the vertebrae is sufficient for the desired antedisplacement (Fig. 2.5.2).

After that, two screws are inserted into each vertebral body to be hoisted flush with the plate (Fig. 2.5.3).

The screws aim to stabilize the VOC, and the surgeon should not attempt to hoist the VOC forward by tightening screws before the VOC is completely isolated.

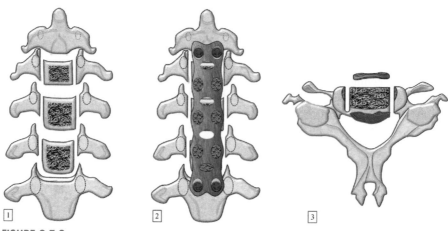

FIGURE 2.5.2

Preparation for the hoisting with bilateral screws, and placement of plate and screws.
(1) Front view of the cervical spine with a complete trough on the surgeon's opposite side and an incomplete trough on the surgeon's side with the bone at the bottom yet to be removed;
(2) Plate properly placed and screws inserted on both sides;
(3) Cross-section view of the vertebrae to be hoisted, with the bone at the bottom of the trough of the surgeon's side not removed yet. Screws are inserted but not entirely in place, and advancement should not be attempted for the moment.

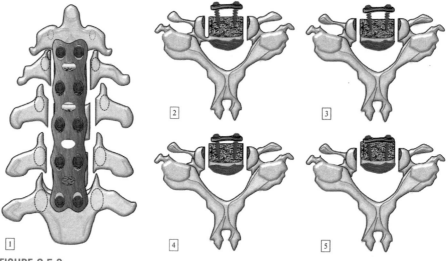

FIGURE 2.5.3

Illustration of ideal simultaneous hoisting via bilateral screws.
(1) Front view;
(2) Plate and screw placed, with the bottom of the surgeon's side trough still connected;
(3) VOC adequately isolated as the bone at the bottom of the surgeon's side trough removed;
(4) Screws in the segments to be hoisted sequentially tightened;
(5) VOC advancement completes as it contacts the plate.

After placement of the plate and screws, an ipsilateral osteotomy was performed for complete isolation of the VOC trough isolate.

The screws are tightened simultaneously with a screwdriver on each one of them. Screws on each side are tightened simultaneously or sequentially to provide robust advancement.

The downside of this method is demonstrated in cases with narrower VOC. When the two screws on the vertebrae are too convergent, they may interfere with each other and terminate the antedisplacement process prematurely (Fig. 2.5.4).

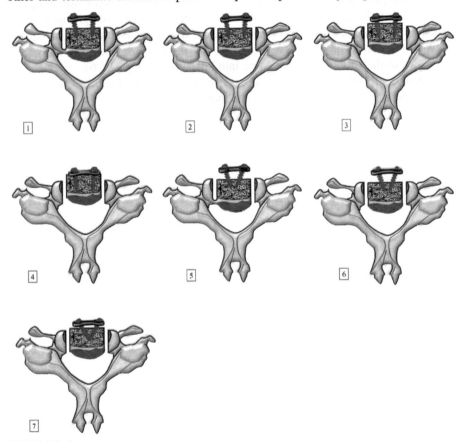

FIGURE 2.5.4

Comparison of optimal and suboptimal situations of hoisting achieved with bilateral screws.
(1) Plate and screws place, and the bottom of the surgeon's side trough still connected;
(2) VOC isolated as the surgeon's side trough completed;
(3) Screws are tightened sequentially to hoist the complex;
(4) VOC contacts the plate, achieving full antedisplacement;
(5) Plate and screws placed, with converging screws and the bottom of the surgeon's side trough still connected;
(6) VOC isolated as the surgeon's side trough completed;
(7) As the screws tightened, the converging screws engage with each other and allow no more advancement. As the VOC cannot contact with the plate, this results in incomplete antedisplacement.

Hoisting with unilateral screws

To avoid incomplete antedisplacement encountered in the bilateral screw plan described above, hoisting the VOC with unilateral screws serves as another option in cases with a narrow OPLL (Fig. 2.5.5).

The plate and screws on the caudal and cephalad vertebrae are in place. Each vertebral body to be hoisted is inserted with one screw on the right or left side, depending on the size of the gap beneath the screw holes on the plate.

After the plate and screws are placed, the bottom of the surgeon's side trough is disconnected to isolate the VOC. Screws on the vertebral bodies are tightened simultaneously with a screwdriver on each of them. After the VOC antedisplacement, screws on the other side of the vertebrae are put in place. As such, the screws on both sides of the vertebrae do not come into interference (Fig. 2.5.6).

The risks of VOC rotation and tilting carried by this method will be discussed in greater detail in the "Hoisting Instrument" part in this section.

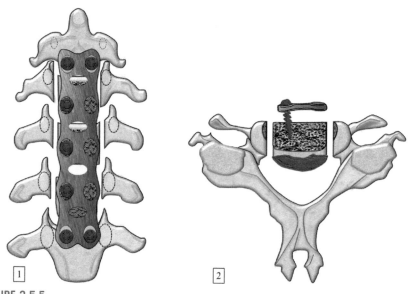

FIGURE 2.5.5

Screws that stabilize the VOC on one side of the segments to be hoisted. The bottom of the surgeon's side trough still connected, screws installed but not entirely in place, and antedisplacement should not be attempted at this moment.
(1) Front view;
(2) Cross-section view.

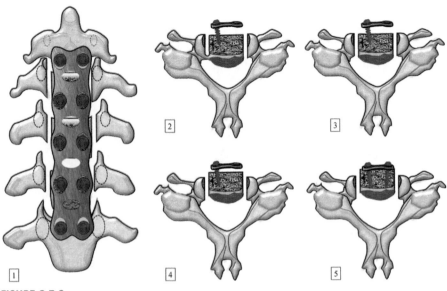

FIGURE 2.5.6

Illustration for hoisting with screws on one side of the segments to be hoisted.

(1) Front view;

(2) After the plate and screw installation, the bone at the bottom of trough ipsilateral to the surgeon is not disconnected;

(3) VOC adequately isolated as the bone at the bottom of the surgeon's side trough removed;

(4) Screws in the segments to be hoisted sequentially tightened;

(5) VOC advancement completes as it contacts the plate. Screws of the other side are then inserted to avoid screw interference during VOC advancement.

Screw technique on the caudal and cephalad vertebrae—sequence

During the ACAF technique, the first screws are placed in the cephalad and caudal vertebral bodies of the desired levels to stabilize the plate. However, if the screws are tightened in the first place, there is little room for adjusting the cervical curvature and disc heights, which will have a potential impact on the hoisting maneuver (Fig. 2.5.7) (see "Strategies to Avoid Incomplete Antedisplacement" below).

Therefore, the following sequence of screw placement is recommended: two screws are placed on the caudal vertebrae to stabilize the plate, followed by screw placement on the segments to be hoisted (Figs. 2.5.8 and 2.5.9).

After being isolated, the VOC is displaced ventrally as the screws on each segment are tightened. Since the plate is not anchored to the cephalad vertebrae yet, the cervical curvature and intervertebral height can be adjusted while VOC antedisplacement.

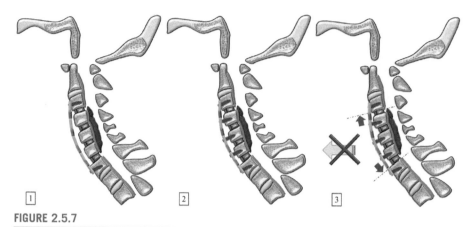

FIGURE 2.5.7

Suboptimal VOC advancement with the plate fixed to the cephalad and caudal vertebrae in the first place.

(1) Plate fixed to C3 and C7, or the cephalad and caudal vertebrae in the first place;

(2) Plate connected to the segments to be hoisted by screws;

(3) VOC advancement maneuver ending up with incomplete antedisplacement. With the plate fixed to the cephalad and caudal vertebrae, the length of the construct is set. Worsen by the interference between the endplates and cages, the VOC ends up unable to contact with the plate.

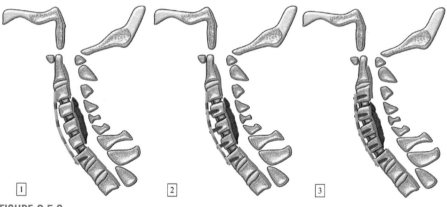

FIGURE 2.5.8

Illustration of the procedure where the plate is fixed to the cephalad vertebrae after twisting screws at the head end after hoisting.

(1) Intervertebral cages are in place, and the plate stabilized to C7, or the caudal vertebrae, with screws;

(2) Screws placed on the segments to be hoisted;

(3) Cervical curvature corrected and VOC contacts with the plate as screws are tightened, followed by screws inserted on the cephalad vertebrae.

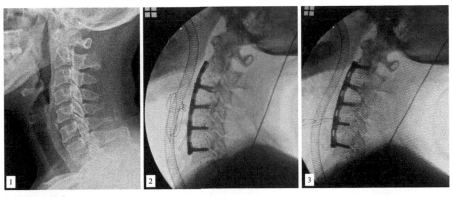

FIGURE 2.5.9

A case of where the plate is fixed to the cephalad vertebrae after VOC hoisting.
(1) The preoperative lateral X-ray film showing narrow C2/3 disc space that may interfere with the antedisplacement of the C3 vertebral body;
(2) Intraoperative fluoroscopy demonstrating plate and screws placed on C6 vertebrae, or the caudal level, but not C2. This allows freedom of adjustment to the intervertebral height and cervical curvature from C2 – C6 segments;
(3) Screws placed on C2, or the cephalad vertebrae, after VOC advancement.

After the antedisplacement is finished, the two screws are placed on the cephalad vertebrae.

Screw technique on the caudal and cephalad vertebrae—compression and stretching

Similar to the compression plate used in managing extremity fractures, the anterior cervical plate can stretch or compress the cephalad and caudal vertebrae. To reduce resistance to the hoisting procedure, smaller intervertebral cages are usually applied in ACAF technique. However, mobile cages can be found in some cases after VOC advancement.

This usually occurs in the disc space of the cephalad or caudal vertebrae and can be managed by compression of the screws in the cephalad and caudal vertebrae (Fig. 2.5.10).

Before placing the cephalad and caudal screws, the vertebral cortex is punched through the screw holes of the plate by using the drill.

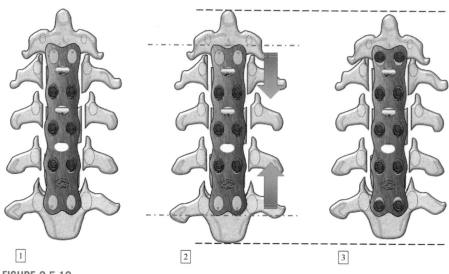

FIGURE 2.5.10

Screws in the cephalad and caudal vertebrae inserted per the principle of compression to narrow down disc spaces.

(1) Before placing the cephalad and caudal screws, the vertebral cortex is punched through the screw holes of the plate;

(2) The cervical spine compressed (blue dotted lines and arrows) between the cephalad and caudal vertebrae guided by the screw and plate construct as the screws purchasing the vertebral bone;

(3) Reduced disc heights (shown with black dotted lines above C2 and below C6).

The cervical spine is compressed between the cephalad and caudal vertebrae guided by the screw and plate construct as the screws purchase the vertebral bone, which results in reduced disc heights in the construct.

Conversely, if excessive resistance is encountered during VOC advancement, the cephalad and caudal disc spaces can be distracted with screws to diminish the friction between the cages and the endplates (Fig. 2.5.11).

Before placing the cephalad and caudal screws, the vertebral cortex is punched through the screw holes of the plate.

The disc spaces are distracted, guided by the screw and plate construct as the screws are tightened into the cephalad and caudal vertebrae.

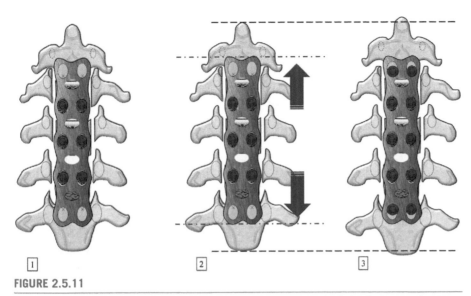

FIGURE 2.5.11

Screws in the cephalad and caudal vertebrae inserted per the principle of compression to distract disc spaces.
(1) Before placing the cephalad and caudal screws, the vertebral cortex is punched through the screw holes of the plate;
(2) The cervical spine is distracted between the cephalad and caudal vertebrae (red dashed lines and arrows) guided by the screw and plate construct as the screws are tightened the vertebral bone, which results in increased disc heights in the construct;
(3) Increased disc heights (shown with black dotted lines above C2 and below C6).

Strategies to avoid incomplete antedisplacement

The vertebral body advancement by the plate and the screws construct avoids the adverse motion seen in free-hand advancement and facilitates a controllable advancement process and neural safety. However, this method is not immune to risks (Figs. 2.5.12 and 2.5.13). In the authors' team's practice, some cases encountered suboptimal antedisplacement during the ACAF procedure and ended up with incomplete antedisplacement. This is represented by the vertebral bodies' inability to contact the plate during the operation, and a gap between them is observed on postoperative CT and lateral X-ray films. The authors have analyzed these cases to determine the causes and impact of incomplete antedisplacement [1].

Definition of incomplete antedisplacement

An incompletely advanced vertebral body is defined as a gap of 1 mm or broader between the vertebral body and the plate after VOC advancement observed on postoperative CT images. And incomplete antedisplacement is defined as the presence of more than one incompletely advanced vertebral bodies.

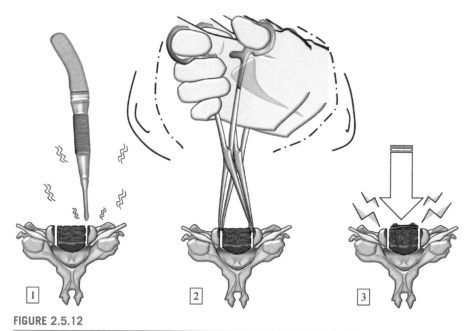

FIGURE 2.5.12

Illustration of free-hand antedisplacement.
(1) VOC vibration or translation during isolation with a burr or rongeur, worsening the spinal cord injury;
(2) The spinal cord subjected to jerks as the surgeon tries to hold and VOC with an Allis forceps for antedisplacement;
(3) The spinal cord subjected to further injury as the surgeon tries to place the plate and screws on the isolated and advanced VOC.

The vertebrae-plate gap is the distance between the ossifications and the plate at the narrowest level observed on postoperative CT or lateral X-ray film (Fig. 2.5.14).

1 mm in the definition is set only for the purpose of description and analysis, and it does not mean that a vertebrae-plate gap of 0.9 mm is categorized as a complete antedisplacement.

Clinical data of incompletely advanced vertebral bodies

A clinical review showed that 21.7% of patients after ACAF had incompletely advanced vertebral bodies with imaging evidence, and such vertebral bodies accounted for 12.1% of the antedisplacement complex on average.

In terms of the vertebrae involved in incomplete antedisplacement, C3 accounted for 50% while C5 to C7, only 16.7%. The cephalad vertebrae were more prone to incomplete antedisplacement than the caudal ones.

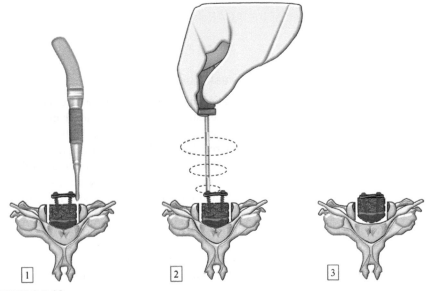

FIGURE 2.5.13

Illustration of the antedisplacement process in the ACAF technique with plate and screw system.

(1) The spinal cord free of secondary injury with the instrumented VOC. Stabilized with the plate and screws, the VOC stays still against the vibration from the burr or rongeur during VOC isolation;

(2) The spinal cord protected from the unintended motion of the VOC. As the surgeon tightens the screws, the isolated VOC is advanced in a manner much more controllable than in the free-hand procedure;

(3) Antedisplacement completed.

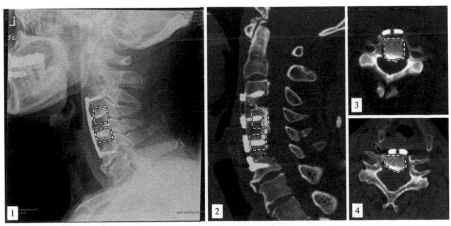

FIGURE 2.5.14

Postoperative imaging of a patient with incomplete antedisplacement.

(1) Postoperative lateral X-ray;

(2) Postoperative sagittal CT;

(3) Postoperative axial CT image at C4;

(4) Postoperative axial CT image at C5. C4 and C5 (outlined with dashes) have been displaced forward. C5 contacts with the plate, but a gap is present between C4 and the plate.

The roles of hoisting force and resistance in antedisplacement

Essentially, the process of vertebral antedisplacement is the one where the VOC is drawn closer and closer to the plate until resistance becomes greater than the hoisting force. Therefore, to account for incomplete antedisplacement, both the hoisting force and the resistance should be considered. In the ACAF technique, the force that hoists the vertebral body comes from the screw purchase in the vertebrae, while the resistance roots in the friction between the endplate and intervertebral cage and the impingement between the vertebral body and the surrounding bone (Fig. 2.5.15).

Friction between intervertebral cages and endplates

In the ACAF technique, in the disc space between an advancing vertebral body and the nonadvancing one above or below it, as an endplate advances in relation to the opposing one that stays still, friction is generated between the advancing endplate and the intervertebral cage. In the case of antedisplacement of multiple vertebral bodies, when the vertebral bodies are advanced in a synchronized manner, relative displacement is present only in the caudal and cephalad disc space but not those within the VOC (Fig. 2.5.16). Therefore, all the VOC vertebral bodies are advanced simultaneously with screw tightening to avoid epactal friction.

The friction is mainly affected by the pressure between the endplate and intervertebral cage.

Therefore, we use an intervertebral cage with the same height as the height of each disc space to avoid excessive pressure and friction during the hoisting procedure.

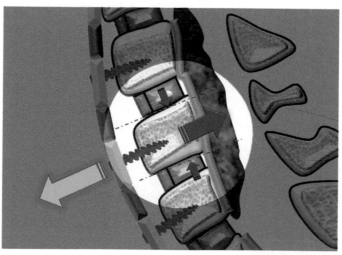

FIGURE 2.5.15

Hoisting force and resistance during vertebral body antedisplacement.
The hoisting force (blue arrow) and the resistance (red arrow). When the resistance is equal to the hoisting force, the vertebral body stops advancing forward.

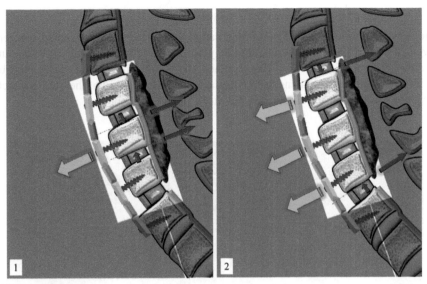

FIGURE 2.5.16

Comparison of the friction generated between the separated and simultaneous antedisplacement in the multisegment ACAF procedure.

(1, 2) The hoisting force (blue arrows) and the resistance (red arrows).

(1) When advanced individually, the C5 vertebral body is subjected to friction in the C4/5 and C5/6 disc spaces where relative displacement occurs;

(2) When advanced simultaneously, the C4—C5—C6 complex is subjected to friction only in the C3/4 and C6/7 disc spaces.

When cases were compared by the categories of incompletely advanced and completely advanced vertebral bodies, the former group had a disc height of 3.7 ± 0.4 mm on average, significantly narrower than the latter group, with 5.5 ± 0.6 mm in disc height. Narrower disc space is prone to increased friction after cage placement. Given the minimum height of 4 mm currently available among cages, a disc space narrower than 4 mm will inevitably sustain greater friction against antedisplacement. Preoperative measurement of the disc height helps predict the difficulty of antedisplacement. For a disc space less than 4 mm high, the upper and lower endplates are carefully prepared and distracted properly to ensure appropriate disc height and stress between the cage and the endplate.

A disc space narrower than 4 mm means that even the smallest cage currently available (4 mm) will generate stress and friction in relation to the endplates.

If a disc space is measured narrower than 4 mm before the operation, its upper and lower endplates are specifically prepared during the operation.

The mechanism explained above accounts for why the cephalad and caudal segments are more vulnerable to incomplete antedisplacement.

Analysis of blockage of antedisplacement

The postoperative CT studies of the cases with incomplete antedisplacement revealed contact between the incompletely advanced vertebral bodies and the surrounding bones (Fig. 2.5.17). Bony contacts that should have been clear could be an important cause of challenged antedisplacement. The pattern of the bony contacts represents a relevant pitfall during operation.

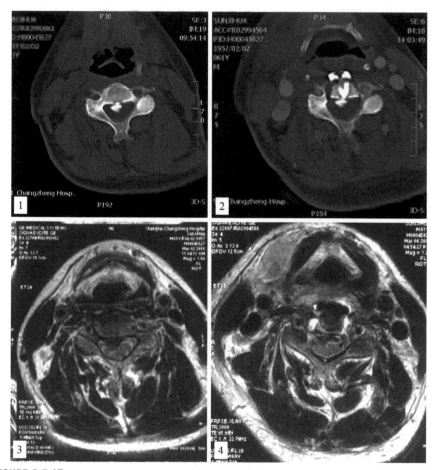

FIGURE 2.5.17

Imaging data of a case with incomplete vertebral antedisplacement caused by oblique troughs.

(1) Preoperative CT with circumscribed OPLL behind C4;

(2) Postoperative CT showing contact of VOC with the lateral wall of the left trough at C4, resulting in a gap greater than 1 mm between the VOC and the plate;

(3) Preoperative MRI with signal changes in the spinal cord due to the ventral osseous indentation at C4;

(4) Postoperative MRI where the intramedullary signal changes at C4 improved as the spinal cord has been free of the ventral compression.

For the incompletely advanced vertebral bodies, the most common pitfall is bone trough obliquity (Fig. 2.5.18).

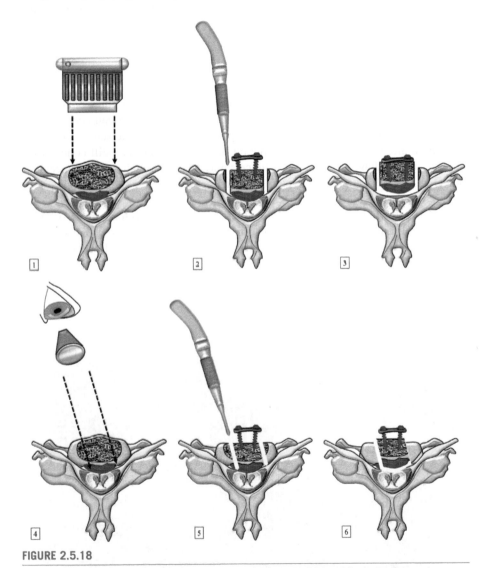

FIGURE 2.5.18

Illustration of incomplete vertebral antedisplacement caused by oblique bone troughs.
(1) Field of view of the surgical microscope perpendicular to the cervical spine and the desired location of troughs (dashed arrow);
(2) Trough developed vertically with a high-speed burr;
(3) Vertebral body adequately advanced;
(4) Line of view where the surgeon uses a head-mounted magnifier;
(5) Trough developed with the high-speed burr tilted to one side;
(6) Incompletely advanced vertebral body as it is obstructed by the lateral wall of the left trough.

In the ACAF technique, a correctly located trough that has deviated causes problems not during the initial phase of advancement but later. Toward the end of the advancement, the VOC yields to the surrounding bone blockage, resulting in incomplete antedisplacement.

Bony connection between the vertebral bodies and surrounding bone

The vertebral body should be thoroughly dissected from the surrounding bone before it can be moved forward. Misjudgment of a thorough dissection can occur due to poor visualization of the trough bottom deep in the wound. If the screws are tightened in an attempt to advance the vertebral body when there are still connections with the surrounding bone, the screw tunnels may be cut through, and advancement fails (Fig. 2.5.19). Due to poor results of decompression, revision is often required, although such a scenario rarely occurs.

The trough width should be maintained at 2.5 ~ 3 mm. If it is too narrow, one will have difficulty assessing whether its bottom has been completely disconnected.

A slight pop sound may be heard when the trough is dissected at the bottom, which suggests the completion of the trough.

Before moving the VOC forward, it is confirmed to be thoroughly isolated from the surrounding structure with a nerve hook.

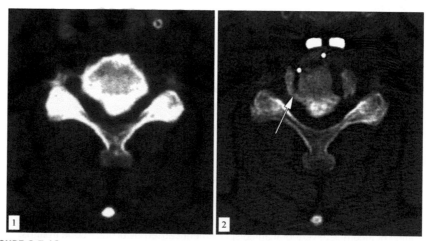

FIGURE 2.5.19

Incomplete advancement due to bony connection between the vertebral body and the surrounding bone.
(1) Preoperative CT;
(2) Postoperative CT showing the insufficiently advanced VOC due to the bony connection at the bottom of the right trough (arrow).

During advancement, the screws are tightened slowly with vigilant monitoring. Once resistance is felt, the screw tightening should be stopped in case of the screw cutting through the tunnel and fail the advancement.

Ring epiphysis along the anterior or posterior vertebral borders

As typical anatomical structures, ring epiphysis is present on the anteroinferior and the posterosuperior edges of the vertebral bodies. It is more protuberant on the upper cervical vertebrae then the lower ones, with the most typical one on the anteroinferior border of C2. In the conventional ACDF procedure, endplates of the disc space of interest are prepared by removing the anterior and posterior overhanging lip. Similarly, endplates are prepared to be parallel and anterior and posterior overhanging lip removed in the ACAF procedure to prevent collision with the advancing cage, blockage of advancement, or excessive friction (Fig. 2.5.20).

Case reviews showed that more than 70% of the incompletely advanced VOCs were associated with overhanging lip.

The C2/3 disc space is carefully prepared as the anteroinferior overhanging lip of C2 is more protuberant.

O-arm X-ray is used intraoperatively for the 3D CT reconstruction to assess whether anterior or posterior bony protuberance is sufficiently removed lest hampering advancement.

Impact of osteoporosis on antedisplacement

As the anterior cortex and a part of the cancellous bone of the vertebral body are removed in the ACAF technique, the screws inserted are purchasing the cancellous bone. Without the anterior cortex, the screw purchase in the vertebral body is significantly diminished, which can be worsened in the case of osteoporosis.

By comparing patients with and without incomplete antedisplacement, the author team found that there had been more osteoporotic patients in the group with insufficient advancement than the other one (Fig. 2.5.21), indicating that osteoporosis is a significant risk factor for incomplete antedisplacement.

Impact of incomplete antedisplacement on the neurological recovery

To investigate the relationship between the outcome of VOC antedisplacement and the neurological recovery, the authors analyzed two groups of patients.

Patients with incomplete antedisplacement were observed with an average improvement of $68.3\% \pm 11.8\%$ in JOA, not significantly different from that documented in the group with adequate antedisplacement, which was $70.7\% \pm 8.2\%$.

The former group was further analyzed and stratified by if the gap between the vertebral body and plate was within or above 6 mm (Figs. 2.5.22 and 2.5.23).

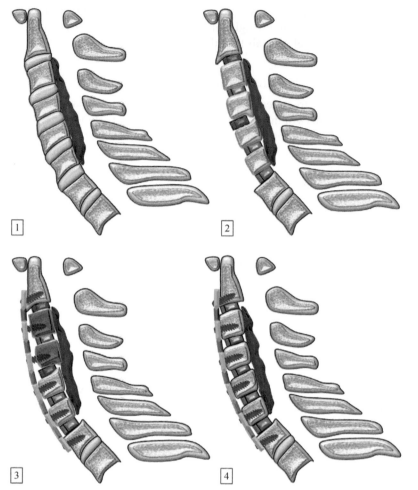

FIGURE 2.5.20

Illustration of incomplete vertebral antedisplacement due to the unthinned ring epiphysis.

(1) Illustration of the sagittal view of the cervical spine with OPLL;

(2) Discectomy and intervertebral cage placement have been performed through anterior, with residual ring epiphysis on the C2 anteroinferior border and C4 posteroinferior border;

(3) Plate and screws placed, C5 and C6 adequately advanced, and C3 and C4 insufficiently advanced due to the residual ring epiphysis on C2 and C4;

(4) The optimal construct where all levels of the VOC are adequately advanced.

The neurological recovery rate was documented as 36.2% in those with a gap at or above 6 mm, and 69.4% in those with a gap up to 6 mm.

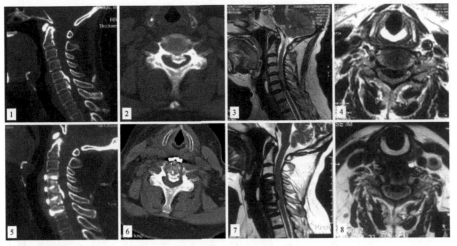

FIGURE 2.5.21

Imaging data of a case with osteoporosis-associated incomplete VOC antedisplacement.

(1) Preoperative CT showing osteoporosis, and OPLL of C5 and C6;

(3, 4) Preoperative MRI showing spinal cord compression due to anterior osseous indentation at C5 and C6;

(5, 6) Postoperative CT showing a gap greater than 1 mm between the VOC and the plate at C5 and C6;

(7, 8) Postoperative MRI showing spinal cord compression at C5 and C6 relieved with CSF effacement.

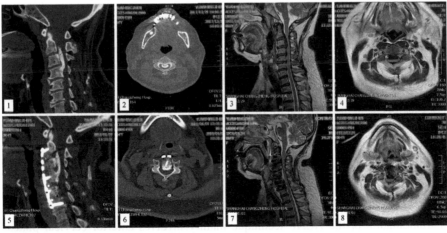

FIGURE 2.5.22

Imaging data of a case with a vertebrae-plate gap above 6 mm.

(1, 2) Preoperative CT showing OPLL from C2 to C4;

(3, 4) Preoperative MRI showing spinal cord compression due to an OPLL of C2/3 to C4 and intervertebral disc protrusion at C5/6;

(5, 6) Postoperative CT showing VOC of C3 to C5 antedisplaced, a vertebrae-plate gap greater than 6 mm at C3;

(7, 8) Postoperative MRI showed that there was still posterior ossification and compression of the spinal cord behind C3.

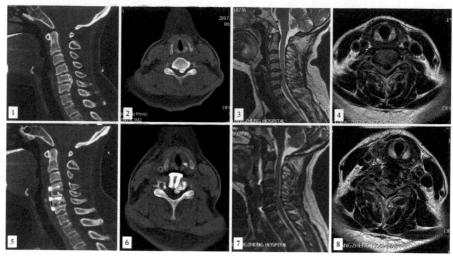

FIGURE 2.5.23

Imaging data of a case with a vertebrae-plate gap below 6 mm.
(1, 2) Preoperative CT showing OPLL at C5 and C5/6;
(3, 4) Preoperative MRI showing spinal cord compression due to anterior indentation from C4/5 to C5/6;
(5, 6) Postoperative CT showing a vertebrae-plate gap <6 mm;
(7, 8) Postoperative MRI showing spinal cord compression at C5 relieved.

Patients with a wider vertebrae-plate gap performed poorer after surgery. With a smaller gap, though still on the side of incomplete advancement, patients seemed to experience unaffected recovery, and they made up the majority of the inadequate cohort. From their practice, the authors attributed most of the blockage to the later phase of advancement when the vertebral body almost contacts the plate. Rarely did blockage occur in the early phase of advancement. Patients ending up with incomplete advancement had an average vertebrae-plate gap of 2.5 ± 0.4 mm, suggesting unlikely cord compression with a 2 mm residual indentation.

Selection of screws and plates

Instrumentation of the ACAF technique mainly involves anterior cervical plates, vertebral body screws, and intervertebral cages. The instrumentation serves three purposes: ① temporary stabilization when VOC is being isolated; ② provision of steady and controllable hoisting force during the antedisplacement of the isolated VOC; and ③ fixation and fusion after completing antedisplacement. These functions are the criteria for the selection of instrumentation construct.

Plate

Function: Intraoperative stabilization for VOC advancement and postoperative fixation.

Design: Most plates come as a thin piece with two screw holes at each vertebral segment. Plates with graft windows of adequate sizes at the disc levels that facilitate bone grafting are preferred.

Preference: Plates with one screw hole at each vertebral level serves the ACAF technique as long as the VOC is thoroughly isolated. Therefore, anterior cervical plates of various designs can be applied in the ACAF technique. However, their design feature may be associated with the technical challenges of operation. With fewer screw holes comes fewer options for the surgeon, and the situation may become unsalvageable if something wrong happens to the several only screw holes. The pattern of the graft window can also affect the operation. The authors use a specific hoisting instrument (see Section 5) that they designed, which enters the vertebral body's center through the graft windows. Therefore, such technique and instrument are better used with plates with more fenestrations. The authors usually use the Skyline plate by Depuy that comes with large windows to visualize vertebral bodies better. The XX by Sofamor provides another good option with four screw holes at the middle segment for entry of the hoisting instrument, instrumentation, or salvage maneuvers (Fig. 2.5.24).

Thickness: The typical 2−2.5 mm plate works well. Though less likely to cause foreign body sensation while swallowing, a thinner plate comes with lower strength, increased pliability, and poor maintenance after being purposefully contoured.

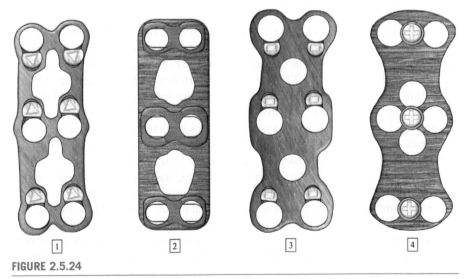

FIGURE 2.5.24

Schematic diagram of 4 common titanium plates.
1. The thickness of this type is relatively thin;
2. This nail hole of this type is attached with a spring device;
3. The area of the bone-graft window is small;
4. Four nail holes are provided in the middle of this type of titanium plate.

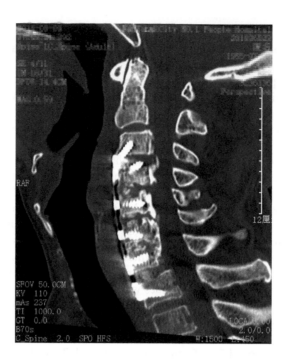

FIGURE 2.5.25

A case of insufficient decompression due to inadequate plate length.

These features are particularly salient in the long thin plates. Therefore, in the long-segment ACAF procedures, the authors prefer plates with higher mechanical strength.

Width: In the ACAF technique, the troughs on both sides of the vertebral body are developed with the plate placed in the bone, and a plate that is too wide will block the bone cut maneuvers. As the average distance between troughs on both sides in the ACAF technique is 16.8—17.9 mm, plates of 16 mm wide are recommended.

Length: The plate's length is tied to the number of surgical segments and the patient's height. Various plate systems offer a range of lengths to address variation among individuals, but not every system provides long anterior cervical plates for multilevel procedure. Hardware-associated morbidities have been significantly correlated to the number of surgical segments in a myriad of basic and clinical studies, which discourages the anterior multisegmental cervical surgeries (more than three vertebral bodies) (Fig. 2.5.25). Consequently, many companies do not always offer some or all of the long anterior cervical plates. The ACAF technique has no problem in achieving a high fusion rate in patients receiving multisegmental advancement of three or more vertebral bodies, according to the authors' investigations, but it is necessary to inquire about the company's size offerings when planning for such a procedure.

Vertebral body screws

Purpose: To provide a reliable force to hoist the vertebral bodies and postoperative fixation.

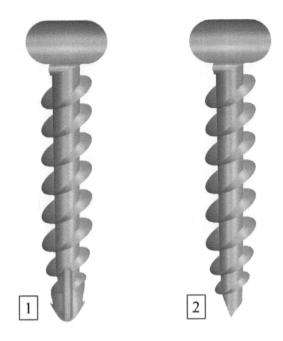

FIGURE 2.5.26

Two types of screws different in the screw tip.
(1) Self-tapping screw with a sharp cutting flute;
(2) Self-drilling screw with a sharp tip.

Types of screws: Screws are generally categorized as self-tapping and self-drilling screws (Fig. 2.5.26). A self-drilling screw comes with a sharper tip than a self-tapping one, making it easier to drill its tunnel and robustly purchases the bone. In contrast, a self-tapping screw comes with a blunt tip, making it difficult to engage the dense OPLL if not pushing it away from the vertebral body (Figs. 2.5.28 and 2.5.29). Therefore, self-drilling screws are usually preferred (Fig. 2.5.27).

Diameter: Screws of two diameters, namely 4.0 and 4.5 mm, are often used in the ACAF technique. The 4.0 mm screw is usually applied first. After advancement is completed, if the screw is determined under fluoroscopy to be so long that it has entered the spinal canal, it is substituted with a shorter screw of 4.5 mm in diameter. Another screw option is those with a blunt and fluteless tip of a larger diameter, usually used for salvage purposes (Fig. 2.5.30).

This patient did not receive the ACAF from the authors' hospital. As the 10-hole plate was the maximum size available from the vendor, the surgeons antedisplaced C5 to C7, the most severe levels, and discectomy of C3/4 disc space where the disease was less severe. Postoperative CT shows that expanded spinal canal at C5 to C7 treated by ACAF technique and residual ossified compressor at C3/4 segment treated by ACDF technique.

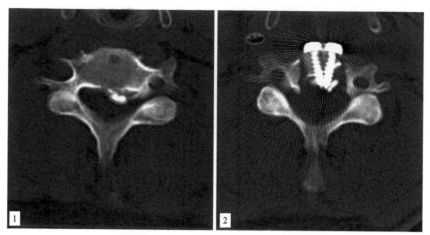

FIGURE 2.5.27

Self-drilling screws engaging the OPLL with its sharp tip.
(1) Preoperative axial CT showing an OPLL;
(2) After ACAF, the screws have engaged in the ossified mass with their tips.

Type of screw head: Restrictive type (fixed-angle) and nonrestrictive type (variable-angle). Both fixed-angle and variable-angle screws work well with plates. Generally, variable-angle screws are used on the upper and lower instrumented vertebrae and fixed-angle ones on the segments in between to ensure consistent hoisting direction (Fig. 2.5.31).

Length: Screw length generally ranges from 12 to 18 mm. Before surgery, the surgical team ensures screws of this range are available, for example, from a vendor. Long screws such as the 16 mm ones are used during advancement. After that, the surgeon confirms if the screws have entered the spinal canal with fluoroscopy. If so, the screws are replaced with those of 12–14 mm long during instrumentation.

Interbody cage

Purpose: To facilitate intervertebral fusion.

Height: The importance of the concordance between the interspace height and the cage height has been discussed above ("Strategies to Avoid Incomplete Antedisplacement").

In the ACAF technique, a cage is of proper size if inserted into the disc space with ease rather than with forceful impaction with a hammer. As the disc space is of fusiform shape sagittally, narrower at the front and back and taller in the middle, an easily inserted cage is clamped tightly by the pincer structure formed by the posterior part of the endplates on both sides between the antedisplaced vertebral bodies. As such, the cage is unlikely to dislodge (Fig. 2.5.32). Even in cases where small

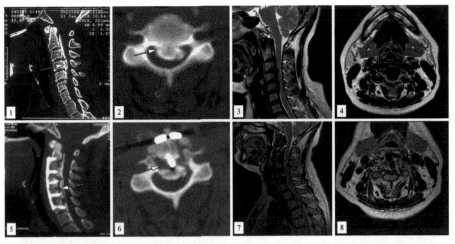

FIGURE 2.5.28

Use of self-tapping screws, not appropriate in this case, resulting in pushing the OPLL away from the vertebral body.

(1) Preoperative sagittal CT showing OPLL at C2 to C5, which is tightly adhered to the C4 vertebral body (arrow);

(2) Preoperative axial CT showing OPLL at C4 tightly adhered to the vertebral body (arrow);

(3) Preoperative sagittal MRI showing spinal cord compression mainly at C3 to C5;

(4) Preoperative axial MRI showing severe spinal cord compression at C4 with intramedullary signal changes;

(5) Postoperative sagittal CT showing antedisplaced C2 to C5 and the ossification away from C4 vertebral body (arrow);

(6) Postoperative axial CT showing antedisplaced C4 vertebral body detached from the ossification (arrow). The screw has gone through the posterior wall of the vertebral body without engaging the OPLL, resulting in insufficient advancement of the ossification;

(7) Postoperative sagittal MRI showing spinal cord decompression partially resolved;

(8) Postoperative axial MRI showing residual spinal cord compression at C4.

cages have been used, no failure of instrumentation has been reported. The most frequently used cages are 5 mm high, followed by the 4 and 6 mm ones.

Length (anteroposterior dimension): The commonly used intervertebral cages are 10–12 mm long. Since an anterior part of the vertebral bodies is resected in the ACAF technique, the endplate's practical sagittal dimension is about 12–16 mm. Therefore, cages of shorter length are recommended.

Width: Cages of width similar to that of the plate are used. Since cages placed before the vertebral bodies are parasagittally cut on both sides, care should be taken to choose cages whose widths fall within the distance between the desired troughs. The most commonly used cages are 12–14 mm wide.

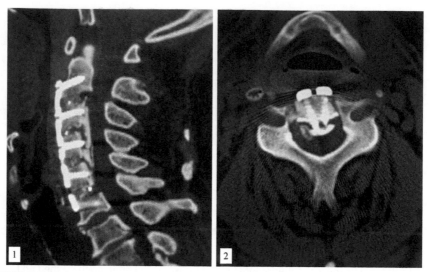

FIGURE 2.5.29

A case where the ossification has been driven off the vertebral body by screws.
(1) Postoperative midsagittal CT showing the OPLL at C4 away from the vertebral body;
(2) Postoperative axial CT at C4 level showing the tip of the screw engaging the ossified mass.

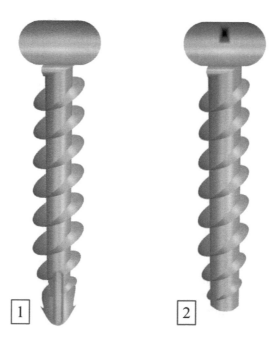

FIGURE 2.5.30

Two types of screws classified by the screw head angulation.
(1) Nonrestrictive or variable-angle screw, which is inserted at an angle chosen within a range and usually applied to the upper and the lower instrumented vertebral bodies;
(2) Restrictive or fixed-angle screw.

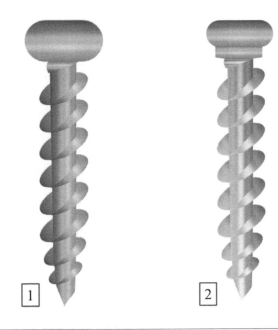

FIGURE 2.5.31

Two types of screws classified by diameter.
(1) A screw with 4.0 mm diameter;
(2) A screw with 4.5 mm diameter, usually used as a salvage screw to substitute a 4.0 mm screw.

Surface texture: The friction between the cage and the endplate constitutes the major friction when the vertebral body is moved forward. According to the law of friction, that under a given load, the lower the surface friction coefficient, the smaller the friction, cages with a low surface friction coefficient, or with smooth surfaces, are recommended.

Material: PEEK or carbon fiber cages are common options, and metal cages, such as titanium alloy, are rarely used. A carbon fiber cage is recommended as it has a similar modulus with that of bone, a protective factor against cage subsidence. On the contrary, the titanium alloy cages are too stiff and prone to artifacts in postoperative CT, affecting postoperative imaging data (Fig. 2.5.33).

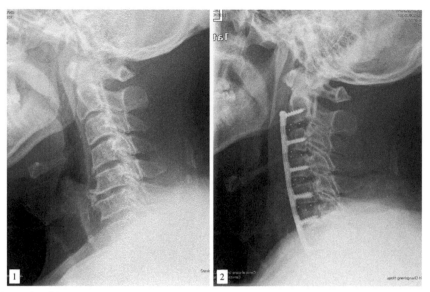

FIGURE 2.5.32

Lateral cervical X-rays before and after the ACAF procedure showing the cages clamped tight by the upper and lower endplates after the vertebral antedisplacement.
(1) Preoperative lateral cervical X-ray showing OPLL at C3 to C6;
(2) Postoperative lateral cervical X-ray showing the antedisplaced C3 to C6 vertebral bodies and cages clamped tight toward the posterior portion of the upper and lower endplates.

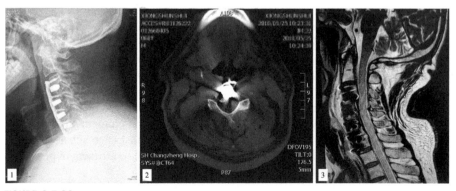

FIGURE 2.5.33

Imaging data of a case with titanium alloy intervertebral cages from an ACAF procedure.
(1) Postoperative lateral cervical X-ray showing dense shadows of titanium alloy intervertebral cages;
(2) Postoperative axial CT showing significant metal artifacts from the titanium alloy cages;
(3) Postoperative sagittal MRI showing uncompromised image quality with the titanium alloy cages.

Hoisting instrument

As described in a previous section, many factors can compromise or fail the vertebral body antedisplacement. To tackle these causes, the authors designed and developed hoisting instruments for definitive, safe, and controllable VOC advancement. The hoisting instrument consists of a rod and a sleeve, and the rod comes with a shaft and a built-in 12 mm vertebral body screw (Fig. 2.5.34).

VOC antedisplacement with the hoisting instrument

The hoisting instrument, rather than a row of screws, can be used to advance the vertebral bodies. The hoisting rod is inserted to the center of the vertebral body, over which the sleeve is dropped down. With a series of rod rotation, the vertebral bodies are drawn ventrally. The antedisplacement is stabilized by placing screws on both sides of the vertebral body (Fig. 2.5.35).

After the discectomy, anterior vertebral bone resection, intervertebral cage placement, vertebral body bone cut, and screw and rod placement at the upper and lower instrumented segments on both sides of the VOC, the hoisting instrument is applied to draw the vertebral bodies ventrally. The use of the hoisting instrument will be described in detail below.

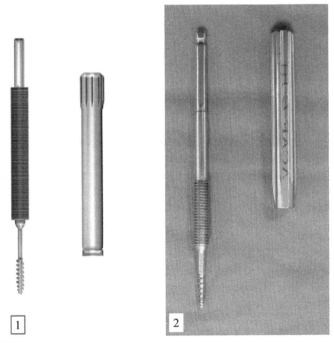

FIGURE 2.5.34

Hoisting instrument.
(1) Illustration of the hoisting instrument made up of a rod and a sleeve;
(2) Picture of hoisting instrument.

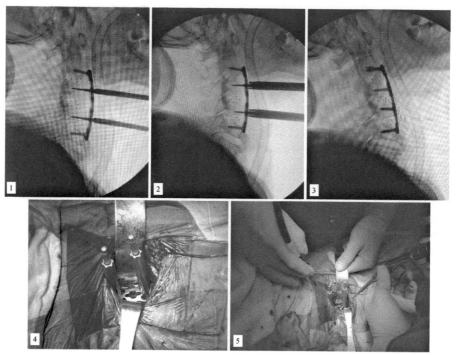

FIGURE 2.5.35

Steps of using the hoisting instrument.
(1) The rods screwed to the vertebral bodies;
(2) The sleeves dropped down over the rods;
(3) Screws placed for instrumentation;
(4, 5) Intraoperative photos of the hoisting instruments.

First, screw the hoisting rod to each vertebral body clockwise through the plate's central grafting windows (Fig. 2.5.36).

Drop the hoisting sleeve over the hoisting rod and turn the sleeve clockwise until it is firmly against the plate. This is repeated on each hoisting rod (Fig. 2.5.37).

As all the sleeves are in place, continue to rotate them clockwise, and the surgeon observes the gaps between the vertebral bodies and the plate are diminishing. The hoisting is completed as the vertebral bodies have been drawn to contact the plate (Fig. 2.5.38).

Remove the hoisting sleeve and insert the screws on each vertebral body. As the construct is stabilized, remove the hoisting rod (Fig. 2.5.39).

Advantages of the hoisting instrument

(1) Enhanced screw holding force in the bone necessary for antedisplacement
The range of screw length options is further narrowed as the screw needs to be long enough to engage the anteriorly thinned vertebral body but not so long as to engage the OPLL or even enter the spinal canal. Given the gap between the

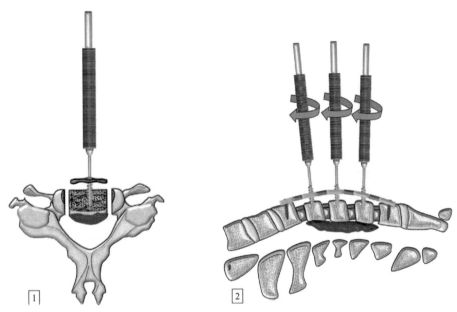

FIGURE 2.5.36

(1) The hoisting rod screwed into the vertebral body;
(2) The hoisting rods placed on each vertebral body.

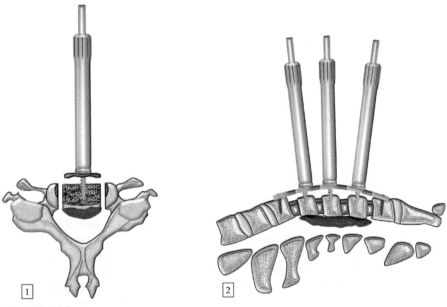

FIGURE 2.5.37

(1) The hoisting sleeve dropped over the hoisting rods;
(2) The hoisting sleeves in place on each vertebral body.

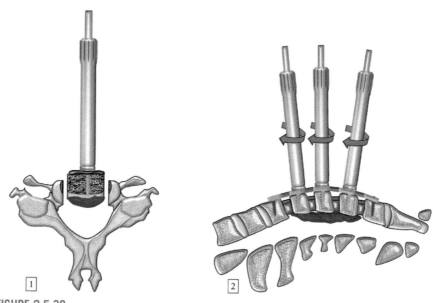

FIGURE 2.5.38

(1) The diminishing gap between the vertebral body and the plate;
(2) Rotating the hoisting sleeves.

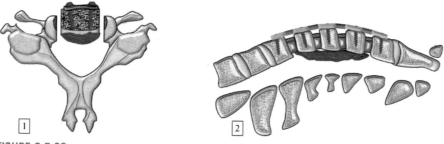

FIGURE 2.5.39

(1) The axial cross-section illustration after vertebral body screw insertion;
(2) The sagittal cross-section illustration after vertebral body screw insertion.

plate and the thinned vertebral body, the screw does not purchase depth in the vertebral body, which is counterproductive since much screw purchase is needed during the initial phase of antedisplacement. Such screws are prone to pull out, in particular in patients with osteoporosis. In contrast, the hoisting instrument holds the vertebral body across its entire 12 mm screw tip and provides a screw holding force robust enough for the initial stage of antedisplacement (Fig. 2.5.40).

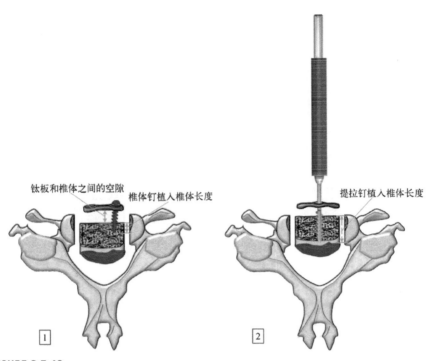

FIGURE 2.5.40

Comparison diagram of the screw purchase profiles between a vertebral screw and the hoisting instrument.
(1) The screw system;
(2) The hoisting instrument system.

Vertebrae-plate gap.
Depth of screw engaged in the vertebral body.
Depth of hoisting screw engaged in the vertebral body.

(2) Avoid problems from antedisplacement with unilateral screws
When unilateral screws are used for hoisting, the other row of screws is inserted for stabilization after antedisplacement. However, the vertebral bodies may tilt (coronal plane, Figs. 2.5.41 and 2.5.43) or rotate (axial plane, Figs. 2.5.42 and 2.5.43) during the advancement step, leading to increased friction between the VOC and the constitutional bony structures during the hoisting process. In contrast, the hoisting instrument readily avoids VOC tilting or rotation as it is placed on the vertebral body's midline.

The hoisting instrument generates a larger amount of screw purchase in the vertebrae than the typical screws during the initial stage of antedisplacement and thus minimizes the risk of screw pull-out. Besides, the rod is placed at the center of the vertebral body, which effectively avoids the downsides of the unilateral screw system.

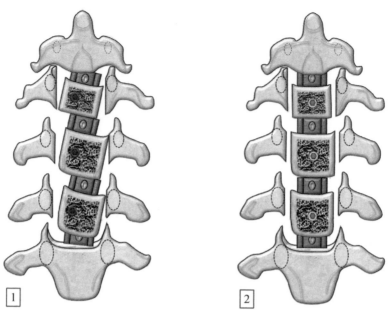

FIGURE 2.5.41

Illustrations comparing vertebral body coronal orientation between the screw system and the hoisting instrument.
(1) Tilted vertebral bodies driven by unilateral vertebral screws;
(2) Vertebral bodies remained centrally oriented after antedisplacement by the hoisting instrument.

Bone grafting

Bone grafting refers to bone tissue placement to the areas with a bone defect or in need of enhancement or fusion in the patient's body. It can be classified as autologous, allogeneic, and artificial bone grafting by the graft materials. In the ACAF technique, two areas need bone grafting: the disc spaces of the surgical segments and the bilateral troughs of the advanced vertebral bodies.

Intervertebral bone grafting

The physiological functions of disc space, where the intervertebral disc locates, include facilitating the motion between the adjacent vertebrae, transmitting load, and limiting excessive translation. Still in its infancy, artificial disc technique bears the unacceptably high incidence of complications such as heterotopic ossification, spontaneous fusion, or recurrent neural impingement. Therefore, interbody fusion remains the standard treatment after discectomy.

Although segmental motion sacrificed, a successful interbody fusion brings the following potential benefits: ① restore intervertebral stability and load distribution

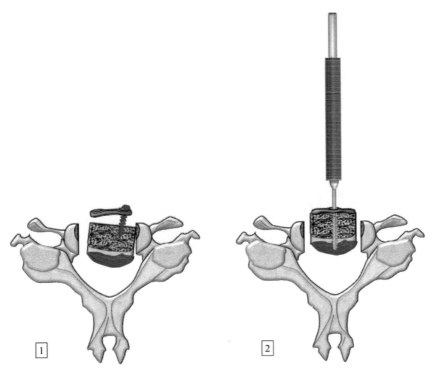

FIGURE 2.5.42

Illustration comparing vertebral body axial orientation between the screw system and the hoisting instrument.
(1) Rotated vertebral body driven by unilateral vertebral screws;
(2) Vertebral bodies remained centrally oriented after antedisplacement by the hoisting instrument.

pattern; ② eliminate intervertebral motion and dynamic compression injury to the spinal cord; ③ avoid abnormal motion that triggers heterotopic ossification or OPLL.

Interspace grafting is often achieved with an intervertebral cage packed with autogenous bone bitten off the anterior part of the vertebral body to be advanced with a triple-joint rongeur and properly shaped. Moderate bleeding from the vertebrae is expected during this bone removal process. Before enough volume of autologous bone is obtained, the use of bone wax for hemostasis should be reduced as much as possible in case it blends with the autologous bone, compromising the fusion result.

Interspaces less than 4 mm high produce excessive distraction and friction after a typical cage is placed. To address this challenge, a piece of bone is removed from the anterior vertebral body with a special rongeur so that the bone removed can be shaped and grafted in the disc space.

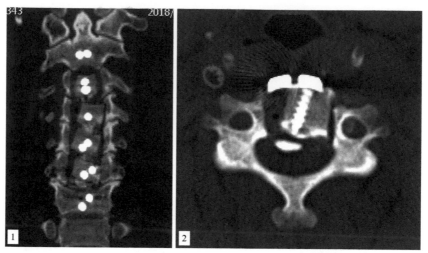

FIGURE 2.5.43

CT images of tilted or rotated vertebral bodies.
(1) Coronal image showing vertebral body tilting;
(2) Axial image showing vertebral body rotation.

Two types of triple-joint rongeurs are relevant to the ACAF technique, which is the vertebral trough rongeur and the vertebral transection rongeur (Fig. 2.5.44).

With aggressive cutting jaws, the vertebral trough rongeur develops troughs of the same width on both sides of the vertebral body. After that, the vertebral transection rongeur can be used to resect a block of bone from the anterior vertebral body. Properly shaped, this block of bone from the anterior vertebral bony can be used as a strut autograft in the disc space (Fig. 2.5.45).

Bone grafting in the bilateral troughs of the vertebral body

The grafting principle of LAM prevails, where bone grafts are placed on the dissected lamina on both sides to ensure bony fusion at the bone defect for the structural integrity of the posterior vertebral ring. Studies have found small defects within a long bone fuse spontaneously, given a stable mechanical environment, and when the bone defect reaches 5 mm, neovascularization activities at the defect site decrease, and bone callus is gradually replaced by fibrous tissue, which end up in pseudarthrosis rather than bony union. In the ACAF technique, the troughs on both sides of the vertebral body are generally 2−3 mm wide, or less than 5 mm, where spontaneously healing is expectable according to the analysis above.

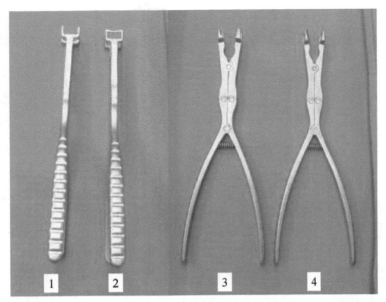

FIGURE 2.5.44

Two types of vertebral rongeurs.
(1, 3) A triple-joint vertebral trough rongeur with a jaw width of 18 mm that produces parasagittal troughs of the same width on both sides of the vertebral body;
(2, 4) A triple-joint vertebral transection rongeur with a blade on the jaws. With the jaws engaging the vertebral body's surfaces by the desired depth, it resects a piece of strut autograft.

However, the trough may be broadened or narrowed if the VOC shifts to one side during advancement (Fig. 2.5.46), leaving spontaneous fusion less predictable on the wider trough as it gets closer to the 5 mm threshold.

Osteogenesis behavior in bone defect of the vertebral body is distinct from that observed in long bone. First, the resected end of the former features cancellous bone, while the latter, cortical bone. Besides, the VOC is deprived of vascular supply except for that from the PLL. Therefore, investigation for the fusion behavior of the vertebral trough in the ACAF technique is awaited. Following up on these patients, the authors found that bony fusion was achieved in some patients while resorption in others (Fig. 2.5.47). Studies are awaited to clarify the bone-healing pattern.

In the ACAF technique, grafting is always recommended for bone troughs, whether broad or narrow. The commonly used bone graft material is autologous

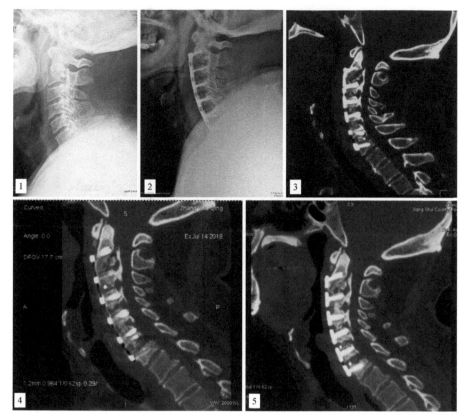

FIGURE 2.5.45

A case of ACAF using a strut autograft in the disc space.
(1) Preoperative lateral cervical X-ray showing OPLL at the levels of C2 to C6;
(2) Postoperative lateral cervical X-ray showing antedisplaced VOC and the C2/3 disc space without a cage;
(3) Sagittal CT on postoperative day one show antedisplaced VOC of C2 to C6, and strut autograft in the C2/3 disc space;
(4, 5) Sagittal CTs three and eight months after the operation, showing satisfactory fusion results in each disc space.

bone from the anterior part of the vertebral bodies. If they have been used up in grafting the interspaces, allogeneic bone can be used in the troughs as a supplement.

Two kinds of allogeneic bone materials are made available (Fig. 2.5.48). One is decalcified tibial cortical slices, reconstituted with normal saline until they become

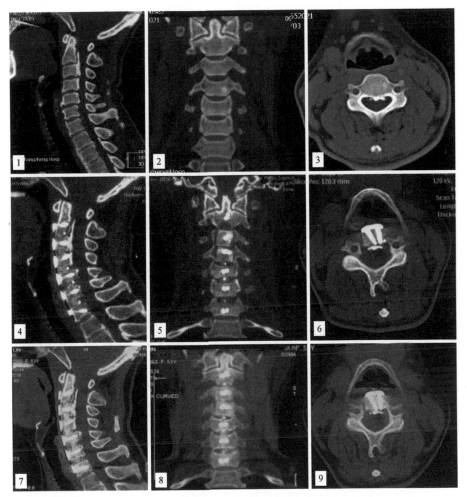

FIGURE 2.5.46

A case with different fusion results in the bone troughs as vertebral bodies have shifted to one side during antedisplacement.

(1–3) Preoperative sagittal, coronal, and axial CTs;

(4–6) The same series of CT images two days after surgery, showing antedisplaced VOC at C3 and C4, discectomy at C5/6 and C6/7, and VOC shifted to the left at C3 and C4, leaving a broader left trough and a narrower right trough;

(7–9) The same series of CT images three months after surgery, showing good fusion on the left trough but suboptimal on the right trough.

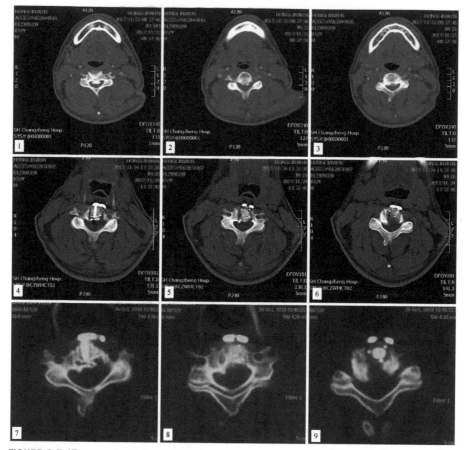

FIGURE 2.5.47

A case of ACAF procedure with a fused right trough and a resorbed left trough;
(1–3) Preoperative axial CT images at three typical levels;
(4–6) The same CT series taken two days after surgery;
(7–8) The same CT series taken one year after surgery.

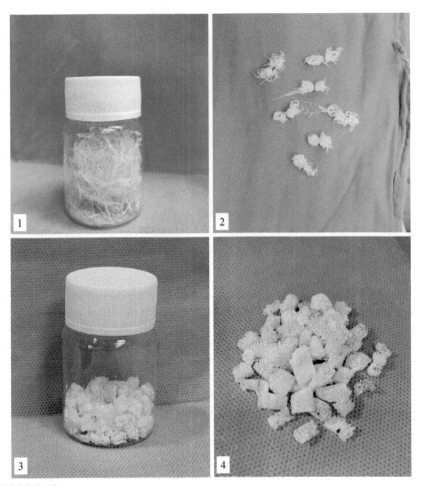

FIGURE 2.5.48

Two commonly used allograft materials for bone grafting in troughs.

(1) Decalcified tibial cortical slices;

(2) The slices soaked with normal saline, grouped in bundles with filament suture to facilitate placement;

(3, 4) Morselized decalcified cancellous bone from the ilium.

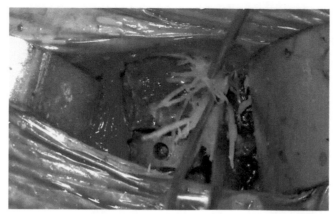

FIGURE 2.5.49

The decalcified tibial cortical slices being placed in the trough of the surgeon's opposite side after it is disconnected.

supple enough to be prepared into bundles and ready for immediate use. After the surgeon's opposite side vertebral trough is completed, the slices are placed in the trough before plate placement (Fig. 2.5.49). Otherwise, the plate obstructs access to the bone trough (Fig. 2.5.50). The other is morselized decalcified cancellous bone from the ilium, which shares a similar structure with the vertebral bone. It applies to the surgeon's side trough after vertebral antedisplacement.

The supple slices of the decalcified tibial cortex are optimal as they do not generate resistance during VOC antedisplacement.

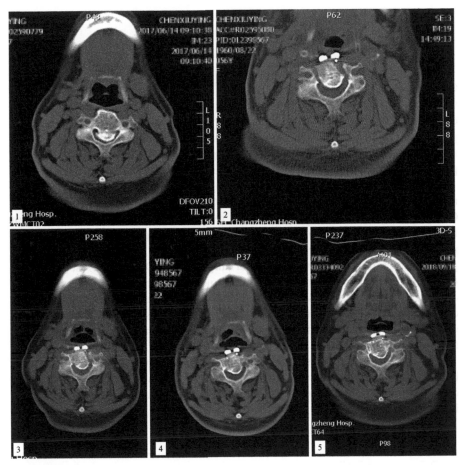

FIGURE 2.5.50

A case where only the right trough has been grafted. During the procedure, the left trough, or the surgeon's opposite side trough, had not been grafted before plate placement. After plate placement and vertebral body antedisplacement, the left trough was covered by the plate, disallowing bone grafting. Therefore, only the right trough was grafted.

(1) Preoperative CT;

(2) CT one day after surgery, showing the left trough blocked by the plate;

(3) CT three months after surgery, showing good bony union in the right trough but soft tissue density in the left trough;

(4) CT eight months after surgery, showing good bony union in the right trough and suboptimal bony union in the left trough;

(5) CT 15 months after surgery, similar to that obtained at eight months.

Reference

[1] Jingchuan S, Kaiqiang S, Yuan W, et al. Quantitative anterior enlargement of the spinal canal by anterior controllable antedisplacement and fusion for the treatment of cervical ossification of the posterior longitudinal ligament with myelopathy. World Neurosurgery 2018;120:e1098−106.

Section 6: Quantitative technique

Computer technologies, including imaging, navigation, and robotics, have been widely used in spinal surgery. The combined use of imaging and navigation technologies enables the surgeon to better visualize the irregular anatomical structures and perform surgeries safer with increased efficiency and accuracy. Although highly potential in spinal surgery, computer technologies are relatively far from everyday practice due to the expensive and necessary auxiliary equipment.

Computer-aided design (CAD) technology has been used in pelvic tumors, maxillofacial surgery, and pelvic fractures. Giovinco et al. reported the usage of CAD in the preparation for the surgical reconstruction of a deformed Charcot foot. This CAD provided an affordable and reproducible, personalized preoperative plan, and allowed the surgeons to practice and refine the surgical approach in the preoperative setting. In pelvic-acetabular surgeries, CAD could be used in simulating the reduction for acetabular fractures and calculating the trajectory and size of the screws using real CT scan data. These studies have demonstrated that surgeons can obtain an optimal operative plan on their computers using the exported CT data of the patients and achieve satisfactory results via an interactive operation planning tool.

Distinct from the conventional techniques, the recently described ACAF and bridge crane techniques require significant precision in isolation and advancement of the ossified mass. In this section, the precise quantification of new techniques is described using the CAD technology in the ACAF and bridge crane techniques.

CAD-based ACAF surgical planning

The treatment principles of ACAF might seem simple, but this surgery often involves several specific and difficult issues. The distance of hoisting VOC depends on the thickness of anterior resection of VB and the curvature of the contoured cervical plate. If the thickness of anterior resection of VB or the curvature of the contoured cervical plate is not enough, it may cause a decrease of the distance of hoisting VOC and incomplete decompression. Conversely, if excessive, it may cause the instability of VB, slip of the screws, dysphagia, and CSF leakage. The lateral border of VOC should be wide enough to include the OPLL. However, the risk of damaging vertebral artery or cervical pedicle would be increased when the border of the VOC was too wide. The amount of resection at each anterior vertebral body is determined by the thickness of the OPLL at each level. All of these data are vital for performing the surgery. However, the OPLL cannot be observed directly in ACAF, and these data are hard to be obtained intraoperatively. Thus, preoperative planning is with paramount importance in ACAF surgery.

With CAD technology, we can now feed it with a patient's preoperative cervical image data to appreciate in detail the ossification, vertebral bodies, and the courses of the vertebral arteries. In this way, the surgeons can plan the amount of bone to be resected from the anterior vertebral body and the distance between the troughs with greater precision and safety, and predict potential pitfall or emergency during operation.

3D modeling

The original patient data were input with the Digital Imaging and Communications in Medicine (DICOM) format, and the thickness of the fault was set as 1 mm to obtain a vivid virtual OPLL cervical spine. The cervical vertebrae were identified semiautomatically based on DICOM data using the MIMICS software. Every level from C2 to C7 of each patient was separated and reconstructed into a 3D model for further parameter calculation. 3D model was created automatically. First, identification of the vertebra was conducted by using a threshold of 226–3071 HU for the detection of bone. Second, each vertebra was detached from the other vertebrae using both axial and sagittal slice images. Third, the region of vertebrae was isolated using the same threshold, and a 3D model was created (Fig. 2.6.1).

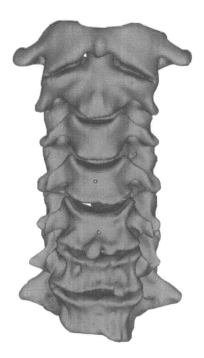

FIGURE 2.6.1

A cervical 3D model established in the MIMICS software based on the patient's cervical CT data.

Virtual surgical planning

All virtual objects with all parts of it can be independently and freely moved, removed, and fixed in a 3D plane. The cervical spine was placed in a supine position. First, bilateral osteotomies for the complete isolation of the VOC were conducted. Second, the VOC was moved ventrally to gain restoration of the AP diameter of the spinal canal. An anterior cervical plate and screws were installed. Resection of the anterior vertebral bodies of the VOC was then performed (Fig. 2.6.2).

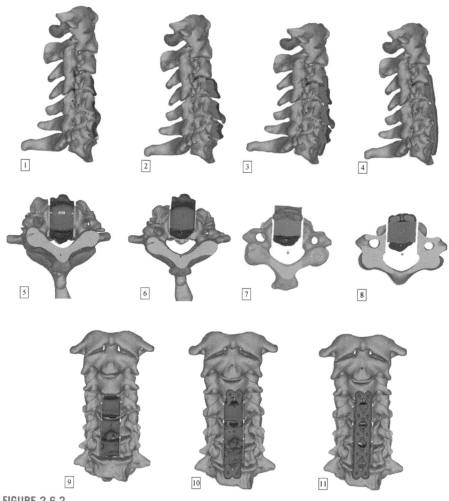

FIGURE 2.6.2

Virtual surgical planning in 3D model.
(1,5,9) Troughs on both sides of the vertebral body develop to isolate the VOC; and VOC ventrally displaced;
(2,6,10) The anteroposterior diameter of the spinal canal restored;
(3, 7) A plate placed on the anterior side of the vertebral bodies;
(4,8,11) The anterior bone of the VOC vertebral bodies resected.

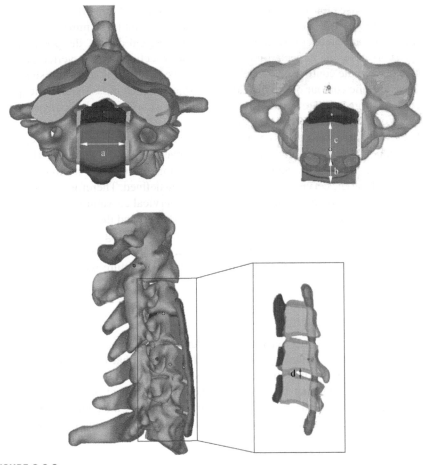

FIGURE 2.6.3

Main parameters.
(1) The VOC width on the axial cross-section between the troughs on both sides measured off preoperative planning;
(2) The thickness of the bone resection from the anterior vertebral body measured on the axial cross-section of the advanced VOC;
(3) The screw length measured on the axial cross-section of the advanced VOC;
(4) The length and contour of the plate to be used measured on a sagittal image.

Main parameters

In the surgical planning model, the width of bilateral osteotomies for VOC isolation, the levels of VOC, height for the intervertebral spacer, thickness of anterior resected VB, length of screws, and anterior plate were recorded (Fig. 2.6.3).

Time spent on software processing

Establishment of the 3D model was the most time-consuming in preoperative planning. The average time used for 3D model establishment was 35.7 min (20–60 min).

The mean time used for the virtual ACAF planning was 17.2 min (10—35 min). The mean time used for measuring the parameters was 5.3 min (4—8 min).

After accurate preoperative measurement and surgical design, the preoperative cervical curvature, the expected amount of bone resection at each vertebral body level, and the plate contour can be obtained. However, there is no established tool that measures the contour of the plate during surgery, which is essential to the quantification of surgery. Therefore, the authors designed a curvature ruler to measure the plate contour during surgery.

The Cobb angle was used to evaluate the total cervical curvature. The reported normal value of the Cobb angle is about 24 (range, 10—34). A study by Harrison et al. reported the C2—C7 angle averaged 35° (range, 16.5—66°). However, the normal or pathologic cervical curvature has not been defined. Therefore, considering the "normal" and "possible pathologic" values of cervical curvature, the tool of CR was designed with curvature angles ranging from 0 to 65 and the length of the measurement line ranging from 120.12 to 126.69 mm. According to the preoperative design about the length and curvature of the plate, we chose the proper-length plate first, and we then contoured the plate to the planned curvature with the aid of CR (Fig. 2.6.4).

Outcomes of application

According to the results, there is a high consistency between the data in preoperative design and the data in actual operation, which indicates that CAD can accurately assist surgery. The CAD may be helpful to reduce the time of operation. The time saving effect of CAD may be caused by the accurate selection of the width of VOC, so as to reduce the time wastage used in osteotomy of the pedicle, hemostasis of the intervertebral foramen vein, and adjustment and replacement of the intervertebral spacer, anterior plate, and screws.

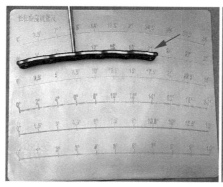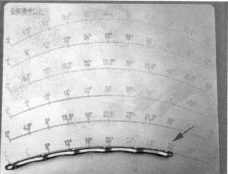

FIGURE 2.6.4

Use of cervical plate contour measuring scale.

The decompression effect of ACAF depends on the extent of anterior-displacement of VOC. In actual operation, intraoperative CT reconstruction can be done with O-arm to confirm the space between the anterior plate and remaining VB is enough for anterior-displacement of VOC. However, effect of radiation for the patient is a big concern for the use of intraoperative CT. In virtual surgery, we can change the sequence of the surgical procedure. First, anterior-displacement of the VOC is conducted. An anterior plate with satisfying length is selected. Thus, the amount of the anterior resection of the VB is naturally determined and served as an important parameter for the intraoperative procedure. The selection of the length of screws in each segment is also an important issue in ACAF operation. To increase the purchase of the screws, we tend to use the longest screw without damaging the spinal cord.

However, the risk of perforating the posterior wall of the VB together with the concern of over exposure of radiation makes the accurate selection of the optimal length of screws difficult. While in the CAD, the length for the screws can be directly measured after the anterior-displacement of VOC and installation of anterior plate. The length for the screws gained from CAD can then be used in the actual operation, which might help decrease the number of intraoperative fluoroscopic imaging and optimize the length of screws.

However, it is important for a surgeon to keep in mind the difference between virtual and real conditions. The difference is mainly due to the difference of body position. Virtual data were obtained from preoperative CT. When CT was taken, the patient was awake and in natural supine position. While during operation, the patient was under general anesthetic. The paraspinal muscles were completely relaxed. Meanwhile, the cervical curvature was adjusted to an over extend position. In this way, the cervical curvature in actual surgery is usually larger than the cervical curvature in CAD. Therefore, the length of anterior plate used in surgery is larger than that in the CAD. Another discrepant data is the height of the intervertebral spacer. Our result is that the height of the intervertebral spacer in actual surgery is 1 mm more than that in the CAD. In addition to the former mentioned increase in the curvature of the cervical spine and the increase in the height of the intervertebral body, the trimming of the end plate is also an important reason for the difference.

Instructional software for ACAF preoperative planning
Software features

To address issues in ACAF technique, we looked to CAD for preoperative planning early on and obtained good results. But this method is not immune to drawbacks. MIMICS, the software for most of the tasks, involves a long learning curve and takes much time in the 3D reconstruction. Clinicians may have to spend much time on learning before they become proficient in using the software. What is more, the challenge with precise VOC advancement still awaits a solution. Although consensus has reached on the contributors of the distance of VOC advancement, namely the amount of bone resected from the anterior vertebral body and the plate contour, the relationship among them remains elusive. Even with a defined bone resection and plate contour before surgery, it is still difficult to calculate the VOC advancement distance. Further impeded by limited surgical access, VOC advancement remains a difficult decision with a high stake: if advanced too much, CSF leak may occur, and if advanced too little, it may leave residual compression. Therefore, this section will introduce a new software for surgical design that focuses on the three most important parameters (plate contour, vertebral advancement distance, and the thickness of anterior vertebral resection) and complicated issues in preoperative planning.

Software rationale

The preoperative cervical sagittal CT images of OPLL patient is input into the Auto-CAD program to simplify the profiles and reformat of the cervical spine and the ossification into a 2D model. Then the ACAF technique is simulated in AutoCAD by two steps (first step: resection of the anterior vertebral bone; second step: VOC hoisting), which integrates the geometric relationship. The geometric relationship is demonstrated here with an example of OPLL involving segments C4 to C6. C4 and C6 were defined as cranial level of VOC and caudal level of VOC, respectively (Fig. 2.6.5, panel 1). S was defined as the required thickness of anterior resection of VB at each level, and S_m was the required thickness of anterior resection in the middle level. Fig. 2.6.5, panel 2 showed some geometric relationships: $\theta = 2 \times (180° - 2\beta)$, $\beta = \tan^{-1}\left(\frac{AB}{2CD}\right)$, $OD = OB = r = \dfrac{l}{2\sin\frac{\theta}{2}}$. We defined the angle θ as the curvature of the contoured cervical plate. In addition, we have another geometric relationship in Fig. 2.6.5, panel 3: $CD = C_m + d - S_m$. C_m was defined as the required distance of hoisting VOC in the middle level. Therefore, we got a formula: $\theta = 2 \times \left(180° - 2\tan^{-1}\frac{l}{2(C_m + d - S_m)}\right)$. It represented the geometric relationship between the required thickness of anterior resection of VB in the middle level, the required distance of hoisting VOC in the middle level, and the curvature of the contoured cervical plate.

According to Fig. 2.6.5, panel 4, the procedure of hoisting the isolated VOC at each level was split into two steps. The isolated VOC at each level was hoisted from the position of VB drawn in a red dotted line to the position of VB drawn in a black dotted line, and then it was hoisted to the position of VB drawn in a solid line. A geometric relationship was easy to get, where C was defined as the required distance of hoisting VOC at each level: $C = C_m - e + f$. Because the required thickness of anterior resection of VB was not necessarily the same at each level, the amount of resection at each anterior VB can be increased or decreased on the basis of S_m according to the thickness of OPLL at each level. Therefore, the

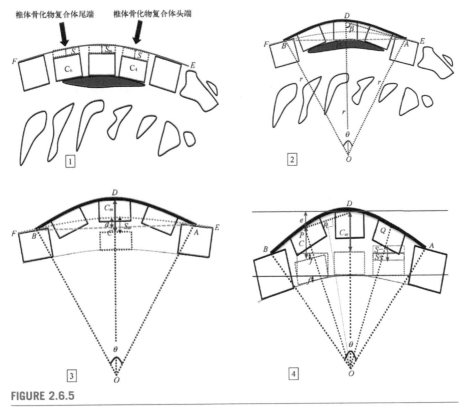

FIGURE 2.6.5

Illustration of the derivation process for the geometric relationships among the plate contour, vertebral hoisting distance, and resection thickness of anterior vertebral bone.
(1) Simplified 2D model of the ACAF technique;
(2) Illustration of the geometric relationship among the plate contour, the chord length of the plate, and the angle measurement of the circle which the plate is fitted;
(3) Illustration of the geometrical relationship among the parameters such as the hoisting distance and the resection thickness of the middle vertebrae;
(4) Illustration of the geometrical relationship among the parameters such as the hoisting distance and the resection thickness of the vertebrae other than the middle one.

geometric relationship can be adapted as shown below: $C = C_m - e + f + S_{\pm}$. The angle θ was divided into $(n + 1)$ parts, each of which was considered as the angle between two adjacent VB, and n was the amount of the hoisted VB (VB was hoisted from C4 to C6 in panel 2, so $n = 3$ and θ was divided evenly into four parts by black dotted lines [$\angle BOP$, $\angle POD$, $\angle DOQ$, and $\angle QOA$]). Accordingly, we got one formula first: $\frac{e}{PD} = \frac{RD}{OD} = \sin\frac{m\theta}{2(n+1)}$. m represented the number of parts between the required VB and midline OD (The angle between C4(C6) and OD was $\angle POD(\angle DOQ)$, so $m = 1$). Second, $OD = OB = r = \dfrac{l}{2\sin\dfrac{\theta}{2}}$ was mentioned above, so $e = \dfrac{l\sin^2\dfrac{m\theta}{2n+2}}{\sin\dfrac{\theta}{2}}$ was deduced. Third, $C = C_m - \dfrac{l\sin^2\dfrac{m\theta}{2n+2}}{\sin\dfrac{\theta}{2}} +$ $S_\pm + f$ was deduced further. Because Fig. 2.6.5 (4) showed the case of $n =$ odd, we also got a formula according to the same principle in the case of $n =$ even.

$C = C_m - \dfrac{l\sin^2\dfrac{(2m-1)\theta}{4n+4}}{\sin\dfrac{\theta}{2}} + S_\pm + f$. Therefore, we came up with the geometric

relationship between the required distance of hoisting VOC at each level, the required thickness of anterior resection of VB at each level, and the curvature of the contoured cervical plate by calculation.

In summary, the following three geometric formulas are obtained:

$$
\begin{cases}
\theta = 2 \times \left(180° - 2\tan^{-1}\dfrac{l}{2(C_m + d - S_m)}\right) \quad (1) \\[4mm]
C = C_m - \dfrac{l\sin^2\dfrac{m\theta}{2n+2}}{\sin\dfrac{\theta}{2}} + S_\pm + f \ (n = \text{odd}) \quad (2) \\[4mm]
C = C_m - \dfrac{l\sin^2\dfrac{(2m-1)\theta}{4n+4}}{\sin\dfrac{\theta}{2}} + S_\pm + f \ (n = \text{even}) \quad (3)
\end{cases}
$$

Application

By measuring the length of affected segments first, cranial level of VOC, caudal level of VOC, and l were determined based on the preoperative sagittal CT images of patient with OPLL. Next, the radiological parameters including d and f were also measured on the CT images. According to the thickness of OPLL in the middle level of VOC, C_m and S_m were initially determined. Second, press Button Initial Calculation, and then θ and C were output in blue area, as shown in Fig. 2.6.6, panel 1. Third, C was further adjusted according to the thickness of OPLL at each level. An increase or decrease of the thickness of anterior resection of VB on the basis of S_m was determined. Input the parameter $S_\pm$ and press Button Adjusted Calculation. C and S were output again, as shown in red and blue area in Fig. 2.6.6, panel 2. Finally, the satisfactory values of each parameter were obtained and a quantitative preoperative design was finished.

Given the complexity of the software process, the team added the teaching function to the program to help users learn the quantitative preoperative design of ACAF technique. Clicking "Teaching Mode," users will enter the teaching module (Fig. 2.6.6 panel 3 and Fig. 2.6.6 panel 4) that guides the steps through calculation,

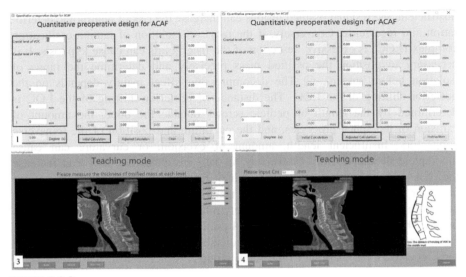

FIGURE 2.6.6

Panels of software operation for ACAF preoperative design.

(1) The first step: input the values in the boxes of the red frames, click "Initial Calculation" to obtain the values in the boxes of the blue frames;

(2) The second step: input the values in the boxes of the red frames, click "Adjusted Calculation" to obtain the values in the boxes of the blue frames;

(3, 4) ACAF preoperative design conducted in the teaching mode.

measurement, documentation, and teaching. The users can conduct the preoperative design step by step under the guidance of the tutorial system.

Outcomes of application

With this software, the authors found that the teaching mode allowed surgeons to learn quickly and proficiently carry out the preoperative planning of ACAF technique. The challenges to operate the software and the amount of time spent on learning are markedly reduced from computer-assisted virtual operation planning system. The crux of VOC hoisting distance calculation is readily managed through the geometric relationships among the three parameters, reducing surgical risks. In addition, the software tackles this complicated clinical crux of the ACAF technique with accuracy comparable to the CAD paradigm, suggesting its value in widespread adoption for the ACAF technique.

Computer-assisted design for the bridge crane technique

Although the bridge crane technique has achieved good results in treating thoracic ossification of the ligamentum flavum (TOLF), the following challenges in clinical practice await better solutions. ① The border of the ossified mass is irregular, and it cannot be observed directly during the operation. If the range of isolation of LOC is insufficient, the residual ossified lesions can increase the risk of neurologic deterioration and recurrence. Conversely, if the range of isolation of lamina-ossification complex (LOC) is excessive, resection of the facet joints can cause kyphosis. It is necessary to position the ossified mass precisely and determine the range of isolation before surgery. ② The decompression effect mainly depends on the posterior shifting of the LOC. The distance of posterior shifting of the LOC is determined by the length of pedicle screws outside the bone, the amount of excision of the spinal processes, and the curvature and position of the transverse connectors. Insufficient length, amount of excision, or curvature can cause incomplete decompression. Conversely, if they are excessive, they can increase the risks of screw loosening and spinal instability. Furthermore, excessive posterior shifting also might led to dural tears and CSF leakage vertebrae. ③ The curvature of the longitudinal rods is closely related to the length of pedicle screws outside the bone at each level and the physiological curvature of thoracic spine. However, the curvature is not usually predictable, and the surgeon has to bend the rods repeatedly for adaption to the screw troughs, which can increase the risk of rod breakage.

Similar to the ACAF preoperative design, the authors also used the computer-based 3D simulations to formulate the preoperative planning of bridge crane technique, which has largely solved the above issues. This virtual surgical planning will be described in detail below.

Establishment of 3D model: The first step, use MIMICS software to reconstruct the 3D model of the surgical thoracic levels (Fig. 2.6.7):

Create a bone mask by setting the bone thresholds (226–2998 HU).

Click "Crop mask" button to select the desired mask area.

Click "Edit mask" to modify the selected mask according to the CT values and anatomical structure.

The thoracic spine mask is completed, and then use the same method to obtain the TOLF mask.

Click "Calculate 3D" button to convert the obtained thoracic spine mask into a 3D object.

Save the 3D model of the thoracic spine in STL format.

The second step, use Pro/Engineer software to obtain the 3D models of pedicle screws and other instruments (Fig. 2.6.8):

Select "mmns_part_solid" as the default mode.

Use the "Extrude and Geometric" tool to draw the surgical instruments according to their actual shapes and sizes, and click "Protrusion" button to draw the threads of the pedicle screw.

Save the 3D models of the surgical instruments in STL format.

Surgical simulation: The thoracic spine and the surgical instruments in STL format are imported into 3-matic software for surgery simulation. Surgical steps are virtually realized by adjusting transparency and resecting or moving the images through clicks on "Transparency," "Trim," and "Interactive Translate" buttons, respectively (Fig. 2.6.9). The procedures of the bridge crane technique in virtual surgery were different from those in real surgery, as shown in Fig. 2.6.10: ① The

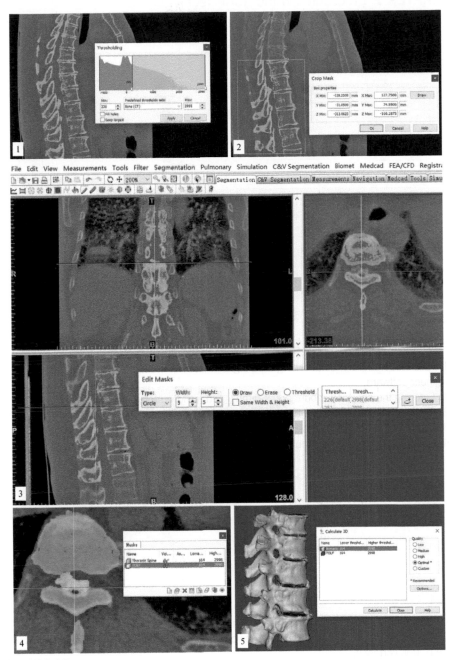

FIGURE 2.6.7

The basic operations of establishing the spine 3D model by using MIMICS software.
(1) Creating a bone mask: press thresholding button;
(2) Selecting the required region: press Crop mask button;
(3, 4) Revising the mask: press edit mask button. Obtaining the revised masks of spine (green) and TOLF (yellow);
(5) Creating the 3D objects of spine and TOLF: press Calculate 3D button.

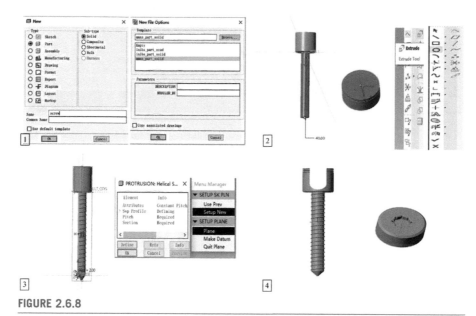

FIGURE 2.6.8

The basic operations of establishing the surgical instrument 3D model by using Pro/engineer software.
(1) Entering the specified mode: press mmns_part_solid button;
(2) Creating the geometry: use extrude tool and Geometric tool;
(3) Inserting the screw threads: press Protrusion button;
(4) Obtaining the screws and nuts.

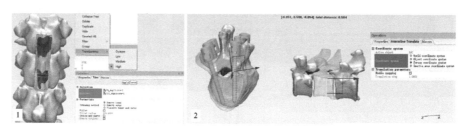

FIGURE 2.6.9

The basic operations of virtual surgery by using 3-matic software;
(1) Visualizing the spine: press transparency button; excising the spinal processes: press trim button vertebral;
(2) Placing the pedicle screws and moving the LOC: press Interactive translate button.

transparency of the 3D model was increased to make the ossified mass visible in the coronal plane. According to the size and shape of the ossified mass, the LOC was safely isolated. ② The LOC was suspended posteriorly based on the evaluation of spinal canal stenosis. ③ The physiological curvature of the thoracic spine was

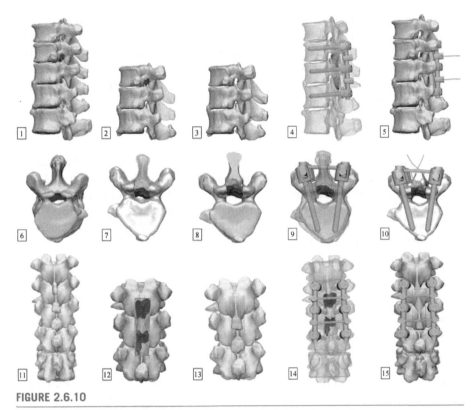

FIGURE 2.6.10

Illustration of the procedures of the bridge crane technique in virtual surgery.
(1, 6, 11) The sagittal plane, axial plane, coronal plane of 3D model;
(2, 7, 12) The isolation of the LOC isolate;
(3, 8, 13) The posterior suspension of the LOC;
(4, 9, 14) The installation of the pedicle screws, longitudinal rods, and transverse connectors;
(5, 10, 15) The excision of spinous processes.

measured in the sagittal plane. Two longitudinal rods were bent with a similar curvature. The pedicle screws were placed in the bone as deeply as possible, and their length outside the bone was not retained. ④ The rods were installed on pedicle screws, and zero-curvature transverse connectors were installed on the rods. ⑤ The spinal processes of the involved laminae were excised and sutures were buried at the base of the LOC.

Finally, if the values of these parameters were not in the appropriate range or could not meet the demand for complete decompression, they would be adjusted in a specific order until satisfactory data were obtained. First, changing the position of the transverse connectors could increase the distance between the LOC and transverse connectors. Second, if satisfactory decompression was not yet met, the amount of excision of the spinal processes would be increased to enlarge the extent of posterior suspension. Third, the length of pedicle screws outside the bone was retained appropriately. The curvature of the longitudinal rods should also be adjusted for adaption to the screw troughs according to the changed length of all the pedicle screws outside the bone at each level. Finally, the curvature of the transverse connectors was also increased if the previous steps did not work.

Main parameters

In the virtual surgery simulation for the bridge crane technique, the authors measured and recorded the following parameters: the length and width of LOC, the length of pedicle screws outside the bone, the amount of excision of the spinal processes, the height of posterior suspension of the LOC, the curvature of the transverse connectors, the curvature of the longitudinal rods, and the position of the transverse connectors (Fig. 2.6.11).

Intraoperative application

During the actual surgery, the spinal processes were first excised according to the amount of excision in CAPP. Then, the positioning screws were placed into the pedicles. By using the positioning screws as a reference, the range of LOC isolation was determined according to the preoperative width and length of the LOC. The positioning screws were removed, and the pedicle screws were placed according to the preoperative length outside the bone. Two longitudinal rods and the transverse connectors were bent with a planned curvature. The planned positions of the transverse connectors installed on the rods were marked, and then the longitudinal rods and the transverse connectors were installed on the pedicle screws successively, which were fixed by nuts. Finally, the sutures were tied to the transverse connectors, and the LOC was successfully suspended. The caliper and specially made curvature ruler were used for parameter measurement to ensure that the operation was performed according to the preoperative plan.

Outcomes of application

By comparing the parameters' results of the preoperative design and those in the actual operation, the authors found no unacceptable errors, which proved the reliability and effectiveness of computer-aided preoperative planning. The key procedure of the bridge crane technique is longitudinal and transverse osteotomy, and posterior suspension of the isolated TOLF. The range of longitudinal and transverse osteotomy (width and length of the LOC) determines whether the TOLF can be isolated completely, and the decompression effect depends on the distance of posterior suspension of isolated LOC (the combination of four parameters). Any inappropriate value or combination of the parameters can increase the risk of complications. Due to the invisible surgical procedure, complete isolation and precise posterior

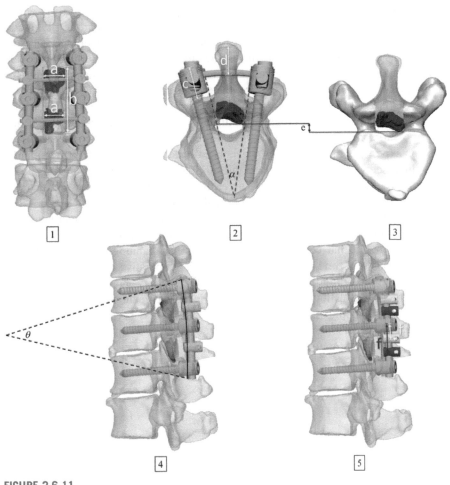

FIGURE 2.6.11

Main parameters.

(1) Width (a) and length (b) of isolate LOC;

(2, 3) Length of pedicle screws outside the bone (c), amount of excision of the spinal processes (d), curvature of the transverse connectors (α), and height of posterior suspension of LOC (e);

(4) Curvature of the longitudinal rods (θ);

(5) Position of the transverse connectors (distance between the cranial neighboring pedicle screw and the transverse connector) (f).

suspension can be a challenge for surgeons. To solve the above problems as much as possible, CAD was used in our preoperative planning. In the process, the 3D models of thoracic spine and surgical instruments were reconstructed by using MIMICS and Pro/Engineer software based on the actual CT data and physical data. The precision of reconstruction has been widely recognized and has been reported in previous studies. Then, the transparency of the spine model was increased, and TOLF hidden in the spinal canal was revealed. The visualization of the 3D model can help surgeons precisely position and isolate the ossified mass completely. Furthermore, surgeons can also change the surgical sequence to obtain an optimal planning for precise posterior suspension. In practice, the distance of posterior suspension of isolated LOC is easily determined according to the thickness of the TOLF, but the amount of excision of spinal processes is difficult to determine at first. In actual surgery, the surgeons can only estimate the amount of excision of spinal processes based on experience and then roughly evaluate the decompression effect by reduplicated fluoroscopy, which can increase the surgical risks and radiation exposure of patients. In virtual surgery, surgeons can easily determine the suspension distance and then adjust other parameters based on the suspension situation. In addition, the specially made measurement tools and intraoperative procedure can help surgeons perform the operation accurately according to the preoperative planning.

We also found that computer-aided preoperative planning can help surgeons minimize operation time by avoiding repeated intraoperative attempts and operations, including bending the rods, performing fluoroscopy, and adjustment of other parameters, as well as minimizing radiation exposure of patients.

To sum up, computer-aided preoperative planning has been feasible and clinically meaningful for the bridge crane surgery for TOLF as a valuable solution for surgeons to develop an optimal surgical plan.

Section 7: Determinants of ACAF technical challenges

As a new technique guided by concepts of vertebra-ossification complex (VOC) and theory of in situ spinal cord decompression, the ACAF technique boasts unique surgical procedures and operative skills. The adoption of any new technique should be a step-wise process where surgeons start with straightforward cases before taking on the challenging ones. The correct estimate of surgical challenge is paramount to the selection of surgical techniques and the preoperative preparations. As such, the determinants of ACAF technical challenges are laid out in this section in terms of surgical approach, incision, and width of the ossified mass.

Surgical approach

Good exposure is the basis for successful surgery. The approach is an integral part when assessing surgical challenges. Upon the first impression, one can tell the width and length of the patient's neck (Fig. 2.7.1).

Neck thickness

The thickness of the neck reflects the thickness of the soft tissue, which depends on the robustness of the paravertebral muscles and the amount of subcutaneous adipose tissue. Regardless of the cause, thick necks require more fascial dissection and produce greater tension upon retraction.

Neck length

Neck accessibility hinges upon two potential barriers: the mandibular for the upper levels and the shoulders for the lower (Fig. 2.7.2).

(1) When access to C2 or C3 is expected in a surgery, surgeons pay special attention to the patient's preoperative extension X-ray to identify the vertebral segments correlating with the mandible. If the lower border of the mandible corresponds to C3, it may pose challenges to C2 exposure. It should be noted that the potential obstruction by the mandible cannot be determined through physical appearance, so the preoperative extension X-ray is essential to evaluate the challenge of C2 exposure.

(2) Patients with high-riding shoulders and short necks may present challenges to the presentation of C6 and vertebrae below on intraoperative lateral fluoroscopy.

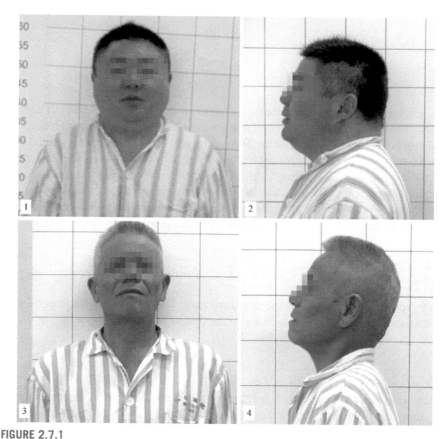

FIGURE 2.7.1

Comparison of the short, thick neck (panel 1 and 2) and slender neck (panel 3 and 4).

Incision options and their challenges to the operation

The level of the surgical segment is undoubtedly tied to the difficulty of exposure. It is straightforward to expose only C4 to C6 but more difficult to expos C2 to C3 or C6 to T1. The direction of the incision also affects the difficulty of exposure. The longitudinal incision allows for more extensive exposure and easier retractor placement, especially for long-segment surgeries or when C2 to C3 or C6 to T1 is involved, though it is less cosmetically suitable. A more cosmetic option is a transverse incision, but it allows for a more difficult exposure when more than three vertebrae are to be hoisted during ACAF (Fig. 2.7.3). When up to four vertebrae are to be hoisted, the dual transverse incisions are recommended.

The transverse incision facilitates antedisplacement with ease and cosmetic.

A transverse incision for hoisting two vertebrae is more difficult than to hoist just one vertebra but still manageable.

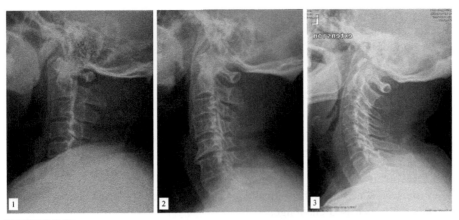

FIGURE 2.7.2

Comparison of the lateral X-ray images of necks of different lengths.

(1) A patient with a short neck, spine shadow superimposed by the shoulders below the lower border of C5;

(2) A patient with a long neck, low-riding shoulders, well-presented C7 vertebra, and the lower border of the mandible corresponding to C2;

(3) Another patient with a long neck, lower-riding shoulders, well-presented T1 vertebra, but the lower border of the mandible corresponding to C3.

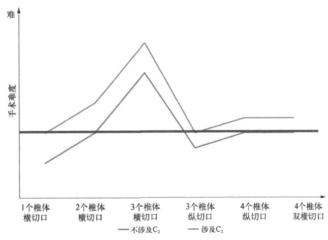

FIGURE 2.7.3

Impact of incision on the surgical challenge.

The area above the benchmark (red horizontal line) represents an increased surgical challenge. The blue curve represents surgeries no involving C2, whereas the orange curve, those involving C2.

Level of surgical challenge.
Challenging.
Straightforward.

1 Transverse incision	Vertebra
2 Transverse incision	Vertebrae
3 Transverse incision	Vertebrae
3 Longitudinal incision	Vertebrae
4 Longitudinal incision	Vertebrae
4 Dual transverse incisions	Vertebrae

C2 not involved.

C2 involved.

A transverse incision is theoretically feasible for three vertebrae hoist but with an exponentially increased challenge.

A longitudinal incision is readily straightforward for a three vertebrae hoist, much less challenging than a transverse incision.

A longitudinal incision for four vertebrae hoist is still feasible, though more difficult than three levels, with difficulty comparable to a transverse incision for two vertebrae hoist.

Dual transverse incisions for four vertebrae hoist, with challenge comparable to a longitudinal incision.

The red line in the graph shows the average challenge of exposure among the patients treated in the author's hospital.

Impact of OPLL width to the surgical challenge

The narrower the OPLL (coronal dimension), the easier the thorough VOC isolation. Does it mean that narrower OPLL poses a little difficulty to the surgery? The concept of the anatomical landmark for grooves has been introduced in the previous section "Anatomical Study on Groove Positions," which describes a reference landmark of the anterior base of the uncinate process. With the uncinate process as a reference, ossified masses are grouped into three categories by the position of their edges: medial to, at, or lateral to the uncinate process. When the horizontal width of the ossified mass is smaller than the distance between the uncinate processes on both sides, the standard method of grooving is used. When these two parameters are equal, the grooves can also be developed with the standard method, and care is taken to ensure the grooves are perfectly parasagittal. When the width of the ossification exceeds the distance between the uncinate processes, the surgery is involved with an increased challenge as the cutting instrument would contact the ossified mass at the bottom of the grooves developed with the standard method. In such a case, the levels of the spine where the ossification extends beyond the uncinate process can be identified on CT preoperative, and when preparing those levels, the grooves should be extended laterally, which poses a greater surgical challenge (Fig. 2.7.4).

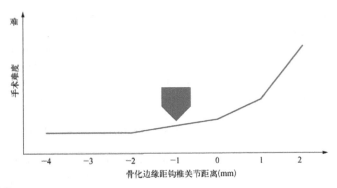

FIGURE 2.7.4

Impact of the ossification width on the surgical challenge.

A slice-by-slice analysis of the preoperative CT scans is paramount to the surgical preparation and estimation of the surgical challenge.

The width of the ossified mass may vary greatly at each level. Strategies should be developed for segments with a wider ossification beforehand in case of surprises during surgery.

The distance between the edge of an ossified mass and the uncinate process reflects the relative ossification's width. This distance is recorded as negative when the edge of the ossified mass is medial to the uncinate process, and positive when it is lateral to the uncinate process.

As long as the edge of the ossified mass does not reach the uncinate process (distance −4 mm to −2 mm), it has little impact on the surgical challenge regardless of its actual width.

Challenging.

Level of surgical challenge.

Straightforward.

−1 mm (the edge is approaching but still medial to the vertebral groove)

0 mm (the edge is at the vertebral groove)

1 mm (the edge is beyond the vertebral groove)

2 mm (the edge is beyond the vertebral groove)

The distance from the ossification edge to the uncinate process.

The level of surgical challenge increases as the edge of the ossified mass extends further beyond the uncinate process. The blue arrow indicates the level of challenge when the edge of the ossified mass is near the vertebral groove. The curve to the left of the blue arrow (representing narrow ossified masses) maintains steady and represents a moderate challenge level.

When the edge of the ossification reaches the uncinate process (distance between −2 and 1 mm), the edge may be encountered when the groove is medialized or deviated. Therefore, ossification of this type is more challenging than that in cases with the edge not reaching the uncinate process.

If the ossification extends beyond the uncinate process (distance over 1 mm), the ossified mass is right at the bottom of the groove developed at the landmark. In these cases, care should be taken to bypass the mass by deviating the groove laterally to avoid complications such as residual ossification or nerve injury. However, to develop an excessively deviated groove may end up in the pedicle or vertebral artery. Therefore, the surgery in such patients is much more challenging than those where the ossification edge is medial to or reaching the uncinate process.

The average distance from the edge of ossification to the uncinate process is between −1 mm and −2 mm among patients treated in the author's department.

Impact of the length of the ossified mass on the surgical challenge

Simply put, the ACAF technique's essence is the mobilization and antedisplacement of the vertebra, so the surgical time is primarily dependent on the length of the ossification, or the number of vertebrae that need to be advanced. Diseases involving more vertebrae involve increased surgical time, more challenges to the exposure, and higher demand for precision in the amount of plate contour and the amount of bone resection from the anterior vertebra (introduced in the section "Quantification Techniques") (Fig. 2.7.5).

The length of the ossification is tied to the number of vertebrae that need to be advanced.

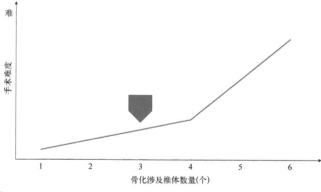

FIGURE 2.7.5

Impact of the number of vertebrae involved in the OPLL on the surgical challenge. The level of surgical challenge increases with the addition of disease segments. The blue arrow represents the level of challenge with a three-level OPLL. The level of challenge rises steadily on the left of the blue arrow but exponentially once the number of vertebrae involved hits four.

Before surgery, CT and MRI studies should be conducted to clarify the vertebrae involved in the OPLL and spinal cord compression levels. These two features are consistent in most cases but not all.

The more vertebrae that need to be advanced, the more challenging the surgery is.

When more than four vertebrae need to be advanced, its level of surgical challenge shoots from those fewer than four due to the lack of proper instrumentation of this length.

The ossifications averagely involve three vertebrae among patients treated in the author's department.

Impact of thickness of the ossified mass on the surgical challenge

In the conventional techniques, the OPLL thickness has an overarching value to evaluating challenges during surgery, and the ratio of spinal canal occupancy of the OPLL is a crucial prognostic predictor in anterior and posterior surgeries. In contrast, the values of the double-layer sign and the nine-portion canal assessment no longer prevail in the ACAF technique, where OPLL resection is not involved. In the ACAF technique, the OPLL thickness mainly affects the distance that the VOC needs to be advanced, which is realized by bone resected from the anterior vertebra and the placement of a precontoured plate. With an increased amount of bone resected from the anterior vertebra, the screw purchase in the vertebra fundamental to antedisplacement decreases. Therefore, with a thicker OPLL comes more challenges and a higher risk of the surgery (Fig. 2.7.6).

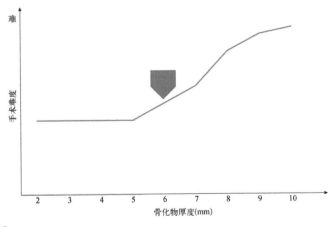

FIGURE 2.7.6

Impact of ossification thickness on the surgical challenge.
The blue arrow indicates the average thickness of OPLL. The curve on its left side indicates that thinner OPLL is less challenging.

Generally, the cervical vertebrae measure between 18 and 22 mm in thickness (anteroposterior dimension), and the commonly used screws, between 12 and 16 mm.

OPLL of thickness below 6 mm has little impact on the surgical challenge.

Otherwise, the anterior part of the vertebra is resected by more than 6 mm deep, so that the remaining vertebra measures less than 12 mm in anteroposterior dimension, where a screw of over 12 mm long may go through its posterior cortex, but a shorter screw provides less screw purchase.

Challenging.

Level of surgical challenge.

Straightforward.

1 vertebra
2 vertebrae
3 vertebrae
4 vertebrae
5 vertebrae
6 vertebrae

Number of vertebrae involved in the OPLL

Challenging.

Level of surgical challenge.

Easy.

Thickness of ossified mass.

Once the OPLL thickness reaches 6 mm, the level of surgical challenge shoots from that point.

The average thickness of ossified mass is 6 ~ 7 mm among patients treated in the author's hospital.

Impact of disc height on the surgical challenge

In describing the factors that may affect antedisplacement in an earlier section, the height of the disc space has been listed as a crucial one. For slightly degenerated disc, discectomy and endplate preparation are completed with ease. On the contrary, severely degenerated disc poses challenges to interbody preparation, bilateral groove development on the vertebra, and vertebral antedisplacement, in addition to the unique challenge of resistance during the antedisplacement process (Fig. 2.7.7).

Challenging.

Level of surgical challenge.

Straightforward.

Disc height.

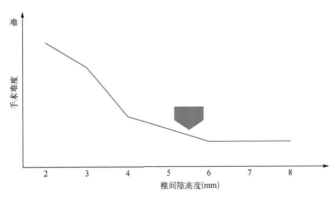

FIGURE 2.7.7

Impact of disc height on the surgical challenge.
The blue arrow indicates the average disc height, and the level of surgical challenge is much lower to the right of the arrow.

Disc height is measured on a lateral cervical X-ray or sagittal CT image before surgery.

In case of a disc space ≤4 mm, care should be taken to thoroughly prepare the endplates lest they generate excessive friction with the cage placed.

Severely degenerated disc space of less than 2 mm high poses an extra challenge to the surgery.

If it does not accept a cage of the proper size, it is prepared, left uninstrumented, and grafted with the morselized bone after VOC antedisplacement through the graft window on the plate.

The disc space among patients treated in the author's hospital measures 5—6 mm high.

Sagittal profile of the ossification on CT

Cervical OPLL can be classified by the sagittal profile on CT into localized, segmental, continual, and mixed types. These categories account for the OPLL length and the presence of any interruption within the ossified mass. The impact of the OPLL length on the surgical challenge has been described above. Does the presence or absence of interruption within the mass affect the surgical challenge? Logics has it that it does not affect surgical challenge as the ACAF technique involves only mobilization but not resection of the ossification. But OPLL that extends to C2 and beyond poses is associated with an exponentially increased challenge. An OPLL extending beyond C2/3 is usually continual from C3. If the VOC ends at C3, the ossification has to be dissected at the C2/3, which may cause complications, including CSF and nerve injury. Alternatively, if the Shelter technique is used to advance the OPLL at C2, the posterior vertebra of C2 is undercut to create a niche to accommodate the advanced ossification at C2. This is a challenging technique as the ossification at C2, or even that at C3, may be inadequately displaced if the niche is too small, resulting in insufficient decompression.

Undercutting decompression

When determining the vertebrae that need to be moved forward, the surgeon looks for those with dorsal compressors, which usually includes all the ossification levels. However, as discussed earlier, the more the surgical segments, the more challenging it is for the surgery. In some situations, undercutting decompression can be adopted to reduce the number of vertebrae that need to be advanced. The undercutting decompression in the ACAF technique is to move the tip of a continuous ossification forward by antedisplacing its adjacent vertebra. When this is done for the ossification at C2, it is called the shelter technique (Fig. 2.7.8).

A prerequisite of the undercut technique is the ossification of the intended undercut level is continuous with that of an adjacent segment.

It should be noted that C4 and C5 are not recommended for the undercut technique because vertebrae at the center of the cervical spine are difficult to access with instruments at any angle of approach.

When the ossification involves more than half of the vertebral height, antedisplacement is preferred to an undercutting decompression.

Undercut decompression is favored in vertebrae with difficult access or unique anatomical features that defy an antedisplacement, such as C2 and T2.

When the ossification spans long (more than four vertebrae), undercutting decompression can be applied for the vertebrae of the cephalad and caudal ends of the disease as a compromise to the unavailability of a longer anterior cervical plate.

Necessary instruments and devices

An ancient Chinese quote has it that "a workman must first sharpen his tools if he is to do his work well." With a complete set of essential instruments and devices, the surgeons complete the procedure with ease. Otherwise, they may struggle through the operation. The specific necessary instruments for the ACAF technique and their purposes are described below.

Burr or piezoelectrical osteotome: With a 3 mm ball tip. It is used for groove development, disc space preparation, and resection of bone from the anterior vertebra (indispensable for the ACAF technique) (Fig. 2.7.9).

Laminectomy rongeur: A 3 mm rongeur is used to prepare disc space and osteophytes (important), a 2 mm rongeur is used for groove development (very

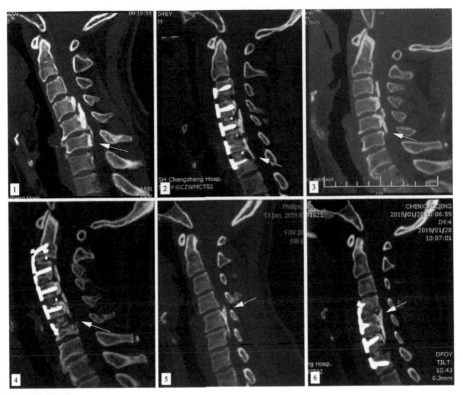

FIGURE 2.7.8

Sagittal CT images of cases receiving undercutting decompression; three cases are presented here.

1, 3, and 5 are images before surgery, and 2, 4, and 6 are the postoperative images. Levels of undercutting decompression are indicated with arrows.

(1, 2) The posterosuperior part of C7 vertebra undercut to contain the ossification antedisplaced as C6 is advanced anteriorly;

(3, 4) The posterosuperior part of C6 vertebra undercut to contain the ossification antedisplaced as C5 is advanced anteriorly;

(5, 6) The posteroinferior part of C4 vertebra undercut to contain the ossification antedisplaced as C5 is advanced anteriorly.

important), and a 1 mm for groove development in challenging situations (important) (Fig. 2.7.10).

Triple-joint curved rongeur is used to resect the anterior vertebra and osteophytes (important) (Fig. 2.7.11).

Titanium plate, screws, and intervertebral cages are used for vertebral antedisplacement (indispensable).

Nerve hook/elevator and bone wax for nerve stripper hemostasis of the bone surfaces surrounding the groove (important) (Fig. 2.7.12).

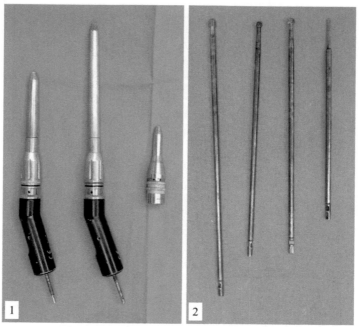

FIGURE 2.7.9

Burrs and drill bits.
(1) Burrs;
(2) Drill bits.

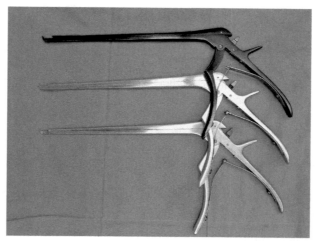

FIGURE 2.7.10

Laminectomy rongeur.

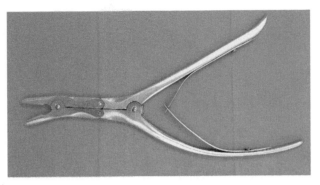

FIGURE 2.7.11

Triple-joint curved rongeur.

Bone wax shaped to peanut size for hemostasis of the bone surface of the resected vertebra, particularly the transected nutrient arteries (optional) (Fig. 2.7.13).

Jaw widths (from top to bottom) are 1 mm, 2 mm, and 3 mm, respectively.

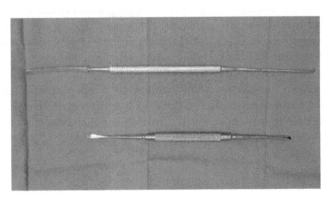

FIGURE 2.7.12

Nerve hook/elevator.

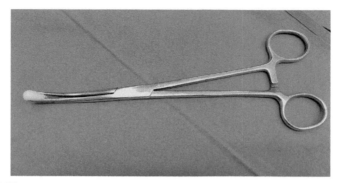

FIGURE 2.7.13

Bone wax shape as peanut size.

Surgical team

Good surgical teamwork helps secure a successful surgery. The success of an ACAF procedure hinges upon not only the surgical expertise in the technique and other skills but also the all-round cooperation of the entire surgical team.

The anesthesiologists assess the patient's risk for anesthesia and determine the intubation system to be used before surgery, maintain the blood pressure and assess patients for transfusion criteria during surgery, and determine the timing of extubation after surgery. The assistant surgeons are tasked with positioning the patient, locating a proper incision, and maintaining an exposure. To maintain the retractors is a challenge to the assistants. Improper retractor placement can easily injure the esophagus, and insufficient exposure can compromise the groove preparation on both sides of the vertebrae. The assistants also contribute significantly to a successful surgery by identifying and managing bleeders and efficiently applying suction devices. Nurses play indispensable roles in the surgery with instrument and supply preparation, patient positioning, and intraoperative cooperation. As the team actively communicates, performs each step with synchronized paces and mutual assistance, and delivers patient-centered care, the team members grow together during each operation and make an excellent surgical team.

Section 8: Shelter technique

Epidemiological of C2 involvement in OPLL

The cervical PLL connects the tectorial membrane around the atlanto-occipital joint cephalad and extends toward the sacral canal. Cervical OPLL is the heterotopic ossification of the PLL. Although C4, C5, and C6 segments are the most frequent sites, C2 involvement is not uncommon, with an incidence reported from 25% to 42%. Wang et al. analyzed OPLL that involved C2 and reported that 73.3% were mixed type, 24.5% and 11.2% were continuous and segmental types, respectively. As the spinal canal at C2 is wider and OPLL of this level is often thinner, the OPLL seldom compresses the spinal cord at C2. However, it does not mean that surgeons can leave it alone. According to the statistics of the authors' cases, 68.8% of patients with OPLL involving C2 develop spinal cord compression at C2/3 disc space, and 89.3% at the level of C3. In terms of the OPLL pattern at C2, 87.5% were not attached to the C2 vertebra, while almost 100% were continuous from the ossification behind C3 vertebra. Therefore, although not the leading cause of cord compression, the OPLL at C2 is tied to the ossified mass at its caudal level. Therefore, surgical decompression cannot be performed without addressing the ossification at C2.

Surgical technique for OPLL at C2

It remains controversial whether decompression to the C2 segment is needed in the surgery for OPLL extending to C2. Some surgeons believe that though without imaging evidence for compression at the C2 segment, a prophylactic procedure for C2 helps prevent spinal canal stenosis and cord compression in the future. Conventional surgical techniques mainly include anterior (through an anterior subtotal corpectomy) and posterior cervical decompression techniques (through laminectomy and LAM).

Given the limited exposure of C2 and the OPLL posterior to its vertebra during the anterior surgery, the surgeons often have to leave the ossified mass behind C2 vertebra just there (Fig. 2.8.1, panel 1 to 3). However, to leave the ossification at C2 unresected, it should be dissected from the rest of the OPLL at C2/3 disc space to ensure the complete decompression of the C3 segment, and the dissection here comes with the risk of CSF leakage. In addition, according to clinical observations, the residual OPLL at C2 may compress the spinal cord in the future among a small number of patients.

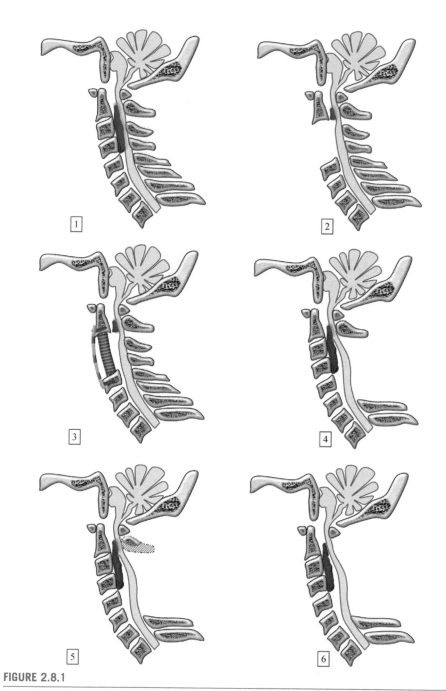

FIGURE 2.8.1

Illustration of conventional anterior and posterior decompression surgeries for OPLL involving C2.

The controversy in treating OPLL with C2 involvement by the posterior technique focuses on the necessity of C2 laminectomy (Fig. 2.8.1, panel 4 to 6). Some surgeons maintain that C2 laminectomy or LAM is necessary for OPLL with cord compression at the C2/3 disc space, and C1 posterior arch is resected additionally when cord compression is found at C2 level as well. As the C2 spinous process bears the attachments for muscles critical to cervical curvature maintenance, such as the semispinalis cervicis and the longissimus capitis, the resection of the C2 lamina and spinous process may lead to cervical kyphosis and neurological deterioration. On the contrary, others hold that decompression can be achieved via sublaminar resection of C2 instead of laminectomy or LAM.

Indeed, surgeons are divided on the proper management of OPLL at C2 in the conventional anterior or posterior decompression surgeries, and the key of the debate can be traced down to the risk-return trade-off between a prophylactic decompression of C2 and the morbidities of CSF leakage and cervical kyphosis. Since OPLL at C2 infrequently causes compression, the surgeon must prudently plan the decompression at this level with minimal unnecessary risk. In the ACAF technique, the surgical strategy for OPLL at C2 has undergone evolvement, which will be discussed in detail below.

Challenges of ACAF in OPLL at C2

The ACAF technique features treating the OPLL and the ventral vertebrae as a whole (i.e., VOC) and dissecting them from the surrounding structure. If the OPLL reaches C2, given the absence of a disc between C1 and C2, it is impossible to include the C2 as a part of the VOC to be mobilized. Since OPLL at C2 rarely causes spinal cord compression, the authors decided to dissect the OPLL at C2/3 early on when performing the ACAF technique (Fig. 2.8.2).

However, such dissection violates the founding intention of avoiding direct manipulation of the ossification in the ACAF technique. Moreover, as the OPLL is dissected through the constrained visualization of and access to the ossification at the C2/3 disc space in such a case, the risk of CSF leakage and neural injuries is higher than in subtotal corpectomy, more so if the OPLL is thick and wide at C2/3 level.

◀─────────────────────────────

(1–3) Anterior cervical subtotal corpectomy;

(1) Sagittal illustration of the cervical spine with OPLL at C2 to C4;

(2) C3 and C4 corpectomies;

(3) Resection of the OPLL behind C3 and C4 vertebrae.

(4–6) Posterior cervical laminectomy;

(4) Laminectomy of C3 to C7;

(5) Laminectomy of C3 to C7 and sublaminar resection of C26;

(6) Laminectomy of C2 to C7.

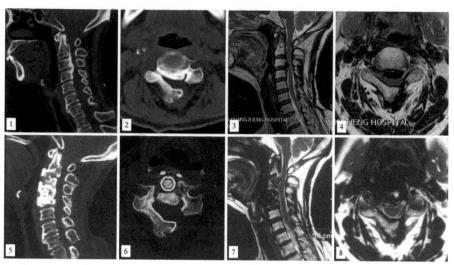

FIGURE 2.8.2

Imaging data of a case of OPLL involving C2 segment treated by ACAF technique.
(1) Sagittal CT before ACAF, showing OPLL from C2 to C4, which is thick at the C3/4 and thin at C2;
(2) Axial CT at the C3/4 of this patient showing a defect in the left lamina and right-deviated spinous process. The patient had undergone single-door laminoplasty from C3 to C7 with poor results;
(3) Cervical MRI before ACAF, showing spinal cord compression at C2 to C2/3;
(4) Axial MRI at C3/4 disc space, showing the spinal cord compression due to OPLL and effacement of the cerebrospinal fluid;
(5) Sagittal CT at one-year follow-up after ACAF, showing antedisplaced VOC from C3 to C3/4, expanded spinal canal, and the OPLL dissected at the C2/3 disc space. CSF leakage occurred during OPLL dissection, and a drain was placed at the lumbar cistern. The wound healed after two weeks;
(6) Axial CT at C3/4 showing antedisplaced VOC;
(7) Cervical MRI at one-year follow-up after ACAF, showing that the spinal cord relieved from compression and recovered cerebrospinal fluid zone;
(8) Axial MRI at the level of C3/4 disc space, showing resumed cerebrospinal fluid zone.

Shelter technique

Shelter technique specifically refers to the undercut technique on the C2 segment in the ACAF technique [1]. The ossified mass behind C2 vertebra is isolated from the posterior wall of C2 vertebra, and bone is resected from the posterior part of the C2 vertebra in the undercut manner. This leaves a niche, or a shelter, behind the residual C2 vertebra that contains the tip of the OPLL at C2 as the VOC is moved forward. According to the dictionary, shelter is a structure that provides cover or protection, for stay animals, for example. Applied in the ACAF, it provides a "house" for "the stray" ossification at C2. As such, the ossification at C2 leaves its original position and away from the spinal cord, and joins the bony reconstruction of the anterior vertebral column.

The technical challenge with the shelter technique lies in developing the niche at the back of the C2 vertebra and the isolation of OPLL at C2 in an undercut manner. Before developing the shelter space, the anterior bone of C3 can be removed to avoid blockage. To start the shelter resection, a 2 mm laminectomy rongeur enters the C2/3 disc space with the jaw pointing cephalad and engaging the plane between C2 vertebra and the OPLL to bite off the posteroinferior border of C2 vertebra. During the shelter resection, the tip of the cutter instrument is maintained slightly upward. Since a surgical microscope does not help with visualization, a head-mounted magnifier and lamp can be used instead. The shelter needs to be roomy enough to contain the C2 OPLL. Note that the residual vertebra and endplate should measure at least 10−12 mm in the anteroposterior dimension to provide sufficient graft receiving area and screw purchase (Figs. 2.8.3−2.8.5).

Surgical pearls

When the laminectomy rongeur is no longer productive due to the limited access, a power cutter (a burr or piezoelectrical osteotome) can be used instead to continue with the cephalad part.

The position of the ossification at C2 is checked with intraoperative X-ray to ensure the border of the shelter space created is beyond that of the ossified mass.

To undercut the posteroinferior part of C2 vertebra, the cutter instrument enters from the C2/3 disc space, engages bone through the plane between the vertebra and the OPLL, and works toward cephalad. In this way, as the OPLL serves as a barrier, the surgeons worry less about entering the spinal canal and injuring nerves.

The shelter border is set beyond the ossification tip longitudinally and beyond the lateral edges of the ossification horizontally (Fig. 2.8.6).

The bilateral borders of the shelter space can be based on the groove landmarks of the C3 vertebra or planned individually on the patient's preoperative CT.

When developing the shelter space, the nerve hook is used to palpate the ossification edges to determine if the boundaries of the shelter space are adequate.

If the proximal or bilateral dimension of the shelter space is within that of the ossification, the ossification cannot enter the space, compromising the antedisplacement and decompression (Fig. 2.8.7).

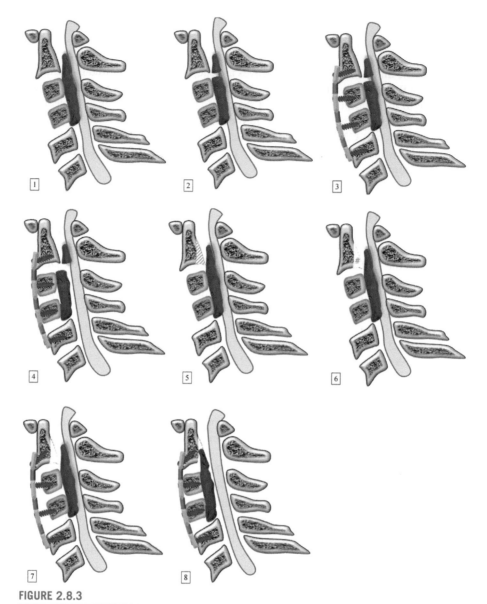

FIGURE 2.8.3

Sagittal illustration of ACAF and shelter techniques for OPLL involving C2 1 ~ 4 ACAF technique.

(1) The anterior parts of C3 and C4 resected;

(2) OPLL dissected at the C2/3 disc space;

(3) With instrumentation in place, VOC is mobilized;

(4) Antedisplaced VOC;

(5–8) Shelter technique;

(5) The anterior parts of C3 and C4 resected, and the desired shelter space indicated on the triangular area in the posterior part of the C2 vertebra;

(6) The shelter developed as bone has been removed (#);

(7) With instrumentation in place, VOC is mobilized;

(8) VOC antedisplaced.

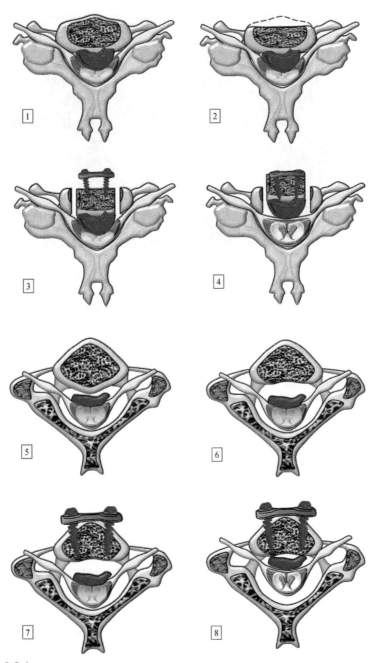

FIGURE 2.8.4

Axial illustration of comparison between ACAF technique and shelter technique.
(1—4) Axial illustration of VOC antedisplacement in ACAF technique;
(1) Axial view of the cervical vertebra, ossified mass, spinal cord, and nerve root at C5 segment;
(2) The anterior part of the vertebra resected;

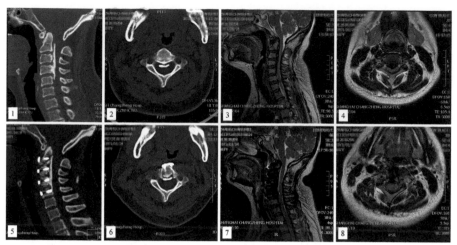

FIGURE 2.8.5

Imaging data of an OPLL case involving C2 segment treated by shelter technique.
(1) Sagittal CT before shelter operation showing OPLL of C2 to C4, which is thicker at the C3/4 disc space;
(2) Axial CT at C2 of this patient showing a thin piece of ossified mass;
(3) Cervical MRI before surgery, showing spinal cord compression at C2/3 to C4/5;
(4) Axial MRI at C3/4 disc space showing spinal cord compression due to the ossified mass and CSF effacement;
(5) Sagittal CT after shelter surgery with antedisplaced VOC from C2 to C4, expanded spinal canal, and OPLL moved ventrally as a whole;
(6) Axial CT at C2, showing antedisplaced ossified mass;
(7) Cervical MRI after shelter surgery, showing the spinal cord free of compression and recovered cerebrospinal fluid zone;
(8) Axial MRI at C3/4 disc space, showing the decompressed spinal cord and resumed cerebrospinal fluid zone.

(3) With instrumentation in place, grooving on both sides of the vertebra, and VOC mobilization;
(4) Antedisplaced VOC;
(5–8) Shelter technique;
(5) Axial view of the cervical vertebra, ossified mass, spinal cord, and nerve root at C2 segment;
(6) The posterior part of C2 resected into a shelter for the antedisplaced ossified mass;
(7) Instrumentation in place;
(8) Antedisplaced ossified mass entering the shelter.

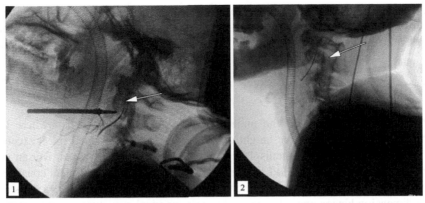

FIGURE 2.8.6

Comparison of shelter dimensions.

(1) The proximal margin of the shelter below the tip of the ossification;

(2) The proximal margin of the shelter leveling with the tip of the ossification (arrow), and a contoured plate in the shelter through the C2/3 disc space for demonstration. ↑.

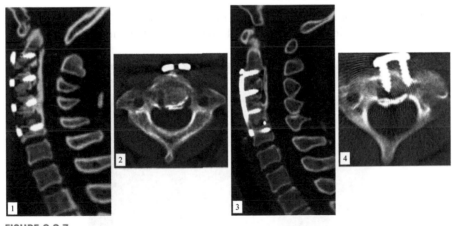

FIGURE 2.8.7

Comparison of antedisplacement with the shelter technique.

(1, 2) The height and width of the shelter exceeding the boundary of the ossification, and the C2 OPLL contained in the shelter as desired;

(3) The proximal border of the shelter below the ossification tip, resulting in their contact and obstruction;

(4) The shelter is not wide enough horizontally, resulting in contact and obstruction on both sides of the ossified mass.

After the shelter is created, the posterior wall of the C2 vertebra is dissected with a burr at the shelter's proximal border, and the presence of any bone ventrally is palpated with a nerve hook. The posterior wall of the C2 vertebra is dissected on both sides in line with the bilateral grooves on the C3 vertebra with the instrument accessing through the C2/3 disc space. As these cuts on both sides join the proximal cut developed in the previous step, the mobilization of OPLL at C2 is completed.

Indications of shelter technique

OPLL mobilization through the undercut technique is recommended where the OPLL extends within half the height of the vertebra. If the ossified mass exceeds half the vertebra's height, antedisplacement of that vertebra is favored over an undercut technique. When the OPLL extends high up at C2, the anatomical constraint is beyond the capability of shelter and undercut technique (Fig. 2.8.8). As the shelter's dimension hinges upon the surgical access, cervical curvature, anteroposterior diameter of the C2 vertebra, and C2/3 disc height, it is difficult to plan for a shelter with accurate measurements before surgery. However, the authors have come up with two practical measurements based on the summary of the previous cases.

Elevation angle of C2 OPLL

To define the limit of shelter technique in managing OPLL at C2, the authors team introduced the elevation angle of C2 OPLL measured on the midsagittal CT image,

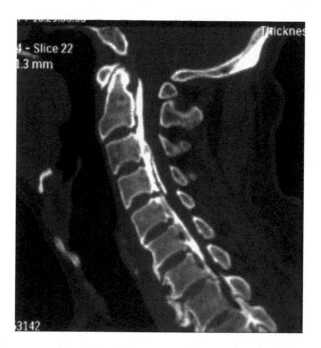

FIGURE 2.8.8

Sagittal CT image of the cervical spine.
The OPLL at the C2 extending too proximal that defies the feasibility of the shelter technique.

defined as the angle between two lines: one line links the point 10 mm posterior to the anterior rim of the C2 inferior endplate and the tip of OPLL at C2, and the other, the line through the anterior and posterior rims of the C2 endplate. Another parameter introduced is the angle of osteotomy at C2 vertebra measured from postoperative sagittal CT, defined as the angle between the shelter's anterior boundary and the C2 endplate (Fig. 2.8.9). In the authors' practice, the angle of osteotomy at C2 vertebra ranges from 24.3° to 70.2° with the mean of 42.4°, and the range between the 40° and 50° represents most of the cases. With this result, the elevation angle of C2 OPLL is measured before surgery, and a result greater than 50° poses more challenges to an intended shelter technique.

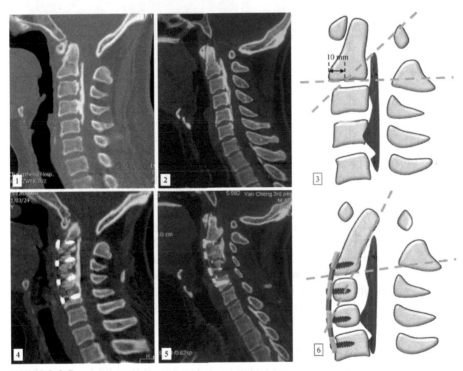

FIGURE 2.8.9

The feasibility of shelter technique for the C2 OPLL assessed from the evaluation of the C2 OPLL.
(1, 2) Preoperative sagittal CT images of two patients;
(3) Elevation angle of C2 OPLL measured before surgery. A line is drawn through the point on the endplate 10 mm from the anterior rim and the OPLL's tip. Another line is drawn between the anterior and posterior rims of the endplate. The angle between the two intersecting lines is the elevation angle of C2 OPLL;
(4, 5) Sagittal CT images of the two patients after the shelter procedure. The OPLL is thoroughly mobilized in 4 but insufficiently in 5;
(6) The angle of osteotomy at the C2 vertebra measured on the postoperative sagittal CT. It is the angle between the line at the shelter border the C2 endplate.

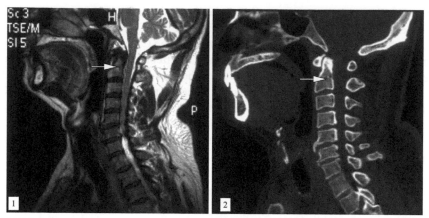

FIGURE 2.8.10

The vestigial disc between the odontoid process and the vertebra of C2 (arrow).
(1) Cervical midsagittal MRI;
(2) Cervical midsagittal CT.

Relationship between the vestigial C2 disc and OPLL

During the development and differentiation of the spine, the odontoid process of C2 gradually fuses with the C2 vertebra, leaving a vestigial disc at the separation site (Fig. 2.8.10). Observing the relationship between the vestigial disc and the OPLL at C2, the authors classified the patients into three groups where: OPLL's tip is above the vestigial disc (OPLL-higher group), below the vestigial disc (OPLL-lower group), and at the vestigial disc (same level group) (Fig. 2.8.11). After analyzing patients' postoperative images in each group, we found that mobilization and antedisplacement of the C2 OPLL were sufficient through the shelter technique in the OPLL-lower group, whereas a residual OPLL tip retained in the spinal canal among all the patients in the OPLL-higher group. And both results are seen in the group with the vestigial and OPLL's tip at the same level.

Based on these results, in the OPLL involving C2, the relations between the OPLL's tip and the vestigial disc are analyzed before surgery. If the OPLL's tip is below the vestigial disc, the shelter technique is feasible. If the OPLL's tip is above the vestigial disc, the less challenging technique of ACAF is favored since the OPLL is dissected in both procedures anyway. If they are of equal height, the surgeon makes the decision based on experience and the elevation angle mentioned above.

Types of OPLL at C2 and C3 and their relations

The authors categorized the relationship between the OPLL at the C2 and C3 into three types to describe the disease in the studies. ① Extensional: the continuous OPLL is attached to the C3 vertebra but clear from the C2 vertebra; ② connective: the continuous OPLL is attached to both the C2 and C3 vertebrae; and ③ separative:

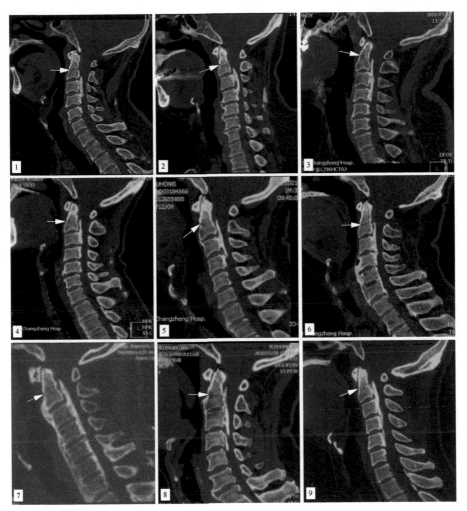

FIGURE 2.8.11

Classification of C2 OPLL based on its relation with the vestigial disc of C2 (arrow); the vestigial disc between the odontoid process and vertebra of C2 (arrow).
(1–3) OPLL-lower group where the OPLL's tip is below the vestigial disc;
(4–6) Same level group where the OPLL's tip is at the same height as the vestigial disc;
(7–9) OPLL-higher group, the OPLL's tip is beyond the vestigial disc.

the interruptive OPLL is attached to both C2 and C3 vertebrae, but the two parts are not joined. Among the patients, 87.5% were extensional, 12.5% connective, and 0% separative (Fig. 2.8.12). In general, the OPLL at C2 and C3 are mostly continuous, and the attachment with the vertebra is predominant at C3 but uncommon in C2. This reflects the development pattern of the OPLL at C2 that, in most cases, it gradually grows from C3 to C2.

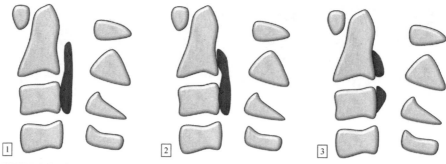

FIGURE 2.8.12

Three types of the relationship of the OPLL at C2 and C3.
(1) Extensional;
(2) Connective;
(3) Separative.

The results presented above provide evidence for the wide adoption of the shelter technique. In the shelter technique, to enable the OPLL at C2 to move anteriorly with VOC's antedisplacement at and below C3, the continuity of the disease between C2 and C3 is a prerequisite. This criterion is consistently met as none of the cases that the authors analyzed had an OPLL with an interruption between C2 and C3 or involving only C2 but not C3.

Reference

[1] Jingchuan S, Kaiqiang S, Shunmin W, et al. "Shelter Technique" in the treatment of ossification of the posterior longitudinal ligament involving the C2 segment. World Neurosurgery 2019;125:e456—64.

Section 9: Thoracic anterior controllable antedisplacement and fusion (TACAF)

Overview

Thoracic OPLL (T-OPLL) is characterized by paresthesia and motor dysfunction of extremities as well as visceral autonomic neuropathy due to spinal cord and/or nerve root compression from the ossified PLL (Fig. 2.9.1), first reported by Tsukimoto in 1960. It occurs less frequently than cervical OPLL with an incidence reported between 1.9% and 4.3% in Japan. The epidemiological study conducted by Ohtsuka et al. showed that the prevalence of T-OPLL is only 1/4 of that of cervical OPLL. Among thoracic spinal pathologies, however, T-OPLL features the worst postoperative symptom improvement and high morbidity. It has a predilection at midthoracic levels among middle-aged women. Rarely involving the thoracic levels alone, T-OPLL frequently comes with concomitant cervical OPLL and ossification of the ligamentum flavum (OLF). Dynamic factors have a minimal role in the pathogenesis of T-OPLL since the movement has been limited by ribs, which sets

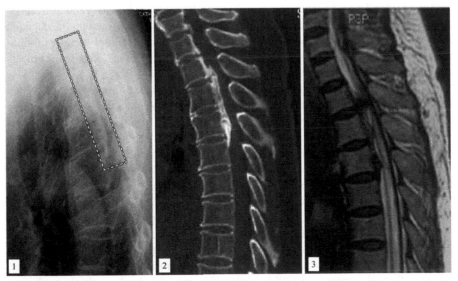

FIGURE 2.9.1

Imaging studies of t-OPLL.
(1) On X-ray, OPLL indicated with the dotted frame.
(2) Midsagittal CT image.
(3) Midsagittal MRI image.

T-OPLL apart from cervical or lumbar OPLL. At midthoracic levels, the spinal cord is more vulnerable to impingement due to the physiological kyphosis, the predilection of T-OPLL in this region, and poor vascular supply.

It does not take long for a clinically incipient T-OPLL to deteriorate, gradually in most patients but rapidly in others. Preceding clinical thoracic myelopathy, some patients may experience tightness and stiffness of the trunk and tingling that radiates to the scapular areas with severity correlated to the extent of cord impingement. On the other hand, pain and/or numbness of lower extremities may precede myelopathy in some patients, followed by tightness and stiffness of the trunk and lower extremities when the myelopathy becomes severe.

Patients usually demonstrate deep tendon hyperreflexia and pathological reflexes in hypertonic lower extremities with gait disturbance on neurological examination. As the myelopathy progresses, their lower extremities become atrophic and decreased in strength, which leads to spastic pain, gait instability, and even inability to walk. However, when the OPLL occurs in the lower thoracic levels or thoracolumbar junction, the compression affects epiconus and/or conus medullaris and injures both the upper and lower motor neurons. The patient may present with the so-called mixed-type paralysis with the pyramidal sign and flaccid paresis with diminished or absent knee or ankle reflexes and muscular atrophy.

The compression level in T-OPLL is usually reliably reflected by the distribution of sensory disturbance, namely impaired superficial and deep sensation and diminished or indifferent superficial reflexes. The myelopathy manifests as brisk tendon reflexes of the lower extremities and the presence of patella and ankle clonus and pathological reflexes. In severe cases, sphincter dysfunction is also noted as dysuria, atonic bladder, incontinence, sexual dysfunction among male patients, and cauda equina syndrome characterized by atonic anal sphincter on digital rectal examination. When OPLL develops in combination with OLF, dorsal cord syndrome is also noted, such as gait disturbance.

In addition, T-OPLL usually associates with cervical and lumbar disease. When OPLL is distributed in the thoracic and cervical spine, dizziness, nausea, emesis, and pain on lower limbs also develop.

The incidence of OPLL is similar between the upper thoracic spine and the middle and lower part, as reported by Epstein et al. Plain radiography has a limited role in locating the OPLL lesion and establishing clinical diagnosis due to the ribcage. However, it helps with screening and evaluation of spinal alignment and kyphosis. 3D-CT and MRI studies are essential to the diagnosis of T-OPLL. CT scans demonstrate the levels that the OPLL affects on axial and sagittal images, the type of ossification, the extent of canal stenosis, and the presence of OLF, information fundamental to the decision-making on surgical technique. MRI provides valuable information as to the extent of cord compression, intramedullary signal intensity, and the affected segments. T-OPLL is classified into flat, beak, multiple-beak, and continuous described by the investigation committee on the Ossification of the Spinal Ligaments of the Japanese Ministry of Public Health and Welfare. In particular, beak type of single or multiple levels is usually associated with grave thoracic

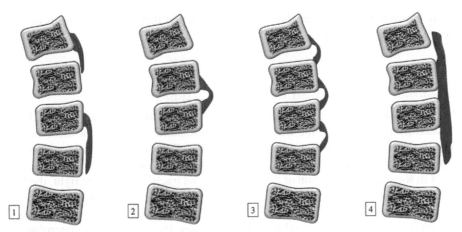

FIGURE 2.9.2

Classification of thoracic ossification of posterior longitudinal ligament.
(1) Flat type.
(2) Beak type.
(3) Multiple-beak type.
(4) Continuous type.

myelopathy. Furthermore, Matsumoto et al. described mixed-type OPLL as those with two types or more (Fig. 2.9.2).

Conventional surgical options

Characterized by prolonged courses and pronounced symptoms, T-OPLL carries increased surgical risk, technical demand, and suboptimal prognosis. Patients with radiological canal stenosis associated with T-OPLL can maintain the extent of symptoms without deterioration for a long time. Mild symptoms are managed with conservative treatment with antispasmodic and antiinflammatory agents, analgesics, and muscle relaxants. Neuroprotective agents can be used for neurologic symptom improvement.

When developing to a certain extent, T-OPLL causes grave myelopathy and acutely progressing clinical symptoms. Paralysis of lower limbs and sphincteric dysfunction even develop rapidly. Surgical management should set in as soon as the clinical diagnosis is established since it is the only solution to resolve compressing structures and restore neural function. The surgical treatment principles are to relieve cord and nerve root impingement from the OPLL and provide a favorable biological and biomechanical environment for cord and nerve recovery. Three surgical approaches are available to T-OPLL, namely the anterior approach that allows for direct decompression, the posterior approach that provides indirect decompression, and a combined anterior and posterior approach. All three approaches have been shown with clinical benefits and downsides, and there is no consensus on the best approach for T-OPLL.

Decompression via an anterior approach

Decompression is performed via anterior sternal splitting approach for T-OPLL located from T1 to T3 while transthoracic anterolateral approach for those below T4. In the sternal splitting approach, the spine is accessed for decompression via a midline split on the sternum, combined with resection of the left sternoclavicular joint in some cases, retraction of the esophagus and trachea toward the right, the left common carotid artery to the left, and the brachiocephalic trunk inferiorly (Fig. 2.9.3).

With the patient in a lateral decubitus position, the transthoracic anterolateral approach is performed by an oblique incision along the rib's course from the anterior edge of the latissimus dorsi muscle to the costochondral junction. In addition, the scapular elevation is performed when accessing upper thoracic levels, whereas the diaphragm is transected along the peripheral margin in some cases when exposing the thoracolumbar segments. Upon visualizing the vertebrae, the parietal pleura is exfoliated from the chest wall; resect the costotransverse and costovertebral joints to facilitate the anterior transposition of the rib, the posterior 1/3 of the vertebrae, pedicles, facet joints, and a part of the ribs of the affected levels before thinning the ossification mass until the ventral side of the dural sac is exposed (Fig. 2.9.4). The resected rib is then used as intervertebral graft material.

The conventional anterior procedures enable direct cord decompression by removal of the ossified mass but are technically demanding and come with exposure-related complications, such as major vascular injuries, chyle leak, injury of the recurrent laryngeal nerve and intercostal nerve, and pulmonary dysfunction;

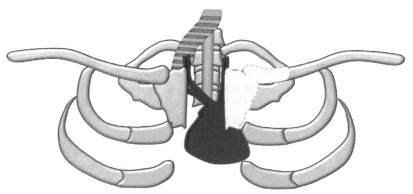

FIGURE 2.9.3

Illustration of sternal splitting approach.

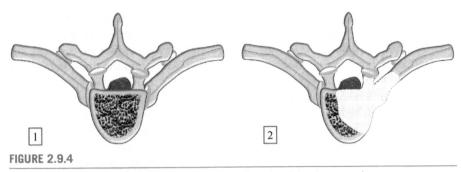

FIGURE 2.9.4

Illustration of decompression by the transthoracic anterolateral approach.
(1) The ossification in the thoracic spine before surgery.
(2) The extent of bony resection.

and postoperative complications including neurological deterioration, CSF leakage, and epidural hematoma.

Circumferential decompression

Anterior surgeries provide the best resolution to thoracic myelopathy induced by OPLL. Their success lies in whether the OPLL is removed or allowed to float with safe and straightforward surgical maneuver, a precarious step, in particular in cases of bulky OPLL or with concomitant OLF. For this challenging group of patients, a circumferential decompression via a combined anterior and posterior approaches has been described.

This technique includes a stage-one procedure of posterior laminectomy that resolves posterior impingement on the cord and provides room for the cord's posterior shift during the second stage procedure. Other preparatory steps for the second stage surgery include thinning the medial part of the facet joints and pedicles, developing grooves of around 1 cm deep on both sides of the vertebrae, mobilizing the adhesion between the OPLL and the dura (Fig. 2.9.5), pedicle screw insertion, and thoracic dekyphosis of 5 ~ 10 degrees. A second stage procedure is arranged three weeks

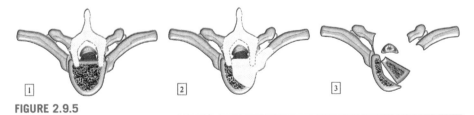

FIGURE 2.9.5

Illustration of circumferential decompression.
(1) Laminectomy via posterior approach in the stage-one procedure.
(2) Bony resection via anterior approach in the stage-two procedure.
(3) Fusion achieved with morselized cancellous bone from the ilium.

later if the patient does not fully resume neurological function. Using the grooves from the stage-one procedure as landmarks, the width and extent of the vertebra to be resected are defined, 1/3 of the vertebra and the ossification are resected via an anterior approach before morselized cancellous bone from the ilium is inserted for fusion.

The circumferential decompression by a combined anterior and posterior approach requires higher surgical expertise with a higher incidence of complications while delivering adequate cord decompression. Circumferential decompression, all performed with a posterior approach alone, was thus introduced.

Satoshi Kato et al. reported ossification removal through a posterior procedure that provides visualization and access to the ventral area of the spinal cord via extensive posterior column resection (including the spinous processes, laminae, transverse processes, and pedicles on both sides) and the ligation and elevation of the nerve roots at the levels of anterior decompression (Fig. 2.9.6). All three cases reported regained cord function without deterioration. No intra- or postoperative complications occurred except for a dural tear in one case. Since the posterior spinal structure has been extensively removed, if complete removal of ossification proves impossible or the spinal cord is still encroached despite a complete lesion resection, further decompression can be gained by dekyphosis. However, the risk of ischemic spinal cord injury from the ligation of bilateral nerve roots has constrained this technique to OPLL of fewer than three levels.

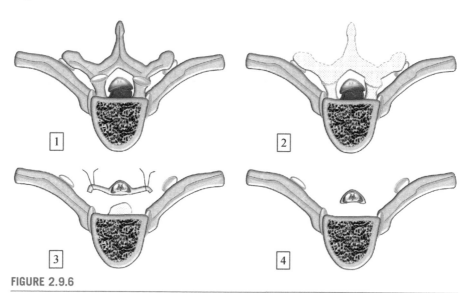

FIGURE 2.9.6

Illustration of the technique described by satoshi Kato.
(1) The ossification in the thoracic spine before surgery.
(2) The posterior structure of the spinal canal removed from the posterior procedure.
(3) Nerve roots ligated and lifted, and ossification removed.
(4) The final structure after surgery.

A "cave-in" type of circumferential decompression, described by Xiaoguang Liu with Peking University, China, starts with the resection of the posterior wall of the spinal canal. If the spinal cord is still compressed from the front, as assessed by intra-operative B ultrasonography, the bilateral bony resection is carried forward along the pedicles' medial walls and 60° toward the midline when reaching the roots of the pedicles. The bone tunnel on both sides become communicated and form a cave, which results in resection of cancellous bone 1/4 to 1/3 of the vertebra volume. The ossification on the ventral side of the dura and the posterior wall of the vertebra constitutes the ceiling of the cave. The anterior decompression is completed with the ossification's release off the ceiling of the cave and removal from either side (Fig. 2.9.7). That case series had improved cord function after surgery with a low incidence of neurological deterioration but a high incidence of postoperative CSF leak (58.3%). What is more, this technique is constrained to diseases of three levels or fewer in the case of cord ischemia.

Posterior decompression

Direct decompression through an anterior approach provides good results for T-OPLL of circumscribed or beak type while being too challenging and risky for multisegmental diseases. In such cases, LAM through a posterior approach that

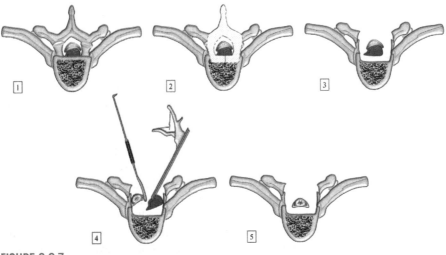

FIGURE 2.9.7

Illustration of the "cave-in" circumferential decompression.
(1) The ossification in the thoracic spine before surgery.
(2) The posterior wall of the spinal canal and posterior cancellous bone of the vertebra removed, and the path of bone resection joined, forming a cave.
(3) A completed "cave" structure.
(4) Release of the ossification off the spinal cord from the side with gentle elevation of the spinal cord.
(5) The final structure after surgery.

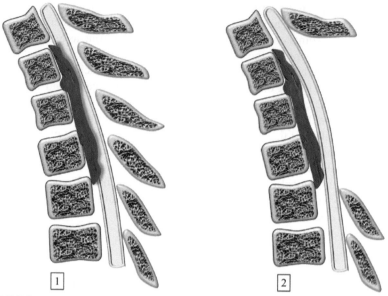

FIGURE 2.9.8

Illustration of posterior procedures.
(1) The ossification in the thoracic spine before surgery.
(2) Final result after laminectomy.

expands the central canal (Fig. 2.9.8) becomes the procedure of choice, particularly in diseases of the cervicothoracic junction.

However, either laminectomy or LAM through a posterior approach provides only moderate benefits when the OPLL is located at the apex of thoracic kyphosis or in hyperkyphotic thoracic spines (Fig. 2.9.9).

Indeed, posterior techniques weaken the tension band effect contributed by the posterior structure and predispose the thoracic spine to hyperkyphosis. The risk of hyperkyphosis can be assessed with ossification-kyphosis angle, a parameter described by Yasuaki Tokuhashi, that when this angle is above 20°, hyperkyphosis may develop and cause neurological deterioration, demonstrated by Norihiro et al. In a retrospective review by Sugita and Shurei et al., all the nine cases who had received posterior decompression with instrumentation saw 100% growth of the ossification at final follow-up, but none reported symptom aggravation. A case presented by Hiroaki Kimura et al. features a patient receiving posterior instrumentation alone without decompression who reported not only good immediate results but also shrinking ossification at the final follow-up. The team attributed the growth ceasing effect to the stabilized disc space in an instrumented spine with preserved anatomy dorsal to the spinal canal, which is consistent with the observation of Matsuyama et al.

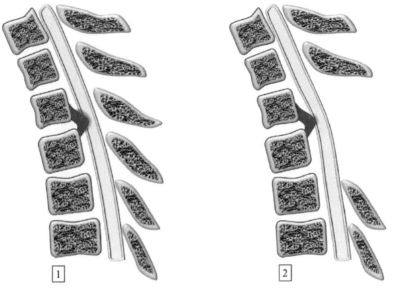

FIGURE 2.9.9

OPLL at the apex of thoracic kyphosis.
(1) The ossification in the thoracic spine before surgery.
(2) Sustained cord compression despite laminectomy.

Among others who have attempted to address multisegmental T-OPLL from the posterior, Zhongqiang Chen, a Chinese surgeon, described a technique of resection of the posterior walls of thoracic vertebrae combined with dekyphosis. Upon completing the resection of the posterior walls of vertebrae, circumferential decompression is performed, and bilateral facet joints are removed at the level of maximum compression. After removing the ossification, dekyphosis is performed via compression of the construct over the set screws, both cephalad and caudal, to the level of decompression to reduce local kyphosis (Fig. 2.9.10). Good surgical results were obtained in all the five cases reported though four out of five had postoperative CSF leakage, and one developed epidural hematoma that required emergency debridement surgery.

Surgical results and complications

The benefit of surgery in OPLL-induced myelopathy in the thoracic spine is usually mediocre, unlike in other thoracic pathologies. According to a multicenter study by Shiro Imagama et al., the most frequent postoperative complication from thoracic surgery for OPLL is worsened neurological deficit, whose incidence and time to recovery are associated with the combination of OLF, severe compressive myelopathy before surgery, radiological evidence of cord indentation, surgical manipulation of

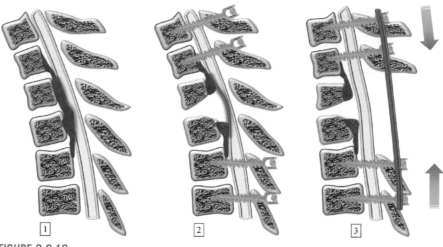

FIGURE 2.9.10

Illustration of the dekyphosis technique.
(1) The ossification in the thoracic spine before surgery.
(2) Circumferential decompression completed.
(3) Straightened thoracic spine upon compression on screws cephalad and caudal to the level of decompression.

the spinal cord, and incomplete decompression. Meanwhile, the impact of surgical time and technique is also worthy of our attention. The comparison of several multicenter studies (Table 2.9.1) of different periods indicates that surgical results have been on the rise over time but concurrent with a growing incidence of complications and worsening neural deficits. This might be partly accounted for by the suboptimal design of studies.

Higher risk of complication has been found associated with the level of surgery, preoperative JOA score, the clinical and radiological profile of myelopathy, positive result of prone and supine position test (PST), surgical time, and intraoperative variation of spinal cord pulsation assessed with ultrasound. Therefore, surgical management preceding severe myelopathy provides a lower incidence of perioperative morbidities, fewer spinal cord manipulation, and better decompression results. A

Table 2.9.1 Comparison of the reported surgical results of T-OPLL.

Neurological deterioration	JOA score recovery rate	
Matsumoto M et al., 2008 (multicenter study)	11.7%	36.8%
Matsumoto M et al., 2011 (multicenter study)	26.3%	45.4%
Xu N et al., 2015 (literature review)	13.9%	50.4%
Imagama S et al., 2018 (multicenter study)	32.2%	55%

positive PST result, produced when the spinal cord compression worsens as the patient changes their position, suggests significant neurological deficits.

A comparison between direct and indirect surgical decompression revealed, counterintuitively, that indirect decompression was associated with greater neurological improvement than direct decompression (63.4% vs. 44.4%) and lower incidence of complication.

Antedisplacement of the thoracic vertebrae

From the review above, there are many surgical procedures derived from direct and indirect decompression for T-OPLL. The benefit is achieved with direct decompression from the anterior or posterior approach and indirect decompression from the posterior, but their incidence of complication remains high. The complicated anatomy involved in anterior surgeries constitutes a constraint of its wider adoption. Posterior surgeries are safer than the anterior ones, but direct decompression via a posterior approach is still technically demanding with a continuously high incidence of complications such as neurological deterioration and CSF leak. Technically easier, though, posterior surgeries have been reported to be associated with the ossification's continuous growth since it is left in place. Therefore, a safer and less complicated technique for T-OPLL is still urgently needed.

As such, the author and his team have described an antedisplacement technique for cervical vertebrae where direct cord decompression is achieved with antedisplaced vertebra and ossification without the risk of intraoperative complication due to surgical manipulation around the dural sac. The team then replicated the procedure for T-OPLL. While an anterior approach in the thoracic spine bears enormous technical challenges due to the complex organ and vascular anatomy in the front and requires particularly skillful maneuvers, the team attempted the vertebra antedisplacement from posterior. This procedure allows decompression in situ as the vertebra ossification complex (VOC) is ventrally displaced with rods and screws and carries a lower risk of postoperative complications, given the safer and more controllable decompression compared with the anterior decompression from posterior described earlier.

Surgical setup
Plaster table

The patient is placed on a plaster table to eliminate movement that increases surgical risk.

Intraoperative neurophysiological monitoring (IONM)

IONM is essential in determining the distance of vertebra antedisplacement. It facilitates the proper antedisplacement as it gives off alert soon after the VOC is excessively antedisplaced.

Piezoelectrical osteotome

Easy to use, a piezoelectrical osteotome prevents heat-induced neurological compromise from a burr during the dissection of the ribs and the posterior vertebral structure.

O-arm X-ray system

An O-arm X-ray system provides a better idea of the extent of thoracic vertebra antedisplacement than a C-arm unit as it also addresses the interference of bony structures around the shoulder. In quantifying the antedisplacement, however, the surgeon assesses from the length of the screw to be inserted rather than the images provided by the O-arm.

Preparation for antedisplacement

How much a spinal cord recover from myelopathy depends on the extent of antedisplacement, which requires meticulous planning before surgery. A complete set of imaging studies is thus essential to the measurement of the planned antedisplacement. X-ray defines thoracic spinal curvature, CT delineates the dimension and extent of the ossification, and MRI pinpoints the severity and levels of cord compression.

X-ray is reviewed first to locate the ossification on both anteroposterior and lateral views of the whole spine.

The profile of the OPLL is then appreciated on CT images and measured for thickness at every involved level. The extent of antedisplacement is equal to the OPLL thickness at the level of maximum canal stenosis.

With the extent of antedisplacement and the pitch of the vertebra screws, the number of threads left between the plate and the vertebra is determined to reflect that extent.

The curvature measurements will be used during surgery during rod contouring with the rod gauge.

When displacing the vertebra anteriorly with titanium rods, care should be taken to prevent an incomplete displacement due to nonsynchronous movement of the vertebra on both sides.

Anesthesia and patient positioning

After general anesthesia, the patient is placed supine on a gurney. When the plaster table is ready, the patient is transferred to the plaster table in a prone position with the anesthesiologist's assistance. Sandbags are placed at the foot of the plaster table and the patient's arms immobilized with bandages to minimize motion.

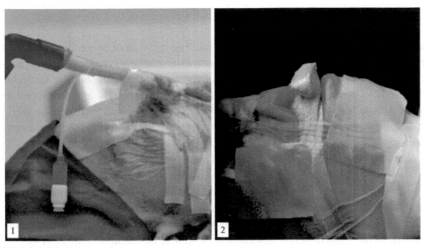

FIGURE 2.9.11

Well-padded skin of the patient's face.
(1) The padded frontal.
(2) The padded jaw.

Algoplaque hydrogel is applied to the patient's face to prevent pressure injuries (Fig. 2.9.11).

Soft pads are placed around the patient on the plaster table to prevent pressure-induced skin damage in the prolonged prone position.

When an OPLL involves the cervicothoracic junction, proper traction is applied to the shoulders for better visualization under fluoroscopy (Fig. 2.9.12).

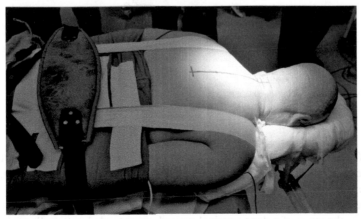

FIGURE 2.9.12

Proper traction applied on the shoulders to improve intraoperative fluoroscopy.

Exposure

According to the levels of the procedure, a midline incision of proper length is made. Paraspinal muscles are dissected off the posterior vertebral structure in a caudal to cephalad manner when hemostasis is achieved with bovie and bipolar coagulator (Fig. 2.9.13). When the exposure is complete, screw tunnels are developed and placed with markers in the pedicles of vertebrae to be antedisplaced as well as two levels above and below to confirm the levels of instrumentation and screw trajectory.

When an accurate level identification is not achieved before the surgery or in less experienced hands, the level identification process can precede skin incision.

Although a more extensive surgical field is warranted for thoracic antedisplacement, the surgeon should withhold from exposing too extensively before level confirmation with markers. For segments not included in antedisplacement, limited exposure to the pedicle screw insertion sites should be enough (Fig. 2.9.14).

Since the antedisplacement procedure is more applicable to cases with extensive T-OPLL, a stronger construct is established with the instrumentation of two levels caudal and cephalad to the LOC.

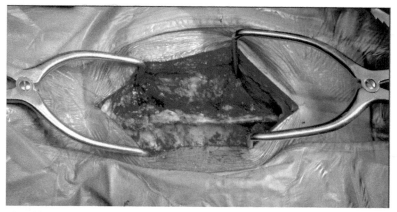

FIGURE 2.9.13

Posterior vertebral structures exposed.

Dissection of ribs on both sides

At the LOC levels, the exposure is expanded laterally to the ribs, which are then cut with a piezoelectrical osteotome at 5 mm lateral to the transverse costal facet. A neural probe is used to validate the dissection on both sides (Fig. 2.9.15).

To facilitate this step, a piezoelectrical osteotome with a curved cutter is recommended. In the cases of a deep surgical wound, an extended cutter allows for easier access.

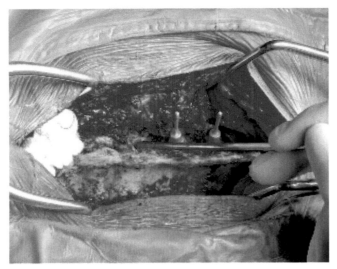

FIGURE 2.9.14

Limited exposure of the levels not to be antedisplaced for pedicle screw insertion only.

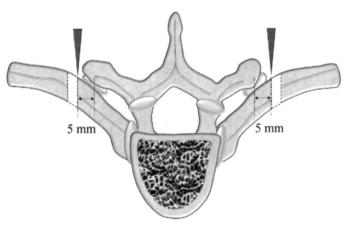

FIGURE 2.9.15

The ribs on both sides cut with piezoelectrical osteotome at 5 mm lateral to the transverse costal facet.

VOC dissection

A plate is placed on each side of the spine at the base between the lamina and spinous process to stabilize the mobilized laminae. One of the plates is fixed one level higher than the other. A groove is developed with a piezoelectrical osteotome at the junction between the lamina and articular process, or the medial wall of the pedicle, on each side of the spine to mobilize the lamina (Fig. 2.9.16). The

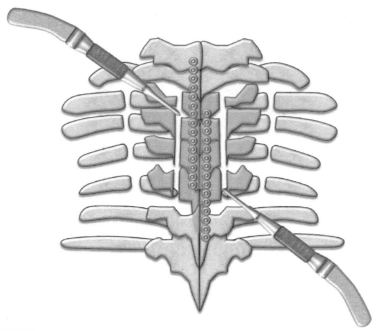

FIGURE 2.9.16

Stabilization plates, one of which is fixed one level higher than the other.
A groove developed with piezoelectrical osteotome at the junction between the lamina and articular process, or the medial wall of pedicle, on each side of the spine.

intervertebral discs on both ends of the VOC are removed and inserted with cages. As such, the VOC is mobilized.

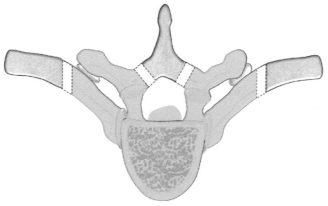

FIGURE 2.9.17

Thoracic VOC composed of the vertebra, ossification, and part of the ribs.

VOC in the thoracic spine is distinct form the cervical one as it includes the vertebra, ossification, and parts of the ribs (Fig. 2.9.17).

When developing the bilateral grooves along the laminae, care should be taken to ensure visualization by effective hemostasis and prevent dural injury with gelfoam and gauze swab.

Pedicle screw insertion

Posted pedicle screws are fully inserted in the prepared tunnels and prebent titanium rods fitted into the tulip of the screws. The rod contour can be fine-tuned in situ. Then the screws on the VOC are backed out by the number of threads calculated preoperatively and locked with set screw (Fig. 2.9.18).

The use of posted pedicle screws is recommended to accommodate rod and set screw insertion on screws backed out after VOC antedisplacement.

Antedisplacement of VOC

Set screws are placed on levels above and below the VOC but not seated. Multiple screwdrivers are mounted to tighten the set screws in a synchronized manner so that

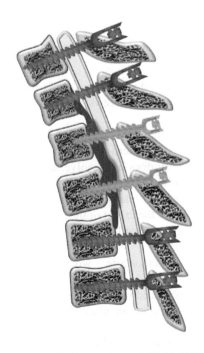

FIGURE 2.9.18

Posted pedicle screws fully seated in the vertebrae cephalad and caudal to the VOC. Pedicle screws with short post inserted in the VOC and backed out by the number of threads that represents the distance of antedisplacement.

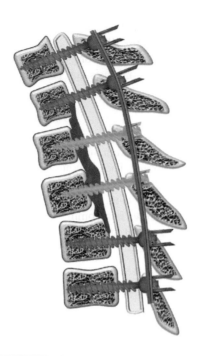

FIGURE 2.9.19

Illustration of VOC antedisplacement in the thoracic spine.

the VOC is pushed ventrally with the lever-arm effect of the rods (Fig. 2.9.19). The extended part is broken off the posted screws. A small plate can be used on the ribs along the edge for stabilization.

During antedisplacement, attention is paid to the INOM and stop the maneuver immediately upon any abnormal pattern and resume until signals become normal again. If the signal abnormality does not resolve, the VOC is reduced posteriorly and the spinal cord soaked in warm normal saline.

In cases with bulky lesions, fluoroscopy by O-arm can be performed after antedisplacement maneuver to verify the extent of the displacement. The compression of the posterior construct can be performed to gain extra decompression via dekyphosis if more displacement is wanted.

Bone graft placement, hemostasis, wound closure, and postoperative immobilization.

The bone graft material is placed in the bilateral grooves. After adequate hemostasis and irrigation, one or two drains are placed before the wound is closed layer by layer.

The commonly used graft material includes allograft or synthetic bone chips or pliable threads. The hemostatic hydrogel can be injected on the grooves if they become too oozy after autograft placement.

Active bleeders are always carefully managed with a bipolar coagulator.

Case presentation

(1) Highlights of the case

A middle-aged woman came in with weakness of lower limbs, tightness around the chest and abdomen, and bladder and bowel dysfunction for six months and aggravated over the past two months.

Physical exam was noted for an impaired sense of light touch, temperature, and pain in the trunk below the sternal angle, genital area, and lower extremities. Muscle strength was measured at 3/5 on the anteromedial muscles of the thighs and the anterior and posterior muscles of the lower legs, and 4/5 on the plantar and dorsal muscles of the feet. Hyperreflexia was elicited from bilateral knees and ankles while diminished anal wink was present. Pathological signs were not elicited. Thoracic JOA was cored 3 out of 11.

Image findings:

X-ray: OPLL from C7 to T5 vertebra (Fig. 2.9.20).

CT: OPLL from C7 to T5 of 9 mm thick. Maximum canal stenosis of 84% and minimum anteroposterior dimension of the canal 4.6 mm (Fig. 2.9.21).

MRI: Severely compressed cord from T2 to T5 (Fig. 2.9.21).

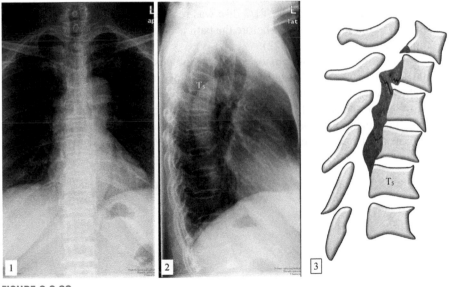

FIGURE 2.9.20

Preoperative X-ray.

(1) Anteroposterior view.

(2) Lateral view.

(3) Schematic representation of the OPLL.

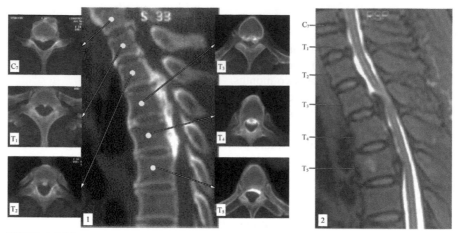

FIGURE 2.9.21

(1) Preoperative CT.
(2) Preoperative MRI.

(2) During surgery

After general anesthesia, the T1/2 disc was resected from anterior with the patient in the supine position before the patient was flipped to a prone position on a plaster table (Fig. 2.9.22).

A midline incision was made to expose the posterior structures from C7 through T7 and expanded laterally to the costovertebral joints. Pedicle screw tunnels were drilled from C7 to T7. The ribs from T2 to T5 on both sides were cut with piezoelectrical osteotome lateral to the costovertebral joints to facilitate the antedisplacement of T2 to T5. The laminae, spinous process, and ligaments at the levels caudal and cephalad to the VOC were removed, and two

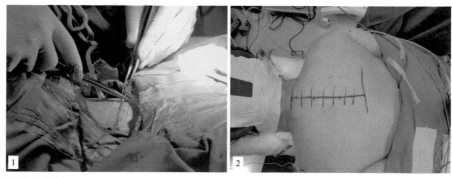

FIGURE 2.9.22

(1) The T1/2 disc material released from an anterior approach.
(2) Patient placed prone on a plaster table.

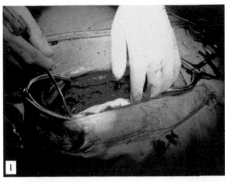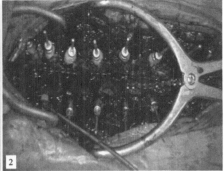

FIGURE 2.9.23

(1) Posterior spinal structures from C7 through T7 exposed.
(2) Prepared screw tunnels and two plates along the spinous process, one of which being one level higher than the other.

plates were inserted along the base of the spinous process on both sides for stabilization, with one being a level higher than the other (Fig. 2.9.23).

The laminae from T2 to T5 were dissected with a groove medial to the medial wall of the pedicles. As such, the VOC was fully mobilized from the laminae and ribs. Standard tulip pedicle screws were used on the planned VOC from T2 to T5 while posted screws were inserted at caudal and cephalad levels. The 9 mm height difference of the heads of these two groups of screws represents the distance of antedisplacement. Prebent titanium rods were fitted, T5/6 disc space released, and set screws on T2 through T5 tightened. The construct was then ready for the antedisplacement maneuver. As the set screws on both ends of the construct tightened gradually, the vertebrae of T2 through T5 were pushed forward through the lever effect of the rods and screws until the screw ends were of the same height (Figs. 2.9.24 and 2.9.25).

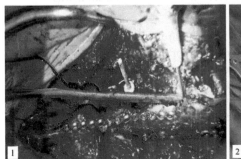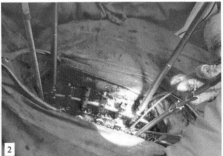

FIGURE 2.9.24

(1) Grooves developed on the laminae medial to the medial wall of the pedicles;
(2) Set screws on the caudal and cephalad ends tightened and vertebrae of T2 to T5 antedisplaced.

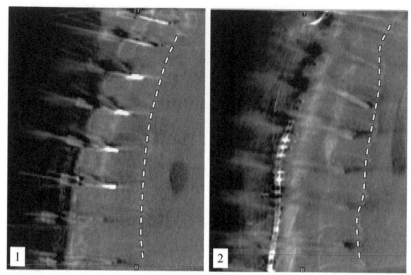

FIGURE 2.9.25

The extent of antedisplacement verified on intraoperative fluoroscopy with O-arm.
(1) Sagittal view prior to antedisplacement where the dotted line indicates the anterior margin of the thoracic vertebrae;
(2) Sagittal view after antedisplacement with a significant shift of the dotted line.

At finishing, bone graft material was placed on the grooves and intervertebral spaces followed by irrigation, hemostasis, drain placement, and layer-by-layer wound closure.

(3) Rehabilitation and follow-up

On postoperative day 1, the patient no longer felt the sense of tightness. Muscle strength of the lower extremities improved to 4+/5 and bladder and bowel control resumed. Thoracic JOA score was tested at 9/11, representing a 75% improvement. There was tenderness over the ribs, but respiration was unaffected.

On imaging studies, the maximum stenosis of the spinal canal was reduced from 84% to 46%, and its minimum anteroposterior dimension increased from 4.6 to 10.0 mm. A small amount of pleural effusion was noted (Figs. 2.9.26 and 2.9.27).

Three months after surgery, the patient went up or down the stairs without having to hold the handrail. Thoracic JOA was scored at 10, an improvement from 9 recorded previously. The ribs were nontender upon palpation (Fig. 2.9.28).

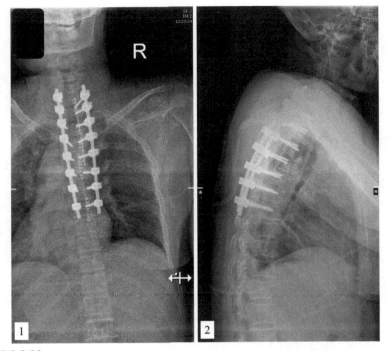

FIGURE 2.9.26

X-ray three days after surgery.
(1) Anteroposterior view.
(2) Lateral view.

On image studies, instrumentation was well positioned and spinal canal volume was restored. The spinal cord resumed its shape and curvature, surrounded by adequate CSF (Figs. 2.9.28−2.9.31).

Well-positioned instrumentation and resumed spinal canal volume.

Discussion

Compared with conventional techniques, thoracic VOC antedisplacement via a posterior approach described above obviates the high-risk step of ossification removal and avoids dural and cord injuries. Instead, the VOC is pushed away from the spinal cord under IONM with the lever effect of the screw-and-rod system, a safe and controllable process of cord decompression without sacrificing the anatomical course of the spinal cord. One of the challenging steps in this technique is VOC's

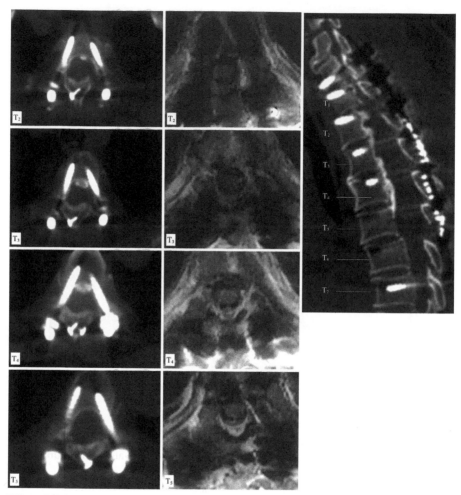

FIGURE 2.9.27

CT and MRI images three days after surgery.

mobilization via bilateral rib dissection, as this may run the risk of intercostal neural or vascular injury. In effect, such injury is rare. Based on existing reports and our experience, the rarity of this injury is attributable to anatomical features and surgical techniques: (1) intercostal nerves and vessels course along the rib interspaces, away from the bony structure, and subperiosteal elevation reduces hemorrhage; (2) with the anterior cortex of the rib yet to be disconnected, a laminectomy rongeur is

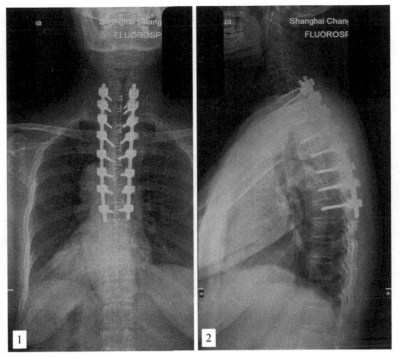

FIGURE 2.9.28

X-ray three months after surgery.
(1) Anteroposterior view.
(2) Lateral view.

used instead of the piezoelectrical osteotome, which further lowers the risk of parietal pleural or vascular injuries.

Postoperative follow-up results demonstrate that neurological improvement was valid among T-OPLL patients receiving antedisplacement procedure, in particular when measured with m-JOA. Adequate cord decompression is validated from imaging evidence. Except for minimal pleural effusion, no other complication occurred after the surgery, which sets this technique aside from the conventional ones with the high incidence of dural tear, CSF leak, and worsened neurological deficits.

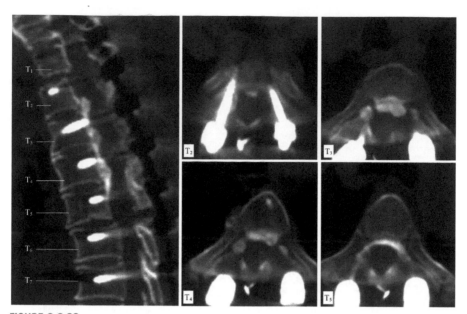

FIGURE 2.9.29

CT images three months after surgery.

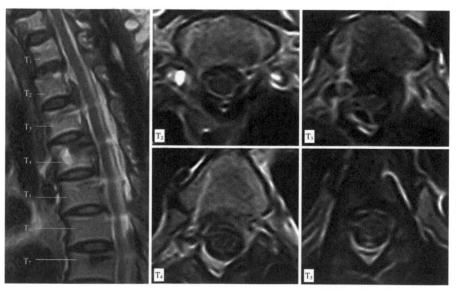

FIGURE 2.9.30

MRI images three months after surgery.
Spinal cord in its natural curvature surrounded by CSF.

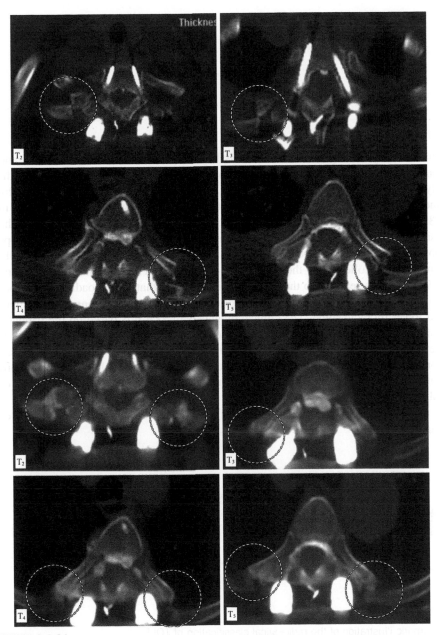

FIGURE 2.9.31

Progress of bone healing in the ribs. The images of the ribs three days after surgery are presented in the upper four panels, while those at three months are in the lower four panels. A continuous callous is evident along the dissection interface without angulation between both ends of the interface.

Section 10: Bridge crane technique

Overview

Anatomically, the ligamentum flavum is located posterior to the spinal canal and constitute its posterior wall with the laminar parts laterally and capsule part medially. TOLF has been recognized as one of the major causes of thoracic myelopathy since its first description by Polgar in 1920 on lateral radiography. TOLF occurs in 3.8%–26% of the general population, much rarer than OPLL, and more often in the Asian population, such as people in Japan, China, and South Korea. OLF develops most frequently to the upper 1/3 or lower 1/3 of the thoracic spine (38.5%), usually symptomatic, followed by the lumbar spine (26.5%) and rarely in the cervical spine (0.9%). This is relevant to the biomechanical finding that stress loading during activities is higher on the cervicothoracic and thoracolumbar regions, or the upper and lower thoracic spine. The clinical diagnosis of TOLF is based on the patient's complaint, symptoms, and radiological findings. CT provides a straightforward profile of the canal structure and the OLF lesion, including its span, shape, and dimensions. MRI is better in conveying the health of the spinal cord, the presence of cord compression, injuries, and even myelopathy, which are essential to the prognosis of individual cases.

Sato T et al. categorized TOLF into five types based on the axial CT images (Fig. 2.10.1).

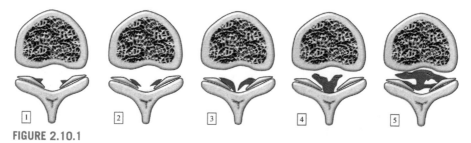

FIGURE 2.10.1

Schematic illustration of the radiological classification of TOLF.
(1) Lateral type;
(2) Extended type;
(3) Enlarged type;
(4) Fused type;
(5) Tuberous type.

1. Lateral type: the ossification affects the part of ligamentum flavum on the facet joint capsule.
2. Extended type: the ossification extends medially and remains to be relatively thin.
3. Enlarged type: the ossification extends medially like in the extended type and thickens and occupies the posterior region of the spinal canal.
4. Fused type: the ossification presenting in a similar pattern as in the enlarged type, but the lesions on both sides join at the midline.
5. Tuberous type: the OLF lesions on both sides join at the midline, form a tuberous mass, and protrude into the spinal canal.

TOLF tends to cause cord impingement and usually manifests as paresis of the lower limbs, bladder and bowel dysfunction, and even impaired mobility. As symptoms develop insidiously and slowly, it is difficult to diagnose in an early stage when patients are largely minimally symptomatic. Once they notice the symptoms, however, the disease is already in an advanced stage when conservative treatment usually fails, and surgical decompression is recommended.

Conventional surgical techniques

In cases where conservative treatment fails, or the ossification is too large, surgical decompression is advocated. What is more, many clinical studies have suggested that the earlier the patients receive surgery, the more benefit they gain since the resolved compression protects the spinal cord against sheer force during motion. Conventionally, TOLF surgeries are performed mainly via posterior approaches, such as LAM, French-door laminectomy, and en bloc laminectomy.

Specifically, LAM and French-door laminectomy, performed via safe midline access in the laminae, are indicated for OLF that spares the lamina's central part, namely lateral, extended, and enlarged TOLF. This midline access is particularly difficult when the OLF extends to the midline or when ossification or adhesion develops on the dura mater. In such a case, dissecting the ossification may injure the dura mater and cause CSF leak. With the inherent risk of spinal cord damage, French-door laminectomy is particularly risky in TOLF with markedly stenosed spinal canal where instrument-induced cord injury is much concerned. Epidural hematoma, another common complication, may also result in degradation of cord impingement and neural function.

En bloc laminectomy is indicated in TOLF where the disease involves the midline area, namely fused or tuberous types. Similar to French-door laminectomy but obviating the midline access, en bloc laminectomy is commonly applied with good results of decompression but not free of early postoperative complications. Also, ossification or adhesion of the dura mater is more likely to be present in the fused or tuberous-type TOLF. In such a case, the attempt to dissect the dura mater off the ossification while maintaining its integrity is usually impossible if not adversely causing a tear of the dura or even arachnoid mater, CSF leak, epidural hematoma, and even cord injury. En bloc laminectomy includes a time-consuming component with the use of a synthetic or fascial patch that substitutes the resected dura mater. Therefore, the procedure that floats the ossified dura mater without dissection was described, but it may leave residual compression. What is more, given the predilection of TOLF on cervicothoracic and thoracolumbar regions, adjacent segment disease may develop more frequently due to the local instability after surgery. Later in the modified en bloc laminectomy described by Jia et al., resection is performed along with the ossification and include the whole block of OLF and laminae. This modified technique is neurologically safer since the laminae are resected en bloc instead of in a piecemeal fashion and that the need to work through the spinal canal with instruments is obviated. Among the 36 patients analyzed, JOA recovered by 33%−100%, and three patients received dura mater repair. However, this technique has not been widely adopted as it is technically demanding, and care should be taken to avoid injuring the spinal cord via the seesaw effect when lifting the lamina on one side. A segmental en bloc laminectomy technique has also been reported to achieve posterior decompression while preserving stability. However, it is not readily applicable in the continuous type of OLF with significant occupancy, and its long-term result is still under investigation.

Bridge crane technique

The bridge crane technique has been developed on the idea of "in situ spinal cord decompression" upheld by Shi Jiangang. This idea advocates the restoration of the spinal cord back to its natural physiological status via decompression. This objective is often missed in the conventional laminectomy or LAM where the posteriorly expanded spinal canal may allow the spinal cord to shift posteriorly, a status that is neither natural or conducive to a full neurological recovery. With this concept of in situ cord decompression, after describing ACAF for cervical OPLL, Prof. Shi Jiangang, with Changzheng Hospital, Shanghai, China, carries the idea forward and introduced the novel bridge crane technique that manages advanced T-OPLL with in situ decompression [1].

The key steps of the technique are described below:

1. Anesthesia, patient positioning, and exposure
   After general endotracheal anesthesia, the patient is placed in the prone position. As the target levels are confirmed under intraoperative radiography, a midline incision is developed on the back and subcutaneous tissue dissected to reveal the spinous processes, sides of laminae, and transverse processes (Fig. 2.10.2, panel 1 and Fig. 2.10.3, panel 1).
2. Mobilization of the lamina-ossification complex (LOC) and installation of the "bridge crane"

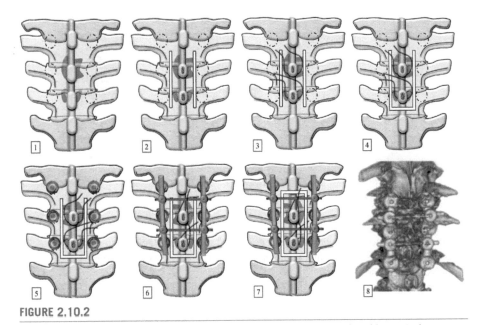

FIGURE 2.10.2

In situ cord decompression with the "bridge crane" technique depicted in posterior view.

(1) Spinous processes and bilateral laminae and transverse processes exposed;

(2) Longitudinal cut along the medial wall of the pedicles;

(3) Spinous processes of the involved lamina resected, bone tunnel developed at the base of the spinous processes with a towel clamp and threaded with a surgical suture for later use;

(4) Longitudinal cuts on both sides joined by a transverse cut between the pedicles of the vertebra caudal to the desired LOC;

(5) Pedicle screws inserted and rods mounted;

(6) Sliding knots tied with the suture to stabilize the LOC;

(7) The other transverse cut developed on the level cephalad to the upper end of the desired LOC;

(8) Reformatted CT image after surgery.

The LOC is mobilized in a way similar to that in laminectomy. The lamina is dissected on both sides, with 2 mm cuts adjacent to the pedicle's medial wall. This cut does not compromise the ligamentum flavum since its natural edge locates more medially (Fig. 2.10.2, panel 2). The spinous processes of the involved laminae are excised. At 5 mm lateral to the base of the spinous processes, a tunnel of 10 mm wide and 5 mm deep is developed on both sides with a towel clamp and threaded with a suture commonly used in thoracic surgery for

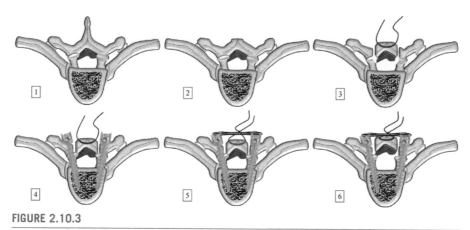

FIGURE 2.10.3

In situ cord decompression with the "bridge crane" technique depicted in axial view.
(1) Spinous processes and bilateral laminae and transverse processes exposed;
(2) Spinous processes excised;
(3) Bone tunnel developed at the base of the resected spinous processes with a towel clamp and threaded with a surgical suture for later use;
(4) Pedicle screws inserted and rods mounted;
(5) Sliding knots tied with the suture to stabilize the LOC;
(6) Surgical knots tied with the same suture after elevation to immobilize the LOC.

later use in the hoisting maneuver (Fig. 2.10.2, panel 3 and Fig. 2.10.3, panel 3). The vertical cuts on both sides are then connected through a transverse cut made at the pedicles of the segment caudal to the LOC (Fig. 2.10.2, panel 4). Pedicle screws are placed in the involved levels on both sides, followed by rods and transverse connectors. The "bridge crane" construct is completed (Fig. 2.10.2, panel 5 and Fig. 2.10.3, panel 4), and the LOC temporarily stabilized with the slide knots on the sutures (Fig. 2.10.2, panel 6 and Fig. 2.10.3, panel 5). As the other transverse cut is made at the segment above the LOC, the LOC is thoroughly mobilized (Fig. 2.10.2 G).

3. Posterior elevation of the LOC
   The mobilized LOC is elevated posteriorly as the sutures are tightened, when decompression is validated by the pulsation of LOC concurrent with that of the dura mater. The distance of LOC elevation is determined by the thickness of the OLF measured preoperatively. Extra room for elevation is obtained with properly contoured transverse connectors and the length of screws in the vertebra. Upon adequate elevation, the LOC is fixed to the bridge crane when the surgical knots are tied with the sutures (Fig. 2.10.3, panel 6). At finishing, the morselized bone from the spinous process is filled into the vertical and

transverse cuts. The patient is under neurophysiologic monitoring during the entire procedure, which includes somatosensory-evoked potentials and motor-evoked potentials.

4. Case presentation

A 58-year-old woman presented to our clinic with numbness and pain of lower extremities, impaired ambulation, and bladder dysfunction for two years that aggravated over the previous month. Radiography revealed dense masses at T9/10 and T10/11, shown to be TOLF of tuberous and enlarged type, respectively, on CT images with the maximum canal occupancy of 71.61% (Figs. 2.10.4 and 2.10.5).

With other necessary work-ups, posterior decompression via the bridge crane technique was performed. The technique involves preparation, exposure, mobilization of the LOC, installation of the bridge crane, and elevation as shown in Fig. 2.10.6. No alert was given off by IONM during the entire procedure (Figs. 2.10.7 and 2.10.8).

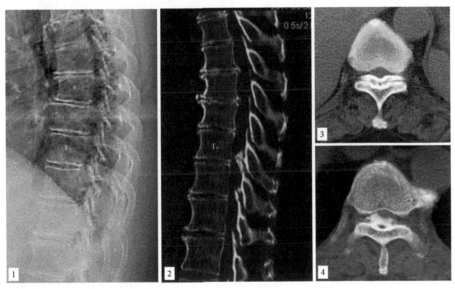

FIGURE 2.10.4

Preoperative imaging studies of the patient.
(1) Lateral X-ray;
(2) Sagittal CT image;
(3) Axial CT image of the T9/10 disc space;
(4) Axial CT image of the T10/11 disc space.

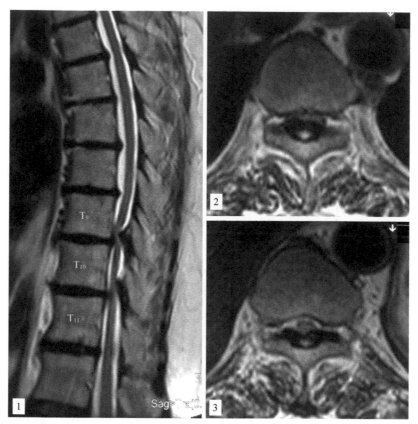

FIGURE 2.10.5

Preoperative imaging studies of the patient.
(1) Sagittal MRI image;
(2) Axial MRI image of the T9/10 disc space;
(3) Axial MRI image of the T10/11 disc space.

The patient had been free of surgical complications over the next six months. She was independently ambulatory again with muscle strength improved from 1/5 to 4/5, marked recovery of motor and sensory function of the lower limbs, and regained bladder control. JOA recovered by 50% and 75% at the third and sixth months, respectively. Adequate decompression and resumed anterior and posterior CSF columns were evident from postoperative imaging studies. The "bridge crane" construct remained in good position and fusion achieved at the grafting sites, as shown on X-ray during the last follow-up.

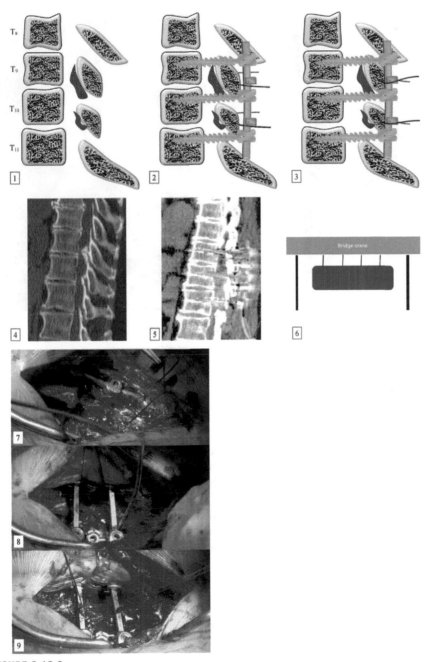

FIGURE 2.10.6

Schematic illustration and intraoperative views of the case.
(1) Ossification of the patient;

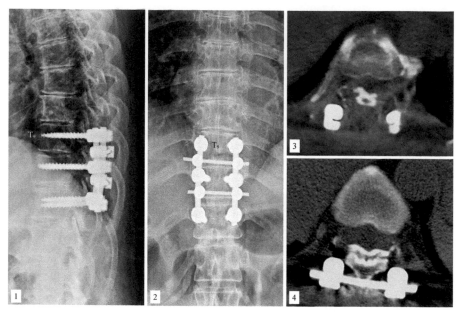

FIGURE 2.10.7

Imaging studies at the six-month follow-up.
(1) Lateral X-ray;
(2) Anteroposterior X-ray;
(3) Axial CT image of the T9/10 disc space;
(4) Axial CT image of the T10/11 disc space.

5. Discussion

The crux of the "bridge crane" technique for in situ cord decompression lies in the mobilization and posterior elevation of the LOC as a whole to generate decompression of the involved levels. Both this technique and the ACAF for cervical OPLL are consistent with Prof. Jiangang Shi's idea of "in situ cord decompression." The distance of elevation for adequate decompression is planned preoperatively and can be adjusted intraoperatively with the total screw length, screw length within the bone, and the contour of the transverse connectors.

(2) Screws and rods inserted and sutures threaded to the construct;
(3) Elevation and knot tying;
(4) Sagittal CT image before surgery;
(5) Sagittal CT image after surgery;
(6) Illustration of the "bridge crane" construct;
(7) Stay sutures placed;
(8) Elevation of LOC;
(9) Final fixation with knot tying.

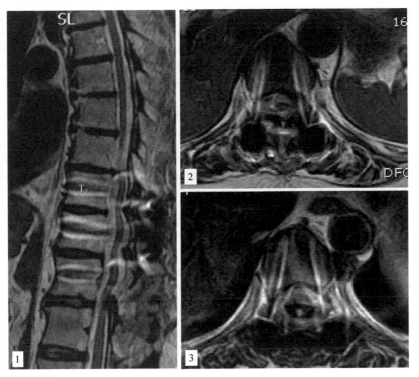

FIGURE 2.10.8

Imaging studies at the six-month follow-up.
(1) Sagittal MRI image;
(2) Axial MRI image of the T9/10 disc space;
(3) Axial MRI image of the T10/11 disc space.

OLF with concomitant dural ossification (DO) constitutes a challenge for conventional techniques. Its incidence was reported at 56% among fused and tuberous-type TOLF by Miyakoshi et al. The challenge comes with the extra steps to address the adhesion of ossification and dural sac, such as repairing the torn dural sac. Decompression via the floating technique was described to obviate the need to resect the OLF, but opinions are divided as to the effect of decompression. The "bridge crane" technique described in this chapter obviates the maneuvers to dissect and excise the ossification by elevating the LOC en bloc. As such, the incidence of dural tear and CSF leak is significantly reduced. Acute neurological deterioration represents a rare complication for a laminectomy, with the incidence reported at 0%—5.5% in cases of cervical stenosis but as high as 14.5% in thoracic stenosis, according to Young et al. It is attributable to the fact that, first, the vascular supply to the thoracic spinal cord is poorer than other regions due to unfavorable anatomical features with a smaller canal volume. Second, according to the theory of Takai et al., thoracic spinal canal stenosis is followed by compensatory vasculogenesis in the ossified tissue and the spinal cord so that resection of the ossification interrupts the venous flow and the local circulation of the spinal cord, resulting in neurological deterioration. In contrast, such vascular risk is minimized in the "bridge crane" technique where the ossification remains intact. Meanwhile, the risk of reperfusion injury of the spinal cord is ameliorated with the gradual and controllable LOC elevation in this technique.

While realizing cord decompression, the "bridge crane" in situ decompression technique preserves the integrity of the thoracic spine structure as much as possible. Based on our practice in the Second Spine Unit of Changzheng Hospital, Shanghai, China, this technique is believed to be safe and effective for patients with TOLF. More efforts will be made to improve the technique and demonstrate its benefit in TOLF with a larger case series.

Reference

[1] Jingchuan S, Kaiqiang S, Jiangang S, et al. The bridge crane technique for the treatment of the severe thoracic ossification of the ligamentum flavum with myelopathy. European Spine Journal 2018;27(8):1846−55.

Case series

Case 1: Ossification of posterior longitudinal ligament (OPLL) of cervical spine C3 to C5/6

Index terms

Antedisplacement of three levels, segmental-type, thickness of ossification 5–7 mm, and occupied ratio below 50%.

History

Patient: A 57-year-old man.

Chief complaint: Numbness of both hands for five weeks.

Physical exam: The patient was noted for unsteady gait; reduced superficial sensation of both hands; muscle strength of upper extremities at 3-/5 and lower extremities 4/5; brisk tendon reflexes of upper limbs with bilateral Hoffmann signs.

Preoperative neurological evaluation: Japanese Orthopedic Association (JOA) score was 15, Nurick score: 1, visual analog scale (VAS): 0, and neck disability index (NDI): 4 (Fig. 3.1.1).

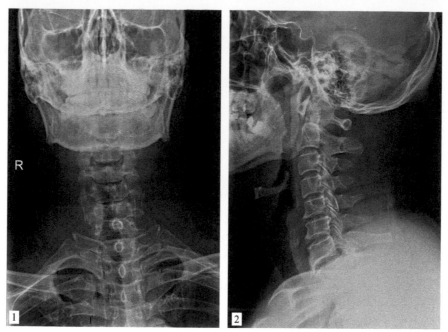

FIGURE 3.1.1

Preoperative X-ray of cervical spine.
(1) Anteroposterior images.
(2) Sagittal images.

Imaging text

C3–C5 ossification of posterior longitudinal ligament (OPLL); C2–C7 Cobb angle was 7.6°, and C2–C6 Cobb angle was 2.6°; K-line (−) (Fig. 3.1.2).

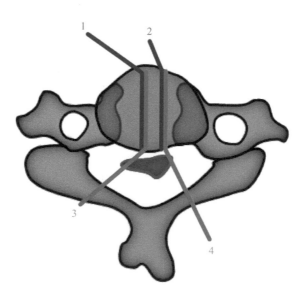

Location of the sagittal images at crossing images

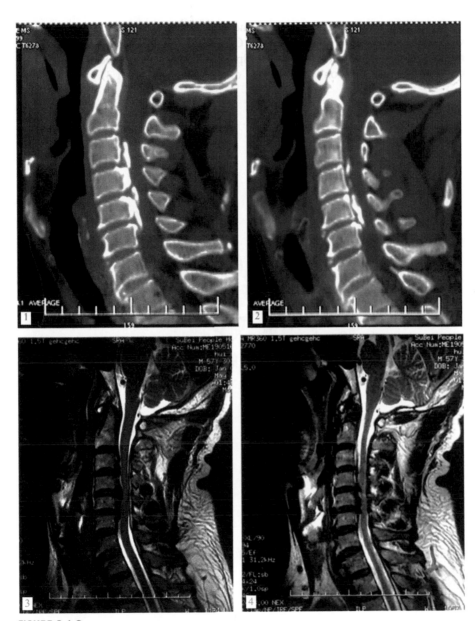

FIGURE 3.1.2

Preoperative sagittal images and location at crossing images.
(1) Midsagittal CT image.
(2) Left paramedian sagittal CT image.
(3) Midsagittal MR image.
(4) Left paramedian sagittal MR image

Preoperative sagittal CT images: Segment-type OPLL at C3 to C6, accompanied with double-layer sign at the levels of C3, C4/5, and C5/6. Preoperative sagittal magnetic resonance imaging (MRI) images: Spinal cord was compressed at C3 to C6 by low signal intensity lesion with kyphosis of spinal cord (Fig. 3.1.3).

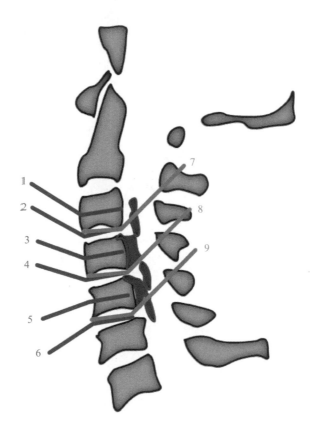

Location of the crossing images at sagittal images

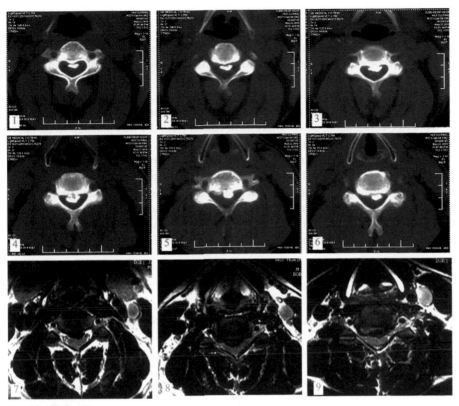

FIGURE 3.1.3

Preoperative axial images and location at sagittal images.

(1) Axial CT image at C3

(2) Axial CT image at C3/4

(3) Axial CT image at C4

(4) Axial CT image at C4/5

(5) Axial CT image at C5

(6) Axial CT image at C5/6

(7) Axial MR image at C3/4

(8) Axial MR image at C4/5

(9) Axial MR image at C5/6

Preoperative axial CT image: A wide-based ossified mass with double-layer sign from C3/4 to C4/5. At C3 level, the thickness and wideness of ossified mass measured were 5.3 mm (OR: 48.6%) and 12.7 mm at C3, 6.2 mm (OR: 42.8%) and 10.5 mm at C4, and 5.9 mm (OR: 44.4%) and 13.6 mm at C4/5. Preoperative axial MR image: Spinal cord was compressed at C3/4 to C5/6 with the shape of spinal cord being boomerang.

Highlights

This patient was diagnosed with segment-type OPLL at levels of C3–C5/6, and double-layer sign present at multiple levels indicated potential prevalence of dural ossification.

Surgical tips

Since this case features segment-type OPLL with double-layer sign and K-line (+), posterior decompression might provide satisfactory outcome with avoiding the occurrence of dural tear.

However, as a poor cervical curvature before surgery, a posterior procedure may aggravate kyphosis and cause recurrence of neural compression from the ossified lesion.

Anterior controllable antedisplacement fusion (ACAF) was planned to be operated that C3 to C5 were ventrally moved.

Considering the ossified mass with huge anteroposterior distances, more bone in the anterior part of the vertebra needs to be removed to provide enough decompression space. Hoisting instruments are recommended to ensure adequate holding force to vertebrae during the process of antedisplacement. Shorter screws are used to fix the plate that avoid screws' break through the posterior wall of vertebra and restrict antedisplacement of vertebrae (Fig. 3.1.4).

Results

Postoperative neurological function: JOA score was 17, Nurick score: 0, VAS: 0, and NDI: 0 (Fig. 3.1.5).

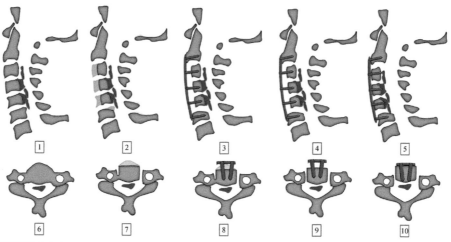

FIGURE 3.1.4

Schematic diagram of operation procedure.

(1, 6) Preoperative imaging of ossification.

(2, 7) The anterior vertebrae from C3 to C5 and posterosuperior part of C6 are resected. On the left side of the vertebra, a 2-mm-wide groove on the lateral side of vertebra, approximately at the medial border of the transverse foramina, was created from C3 to C5. While an incomplete groove was made on the right side with posterior cortical bone preserved.

(3, 8) Titanium plate and screws are installed on C2 to C7.

(4, 9) On the right side of the vertebrae, the remaining cortical bone behind the vertebra was resected, and the vertebrae with OPLL were completely isolated.

(5, 10) Tightening screws hoist the C3 to C5 vertebral bodies.

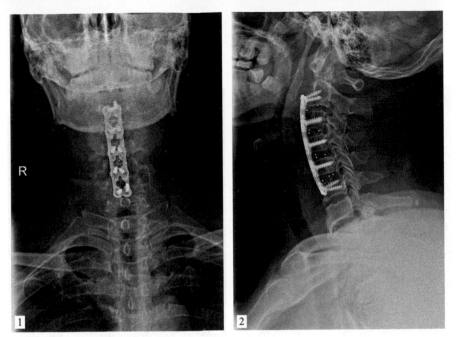

FIGURE 3.1.5

Postoperative cervical X-ray.
(1) Anteroposterior imaging.
(2) Sagittal images.

Cervical curvature was restored, and C2–C7 Cobb was 18.2°.
Postoperative axial images and location at sagittal images (Fig. 3.1.6).

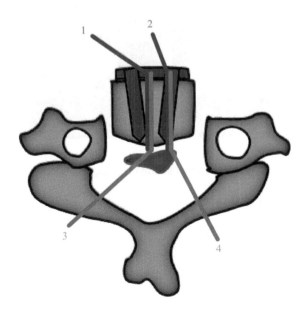

Location of sagittal image at crossing images

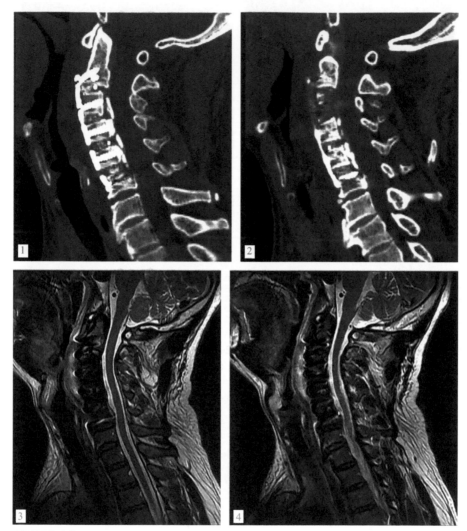

FIGURE 3.1.6

Postoperative sagittal images and location at crossing images.
(1) Midsagittal CT image.
(2) Left paramedian sagittal CT image.
(3) Midsagittal MR image.
(4) Left paramedian sagittal MRI image.

Postoperative sagittal CT images: The area of spinal canal was enlarged as ventrally moved vertebra-OPLL complex (VOC) of C3–C5, and cervical curvature was restored. Postoperative sagittal MRI images: the spinal cord was decompressed completely and recovered to lordosis (Fig. 3.1.7).

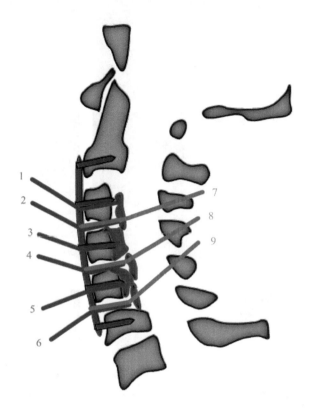

Location of the crossing images at sagittal images

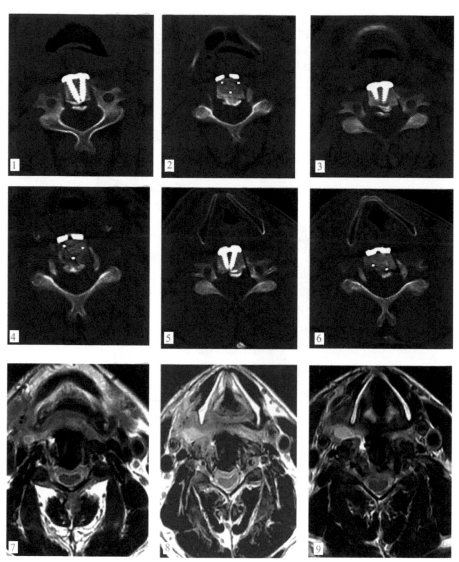

FIGURE 3.1.7

Postoperative cervical axial images and location at sagittal images.
(1) Axial CT image at C3.
(2) Axial CT image at C3/4.
(3) Axial CT image at C4.
(4) Axial CT image at C4/5.
(5) Axial CT image at C5.
(6) Axial CT image at C5/6.
(7) Axial MRI image at C3/4.
(8) Axial MRI image at C4/5.
(9) Axial MRI image at C5/6.

Postoperative axial CT image: Two bone grooves were posted parallel to the anteroposterior direction of vertebra on right and left sides with 20.8 mm wide between both. VOC was forward moved 7.4 mm resulting in OR being 0%. Postoperative MR image: The shape of spinal cord was recovered that it became oval shape.

Discussion

In this case with a narrow ossified mass, would anterior cervical corpectomy and fusion (ACCF) achieve adequate decompression?

The ossified mass was measured within 14 mm in width at all levels in preoperative images. ACCF could achieve satisfied neural decompression allowing the ossified mass being entirely resected.

However, a long segment titanium mesh was required, which comes with higher incidence of implant-related complications.

Moreover, the possible ossified dura at multiple segments, as revealed on preoperative CT images, poses extra risk of dural tear and cerebrospinal fluid (CSF) leakage during resection of ossification.

In comparison, as another anterior approach, ACAF provides direct decompression while keeping the ossified lesion where it is and preserving the adhered ossified lesion and the dura as a whole. Therefore, ACAF constitutes a less technically demanding procedure with lower risk of injury to the dura and spinal cord.

Case 2: Ossification of posterior longitudinal ligament (OPLL) of cervical spine (From C2 to C5)

Index terms

Antedisplacement of fewer than three vertebrae, continuous lesion, wide-based lesion, thickness of ossification 7–9 mm, occupancy ratio between 50% and 60%, shelter technique, and undercut decompression.

History

Patient: A 47-year-old woman.

Chief complaint: Upper back pain for one year that worsened with pain and numbness of upper extremities six months ago.

Physical exam: The patient walked with unsteady gait and experienced paresthesia (pain) over the upper back and the left neck and shoulder; decreased pain, warmth, and cold sensation of the pulp of the right little finger; and Eaten and Spurling signs present on the left side. Muscle strength was measured at 4/5 on upper extremities and 4/5 on lower extremities, with Hoffmann and Babinski signs on both sides.

Preoperative function: JOA score was 14, Nurick score: 1, VAS: 3, and NDI: 12 (Fig. 3.2.1).

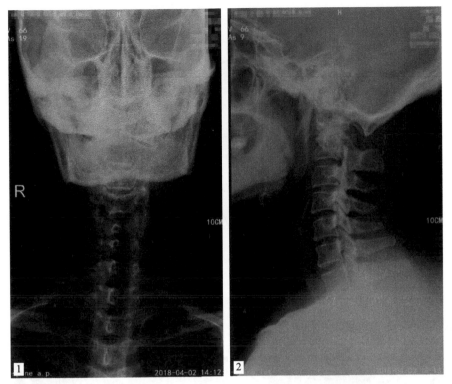

FIGURE 3.2.1

Preoperative X-ray of the cervical spine.
(1) Anteroposterior view.
(2) Lateral view.

Imaging studies

Cobb angle of 12.8° from C2 to C7. A K-line (+) OPLL spanning from C2 to C5 (Fig. 3.2.2).

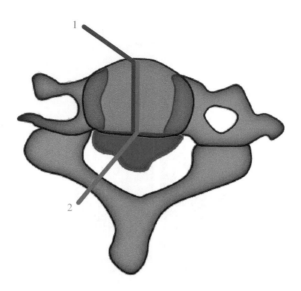

Reference of the sagittal views

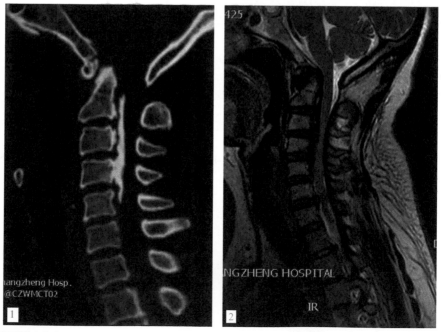

FIGURE 3.2.2

Preoperative sagittal views and their reference on the axial diagram.
(1) Midsagittal CT image.
(2) Midsagittal MRI image.

A plateau-type continuous OPLL spanning from C2 to C5, clear of the vertebral bodies at C2 to C3 and C5, as shown on preoperative midsagittal CT images (panel 1). The spinal cord in a progressive "S" curve. A low signal intensity lesion spanning C2 to C5 has indented the spinal cord and caused myelopathy at C4 level with medullary hyperintensity, revealed on preoperative sagittal MRI images (panel 2) (Fig. 3.2.3).

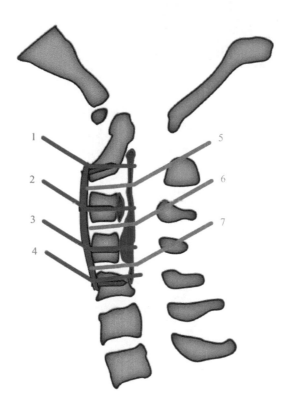

Reference of the axial views

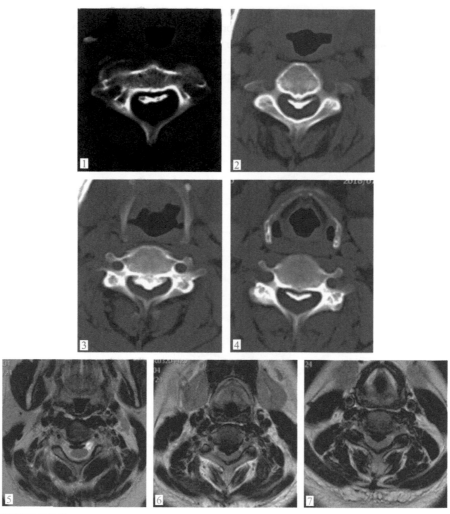

FIGURE 3.2.3

Preoperative axial cervical images and their reference on the sagittal diagram.

(1) Axial CT image along the inferior rim of C2 vertebra.

(2) Axial CT image at C3 vertebra.

(3) Axial CT image at C4 vertebra.

(4) Axial CT image along the superior rim of C5 vertebra.

(5) Axial MRI image at C2/3 disc space.

(6) Axial MRI image at C3/4 disc space.

(7) Axial MRI image at C4/5 disc space.

A wide-based OPLL lesion centered in the spinal canal and clear of the C2, C3, and C5 vertebral bodies that measures 4.3 mm thick and 13.0 mm wide with canal occupancy of 31.2% at C2 level, 6.6 mm thick and 11.4 mm wide with occupancy of 56.4% at C3, 7.2 mm thick and 17.0 mm wide with occupancy of 60% at C4, and 4.5 mm thick and 12.5 mm wide with occupancy of 39.5% across the superior surface of C5 vertebra (panel 1 to 4). The lesion is presented as a low signal intensity mass along the anterior part of the spinal canal, opposing the indented cord in the shape of the boomerang or triangle on axial MRI images.

Highlights

This case features a long, plateau-type, and continuous OPLL that extends into the upper cervical spine. The ossified lesion is adhered to the C4 vertebra but clear of vertebral bodies of the other levels according to preoperative axial CT images.

Surgical planning

This multilevel, continuous, and K-line (+) OPLL that extends into the upper cervical spine has rendered direct decompression via an anterior approach challenging with a noticeable risk of complications. Indirect decompression via a posterior approach provides a less demanding and safer solution, but with suboptimal resection of the upper cervical lesion. What's worse, a decompression procedure involving C2 lamina and spinous process resection may result in kyphosis and progression of neural dysfunction as the insertions of musculatures essential for cervical curvature maintenance, namely semispinalis cervicis and longissimus capitis, are sacrificed in a posterior procedure.

The plan was to perform ACAF with antedisplacement of C3 and C4 vertebral bodies.

Since the ossified lesion was continuous with thickness less than half of the anteroposterior dimension of the vertebra, the decompression of C2 through C5 would involve hoisting of C3 and C4 vertebral bodies, shelter technique at C2, and undercut decompression for the other parts of ossification (Fig. 3.2.4).

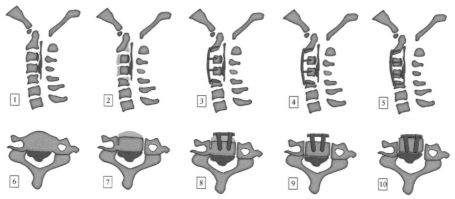

FIGURE 3.2.4

Illustration of the surgical plan on sagittal and axial views.

(1, 6) Illustration of the OPLL on sagittal and axial views.

(2, 7) Resection of the anterior vertebral bodies of C3 and C4, the posteroinferior rim of C2, and the posterosuperior rim of C5. A complete trough on the left and a half one on the right at C3 and C4.

(3, 8) Titanium plate and vertebra screws placed on C2 to C5.

(4, 9) The right trough on C3 and C4 completed.

(5, 10) C3 and C4 vertebral bodies antedisplaced with the tightening of screws.

Results

Postoperative function: JOA was scored at 15, Nurick score: 1, VAS: 2, and NDI: 14 (Fig. 3.2.5).

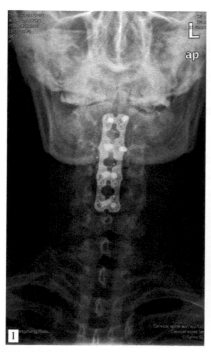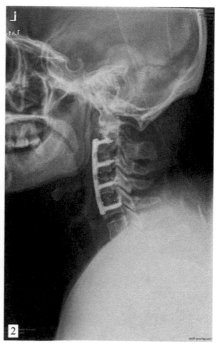

FIGURE 3.2.5

Postoperative X-ray of the cervical spine.

(1) Anteroposterior view.

(2) Lateral view.

Instrumentation from C2 to C5 and antedisplaced C3 and C4 vertebral bodies (Fig. 3.2.6).

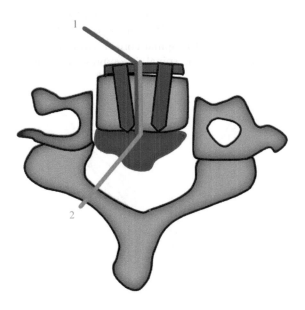

Reference of the sagittal views

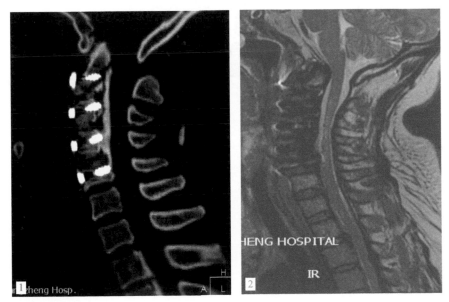

FIGURE 3.2.6

Postoperative sagittal images and their reference on the axial diagram.
(1) Midsagittal view on CT.
(2) Midsagittal view on MRI.

The oblique posteroinferior surface of C2 vertebra from shelter procedure, the ventrally displaced VOC from C2 to C5, and the tip of the OPLL at C2 moved into the shelter at C2 (panel 1). The spinal cord recovers its normal lordosis with CSF around it, evidence of adequate spinal decompression (panel 2) (Fig. 3.2.7).

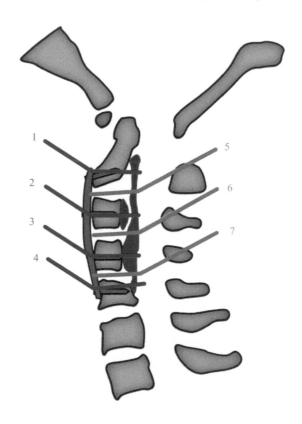

Reference of the axial images

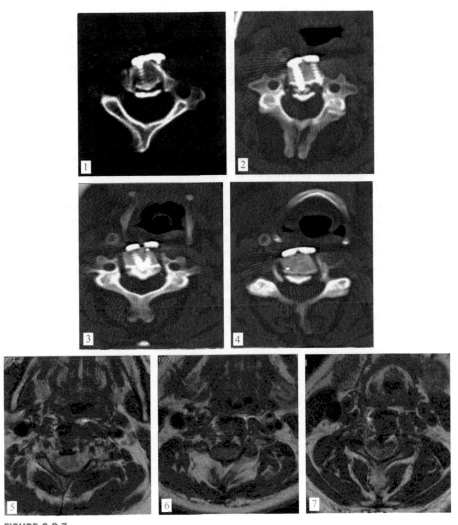

FIGURE 3.2.7

Postoperative axial images and their reference on the sagittal diagram.

(1) Axial CT image across the inferior rim of C2 vertebra.

(2) Axial CT image at C3 vertebra.

(3) Axial CT image at C4 vertebra.

(4) Axial CT image at C5 vertebra.

(5) Axial MRI image at C2/3 disc space.

(6) Axial MRI image at C3/4 disc space.

(7) Axial MRI image at C4/5 disc space.

The vertebral bodies have been dissected with parasagittal cuts on both sides 20.8 mm apart and antedisplaced by 5.8 mm. At C4 where canal stenosis was most severe before surgery, the canal occupancy drops from 60% to 21.2% (panel 1 to 4). The spinal cord has resumed its normal columnar shape surrounded by CSF, as revealed by axial MRI scans (panel 5 to 7).

Discussion

Do we need to dissect the posterior longitudinal ligament (PLL) in the shelter and undercut decompression procedure? If left undissected, does it counteract the decompression result?

As the intact PLL exerts a certain amount of axial tension, it may pull back the vertebrae-ossification complex and even fail the antedisplacement procedure if not dissected at the caudal and cephalad ends at the levels of undercut decompression. As such, in planning the surgery, we intended to dissect the PLL at the cephalad and caudal ends.

During surgical execution, after undercutting the C2 and C5 vertebral bodies, the access to and exposure of the PLL was so minimal that we aborted the dissection step in the case of potential dural or neural injuries. Also, cages of smaller sizes were used to alleviate axial tension on the PLL.

Case 3: Ossification of posterior longitudinal ligament (OPLL) of cervical spine From (C5 to C5/6)

Index terms

Antedisplacement of fewer than three vertebrae, circumscribed (localized) lesion, ossification with foraminal encroachment, thickness of ossification over 9 mm, and canal occupancy ratio of 60%—70%.

History

Patient: A 68-year-old man.

Chief complaint: Nuchal pain as well as pain and numbness of the left upper limb for one month.

Physical exam: It was notable for Eaten and Spurling signs and muscle strength of 3/5 on the left upper limb.

Preoperative function: JOA score was 12, Nurick score: 1, VAS: 7, and NDI: 2 0 (Fig. 3.3.1).

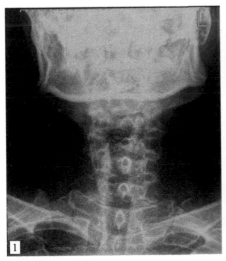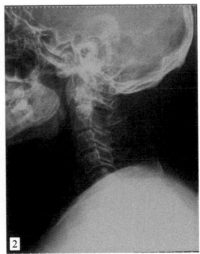

FIGURE 3.3.1

Preoperative cervical X-ray.
(1) Anteroposterior view.
(2) Lateral view.

Imaging studies

Cobb angle of 14.8° from C2 through C7. A K-line (−) disease (Fig. 3.3.2).

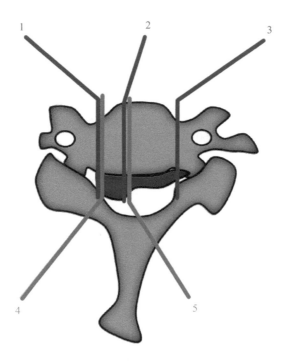

Reference of the sagittal planes

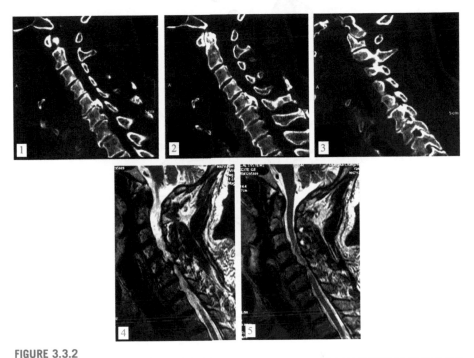

FIGURE 3.3.2

Preoperative sagittal images and their reference on axial diagram.

(1) Sagittal CT of the right uncinate process.
(2) Right paramedian sagittal CT view.
(3) Sagittal CT of the left uncinate process.
(4) Sagittal MRI of the right uncinate process.
(5) Right paramedian sagittal MRI view.

A circumscribed OPLL lesion at C5 and C5/6 (panel 1 to 3). Straightened cervical lordosis, spinal cord compression at C5/6 with signal changes indicating myelopathy, and complete effacement of CSF (panel 4 and 5) (Fig. 3.3.3).

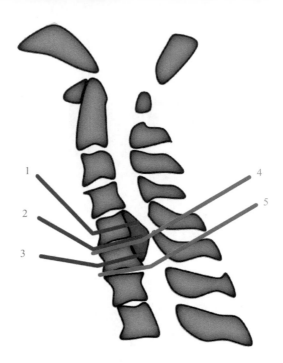

Reference of the axial images

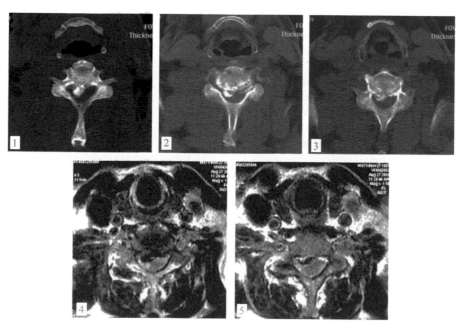

FIGURE 3.3.3

Preoperative cervical axial images and their reference on the sagittal diagram.

(1) Axial CT image at C5 vertebra.

(2) Axial CT image at C5/6 disc space.

(3) Axial CT image at C6 vertebra.

(4) Axial MRI image at C5/6 disc space.

(5) Axial MRI image at C6/7 disc space.

A wide-based lesion at C5/6 extending into the left lateral canal that measures 10.6 mm thick and 25.3 mm wide, with a canal occupancy ratio of 64.5% (panel 1 to 3). The ossification is eccentric to the right, which has resulted in a triangular cord rotating to the left side (panel 4 and 5).

Highlights

This case features a circumscribed OPLL lesion of C5 to C5/6, most protuberant at C5/6 level, with a wide base that extends onto the left lateral canal and impinges the nerve root.

Surgical planning

A K-line (−), circumscribed OPLL of 60% occupancy at maximum makes the case a candidate for the anterior procedure.

The lesion at C5 level renders anterior cervical discectomy and fusion (ACDF) suboptimal in terms of decompression, whereas ACCF with subtotal corpectomy of C5 seems to be an option.

However, with a broad base and double-layer sign comes an elevated risk of dural tear and residual compression at the neural exit foramen. What is more, with the limited medial-lateral dimension of corpectomy, any attempt to further decompress the neural exit foramen would pose an extra risk.

The decision was made on an ACAF with C5 and C6 being hoisted.

In handling wide-based diseases, the locations of the grooves are carefully planned. From preoperative measurement, the lesion was 25.3 mm wide at the C5/6 level, where the medial walls of the bilateral foramina transversarium were 28.4 mm apart.

In developing the parasagittal groove referenced at the anterior base of the uncinate process, the groove is positioned lateral to the margin of the ossification in case of leaving residual lesions with a narrower VOC.

A short lesion does not come with the advantage of decompression gained from curvature restoration. To ensure adequate decompression, the anterior vertebra of the same anteroposterior dimension as the ossification is resected (Fig. 3.3.4).

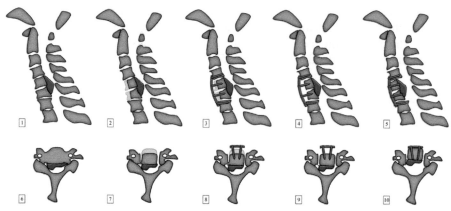

FIGURE 3.3.4

Illustration of the surgical plan on sagittal and axial views.

(1, 6) Illustration of the OPLL on sagittal and axial views before surgery.

(2, 7) Resection of the anterior vertebral bodies of C5 and C6, a left groove, and a right half-groove on C5 and C6.

(3, 8) Titanium plate and screws placed in vertebral bodies from C4 to C7.

(4, 9) Completion of the right groove on C5 and C6.

(5, 10) Antedisplaced C5 and C6 vertebral bodies after screw tightening.

Results

Radicular pain on the left side was alleviated. Negative spurling sign.

Postoperative function: JOA score was 13, Nurick score: 1, VAS: 3, and NDI: 11 (Fig. 3.3.5).

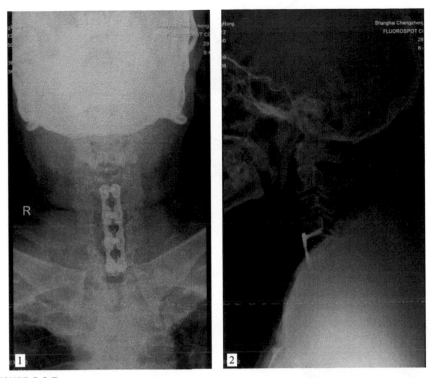

FIGURE 3.3.5

Postoperative cervical X-ray.

(1) Anteroposterior view.

(2) Lateral view.

Instrumentation on C4 through C7 and antedisplaced C5 and C6 vertebral bodies (Fig. 3.3.6).

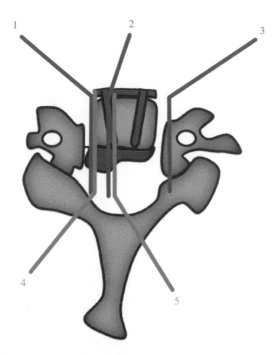

Reference of the sagittal planes

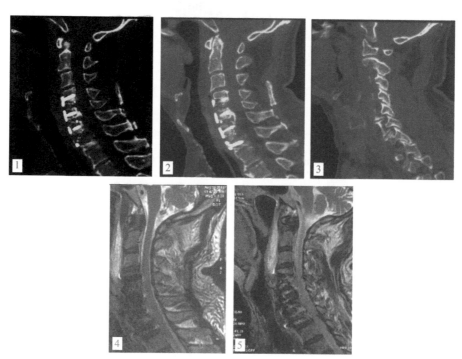

FIGURE 3.3.6

Postoperative sagittal images and their reference on the axial diagram.
(1) Sagittal CT image of the right uncinate process.
(2) Right paramedian sagittal CT image.
(3) Sagittal CT image on the left uncinate process.
(4) Sagittal MRI image of the right uncinate process.
(5) Right paramedian sagittal MRI image.

Antedisplaced VOC from C5 to C6 (panel 1 to 3). Restored lordotic spinal cord of normal signal intensity surrounded by CSF as the anterior indentation is cleared (panel 4 and 5) (Fig. 3.3.7).

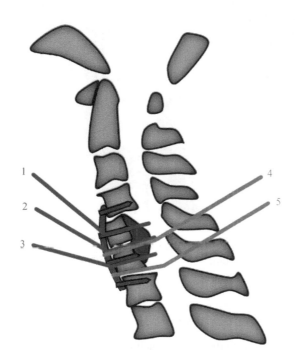

Reference of the axial images

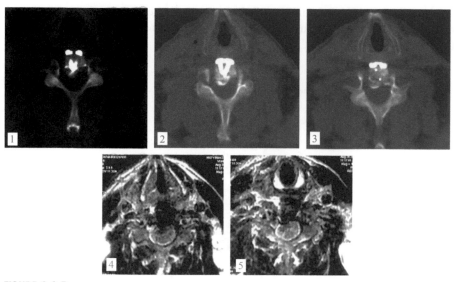

FIGURE 3.3.7

Postoperative axial cervical images and their reference on the sagittal diagram.
(1) Axial CT image at C5 vertebra.
(2) Axial CT image at C5/6 disc space.
(3) Axial CT image at C6 vertebra.
(4) Axial MRI image at C5/6 disc space.
(5) Axial MRI image at C6/7 disc space.

The VOC dissected from the boney structures by cuts on both sides 24.8 mm part and displaced anteriorly by 7.4 mm, expanding the spinal canal anteroposteriorly and reducing the canal occupancy ratio from 64.5% to 24.1% (panel 1 to 3). The spinal cord resumes its elliptical shape at C5/6 with normal CSF around it (panel 4 and 5).

Discussion

What are the challenges of the conventional ACCF technique for this case of OPLL? In comparison, what benefits does the ACAF technique entail?

The subtotal corpectomy of C5 in this case entails several challenges: first, given severe cord indentation and potential dural ossification, as indicated by the double-layer sign of the lesion, the resection of the ossified lesion may result in dural tear and deterioration of cord function after surgery. Second, the typical coronal dimension of subtotal corpectomy performed in ACCF is 12—14 mm, narrower than the OPLL width in this case. This necessitated resection of the residual OPLL on both sides in an undercut fashion, which involves extra risk for the procedure.

In contrast, ACAF allows a wider coronal dimension of the corpectomy, which provides better decompression for wide-based lesions. Meanwhile, the ossification is left in situ, which reduces the risk of complications such as dural tear and CSF leakage.

Case 4: Developmental spinal canal stenosis with Ossification of posterior longitudinal ligament (OPLL) of the cervical spine (From C4 to C5)

Index terms

Antedisplacement of fewer than three vertebrae, segmental OPLL, thickness of ossification within 5 mm, occupancy ratio below 50%, and K-line (−) OPLL.

History

Patient: A 56-year-old man.

Chief complaint: Soreness of the neck and shoulders with numbness of the right upper extremity for 20 days.

Physical exam: Decreased superficial sensation was noted on the lateral side of the arm, radial side of the forearm, thumb, index finger, and palmer side of the middle finger of the right upper extremity. Muscle strength was measured at 4/5 on the left upper extremity and 3/5 on the right upper extremity. All the four extremities were noted as hypertonic, and both lower limbs presented brisk tendon reflexes and Hoffmann and Babinski signs.

Preoperative function: JOA score was measured at 13, Nurick score: 1, VAS: 3, and NDI: 3 (Fig. 3.4.1).

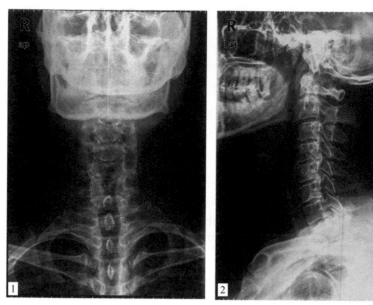

FIGURE 3.4.1

Preoperative X-ray of the cervical spine.
(1) Anteroposterior view.
(2) Lateral view.

Imaging studies

A straightened cervical spine with Cobb of 15.3° from C2 to C7. A K-line (−)OPLL spanning from C4 to C5 (Fig. 3.4.2).

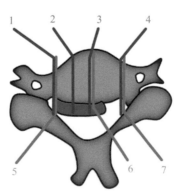

Reference of the sagittal planes

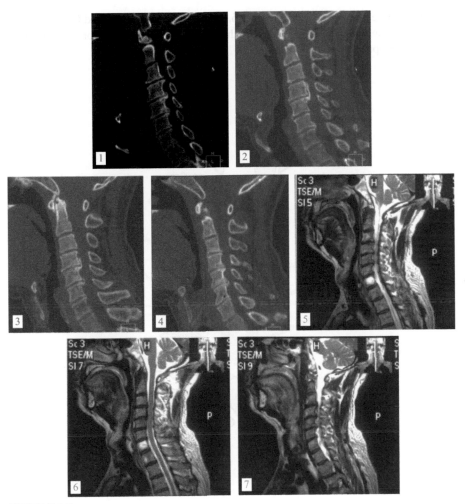

FIGURE 3.4.2

Preoperative sagittal images and their reference on the axial diagram.

(1) Sagittal CT image of the right uncinate process.

(2) Right paramedian sagittal CT.

(3) Midsagittal CT image.

(4) Sagittal CT image of the left uncinate process.

(5) Sagittal MRI image of the right uncinate process.

(6) Midsagittal MRI image.

(7) Sagittal MRI image of the left uncinate process.

An OPLL lesion at C4, C4/5, and C5/6, being segmental at C4 and C4/5 (panel 1 to 4). Spinal stenosis from C3/4 to C5 with obliteration of the anterior and posterior CSF column (panel 5 and 6) (Fig. 3.4.3).

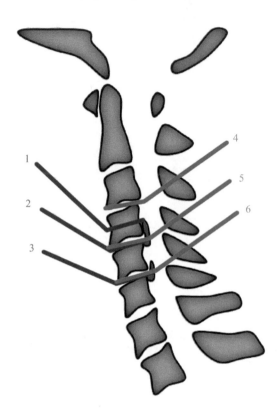

Reference of the axial images

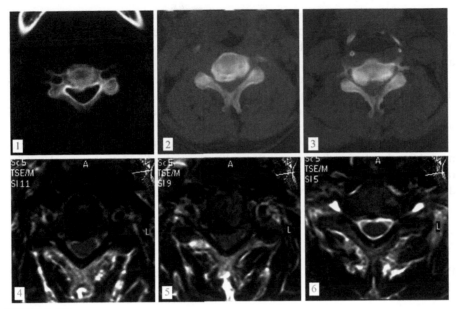

FIGURE 3.4.3

Preoperative axial images of the cervical spine and their reference on the sagittal diagram.
(1) Axial CT image at C4 vertebra.
(2) Axial CT image at C4/5 disc space.
(3) Axial CT image at C5/6 disc space.
(4) Axial MRI image at C3/4 disc space.
(5) Axial MRI image at C4/5 disc space.
(6) Axial MRI image at C5/6 disc space.

The ossification is eccentric to the right at C4/5 and more protuberant around the right neural exit foramen, and this wide-based lesion measures 3.7 mm thick, 16.9 mm wide, and 43% in canal occupancy (panel 1 to 3). An indented triangular cord with encroachment at the right neural exit foramen at C4/5 (pane 4 to 6).

Highlights

This case features a wide-based circumscribed OPLL lesion from C4 to C6 of 16.9 mm wide eccentric to the right that extends into the right neural exit foramen.

Surgical planning

A K-line (−) circumscribed OPLL can be addressed from anterior.

ACCF is not an option in this case since it does not readily remove the lesion dorsal to C4 vertebra. Among the conventional procedures, ACCF at C4 alone and ACDF of C5/6 would be considered. ACCF at C4 and C5 also provides an alternative.

However, with the groove developed in the ACCF procedure, one may risk having residual lesions when handling a wide-based OPLL.

The decision was made to perform ACAF with antedisplacement of C4 and C5 vertebral bodies.

Caution was exercised while ossification removal at the right neural exit foramen. After developing the grooves, the ossification extending into the neural exit foramen was removed with a curette. The decompression maneuvers should not be directed far lateral to avoid venous hemorrhage (Fig. 3.4.4).

Results

Postoperative function: JOA was scored at 17, Nurick score: 0, VAS: 1, and NDI: 2 (Fig. 3.4.5).

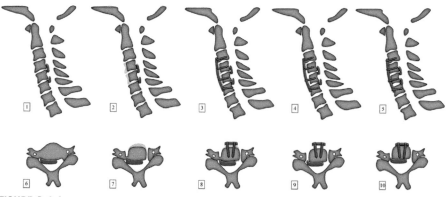

FIGURE 3.4.4

Illustration of the surgical plan on sagittal and axial views.

(1, 6) Illustration of the OPLL on sagittal and axial views before surgery.

(2, 7) Resection of anterior vertebral bodies of C4 and C5, a complete groove on the left and a half one on the right.

(3, 8) Titanium plate and vertebra screws placed from C3 to C6.

(4, 9) A completed groove on the right on C4 and C5 vertebral bodies.

(5, 10) Antedisplaced C4 and C5 vertebral bodies as the screws were tightened.

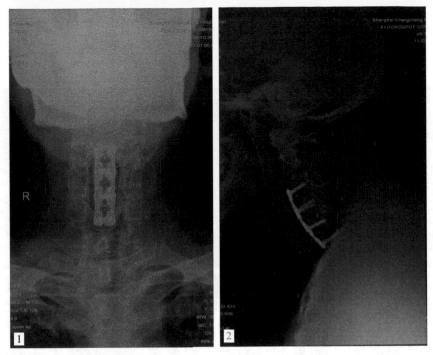

FIGURE 3.4.5

Postoperative X-ray of the cervical spine.

(1) Anteroposterior view.

(2) Lateral view.

   Instrumentation from C3 to C6 with antedisplaced C4 and C5 vertebral bodies (Fig. 3.4.6).

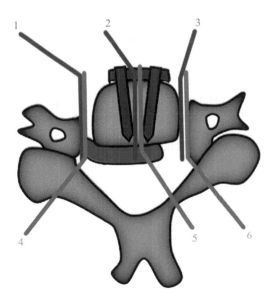

Reference of the sagittal planes

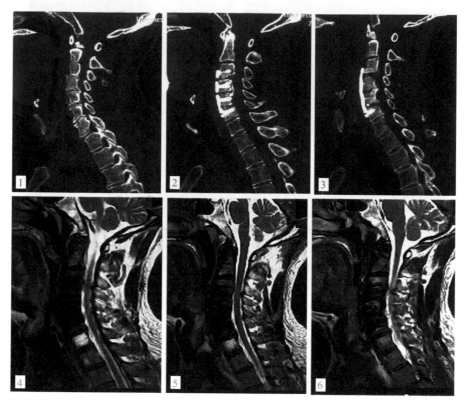

FIGURE 3.4.6

Postoperative sagittal images of the cervical spine and their reference on the axial diagram.

(1) Sagittal CT image of the right uncinate process.

(2) Midsagittal CT image.

(3) Sagittal CT image of the left uncinate process.

(4) Sagittal MRI image of the right uncinate process.

(5) Midsagittal MRI image.

(6) Sagittal MRI image of the left uncinate process.

The vertebra-ossification complex of C4 to C5 has been antedisplaced by 4.7 mm (panel 1 to 3). The spinal cord is in the expanded spinal canal surrounded by CSF (panel 4 to 6) (Fig. 3.4.7).

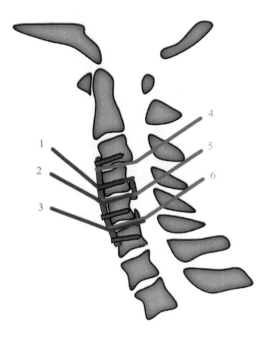

Reference of the axial images

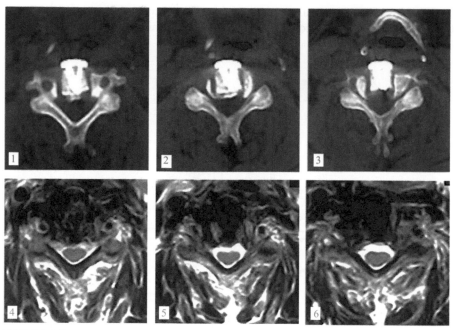

FIGURE 3.4.7

Postoperative axial images and their reference on the sagittal diagram.
(1) Axial CT image at C4 vertebra.
(2) Axial CT image at C4/5 disc space.
(3) Axial CT image at C5/6 disc space.
(4) Axial MRI image at C3/4 disc space.
(5) Axial MRI image at C4/5 disc space.
(6) Axial MRI image at C5/6 disc space.

The vertebral bodies have been dissected with cuts parallel to the sagittal plane 20.3 mm apart, reducing the spinal canal occupancy to 22% (panel 1 to 3). The spinal cord resumes its elliptical shape on cross-section and the right neural exit foramen is free of obstruction (panel 4 to 6).

Discussion

Is it possible to antedisplace the C4 vertebra alone?

As the ossification involved C4, the superior rim of C5, and C5/6 disc space, indicated by imaging studies, the surgical procedure was directed from C4 to C5/6.

Since the disease involved less than half the height of the C5 vertebra, one way to perform the procedure is to selectively preserve the C5 vertebra by undercut decompression of its superior rim.

On the other hand, as the C4/5 disc space was severely collapsed and degenerated with calcification of the disc, the undercut decompression of the C5 superior rim would be performed together with C4/5 disc space decompression. This surgery would be time-consuming and technically demanding.

As such, the decision was made to antedisplace both C4 and C5 vertebral bodies for decompression, so that all the surgeon needs to do for C4/5 disc space is to prepare the endplates for the cage. This surgery would be less time-consuming and more comfortable and provide adequate decompression.

Case 5: Ossification of posterior longitudinal ligament (OPLL, C3/4) and hyperextension injury of the cervical spine

Index terms

Antedisplacement of fewer than three vertebrae, circumscribed (localized) lesion, thickness of ossification within 5 mm, occupancy ratio between 50% and 60%, and history of hyperextension injury.

History

Patient: A 68-year-old man.

Chief complaint: Trauma-related nuchal and shoulder pain with numbness of upper limbs for 20 days.

Physical exam: The patient presented with periorbital bruise and scratches on the forehead and face, unsteady gait, hypertonic extremities, and pain on the neck and both shoulders. Muscle strength was measured at 2/5 on the left upper limb and 3/5 on the right upper limb. He experienced brisk tendon reflexes on all four extremities, Hoffmann and Babinski signs on both sides, and urinary dysfunction.

Preoperative function: JOA score was 10, Nurick score: 2, VAS: 4, and NDI: 21 (Fig. 3.5.1).

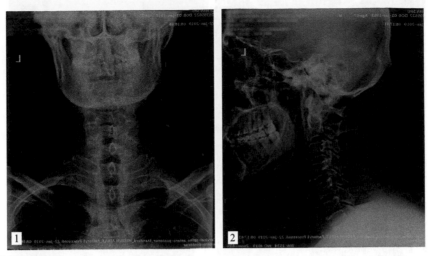

FIGURE 3.5.1

Preoperative X-ray of the cervical spine.
(1) Anteroposterior view.
(2) Lateral view.

Imaging studies

Cobb angle of 20.6° from C2 to C7 and a K-line (+) OPLL from C3 to C4 (Fig. 3.5.2).

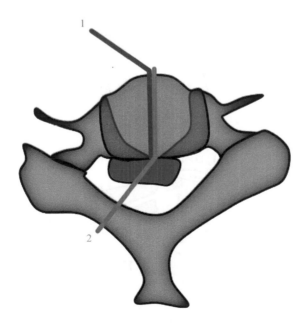

Reference of the sagittal planes

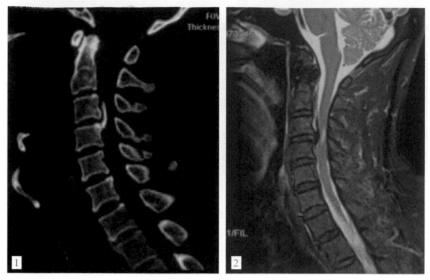

FIGURE 3.5.2

Preoperative sagittal images and their reference on the axial diagram.
(1) Midsagittal CT image.
(2) Midsagittal MRI image.

A circumscribed (localized) OPLL lesion from C3 to C3/4 (panel 1). The spinal cord being compressed at C3/4 level with high medullary signal intensity and complete effacement of CSF (panel 2) (Fig. 3.5.3).

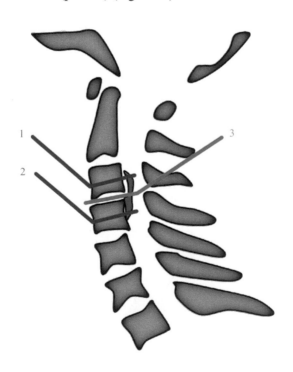

Reference of the axial images

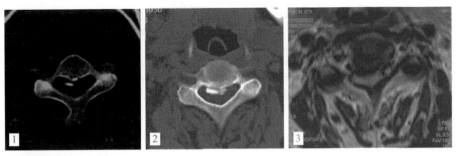

FIGURE 3.5.3

Preoperative axial images and their reference on the sagittal diagram.
(1) Axial CT image at C3 vertebra.
(2) Axial CT image at C4 vertebra.
(3) Axial MRI image at C3/4 disc space.

A plateau-type, mushroom-shaped ossification lesion of 13.6 mm wide and 4.2 mm thick centered in the spinal canal with 53.8% occupancy at C3/4 (panel 1 and 2). An indented spinal cord of boomerang shape with a high medullary signal at C4/5 (panel 3).

Highlights

This case features a circumscribed OPLL lesion dorsal to C3 vertebra and on C3/4, wide-based, plateaued, and centered in the spinal canal with a double-layer sign. The hyperextension injury that the patient sustained earlier worsened the cord impingement, evidenced by the medullary signal hyperintensity due to myelopathy and edema.

Surgical planning

Conventionally, this patient could be treated with ACCF on C3 alone. Since the disease is also on the posterosuperior rim of the C4 vertebra, the procedure would also include dissection of the disease at C3/4 and undercut decompression of the posterosuperior rim of the C4 vertebra. This would be a more demanding surgery with the risk of suboptimal decompression.

Alternatively, ACCF could be performed from C3 to C4 with bonier resection and a longer construct, which increases the risk of device-related complications.

The decision was made on ACAF with antedisplacement of C3 and C4 vertebral bodies.

Though the disease was eccentric to the right at the level of C4 superior rim, grooves were developed at the anterior bases of uncinate processes on both sides 19.5 mm apart for satisfactory antedisplacement.

The VOC was hoisted by the same distance as the thickness of the OPLL since the attempt to restore cervical curvature and allow extra decompression with a bent plate does not work well in short-segment diseases (Fig. 3.5.4).

Results

Postoperative function: JOA was scored at 10, Nurick score: 2, VAS: 4, and NDI: 21 (Fig. 3.5.5).

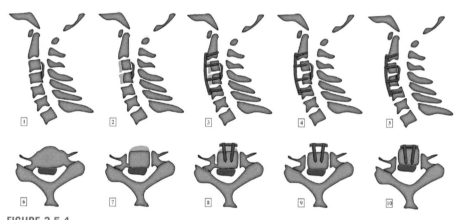

FIGURE 3.5.4

Illustration of the surgical plan in sagittal and axial views.

(1, 6) Illustration of the OPLL on sagittal and axial views before surgery.

(2, 7) Resection of anterior vertebral bodies of C3 and C4, a complete groove on the left and a half one on the right.

(3, 8) Titanium plate and vertebra screws placed from C2 to C5.

(4, 9) The right groove on C3 and C4 completed.

(5, 10) Antedisplaced C3 and C4 vertebral bodies as the screws were tightened.

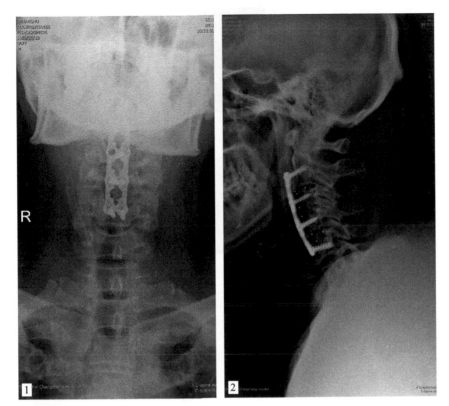

FIGURE 3.5.5

Postoperative X-ray of the cervical spine.
(1) Anteroposterior view.
(2) Lateral view.

Instrumentation from C2 to C5 with antedisplaced C3 and C4 (Fig. 3.5.6).

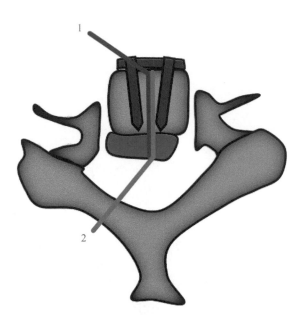

Reference of the sagittal planes

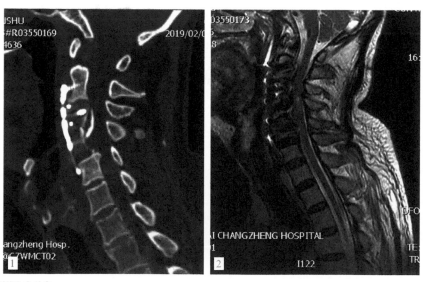

FIGURE 3.5.6

Postoperative sagittal images and their reference on the axial diagram.
(1) Midsagittal CT image.
(2) Midsagittal MRI image.

Antedisplaced C3 and C4 as evidenced by their shifted posterior borders on sagittal CT images (panel 1). Cord impingement resolved with an expanded spinal canal (panel 2) (Fig. 3.5.7).

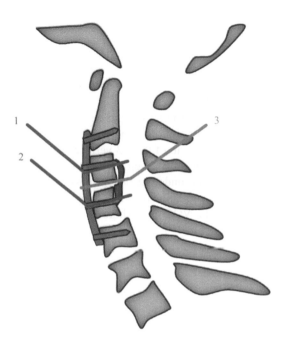

Reference of the axial images

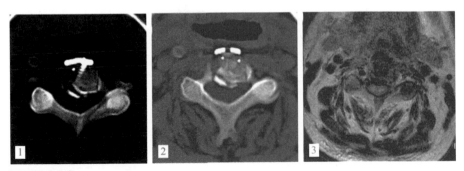

FIGURE 3.5.7

Postoperative axial images of the cervical spine and their reference on the sagittal diagram.
(1) Axial CT image at C3 vertebra.
(2) Axial CT image at C4 vertebra.
(3) Axial MRI image at C3/4 disc space.

With grooves on both sides 19.5 mm apart and the VOC antedisplaced by 4.5 mm, spinal canal occupancy is reduced to 23% (panel 1 and 2). The spinal cord resumes its normal elliptical shape on cross-section with improved signal intensity (panel 3).

Discussion

Is a complete decompression achievable with single-level antedisplacement of C3 or C4 alone and undercut decompression?

Seemingly spanning from C3 to the superior rim of C4, the OPLL lesion in this case was adhered to the superior rim of C4 but clear of C3 with the maximum stenosis at C3/4. The antedisplacement of the C3 vertebra alone, therefore, may cause incomplete displacement, if not failed. Neither would the antedisplacement of the C4 vertebra alone works as the undercut decompression may fail to address the lesion at C3 as it involved more than half of its vertebral height. Therefore, it takes both C3 and C4 to displace the VOC as a whole.

Case 6: Ossification of posterior longitudinal ligament (OPLL) of cervical spine (From C3 to C4)

Index terms

Antedisplacement of more than three vertebral bodies, circumscribed lesion, thickness of ossification 5—7 mm, occupancy ratio below 50%—60%, and partial antedisplacement.

History

Patient: A 35-year-old man.

Chief complaint: Numbness of both hands for one year, and numbness and pain of both lower limbs for five months.

Physical exam: The patient presented with the reduced tactile sensation of the palmar and dorsal side of both hands, hyperalgesic lateral side of the left arm, and decreased superficial sensation of the dorsal skin of both feet. The muscle strength of all four extremities was measured at 4/5. Biceps reflex and tendon reflex of the lower limb on both sides were brisk.

Preoperative function: JOA score was 12, Nurick score: 1, VAS: 1, and NDI: 4 (Fig. 3.6.1).

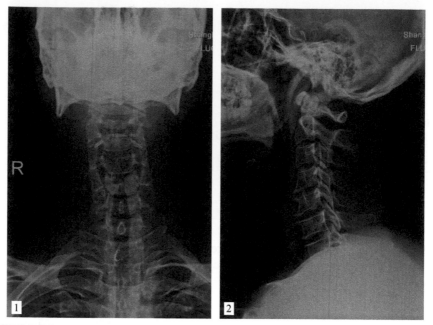

FIGURE 3.6.1

Preoperative X-ray of cervical spine.
(1) Anteroposterior view.
(2) Lateral view.

Imaging studies

Straightening of the cervical lordosis, with Cobb angle 7.3° from C2 through C7. A K-line (+)OPLL spanning from C3 to C4 (Fig. 3.6.2).

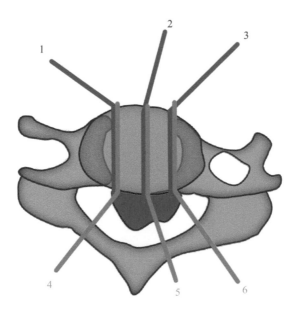

Reference of the sagittal planes

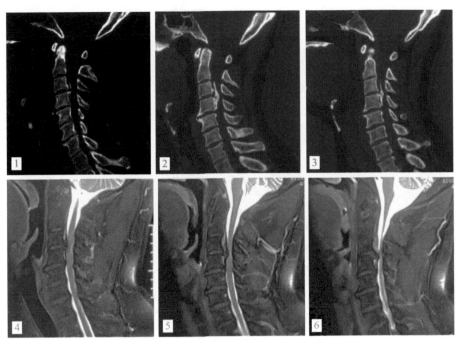

FIGURE 3.6.2

Preoperative sagittal images and their reference on the axial diagram.
(1) Paramedian sagittal CT image of the right.
(2) Midsagittal CT image.
(3) Paramedian sagittal CT image of the left.
(4) Paramedian sagittal MRI image of the right.
(5) Midsagittal MRI image.
(6) Paramedian sagittal MRI image of the left.

A circumscribed (localized) OPLL lesion of C3 to C4, which peaks and encroaches the spinal canal at C3/4 (panel 1 to 3). Anterior indentation of the cervical cord at C3 to C3/4, more severe at C3/4; complete effacement of CSF; and intramedullary signal hyperintensity of the cord (panel 4 to 6).

Highlights

This case features a circumscribed (localized) OPLL lesion from C3 to C4, with a double-layer sign at C3 and encroachment at C3/4 at the peak of the lesion. Intramedullary signal hyperintensity is noted due to compression (Fig. 3.6.3).

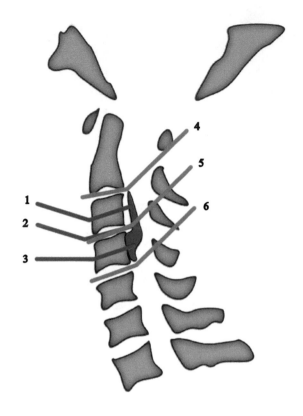

Reference of the axial planes

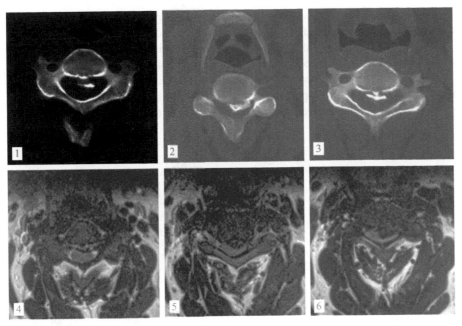

FIGURE 3.6.3

Preoperative axial images of the cervical spine and their reference on the sagittal diagram.

(1) Axial CT image at C3 vertebra.
(2) Axial CT image at C3/4 disc space.
(3) Axial CT image at C4 vertebra.
(4) Axial MRI image at C2/3 disc space.
(5) Axial MRI image at C3/4 disc space.
(6) Axial MRI image at C4/5 disc space.

The double-layer sign at C3 where the ossification measures 6 mm thick (anteroposterior), 10 mm wide (coronal), and 41.7% in canal occupancy. It is 5 mm thick, 11 mm wide, and 50% in canal occupancy at C3/4 disc space. The lesion becomes narrow-based and eccentric to the left at C4 and measures 5 mm thick, 15 mm wide, and 50% in canal occupancy (panel 1 to 3). The indented spinal cord appears in the shapes of boomerang and crescent with signal hyperintensity (panel 4 to 6).

Surgical planning

A short-segment, hill-shaped, and K-line (−) OPLL lesion could be managed with direct anterior decompression. An ACCF procedure may facilitate a complete resection of the lesion as it is narrow in the mediolateral dimension.

The double-layer sign within the lesion indicates possible involvement of the dura that requires meticulous dissection of the dura and the lesion.

To prevent dural tear and CSF leakage during the dissection, the ACAF procedure is planned with the antedisplacement of C3 and C4 vertebral bodies.

The left paracentral lesion at C3/4 disc space may leave the resection incomplete if a sagittal groove is developed on the anterior base of the left uncinate process. The groove needs to be lateralized to facilitate a complete resection (Fig. 3.6.4).

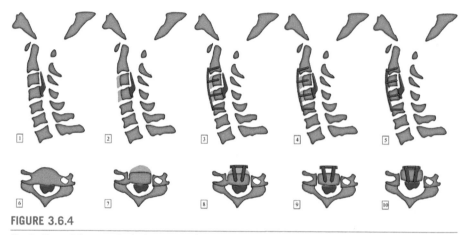

FIGURE 3.6.4

Illustration of the surgical plan on sagittal and axial views.

(1, 6) Illustration of the OPLL on sagittal and axial views before surgery.

(2, 7) Resection of anterior vertebral bodies of C3 and C4, a complete groove on the left and a half one on the right.

(3, 8) Titanium plate and vertebra screws placed from C2 to C5.

(4, 9) A completed groove on the right on C3 and C4 vertebral bodies.

(5, 10) Antedisplaced C3 and C4 vertebral bodies as the screws were tightened.

Results

Postoperative function: JOA was scored at 15, Nurick score: 1, VAS: 0, and NDI: 4 (Fig. 3.6.5).

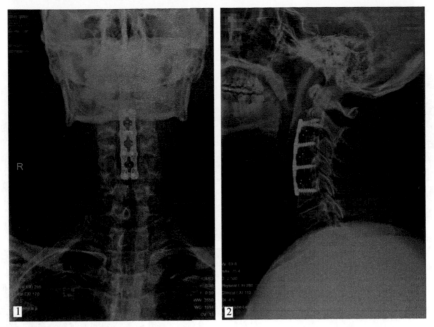

FIGURE 3.6.5

Postoperative X-ray of the cervical spine.
(1) Anteroposterior view.
(2) Lateral view.

Instrumentation from C2 to C5 with antedisplaced C3 and C4 vertebral bodies (Fig. 3.6.6).

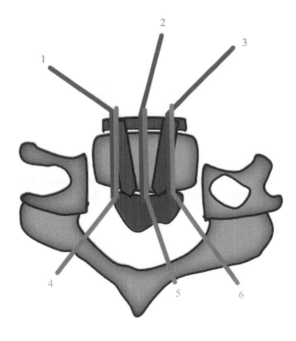

Reference of the sagittal planes

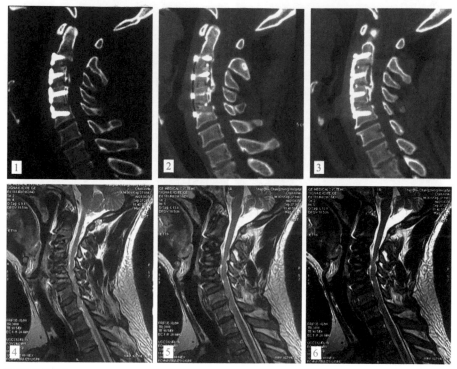

FIGURE 3.6.6

Postoperative sagittal images of the cervical spine and their reference on the axial diagram.

(1) Right paramedian sagittal CT image.

(2) Midsagittal CT image.

(3) Left paramedian sagittal CT image.

(4) Right paramedian sagittal MRI image.

(5) Midsagittal MRI image.

(6) Left paramedian sagittal MRI image.

Restored cervical curvature and central canal volume and antedisplaced VOC of C3 to C4 (panel 1 to 3). The spinal cord free of compression surrounded by CSF without signal hyperintensity (panel 4 and 5) (Fig. 3.6.7).

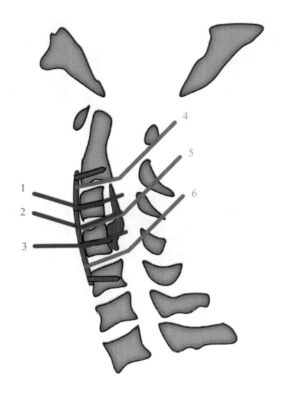

Reference of the axial planes

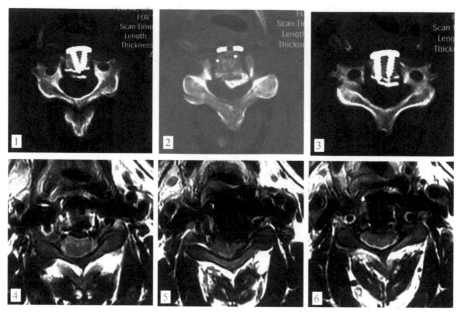

FIGURE 3.6.7

Postoperative axial cervical images and their reference on the sagittal diagram.

(1) Axial CT image at C3 vertebra.
(2) Axial CT image at C3/4 disc space.
(3) Axial CT image at C4 vertebra.
(4) Axial MRI image at C2/3 disc space.
(5) Axial MRI image at C3/4 disc space.
(6) Axial MRI image at C4/5 disc space.

The vertebral bodies have been dissected with parasagittal cuts on both sides 21 mm apart and VOC antedisplaced by 4 mm. Canal occupancy has been reduced to 0% at C3, 15.4% at C3/4, and 30.4% at C4 (panel 1 to 3). The spinal cord has resumed its normal columnar shape surrounded by CSF, as revealed by axial MRI scans (panel 4 to 6).

Discussion

What are the cautions when planning and developing the grooves for cases with the lateral-deviated type of lesion.

A paracentral lesion may encroach the neural exit foramen even when it is relatively narrow. As such, the surgeon should note the relations between the planned groove and the lateral border of the ossification and prevent inadequate decompression of the eccentric lesion.

The left paracentral and narrow-based lesion of 15 mm wide at C3/4 laterally extended beyond the level of the uncinate process.

In such a case, a parasagittal groove developed off the uncinate process at C3/4 may cause incomplete resection.

Therefore, while developing the groove along uncinate processes with a burr, the dissection is directed laterally along the bottom of the groove at C3/4 to mobilize the lateral paracentral lesion.

Case 7: Ossification of posterior longitudinal ligament (OPLL) of cervical spine (From C3 to C5)

Index terms

Antedisplacement of three vertebral bodies, segmental lesion, wide-based lesion, thickness of ossification 5−7 mm, occupancy ratio of 50%−60%, and ACAF + ACDF combined technique.

History

Patient: A 52-year-old man.

Chief complaint: Numbness on both hands and gait instability for two months.

Physical exam: The patient walked with an unsteady gait. The tactile sensation was decreased on all fingers. Muscle strength was measured at 3/5 on the left deltoid, 4-/5 on both hands, and 4-/5 on both lower limbs. Tendon reflexes were brisk on the left triceps and both lower limbs, with bilateral Babinski sign.

Preoperative function: JOA score was 8, Nurick score: 3, VAS: 0, and NDI: 26 (Fig. 3.7.1).

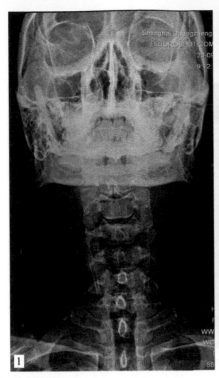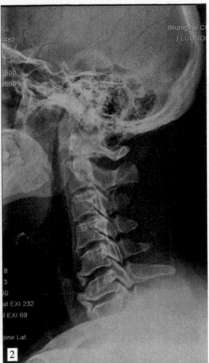

FIGURE 3.7.1

Preoperative cervical X-ray.
(1) Anteroposterior view.
(2) Lateral view.

Imaging studies

A straightened cervical spine with Cobb of 7.4° from C2 to C7 and Pavlov ratio below 0.75 from C3 to C5. A K-line (+)OPLL from C3 to C5 (Fig. 3.7.2).

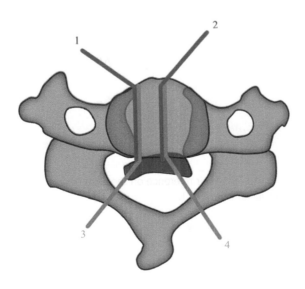

Reference of the sagittal planes

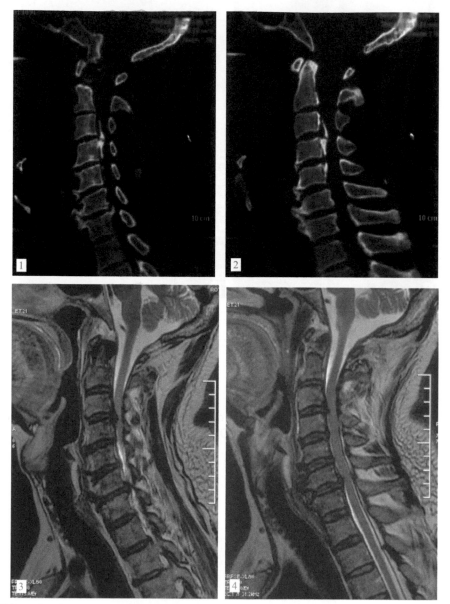

FIGURE 3.7.2

Preoperative sagittal images and their reference on the axial diagram.

(1) Right paramedian sagittal view on CT.

(2) Midsagittal view on CT.

(3) Right paramedian sagittal view on MRI.

(4) Midsagittal view on MRI.

A segmental OPLL from C3 to C5, with the peak encroaching the central canal at C3/4 and osteophytes at C6/7 (panel 1 and 2). Cord compression from C3 through C6/7 with complete effacement of CSF, in particular at C3/4 and C6/7; and intramedullary signal hyperintensity at the level of maximum cord compression of C3/4 and C6/7 (panel 3 and 4) (Fig. 3.7.3).

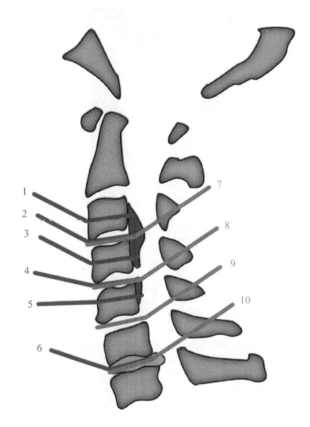

Reference of the sagittal planes

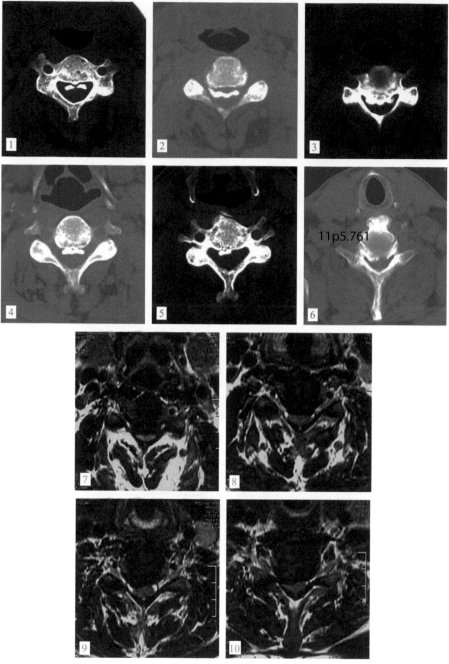

FIGURE 3.7.3

Preoperative axial images of the cervical spine and their reference on the sagittal diagram.
(1) Axial CT image at C3 vertebra.
(2) Axial CT image at C3/4 disc space.
(3) Axial CT image at C4 vertebra.
(4) Axial CT image at C4/5 disc space.
(5) Axial CT image at C5 vertebra.
(6) Axial CT image at C6/7 disc space.
(7) Axial MRI image at C3/4 disc space.
(8) Axial MRI image at C4/5 disc space.
(9) Axial MRI image at C5/6 disc space.
(10) Axial MRI image at C6/7 disc space.

A segmental OPLL with a double-layer sign present from C3 to C3/4. At C3 level, the OPLL measures 5 mm thick (anteroposterior) and 14 mm wide (mediolateral), occupying 41.7% of the spinal canal. At C3/4 level, it appears wide-based and measures 6 mm thick and 21 mm wide with occupancy of 50%. At C4/5 level, it is 5 mm thick and 16 mm wide with occupancy of 41.7% (panel 1 to 6). The indented spinal cord at C3/4 and C6/7 in the shape of a crescent or boomerang with signal hyperintensity while maintaining the oval shape at C4/5 and C5/6 (panel 7 to 10).

Highlights

This case features a straightened cervical spine with segmental OPLL from C3 through C5 and concurrent protrusion and calcification of the C6/7 disc. The ossified mass peaks at C3/4 and encroaches the central canal. The right paracentric, calcified, and protruded disc of C6/7 is in the neural exit foramen.

Surgical planning

This case features a multisegmental yet noncontinuous lesion composed of OPLL from C3 through C5 and osteophytes at C6/7 disc space.

For a multisegmental K-line (+) case, indirect decompression via a posterior approach serves as an option but involves significant surgical insult. What is more, a motion-preserving posterior procedure may aggravate the ossification disease in the front and the intervertebral disc degeneration, which compromise neural function further down the road.

Direct decompression via an anterior procedure remains an option despite multiple segment disease. One may consider ACCF at C3 through C4 combined with ACDF at C4/5 and C6/7 with the ossified lesion at the posterosuperior rim of C5 resected. In such a case, the C5/6 disc space spared from instrumentation may succumb to degeneration soon.

The decision was made to perform ACAF for C3 through C5 and ACDF for C6/7.

As the OPLL lesion extends beyond the uncinate processes bilaterally, the parasagittal grooves alone may not produce complete resection. The grooves toward the bottom should be directed laterally on both sides to ensure resection of all impinging structures.

As the use of plate that restores cervical lordosis contributes to decompression as well, we planned to resect the anterior bony structure of depth smaller than that of the VOC to spare vertebral bone stocks (Fig. 3.7.4).

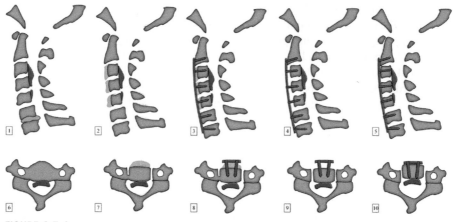

FIGURE 3.7.4

Illustration of the surgical plan on sagittal and axial planes.

(1, 6) Illustration of the disease on sagittal and axial views before surgery.

(2, 7) The C3 to C5 vertebrae are partially resected from anterior. A complete trough is developed on the left vertebral bodies from C3 to C5 while a half one is made on the right side with the posterior cortex yet to be dissected. The degenerated soft tissue at C6/7 disc space is removed.

(3, 8) Plate and screws placed on vertebral bodies from C2 through C6 and cages in place.

(4, 9) The bottom of the right half-groove on C3 through C5 dissected.

(5, 10) Screws are tightened to hoist the C3 to C5 vertebral bodies.

Results

Postoperative function: JOA score was 13, Nurick score: 1, VAS: 0, and NDI: 21 (Fig. 3.7.5).

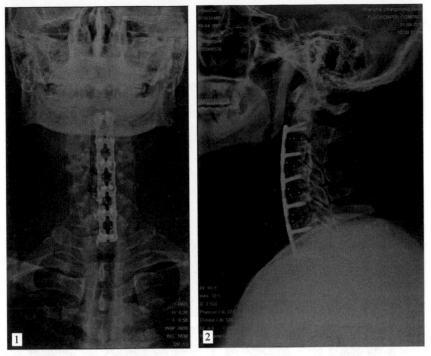

FIGURE 3.7.5

Postoperative cervical spine X-ray.
(1) Anteroposterior view.
(2) Lateral view.

Restored cervical curvature with Cobb of 25.8 from C2 through C7, instrumentation from C2 through C7, and antedisplaced C3 to C5 vertebral bodies (Fig. 3.7.6).

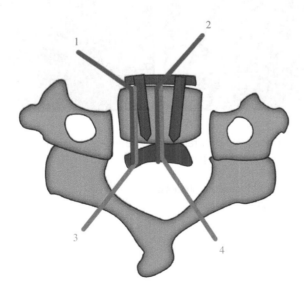

Reference of the sagittal planes

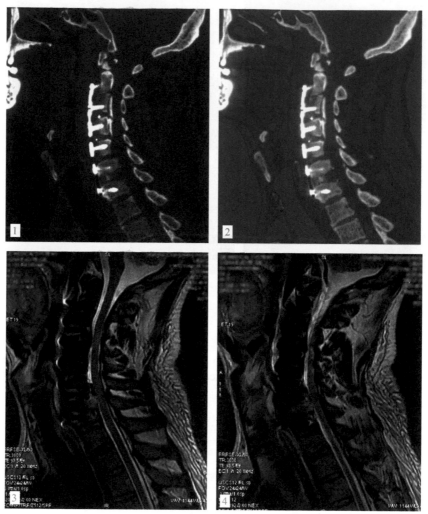

FIGURE 3.7.6

Postoperative sagittal views and their reference on the axial diagram.
(1) Sagittal CT of the right uncinate process.
(2) Midsagittal CT image.
(3) Sagittal MRI of the right uncinate process.
(4) Midsagittal MRI image.

Ventrally displaced VOC from C3 to C5 and C6/7 lateral canal free of osteophytes (panel 1 and 2). The spinal cord from C3 to C5 is fully surrounded by CSF and free of compression at C6/7 disc space, and the area of signal hyperintensity becomes ill-defined at C3/4 and absent at (panel 3 and 4) (Fig. 3.7.7).

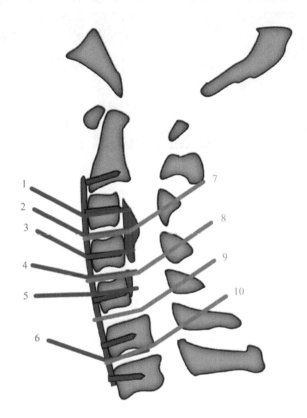

Reference of the axial images

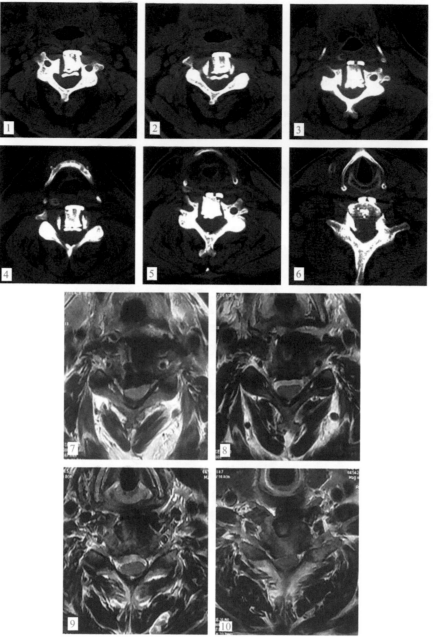

FIGURE 3.7.7

Postoperative axial cervical images and their reference on the sagittal diagram.

(1) Axial CT image at C3 vertebra.
(2) Axial CT image at C3/4 disc space.
(3) Axial CT image at C4 vertebra.
(4) Axial CT image at C4/5 disc space.
(5) Axial CT image at C5 vertebra.
(6) Axial CT image at C6/7 disc space.
(7) Axial MRI image at C3/4 disc space.
(8) Axial MRI image at C4/5 disc space.
(9) Axial MRI image at C5/6 disc space.
(10) Axial MRI image at C6/7 disc space.

The VOC dissected from the boney structures on both sides from C3 to C5 with grooves 19 mm apart and displaced anteriorly by 4 mm, resulting in canal occupancy decreased to 16.7% at C3/4, the level of maximum compression (panel 1 to 6). The spinal cord resumes its oval shape at C3/4 and C6/7, the levels of maximum compression, with normal CSF around it (panel 7 to 10).

Discussion

Shall the C6 vertebra be included in the antedisplacement in this case? Why was it spared during surgical execution?

The OPLL involved C3 through C5 while the cord compression at C6/7 was attributable to osteophytes on the right of the central canal that measured 12 mm wide and 3.6 mm thick and occupied 20.7% of the central canal.

C6 was not a part of the OPLL disease, and its Pavlov ratio stood at 0.75 before surgery.

Cord compression was maximum at C6/7 where disc height was preserved, and a complete decompression was expectable.

Therefore, the ACAF procedure was directed from C3 through C5, sparing the C6, and an ACDF technique was used to decompress the spinal cord at C6/7.

Case 8: Ossification of posterior longitudinal ligament (OPLL) of cervical spine (From C4 to C6)

Index terms

Antedisplacement of three vertebral bodies, segmental ossification, wide-based lesion, the thickness of ossification 7—9 mm, occupancy ratio above 70%, cervical kyphosis, K-line (−) OPLL, and residual ossification.

History

Patient: A 64-year-old man.

Chief complaint: Numbness and weakness of lower limbs with gait instability for 20 years that became worse over the past six months.

Physical exam: The patient experienced reduced tactile, pain, warmth and cold sensation in lower limbs, and walked with hypertonic and unsteady gait. Muscle strength was measured at 4/5 on both upper limbs and 3/5 on both lower limbs. Both lower limbs had brisk tendon reflexes, ankle clonus, and Hoffmann and Babinski signs.

Preoperative function: JOA score was 9, Nurick score: 5, VAS: 3, and NDI: 26 (Fig. 3.8.1).

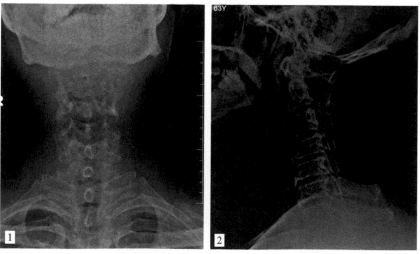

FIGURE 3.8.1

Preoperative X-ray of the cervical spine.
(1) Anteroposterior view.
(2) Lateral view.

Imaging studies

A kyphotic cervical spine with a Cobb angle of $-5.8°$ from C2 through C7, Pavlov ratio of 0.57, and a K-line $(-)$ OPLL from C4 to C5 (Fig. 3.8.2).

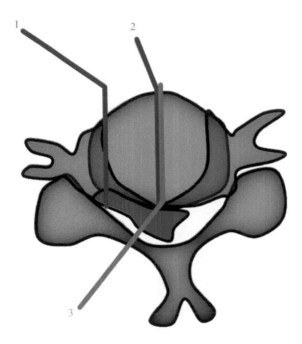

Reference of the sagittal planes

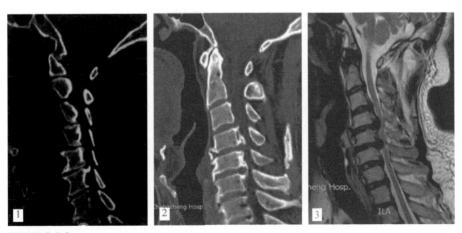

FIGURE 3.8.2

Preoperative sagittal images and their reference on axial diagram.
(1) Sagittal CT image of the right uncinate process.
(2) Midsagittal CT image.
(3) Midsagittal MRI image.

A segmental OPLL spanning from C4 to C5/6, thickest at C5/6 (panel 1 and 2). Anterior indentation from C3/4 to C5/6 with complete effacement of CSF and straightening of the spinal cord, with maximum cord compression at C4/5 and C5/6 (panel 3) (Fig. 3.8.3).

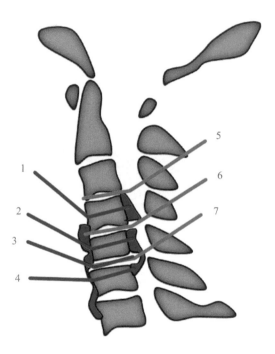

Reference of the axial images

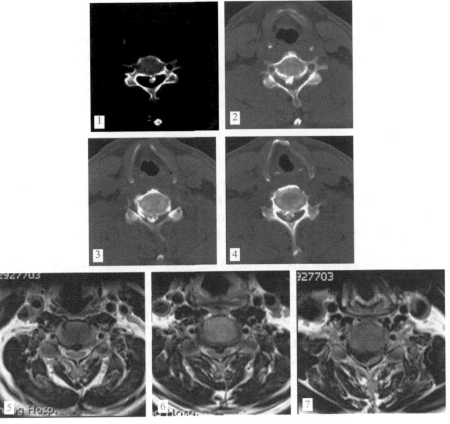

FIGURE 3.8.3

Preoperative axial images of the cervical spine and their reference on the sagittal diagram.

(1) Axial CT image at C4 vertebra.
(2) Axial CT image at C5 vertebra.
(3) Axial CT image at C5/6 disc space.
(4) Axial CT image at C6 vertebra.
(5) Axial MRI image at C3/4 disc space.
(6) Axial MRI image at C4/5 disc space.
(7) Axial MRI image at C5/6 disc space.

The ossified mass appears narrow-based at C4 vertebra 6.8 mm thick (anteroposterior), 7.3 mm wide (mediolateral), and 62.4% in canal occupancy. It becomes wide-based and eccentric to the right at C5/6 disc space 8.0 mm thick, 20 mm wide, and 80% in canal occupancy. MRI reveals a boomerang spinal cord at C4 due to the right-anterior indentation.

Highlights

This case features abnormal cervical curvature, developmental central canal stenosis, OPLL, and degenerative protrusion of soft tissue in the disc space. Cord compression is noted from C3/4 through C5/6. At C5/6, the ossified lesion is wide-based, eccentric to the right, traversing the right neural exit foramen, and flush with the medial rim of the transverse foramen.

Surgical planning

In this K-line (−) OPLL with over 60% of canal occupancy, a direct decompression with ACCF of C4 to C5 or C4 through C6 provides an option. Given the right-deviated ossified mass with neural exit foramen involvement, however, there is a higher risk of residual compression due to partial resection as the grooves are closer in subtotal corpectomy in ACCF.

The decision was made to perform ACAF that hoists C4 through C6 vertebral bodies.

The ossified anterior longitudinal ligament from C2 to C5 would be resected referenced off the anterior rim of the nonossified vertebral bodies to ensure accurate measurement and resection of the anterior partial resection of the vertebral bodies with OPLL.

Sagittal grooves would be developed referenced off the anterior root of uncinate processes. The grooves would be extended laterally at the disc space levels.

Since the restoration of cervical curvature expands the central canal to some extent, the anteroposterior extent of the partial vertebra resection is smaller than that of the ossification (Fig. 3.8.4).

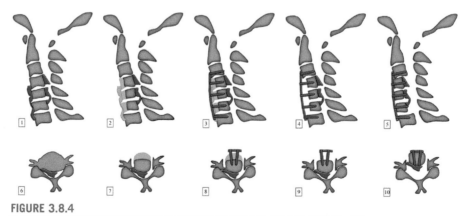

FIGURE 3.8.4

Illustration of the surgical plan on sagittal and axial views.

(1, 6) Illustration of the disease on sagittal and axial views before surgery.

(2, 7) Resection of the anterior part of the vertebral bodies of C4, C5, and C6, a left groove and a right half-groove on C4, C5, and C6.

(3, 8) Titanium plate and screws installed in vertebral bodies from C3 to C7.

(4, 9) Completion of the right groove on C4, C5, and C6.

(5, 10) Antedisplaced C5 and C6 vertebral bodies after screw tightening.

Results

Postoperative function: JOA was scored at 12, Nurick score: 3, VAS: 1, and NDI: 22 (Fig. 3.8.5).

Cobb angle of 6.2° from C2 to C7. Instrumentation on C3 through C7 and ante-displaced vertebral bodies from C4 through C6 (Fig. 3.8.6).

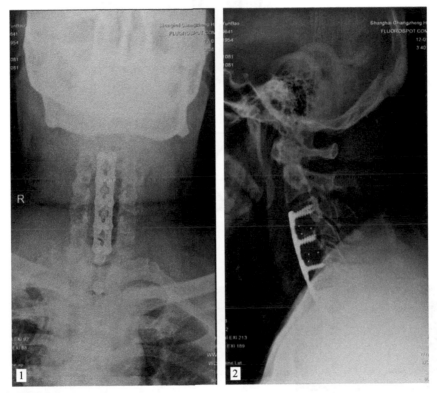

FIGURE 3.8.5

Postoperative cervical X-ray.
(1) Anteroposterior view.
(2) Lateral view.

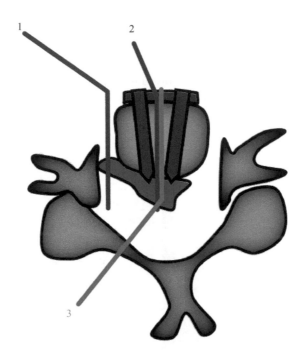

Reference of the sagittal planes

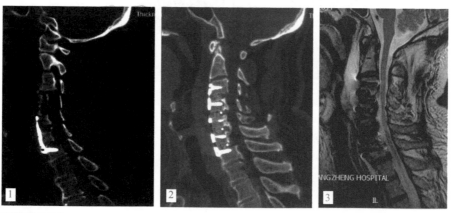

FIGURE 3.8.6

Postoperative sagittal images and their reference on the axial diagram.
(1) Sagittal CT image of the right uncinate process.
(2) Midsagittal CT image.
(3) Midsagittal MRI image.

Forward displaced posterior walls of vertebral bodies from C4 through C6 and resumed anteroposterior dimension of the spinal canal on postoperative sagittal CT images. Decompressed cord surrounded by CSF appreciated on postoperative sagittal MRI images (Fig. 3.8.7).

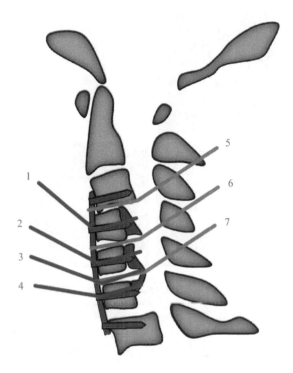

Reference of the axial images

The C4 vertebra and the ossified mass have been dissected with parasagittal cuts on both sides 24.2 mm apart and antedisplaced by 6.6 mm, with canal occupancy reduced to 15.7%, shown on postoperative axial CT images. Satisfactory cord decompression indicated with a triangular cord at C4 on axial MRI image.

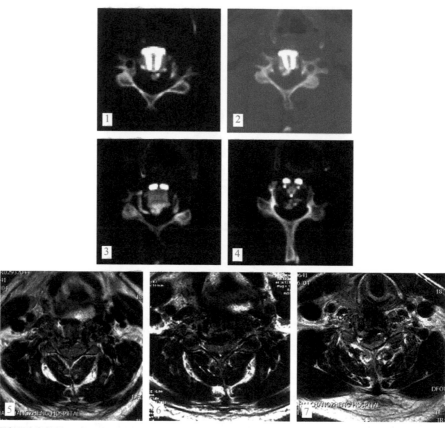

FIGURE 3.8.7

Postoperative cervical axial images and their reference on the sagittal diagram.
(1) Axial CT image at C4 vertebra.
(2) Axial CT image at the inferior surface of C5 vertebra.
(3) Axial CT image at C5/6 disc space.
(4) Axial CT image at the inferior surface of C6 vertebra.
(5) Axial MRI image at C3/4 disc space.
(6) Axial MRI image at C4/5 disc space.
(7) Axial MRI image at C5/6 disc space.

Discussion

Is it possible to manage this case with antedisplacement of C4 and C5 vertebral bodies?

The maximum canal compression is noted at C5/6, with occupancy of more than 80%. Considering the ossified mass at the C5/6 level was not joined with the proximal part, it was impossible to decompress by undercutting the superoposterior part of the C6 vertebra and advancing the VOC.

Even if it is joined as a one-block lesion, dissection of the lesion at C5/6 and undercutting the superoposterior part of C6 vertebra runs the risk of cord injury, let alone the challenge of the technique itself.

What is more, with the imagery evidence of C6/7 disc degeneration and effacement of CSF, setting C6 as the lower instrumented vertebra aggravates the degeneration of C6/7.

The plan, therefore, was to antedisplace C4 through C6 vertebral bodies.

Case 9: Ossification of posterior longitudinal ligament (OPLL) of cervical spine From (C4 to C7)

Index terms

Antedisplacement of three vertebral bodies, segmental OPLL, wide-based lesion, thickness of ossification 7—9 mm, occupancy ratio above 70%, and oblique groove.

History

Patient: A 52-year-old man.

Chief complaint: Numbness and weakness of the four extremities for three months that worsened over the past two months.

Physical exam: The patient experienced gait instability and decreased tactile sensation of extremities. Muscle strength was measured at 3/5 on upper limbs and 4/5 on lower limbs. Brisk tendon reflexes were noted on upper limbs.

Hoffmann and Babinski signs were present on both sides.

Preoperative function: JOA score was 11, Nurick score: 3, VAS: 0, and NDI: 13 (Fig. 3.9.1).

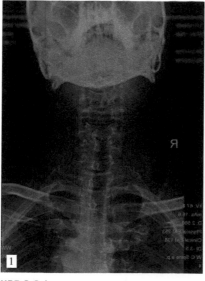 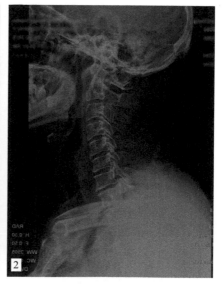

FIGURE 3.9.1

Preoperative X-ray of the cervical spine.
(1) Anteroposterior view.
(2) Lateral view.

Imaging studies

Cobb angle of 19.2° when measured from C2 to C7 and Pavlov ratio 0.835. A K-line (+) OPLL lesion (Fig. 3.9.2).

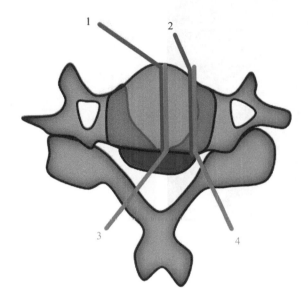

Reference of the sagittal planes

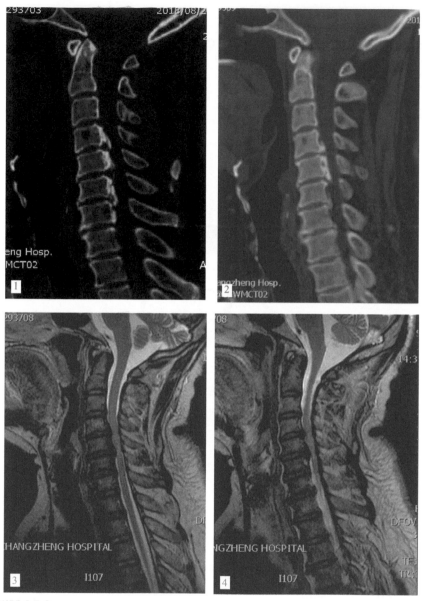

FIGURE 3.9.2

Preoperative sagittal views and their reference on the axial diagram.
(1) Midsagittal CT image.
(2) Left paramedian sagittal CT image.
(3) Midsagittal MRI image.
(4) Left paramedian sagittal MRI image.

A plateau-type segmental OPLL from C4 to C7 (panel 1 and 2). Cord compression from C4/5 through C6/7, most severe at C5/6, CSF effacement, and changes of intramedullary signal intensity (panel 3 and 4) (Fig. 3.9.3).

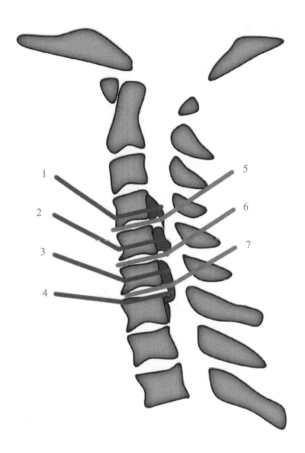

Reference of the axial images

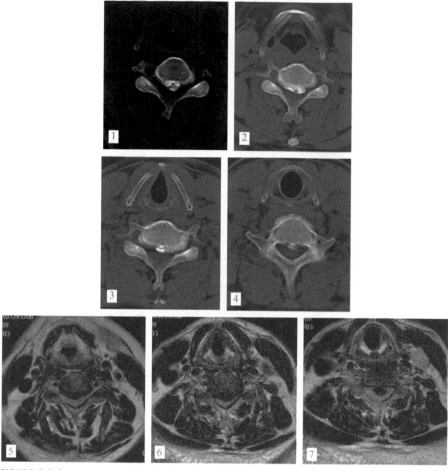

FIGURE 3.9.3

Preoperative axial cervical images and their reference on the sagittal diagram.

(1) Axial CT image at C4 vertebra.

(2) Axial CT image at C5 vertebra.

(3) Axial CT image at C6 vertebra.

(4) Axial CT image at the superior surface of C7 vertebra.

(5) Axial MRI image at C4/5 disc space.

(6) Axial MRI image at C5/6 disc space.

(7) Axial MRI image at C6/7 disc space.

Preoperative axial CT images reveal that the ossified mass measures 5.0 mm thick and 14.5 mm wide at C4. It is eccentric to the right, wide-based, of 17.3 mm wide and 7.3 mm thick, and 70% canal occupancy at C5. At C5/6, this left eccentric mass of 18.6 mm wide and 4.6 mm thick extends into the left neural exit foramen. Of 15.9 mm wide and 6.0 mm thick, it continues to be left paracentral at C6/7 and encroach neural exit foramen. Spinal cord in the shape of boomerang or triangle due to anterior indentation, with signal hyperintensity at C5/6 (panel 5 to 7).

Highlights

This case features central canal stenosis secondary to a wide-based and vertebral midline-centered segmental OPLL from C4 to C7, as revealed on preoperative axial CT images. Intramedullary signal hyperintensity is noted at C5/6, indicating cord myelopathy.

Surgical planning

Indirect decompression via a posterior procedure provides an option for K-line (+) OPLL that spans three vertebrae, as seen in this case.

With significant soft tissue disturbance and motion preservation, a posterior procedure comes with the risk of loss of cervical lordosis and recurrence of cord compression from the growing ossification further down the road.

The decision was made to perform the ACAF technique that antedisplaces the VOC from C4 to C6 and undercutting decompression at C7.

Care should be taken to probe the continuity of the ossified mass at C6/7 to evaluate the feasibility of undercut decompression and hoisting of VOC at C7.

Decompression via lordosis correction seemed unlikely given the unaffected cervical curvature so an anterior part of the vertebrae of the same thickness as the ossification is resected (Fig. 3.9.4).

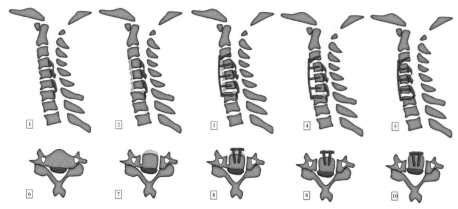

FIGURE 3.9.4

Illustration of the surgical plan on sagittal and axial views.

(1, 6) Illustration of the disease on sagittal and axial views before surgery.

(2, 7) Resection of the anterior part of the vertebral bodies of C4 through C6 and the posterosuperior rim of C7. A complete trough on the left and a half one on the right at C4 through C6 vertebral bodies.

(3, 8) Titanium plate and vertebra screws placed on C3 to C7.

(4, 9) Completion of the right groove on C4, C5, and C6.

(5, 10) C4 through C6 vertebral bodies antedisplaced with the tightening of screws.

Results

Postoperative function: JOA score was 13, Nurick score: 2, VAS: 0, and NDI: 7 (Fig. 3.9.5).

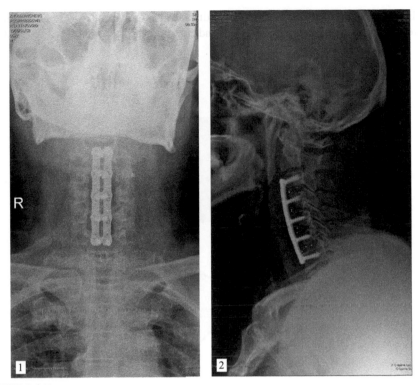

FIGURE 3.9.5

Postoperative X-ray of the cervical spine.
(1) Anteroposterior view.
(2) Lateral view.

Instrumentation from C3 to C7 and antedisplaced C4 through C6 vertebral bodies. Vertebra screws of 14 mm in C3 and C7 and 12 mm in C4 through C6 (Fig. 3.9.6).

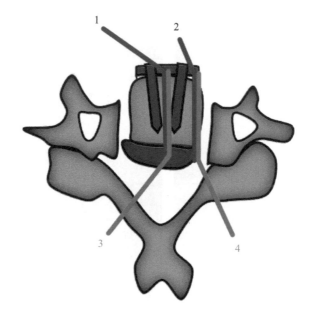

Reference of the sagittal planes

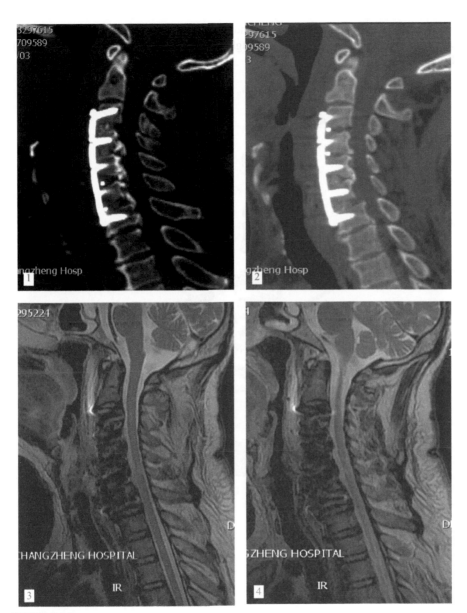

FIGURE 3.9.6

Postoperative sagittal images and their reference on the axial diagram.

(1) Midsagittal CT image.

(2) Left paramedian sagittal CT image.

(3) Midsagittal MRI image.

(4) Left paramedian sagittal MRI image.

Antedisplaced VOC from C4 to C6 and an expanded spinal canal (panel 1 and 2). Decompressed spinal cord from C4 through C6/7 surrounded by CSF (panel 3 and 4) (Fig. 3.9.7).

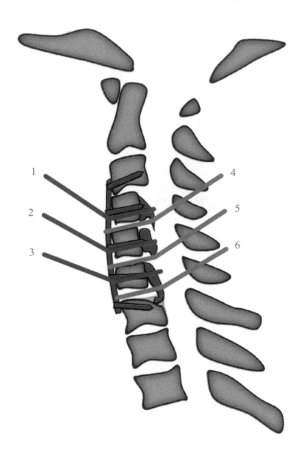

Reference of the sagittal planes

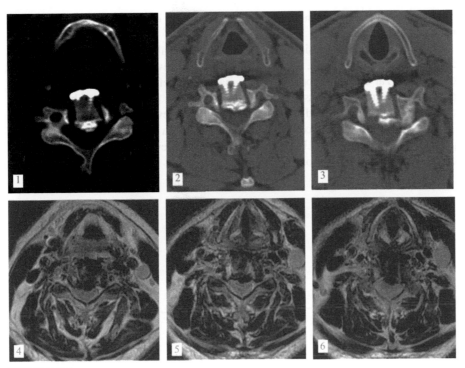

FIGURE 3.9.7

Postoperative axial cervical images and their reference on the sagittal diagram.

(1) Axial CT image at C4 vertebra.
(2) Axial CT image at C5 vertebra.
(3) Axial CT image at C6 vertebra.
(4) Axial MRI image at C4/5 disc space.
(5) Axial MRI image at C5/6 disc space.
(6) Axial MRI image at C6/7 disc space.

The VOC dissected from the boney structures on both sides by grooves 19.3 mm apart and displaced anteriorly by 6.1 mm; the canal occupancy ratio has decreased to 25% (panel 1 to 3). The spinal cord resumes its normal shape with normal CSF around it (panel 4 to 6).

Discussion

Why was undercut decompression not performed before hoisting the VOC even though the ossified mass extended down to C7 from the inferior surface of the C6 vertebra?

Undercut decompression of the superoposterior rim of C7 vertebra was a component of the surgical plan.

Probing the ossified lesion at the disc space revealed a thin distal tip without adhering to the C7 vertebra. In addition, there was no evidence of cord compression of the OPLL at C7 on preoperative MRI images. Therefore, the surgeon aborted the plan of undercut decompression for the superoposterior part of C7 vertebra and went ahead to dissect the ossified lesion at the disc space level.

The VOC was found in contact with the C7 vertebra on postoperative CT images probably because the OPLL was distalized to C7 level as the C6/7 disc space collapsed due to lordosis correction.

Case 10: Ossification of posterior longitudinal ligament (OPLL) of cervical spine (From C5 to C5/6)

Index terms

Antedisplacement of fewer than three vertebral bodies, circumscribed (localized) OPLL, thickness of ossification 7–9 mm, and occupancy ratio between 60% and 70%.

History

Patient: A 53-year-old man.

Chief complaint: Numbness of upper limbs for six months and gait instability for two months.

Physical exam: The patient reported the decreased tactile sensation of the right trunk below the intermammary line and numbness of the index, middle, and small fingers on both sides. Lower extremities were noted for brisk tendon reflexes as well as Hoffmann and Babinski signs.

Preoperative function: JOA score was 8, Nurick score: 3, VAS: 3, and NDI: 17 (Fig. 3.10.1).

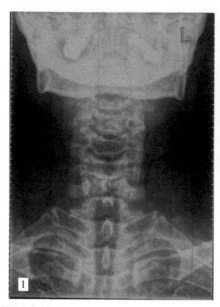
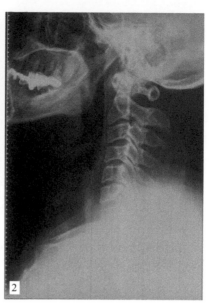

FIGURE 3.10.1

Preoperative X-ray of the cervical spine.
(1) Anteroposterior view.
(2) Lateral view.

Imaging studies

A straightened cervical spine with Cobb of 7.2° from C2 to C7, a K-line (+) OPLL, and kyphosis of C2 through C5 (Fig. 3.10.2).

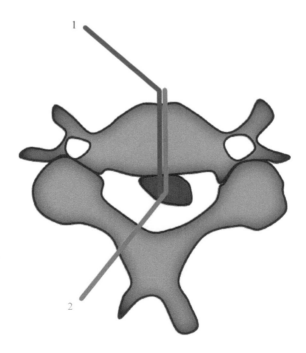

Reference of the sagittal planes

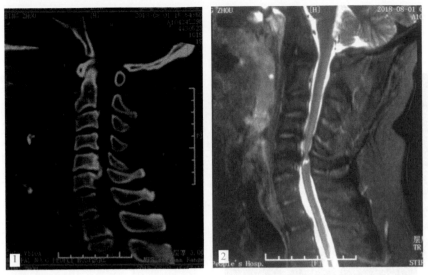

FIGURE 3.10.2

Preoperative sagittal images and their reference on the axial diagram.

(1) Midsagittal CT image.

(2) Midsagittal MRI image.

A circumscribed OPLL from C5 to C5/6, most prominent at C5/6, with a double-layer sign as shown on the preoperative sagittal CT image. Cord compression at C4/5 and C5/6, more severe at C5/6 where intramedullary signal hyperintensity indicates myelopathy (Fig. 3.10.3).

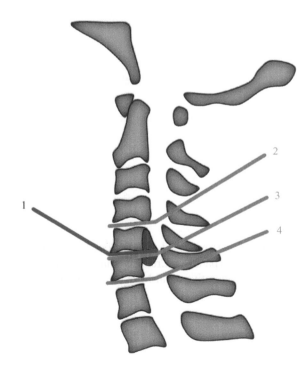

Reference of the axial images

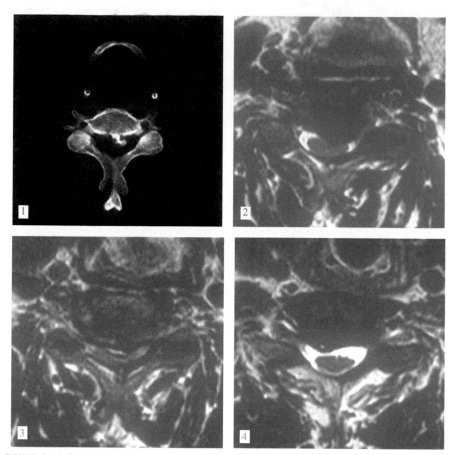

FIGURE 3.10.3

Preoperative axial images of the cervical spine and their reference on the sagittal diagram.
(1) Axial CT image at C5/6 disc space.
(2) Axial MRI image at C4/5 disc space.
(3) Axial MRI image at C5/6 disc space.
(4) Axial MRI image at C6/7 disc space.

A midline-centered and narrow-based OPLL of 8.4 mm thick, 15.6 mm wide, and 61.7% in canal occupancy (panel 1). Crescent-shaped spinal cord due to anterior indentation indicated on preoperative axial MRI images (panel 2 to 4).

Highlights

This case features short-segment circumscribed OPLL spanning C5 and C5/6 complicated with a disc protrusion of C4/5. This circumscribed OPLL is most prominent at C5/6, as shown on preoperative sagittal CT images. A double-layer sign is present within the narrow-based ossified mass, as shown on preoperative axial CT images.

Surgical planning

Direct anterior decompression is applicable in cases of short circumscribed OPLL of 60% or higher canal occupancy.

Since ACDF does not readily resect the ossified mass posterior to the C5 vertebra, C5 ACCF constitutes an alternative. However, the direct resection of the ossified mass may result in dural tear and CSF leakage given the potential dural involvement indicated by the double-layer sign at C5/6 on CT images.

Instead, ACAF provides a safer option for controlled neural decompression via C5 and C6 antedisplacement that obviates dural tear. Restoration of cervical curvature of short OPLL provides a minimal gain of decompression, so the anterior part of the vertebra of the same thickness as the ossification was resected (Fig. 3.10.4).

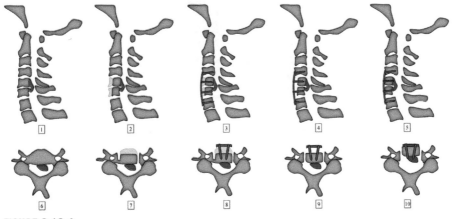

FIGURE 3.10.4

Illustration of the surgical plan on sagittal and axial views.

(1, 6) Illustration of the disease on sagittal and axial views before surgery.

(2, 7) Resection of the anterior part of vertebral bodies, a complete groove on the left, and a half one on the right of C5 and C6.

(3, 8) Titanium plate and vertebra screws placed from C4 to C7.

(4, 9) A completed groove on the right on C5 and C6 vertebral bodies.

(5, 10) Antedisplaced C5 and C6 vertebral bodies as the screws were tightened.

Results

Postoperative function: JOA was scored at 12, Nurick score: 2, VAS: 1, and NDI: 13 (Fig. 3.10.5).

Minimally restored curvature, instrumentation from C4 through C7, and antedisplaced C5 and C6 vertebral bodies (Fig. 3.10.6).

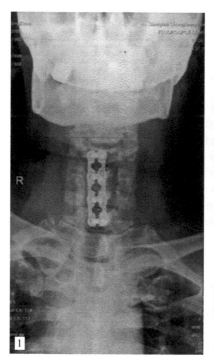 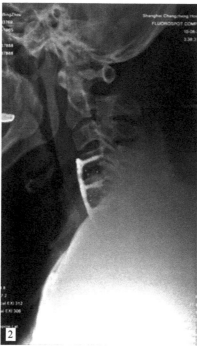

FIGURE 3.10.5

Postoperative X-ray of the cervical spine.
(1) Anteroposterior view.
(2) Lateral view.

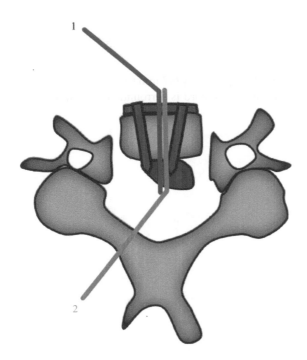

Reference of the sagittal planes

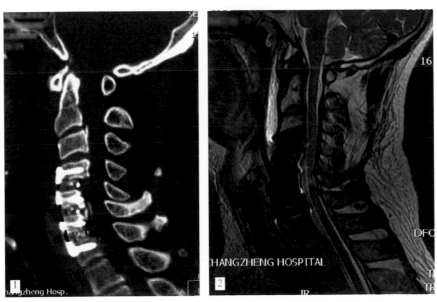

FIGURE 3.10.6

Postoperative sagittal images of the cervical spine and their reference on the axial diagram.
(1) Midsagittal CT image.
(2) Midsagittal MRI image.

VOC of C5 to C6 antedisplaced by 6.7 mm (panel 1). Adequate decompression at C4/5 and C5/6 where the spinal cord is surrounded by CSF (panel 2) (Fig. 3.10.7).

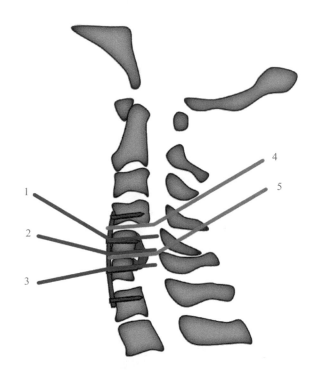

Reference of the axial images

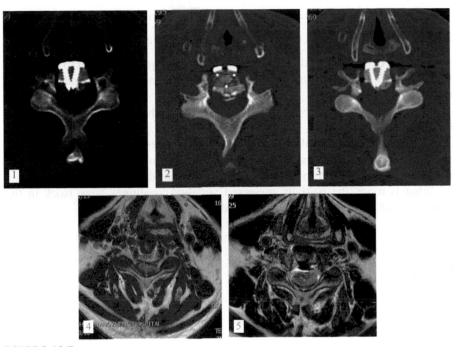

FIGURE 3.10.7

Postoperative axial images and their reference on the sagittal diagram.
(1) Axial CT image at C5 vertebra.
(2) Axial CT image at C5/6 disc space.
(3) Axial CT image at C6 vertebra.
(4) Axial MRI image at C4/5 disc space.
(5) Axial MRI image at C5/6 disc space.

The vertebral bodies have been dissected with cuts parallel to the sagittal plane 25.1 mm apart, reducing the spinal canal occupancy to 0% on axial CT images. The spinal cord resumes its oval shape on cross-section, as shown on axial MRI images.

Discussion

1 What are the challenging components in decompressing C5/6 disc space with ACDF technique in this case?

First, there is risk of partial decompression at C5/6 due to the loss of disc height. The distraction of the disc space during the procedure may result in up-sizing the cage and axial symptoms after surgery.

Another risk of intervertebral decompression via ACDF comes from the potential dural involvement of the OPLL at C5/6 suggested on image studies.

Third, ACDF does not facilitate the resection posterior to C5 vertebra.

2 What are the advantages of ACAF over ACCF in circumscribed OPLL?

Though ACCF of C5 with or without C6 may be an option, the need to dissect the lesion at C5/6 and debulk the lesion posterior to C6 vertebra creates challenge and risk.

Seemingly safer, ACCF of C5 and C6 increases the risk of instrumentation-related complications.

In contrast, ACAF enables indirect neural decompression via antedisplacement of vertebral bodies and less iatrogenic interference to the dura. It obviates the need to dissect the lesion and further reduce the risk of dural tear and CSF leakage.

What is more, the partially preserved vertebra constitutes bone stock in the construct that facilitates the fusion of the disc space.

Case 11: Ossification of posterior longitudinal ligament (OPLL) of cervical spine From C3 through C6

Index terms

Antedisplacement of three vertebral bodies, mixed-type ossification of the posterior longitudinal ligament (OPLL), wide-based OPLL, the thickness of ossification 5−7 mm, occupancy ratio 60%−70%, undercut decompression, cervical kyphosis.

History

Patient: A 54 year-old woman.

Chief complaint: Numbness of both hands for nine years which worsens with pain on shoulders and neck over the past three years.

Physical exam: Walking in steady gait, the patient had a reduced range of motion of the cervical spine. Muscle strength was measured at 5/5 on deltoid, biceps, and triceps of both upper limbs; 4/5 for wrist flexion and extension and 4/5 for hand grips on both upper limbs. Biceps and triceps tendon reflexes and radial periosteal reflexes were diminished on both sides.

Preoperative function: Japanese Orthopedic Association (JOA) score was 15, Nurick score: 1, visual analog scale (VAS): 5, and neck disability index (NDI): 15 (Fig. 3.11.1).

Imaging studies

A kyphotic cervical spine with a Cobb angle of −5.6° measured from C2 through C7, Pavlov ratio of 0.75, and a K-line (−) OPLL lesion spanning from C3 to C6 (Fig. 3.11.2).

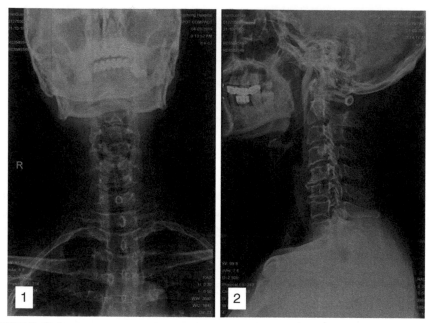

FIGURE 3.11.1

Preoperative X-ray of the cervical spine.

(1) Anteroposterior view.

(2) Lateral view.

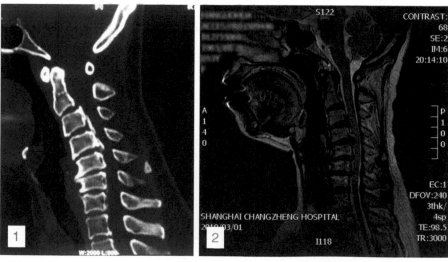

FIGURE 3.11.2

Preoperative sagittal images and their reference on axial diagram.

(1) Midsagittal CT image.

(2) Midsagittal MRI image.

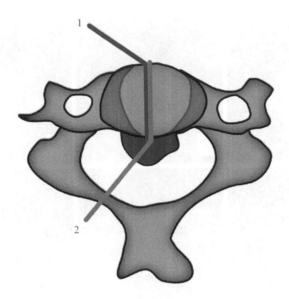

Reference of the sagittal planes

A mixed-type OPLL from C3 to C6, more severe from C4 through C5 (panel 1). Anterior indentation of the cervical cord at C3/4 to C6/7 in a kyphotic cervical spine, mostly at disc spaces. Cord impingement most prominent at C4/5 (panel 2) (Fig. 3.11.3).

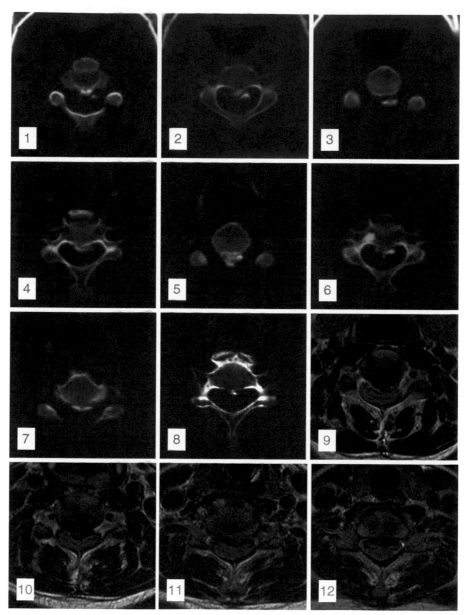

FIGURE 3.11.3

Preoperative axial images of the cervical spine and their reference on the sagittal diagram.

(1) Axial CT image at C2/3 disc space.

(2) Axial CT image at C3 vertebra.

(3) Axial CT image at C3/4 disc space.

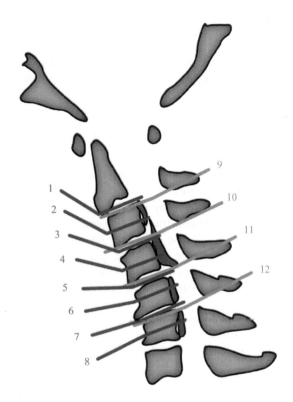

Reference of the axial planes

Preoperative axial computed tomography (CT) images suggest double-layer sign present from C4 to C5 in the narrow-based ossified lesion. The OPLL measures 3 mm thick (anteroposterior), 12 mm wide (mediolateral), and 25% in canal occupancy at C3. It becomes 6 mm thick, 17 mm wide, and 60% in canal occupancy at C3/4. It is 5 mm thick, 14 mm wide, and 41.7% in canal occupancy at C4, and 4 mm thick, 14 mm wide, and 33.3% in canal occupancy at C5 (panel 1 to 8). Impinged spinal cord in boomerang shape at all disc levels from C3/4 to C6/7 (panel 9 to 12).

(4) Axial CT image at C4 vertebra.
(5) Axial CT image at C4/5 disc space.
(6) Axial CT image at C5 vertebra.
(7) Axial CT image at C5/6 disc space.
(8) Axial CT image at C6 vertebra.
(9) Axial MRI image at C2/3 disc space.
(10) Axial MRI image at C3/4 disc space.
(11) Axial MRI image at C4/5 disc space.
(12) Axial MRI image at C5/6 disc space.

Highlights

This case features long-segment mixed-type OPLL in the kyphotic cervical spine with a double-layer sign at multiple levels that indicate the potential involvement of the dura.

Surgical planning

It is known that indirect decompression via a posterior approach has a limited role in kyphotic and K-line (−) OPLL case.

The direct decompression offered by anterior cervical corpectomy and fusion (ACCF) at C4 to C6 with a long construct of instrumentation carries a greater risk of fusion-related complications at disc spaces.

The presence of double-layer sign at multiple levels indicates the potential dural involvement and that the direct resection of the ossification may cause a dural tear.

The decision was made to perform ACAF that antedisplaces C4 through C6 vertebral bodies.

As the use of a plate that corrects cervical kyphosis contributes to cord decompression as well, we planned to resect the anterior bony structure of depth smaller than that of the ossified mass (Fig. 3.11.4).

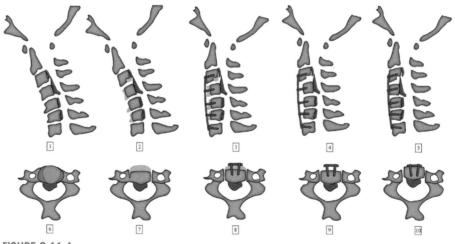

FIGURE 3.11.4

Illustration of the surgical plan on sagittal and axial planes.

(1, 6) Illustration of the disease on sagittal and axial views before surgery.

(2, 7) The C4 to C6 vertebrae are partially resected from anterior and C3 vertebra from inferoposterior. A complete trough is developed on the left vertebral bodies from C4 to C6 while a half one is made on the right side with the posterior bone yet to be dissected.

(3, 8) Plate and screws implanted on vertebral bodies from C3 through C7.

(4, 9) The bottom of the right half-groove on C4 through C6 dissected.

(5, 10) Screws are tightened to hoist the C4 to C6 vertebral bodies.

Results

Postoperative function: JOA score was 17, Nurick score: 0, VAS: 1, and NDI: 5 (Fig. 3.11.5).

Restored cervical curvature with Cobb of 3° measured from C2 through C7 and antedisplaced C4 to C6 vertebral bodies (Fig. 3.11.6).

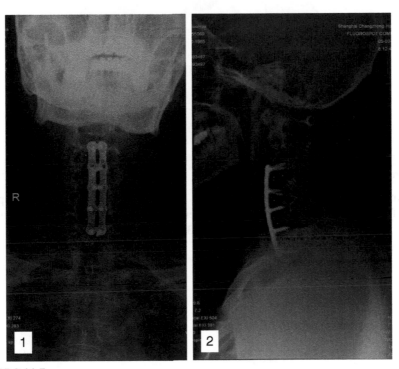

FIGURE 3.11.5

Postoperative cervical spine X-ray.

(1) Anteroposterior view.

(2) Lateral view.

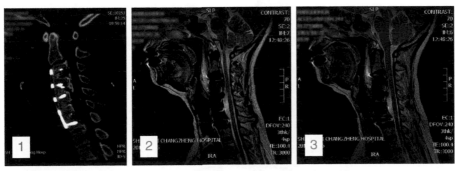

FIGURE 3.11.6

Postoperative sagittal views and their reference on the axial diagram.

(1) Midsagittal CT image.

(2) Paramedian sagittal MRI image of the right uncinate process.

(3) Midsagittal MRI image.

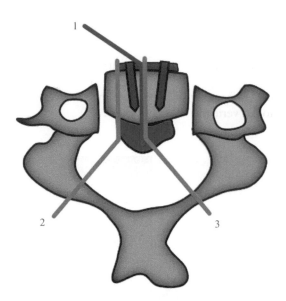

Reference of the sagittal planes

Antedisplaced vertebrae-OPLL complex (VOC) from C4 to C6 (panel 1). Spinal cord free of compression surrounded by cerebrospinal fluid (CSF) in the cervical spine with restored curvature (panel 2 and 3) (Fig. 3.11.7).

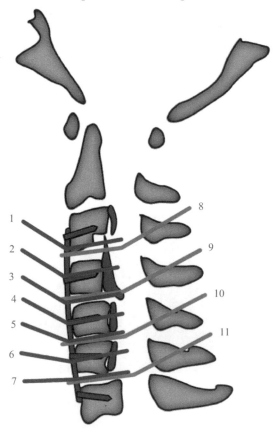

Reference of the axial planes

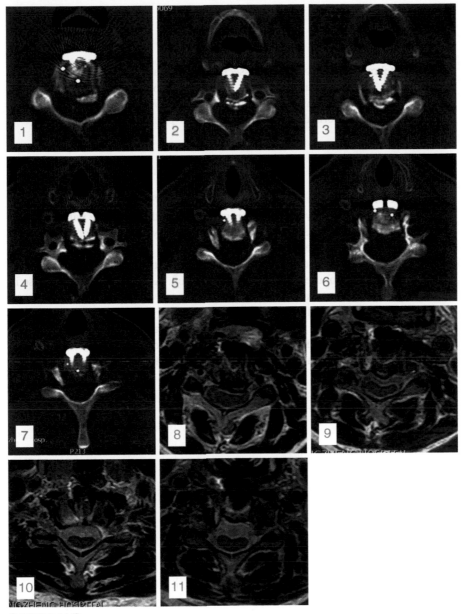

FIGURE 3.11.7

Postoperative axial cervical images and their reference on the sagittal diagram.

(1) Axial CT image at C3/4 disc space.

(2) Axial CT image at C4 vertebra.

(3) Axial CT image at C4/5 disc space.

(4) Axial CT image at C5 vertebra.

(5) Axial CT image at C5/6 disc space.

(6) Axial CT image at C6 vertebra.

(7) Axial CT image at C6/7 disc space.

(8) Axial MRI image at C3/4 disc space.

(9) Axial MRI image at C4/5 disc space.

(10) Axial MRI image at C5/6 disc space.

(11) Axial MRI image at C6/7 disc space.

The vertebral bodies have been dissected with parasagittal cuts on both sides 18 mm apart and VOC antedisplaced by 4 mm, though C4 is only partially advanced, and canal occupancy has been reduced to 18% (panel 1 to 7). The spinal cord has resumed its normal oval shape (panel 8 to 11).

Discussion

Why did the procedure leave the C4 partially advanced?

Since the VOC was fully mobilized from the rest of the vertebrae with complete grooves at all levels and free of lateral shift, it is unlikely that the displacement was obstructed by the rest of the vertebrae.

An oversized cage with excessive friction coefficient is not relevant in this case since spreaders were not used during disc preparation. Also, poor screw purchase is not in play as the patient was clear for osteoporosis.

Ruling out the factors of excessive resistance during antedisplacement and suboptimal hoisting force, our team looked into the direction of the vertebra screws from C4 through C6. Indeed, the two screws in the C4 vertebra were too convergent that they engaged and prematurely terminated the antedisplacement.

Case 12: Ossification of posterior longitudinal ligament (OPLL) of cervical spine From C4 through C6

Index terms

Antedisplacement of fewer than three vertebral bodies, continuous OPLL, wide-based lesion, the thickness of ossification 5–7 mm, occupancy ratio 60%–70%, undercut decompression, and cervical kyphosis.

History

Patient: A 48-year-old woman.

Chief complaint: Pain of the neck and back with weakness of the right extrem ities for 20 days.

Physical exam: The patient, coming in the clinic exam room in a gurney, manifested diminished superficial sensation below the sternal angle and on the perineum; increased pain, warm and cold reactivity on the right extremities but decreased on the left. Muscle strength was measured at 4/5 on the left upper limb, 3/5 on the right upper limb, and 4/4 on both lower limbs. Brisk tendon reflexes were noted with Hoffmann and Babinski signs on lower extremities.

Preoperative function: JOA score was 10, Nurick score: 4, VAS: 1, and NDI: 18 (Fig. 3.12.1).

Imaging studies

A kyphotic cervical spine with a Cobb angle of $-5.7°$ measured from C2 through C7, Pavlov ratio of 0.64, and a K-line (+) OPLL lesion spanning from C5 to C6 (Fig. 3.12.2).

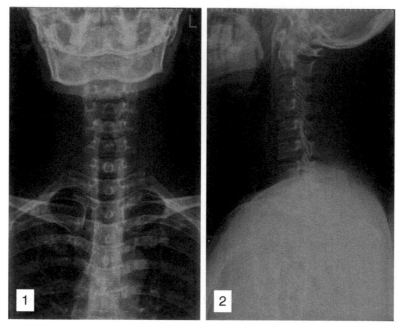

FIGURE 3.12.1

Preoperative X-ray of cervical spine.
(1) Anteroposterior view.
(2) Lateral view.

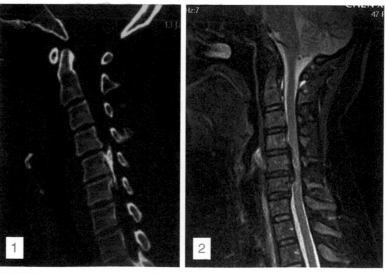

FIGURE 3.12.2

Preoperative sagittal images and their reference on axial diagram.
(1) Midsagittal CT image.
(2) Midsagittal MRI image.

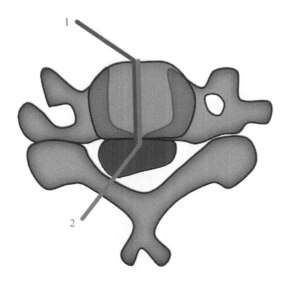

Reference of the sagittal planes

A continuous OPLL from C5 to C6 noted in a straightened cervical spine thickest at C5 and with a double-layer sign at C6 (panel 1). A straightened spinal cord impinged at C4/5 to C5/6, most severe at C5/6, with CSF effacement and intramedullary signal hyperintensity that indicates myelopathy (panel 2) (Fig. 3.12.3).

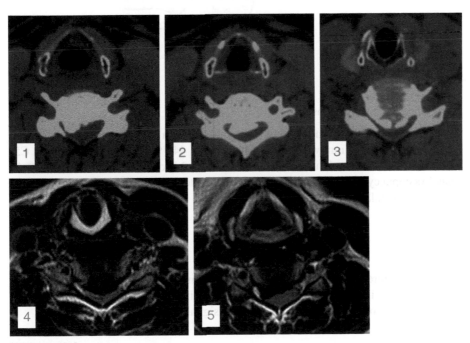

FIGURE 3.12.3

Preoperative axial images of the cervical spine and their reference on the sagittal diagram.
(1) Axial CT image at the inferior surface of C4 vertebra.
(2) Axial CT image at C5 vertebra.
(3) Axial CT image at C6 vertebra.
(4) Axial MRI image at C4/5 disc space.
(5) Axial MRI image at C5/6 disc space.

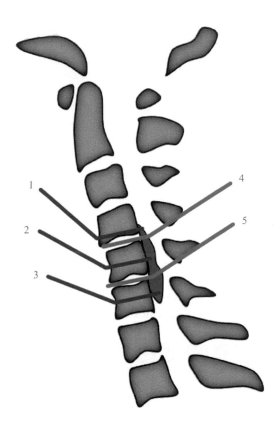

Reference of the axial planes

A narrow-based midline-centered OPLL, thicker on the right side, 5.5 mm thick (anteroposterior), 16 mm wide (mediolateral), and 44.7% in canal occupancy at C5, and it is wide-based and midline-centered 5.7 mm thick, 20.1 mm wide, and 60% in canal occupancy at C6 (panel 1 to 3). Due to anterior indentation, the spinal cord appears triangular or boomerang-shaped (panel 4 and 5).

Highlights

This case features a wide-based, plateau-typed continuous OPLL spanning from C4 to C6 without interruption that appears right-shifted. Myelopathy resulting from cord compression is noted with a change of signal intensity at C5.

Surgical planning

Indirect decompression via a posterior approach provides suboptimal decompression in cases of 60% or higher canal occupancy in a straightened cervical spine. Direct decompression via an anterior approach is thus preferred. The ACCF technique carries a higher risk of residual impingement in wide-based OPLL.

The decision was made, therefore, to antedisplace C5 and C6 vertebral bodies with ACAF technique, undercut the posterior part of C4, and restore cervical lordosis with a prebent plate.

Since the tip of the lesion was small posterior to C4 inferior surface, the infero-posterior part of C4 was undercut just enough till that tip was palpable with a neural probe (Fig. 3.12.4).

Results

Postoperative function: JOA was scored at 12, Nurick score: 2, VAS: 0, and NDI: 17 (Fig. 3.12.5).

Cobb angle of 6.6° from C2 to C7. Antedisplaced vertebral bodies from C4 through C6 (Fig. 3.12.6).

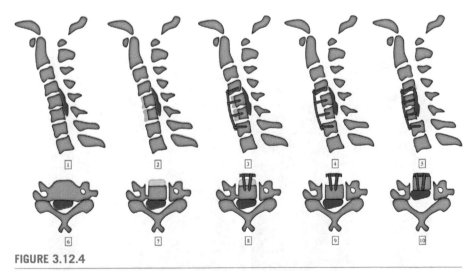

FIGURE 3.12.4

Illustration of the surgical plan on sagittal and axial views.
(1, 6) Illustration of the disease on sagittal and axial views before surgery.
(2, 7) Resection of the anterior part of the vertebral bodies of C5 and C6 and the inferoposterior part of the C4 vertebra, a left groove and a right half-groove on C5 and C6.
(3, 8) Titanium plate and screws placed in vertebral bodies from C4 to C7.
(4, 9) Completion of the right groove on C5 and C6.
(5, 10) Antedisplaced C5 and C6 vertebral bodies after screw tightening.

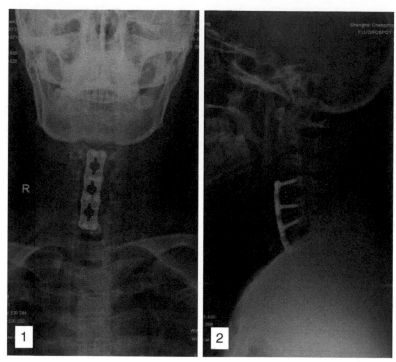

FIGURE 3.12.5

Postoperative cervical X-ray.

(1) Anteroposterior view.

(2) Lateral view.

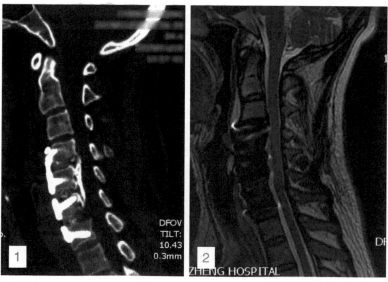

FIGURE 3.12.6

Postoperative sagittal images and their reference on the axial diagram.

(1) Midsagittal CT image.

(2) Midsagittal MRI image.

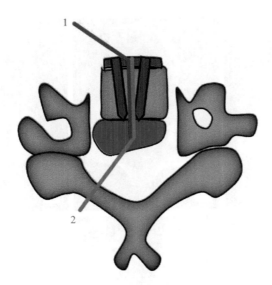

Reference of the sagittal planes

Ventrally displaced VOC from C5 through C6 and the spinal canal of resumed volume (panel 1). Adequate decompression of the spinal cord free of impinging lesions posterior to C5 and C6 vertebral bodies, particularly at C6 of maximum preoperative compression, and the spinal cord surrounded by CSF (panel 2) (Fig. 3.12.7).

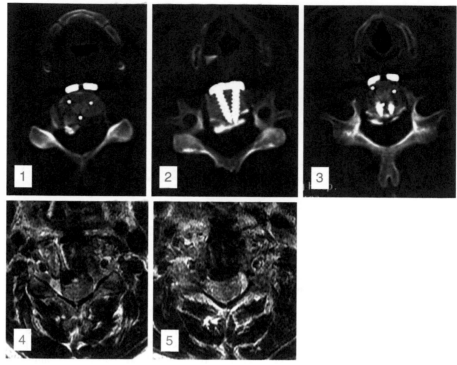

FIGURE 3.12.7

Postoperative cervical axial images and their reference on the sagittal diagram.
(1) Axial CT image at the inferior surface of C4 vertebra.
(2) Axial CT image at C5 vertebra.
(3) Axial CT image at C6 vertebra.
(4) Axial MRI image at C4/5 disc space.
(5) Axial MRI image at C5/6 disc space.

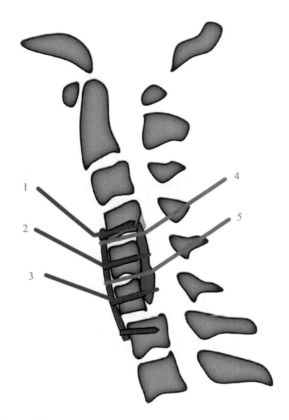

Reference of the axial planes

The C5 and C6 VOC has been dissected with parasagittal cuts on both sides 22.1 mm apart and antedisplaced by 3.5 mm, with canal occupancy reduced to 18% as the anteroposterior dimension of the canal has been expanded, shown on postoperative axial CT images. Satisfactory cord decompression indicated with the oval cord on axial MRI image.

Discussion

For the disease posterior to the C6 vertebra, why was C6 antedisplacement performed instead of undercut decompression?

Undercut decompression works in either tip of a continuous OPLL that involves less than half of the vertebra height.

As the OPLL's distal tip covered more than half of the C6 vertebral height, an undercut decompression would significantly reduce bone volume and endplate dimension and increase the risk of a fusion failure. As such, C6 antedisplacement was performed as a part of the procedure.

Case 13: Ossification of posterior longitudinal ligament (OPLL) of cervical spine From C4 through C7

Index terms

Antedisplacement of four vertebral bodies, mixed-type OPLL, wide-based OPLL, the thickness of ossification 5–7 mm, and occupancy ratio 50%–60%.

History

Patient: A 51-year-old woman.

Chief complaint: Radiating pain of the right upper limb for one year.

Physical exam: Limited range of motion in the cervical spine and preserved gait stability. Tenderness and pain on percussion on spinal processes, interspinous space, and the paraspinal region from C5 to C7. Radiating pain on the ulnar and radial sides of the right upper arm. Spurling sign was positive on the right side. Muscle strength was measure at 4-/5 on the right upper limb, 4/5 on the left upper limb, and 4+/5 on the lower limbs.

Preoperative function: JOA score was 13, Nurick score: 1, VAS: 3, and NDI: 23 (Fig. 3.13.1).

Imaging studies

Cobb angle of 14.7° when measured from C2 to C7 and Pavlov ratio above 0.75. A K-line (+) OPLL lesion from C4 to C7 in a lordotic cervical spine (Fig. 3.13.2).

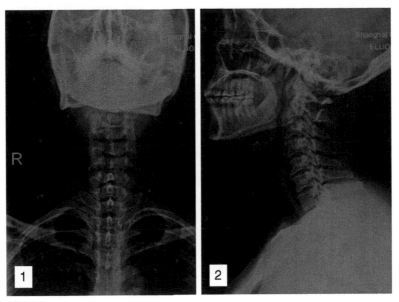

FIGURE 3.13.1

Preoperative X-ray of the cervical spine.
(1) Anteroposterior view.
(2) Lateral view.

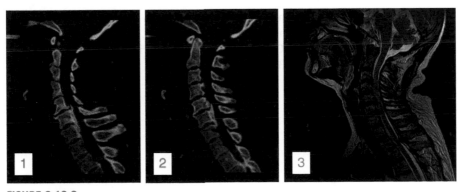

FIGURE 3.13.2

Preoperative sagittal views and their reference on the axial diagram.
(1) Parasagittal CT image at the right uncinate process.
(2) Midsagittal CT image.
(3) Midsagittal MRI image.

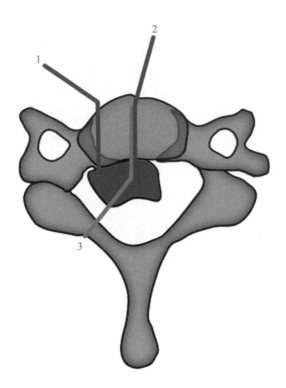

Reference of the sagittal planes

In addition to the predominant mixed-type OPLL from C4 to C7, ossification of the ligamentum flavum is present at T2/3 (panel 1 and 2). Cord compression from C3/4 to C6/7, predominantly at C5 to C6, and changes of intramedullary signal intensity at C5 (panel 3) (Fig. 3.13.3).

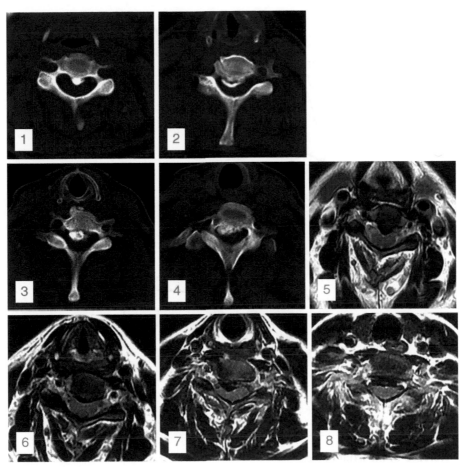

FIGURE 3.13.3

Preoperative axial cervical images and their reference on the sagittal diagram.

(1) Axial CT image at C4 vertebra.

(2) Axial CT image at C5 vertebra.

(3) Axial CT image at C6 vertebra.

(4) Axial CT image at C7 vertebra.

(5) Axial MRI image at C3/4 disc space.

(6) Axial MRI image at C4/5 disc space.

(7) Axial MRI image at C5/6 disc space.

(8) Axial MRI image at C6/7 disc space.

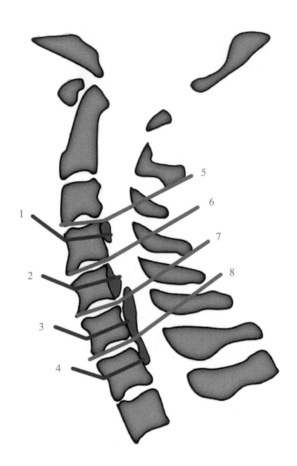

Reference of the axial planes

A wide-based OPLL eccentric to the right, primarily from C5 to C7, that measures 5.0 mm thick (anteroposterior), 9 mm wide (mediolateral), and 39% in canal occupancy at C4. It is 5.9 mm thick, 15.6 mm wide, and 48% in canal occupancy with a double-layer sign at C5; and 5.1 mm thick, 15.7 mm wide, and 56% in canal occupancy at C6. At C7; it has a wider base and measures 5.9 mm thick, and 18.2 mm wide, and 57% in canal occupancy (panel 1 to 4). Spinal cord in the shape of boomerang and triangle on axial MRI images due to anterior indentation, with CSF effacement.

Highlights

This case features an extensive, wide-based, right-eccentric, and mixed-type cervicothoracic OPLL.

Surgical planning

One may consider indirect decompression via a posterior approach for K-line (+) OPLL that spans multiple segments, as seen in this case. However, the patient needs a minimal posterior shift of the spinal cord to prevent nerve palsy, given the prominent cervical lordosis and the cervicothoracic disease.

What is more, a posterior procedure carries greater surgical insult and increased risk of recurrent cord dysfunction resulting from disease aggravation.

The decision was made to decompress the cord with C4 to C7 antedisplacement via the ACAF technique.

To address the disease at the cervicothoracic level, a longitudinal incision or double horizontal incisions can be developed.

The room of decompression from curvature correction is minimal since the patient had preserved cervical lordosis. Therefore, an anterior part of the vertebrae of the same thickness as the ossification is resected (Fig. 3.13.4).

Results

Postoperative function: JOA score was 13, Nurick score: 1, VAS: 2, and NDI: 18 (Fig. 3.13.5).

Instrumentation from C3 to T1 and antedisplaced C4 through C7 vertebral bodies.

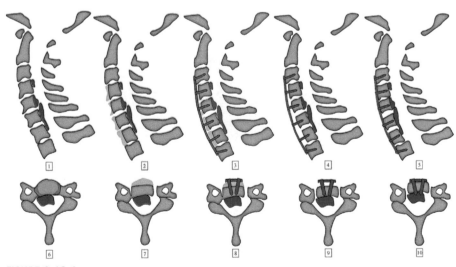

FIGURE 3.13.4

Illustration of the surgical plan on sagittal and axial views.

(1, 6) Illustration of the disease on sagittal and axial views before surgery.

(2, 7) Resection of the anterior part of the vertebral bodies of C4 through C7. A complete trough on the left and a half one on the right at C4 through C7 vertebral bodies.

(3, 8) Titanium plate and vertebra screws installed on C3 to T1.

(4, 9) Completion of the right groove on C4 through C7.

(5, 10) C4 through C7 vertebral bodies antedisplaced with the tightening of screws.

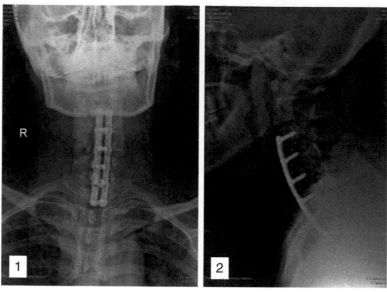

FIGURE 3.13.5

Postoperative X-ray of the cervical spine.
(1) Anteroposterior view.
(2) Lateral view.

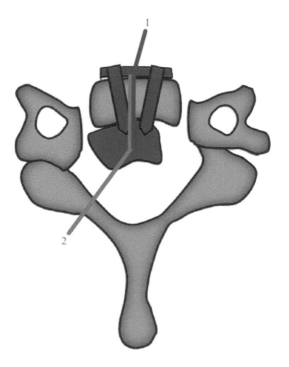

Reference of the sagittal planes

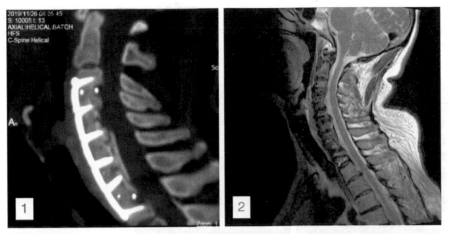

FIGURE 3.13.6

Postoperative sagittal images and their reference on the axial diagram.
(1) Midsagittal CT image.
(2) Midsagittal MRI image.

Antedisplaced VOC from C4 to C7 and expanded central canal (panel 1). Adequately decompressed spinal cord surrounded by CSF (panel 2) (Fig. 3.13.6).

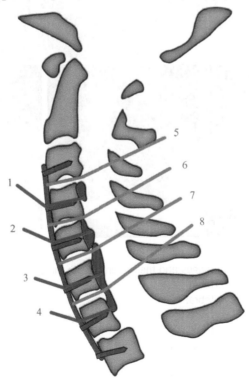

Reference of the axial planes

The VOC displaced anteriorly by 6.3 mm with grooves on both sides 22 mm apart, reducing canal occupancy to 0% (panel 1 to 4). The spinal cord resumes its oval shape on cross-section with normal CSF around it (panel 5 to 8) (Fig. 3.13.7).

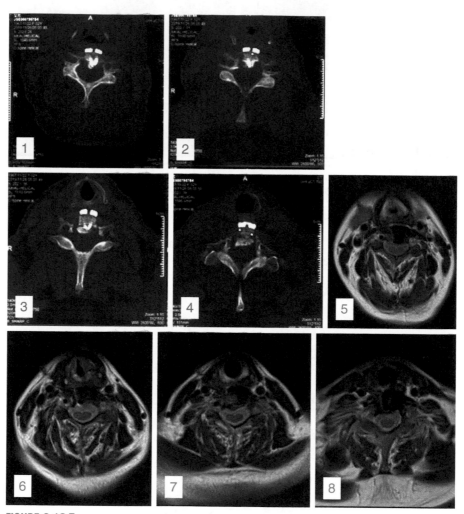

FIGURE 3.13.7

Postoperative axial cervical images and their reference on the sagittal diagram.
(1) Axial CT image at C4 vertebra.
(2) Axial CT image at C5 vertebra.
(3) Axial CT image at C6 vertebra.
(4) Axial CT image at C7 vertebra.
(5) Axial MRI image at C3/4 disc space.
(6) Axial MRI image at C4/5 disc space.
(7) Axial MRI image at C5/6 disc space.
(8) Axial MRI image at C6/7 disc space.

Discussion

As the postoperative CT images reveal bicortical vertebra screws that engage the ossified mass, does it suggest that one should change for shorter screws during final fixation?

A larger anterior part of the vertebrae was resected in this case to provide room for decompression since curvature restoration was not contributory where cervical lordosis was unaffected.

Therefore, the screws on the antedisplaced segments went through the posterior cortex and engaged in the ossified mass. It does not obstruct the antedisplacement of the ossified mass since the mass is closely attached to the posterior vertebral wall.

Indeed, this results in a better purchase of the screw in the VOC. In contrast, in the segments spared from OPLL, long screws going through the posterior cortex may risk canal protrusion. In such a case, the screws are substituted by shorter ones after VOC advancement.

Case 14: Ossification of posterior longitudinal ligament (OPLL) of the cervical spine From C5 to C6/7

Complicated with disc protrusion.

Index terms

Antedisplacement of fewer than three vertebral bodies, segmental OPLL, the thickness of ossification 5–7 mm, occupancy ratio below 50%, ACAF + anterior cervical discectomy and fusion (ACDF), and residual lesion.

History

Patient: A 53-year-old man.

Chief complaint: Pain and numbness of both upper limbs for five years and worsen for one month.

Physical exam: Physical exam was noted for gait disturbance; numbness of the index, middle, and small fingers of the left side; and pain on the neck and right shoulder. Muscle strength was measured at 4/5 on the left upper limb and 3/5 on the right upper limb. Hoffmann sign was present on both sides.

Preoperative function: JOA score was 14, Nurick score: 1, VAS: 3, and NDI: 12 (Fig. 3.14.1).

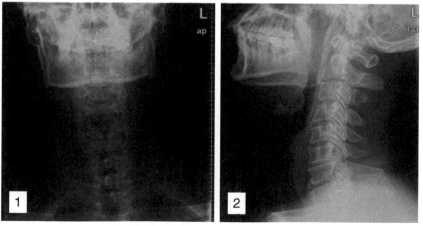

FIGURE 3.14.1

Preoperative X-ray of the cervical spine.
(1) Anteroposterior view.
(2) Lateral view.

Imaging studies

Unaffected cervical curvature, Cobb of 15.3° from C2 to C7, and Pavlov ratio 0.57, 0.73, 0.70, and 0.70 at C3 through C6, respectively. K-line (+) OPLL lesion.

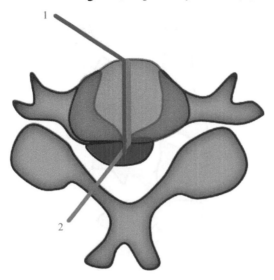

Reference of the sagittal planes

A plateau-type segmental OPLL from C5 through C7 (panel 1). Anterior indentation of the spinal cord from C3/4 to C6/7 with complete obliteration of anterior and posterior CSF column (panel 2) (Fig. 3.14.2).

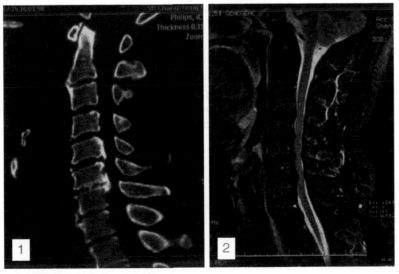

FIGURE 3.14.2

Preoperative sagittal images and their reference on the axial diagram.
(1) Midsagittal CT image.
(2) Midsagittal MRI image.

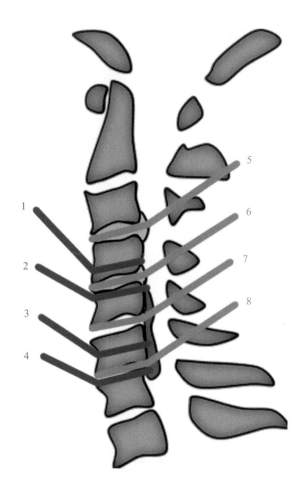

Reference of the axial planes

A narrow-based ossified lesion of relatively small bulk measures 6.0 mm thick, 18.6 mm wide, and 44.4% in canal occupancy at C5/6; and 5.4 mm thick, 20.4 mm wide, and 45% in canal occupancy at C6/7 (panel 1 to 4). The indented spinal cord appears in the shapes of boomerang or crescent (panel 5 to 8) (Fig. 3.14.3).

Highlights

This case features a spinal cord compressed at multiple levels primarily by the protruded C3/4 and C4/5 intervertebral discs and less severely by the OPLL on C5 to C6/7.

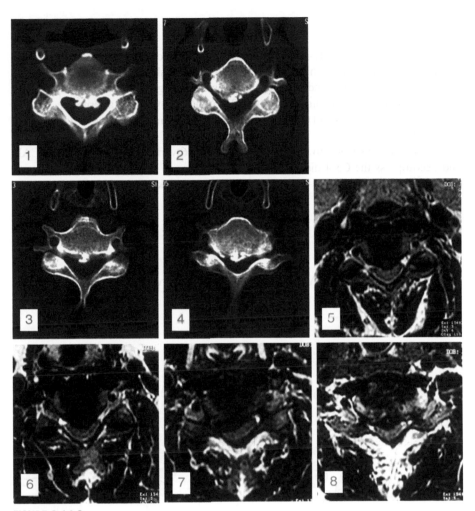

FIGURE 3.14.3

Preoperative axial images of the cervical spine and their reference on the sagittal diagram.

(1) Axial CT image at the inferior surface of C4 vertebra.

(2) Axial CT image at the superior surface of C5 vertebra.

(3) Axial CT image at C6 vertebra.

(4) Axial CT image at the superior surface of C7 vertebra.

(5) Axial MRI image at C3/4 disc space.

(6) Axial MRI image at C4/5 disc space.

(7) Axial MRI image at C5/6 disc space.

(8) Axial MRI image at C6/7 disc space.

Surgical planning

In a case of extensive and K-line (+) OPLL, indirect decompression can be achieved via a posterior approach which, however, carries the risk of a recurrent neurologic deficit as the ossification and disc degeneration may progress further down the road.

ACCF on C5 and C6 combined with C3/4 ACDF provides an alternative, but the wide-based lesion at C5 and C7 superior surface could cause incomplete decompression of ACCF.

A decision was made to antedisplace C5 and C6 vertebral bodies via an ACAF and decompress the C3/4 disc space via ACDF.

An anterior part of the vertebrae of the same thickness as the ossification is resected (Fig. 3.14.4).

Results

Postoperative function: JOA score was 14, Nurick score: 1, VAS: 2, and NDI: 10 (Fig. 3.14.5).

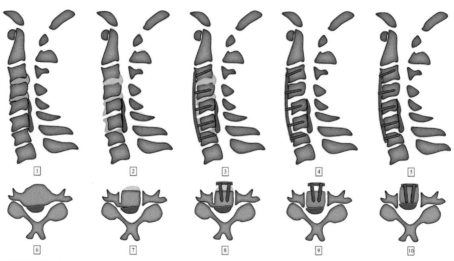

FIGURE 3.14.4

Illustration of the surgical plan on sagittal and axial views.

(1, 6) Illustration of the disease on sagittal and axial views before surgery.

(2, 7) Resection of the anterior part of the vertebral bodies of C5 and C6. A complete trough on the left and a half one on the right at C5 and C6 vertebral bodies.

(3, 8) Titanium plate and vertebra screws placed on C3 to C7.

(4, 9) Completion of the right groove on C5 and C6.

(5, 10) Antedisplaced C5 and C6 vertebral bodies after screw tightening.

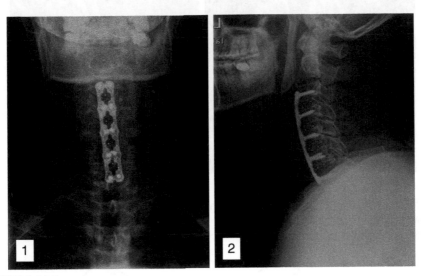

FIGURE 3.14.5

Postoperative X-ray of cervical spine.
(1) Anteroposterior view.
(2) Lateral view.

Cobb angle of 21.3° from C2 through C7. Instrumentation from C3 to C7 and antedisplaced C5 and C6 vertebral bodies.

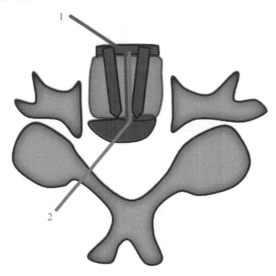

Reference of the sagittal planes

Antedisplaced VOC from C5 to C6 and expanded spinal canal (panel 1). Decompressed spinal cord from C3/4 through C6/7 surrounded by CSF in a patent canal (panel 2) (Fig. 3.14.6).

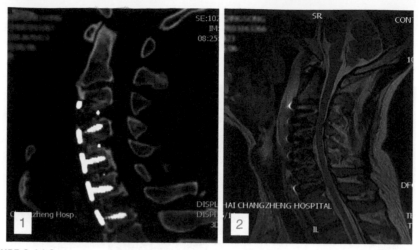

FIGURE 3.14.6

Postoperative sagittal images and their reference on the axial diagram.
(1) Midsagittal CT image.
(2) Midsagittal MRI image.

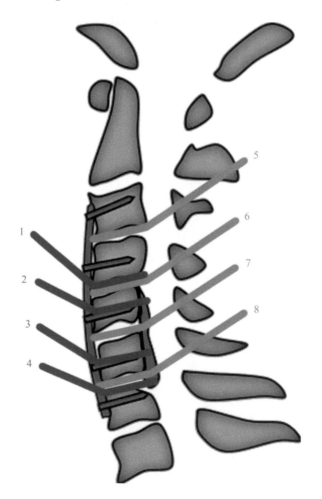

Reference of the axial planes

The VOC dissected from the boney structures on both sides by grooves 19.8 mm apart and displaced anteriorly by 4.9 mm; the canal occupancy ratio decreased to 17%; and residual lesion on the right side in the spinal canal at C5 and C6 vertebra levels (panel 1 to 4). Neural impingement at C3/4 and C6/7 resolved (panel 5 to 8) (Fig. 3.14.7).

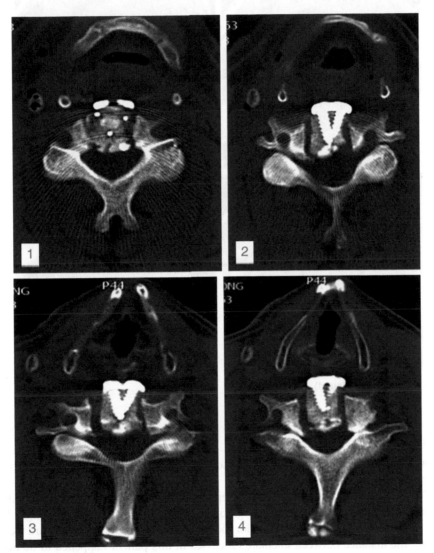

FIGURE 3.14.7

Postoperative axial cervical images and their reference on the sagittal diagram.
(1) Axial CT image at C4/5 disc space.
(2) Axial CT image at C5 vertebra.
(3) Axial CT image at C6 vertebra.
(4) Axial CT image at C6/7 disc space.
(5) Axial MRI image at C3/4 disc space.
(6) Axial MRI image at C4/5 disc space.
(7) Axial MRI image at C5/6 disc space.
(8) Axial MRI image at C6/7 disc space.

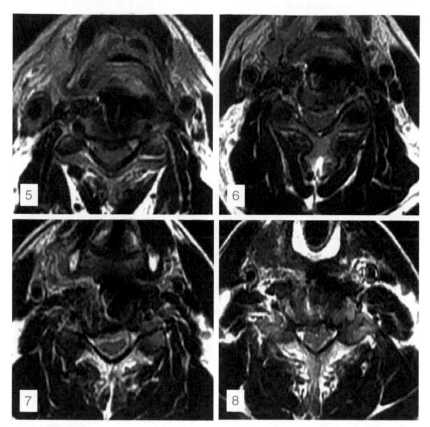

FIGURE 3.14.7 (Continued)

Discussion

How to avoid leaving residual lesions as seen on C5 and C6 around the right groove on postoperative CT scans?

The residual lesions in this case were due to narrow decompression width, defined as the distance between the grooves on the vertebral bodies. Though the grooves were developed off the anterior roots of uncinate processes, a standard technique, the distance between uncinate processes in this patient happened to be narrower, resulting in reduced decompression width.

To avoid this problem, preoperative measurement should involve not only the dimension of the ossified lesion but also the distance between the anterior bases of uncinate processes.

In patients with closer uncinate processes, care should be taken to lateralize the grooves to prevent incomplete resection.

Case 15: Ossification of posterior longitudinal ligament (OPLL) of cervical spine At C3 to C4 and C5 to C6

Index terms

Antedisplacement of four vertebral bodies, mixed-type OPLL, thickness of ossification 7—9 mm, occupancy ratio between 60% and 70%, K-line (−) OPLL, and oblique grooves.

History

Patient: A 68-year-old man.

Chief complaint: Numbness and weakness of both upper limbs for two years that worsen over the past two months.

Physical exam: Physical exam was noted for gait disturbance, diminished superficial sensation on both upper limbs and both soles, and hypertonic upper and lower extremities. Muscle strength was measured at 3/5 on both upper limbs, 4/5 on both lower limbs. Tendon reflexes were brisk on all the limbs.

Preoperative function: JOA score was 9, Nurick score: 3, VAS: 0, and NDI: 9.

Imaging studies

A straightened cervical spine with Cobb of 2.1° from C2 to C7, Pavlov ratio above 0.75, and a K-line (−) OPLL of C3 through C4 (Fig. 3.15.1).

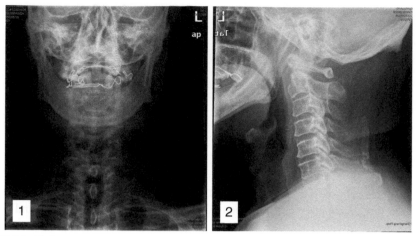

FIGURE 3.15.1

Preoperative X-ray of the cervical spine.
(1) Anteroposterior view.
(2) Lateral view.

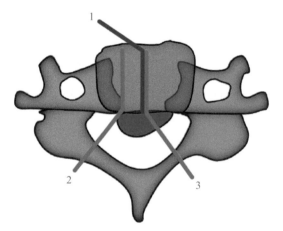

Reference of the sagittal planes

A mixed-type OPLL on C3 to C4 and C6, hill-shaped at C3/4, with canal encroachment and incipient ossification at C5/6 (panel 1). Anterior indentation from C3 to C7 with complete effacement of CSF and straightening of the spinal cord, with maximum cord compression at C3/4 and C5/6 and intramedullary signal change at C5/6 (panel 2 and 3) (Fig. 3.15.2).

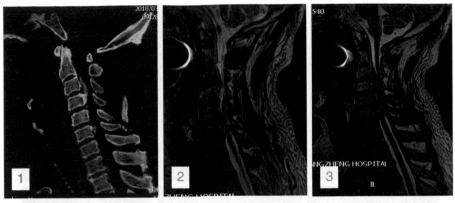

FIGURE 3.15.2

Preoperative sagittal images and their reference on the axial diagram.

(1) Midsagittal CT image.

(2) Right paramedian sagittal MRI image.

(3) Midsagittal MRI image.

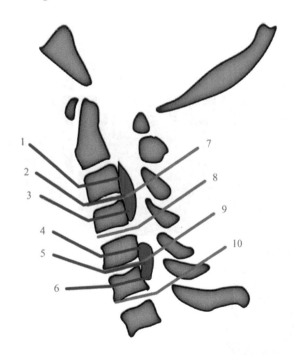

Reference of the sagittal planes

   Incipient ossification at C5/6 to C6. A midline-centered narrow-based OPLL, more prominent on the right side, at C3/4 8.4 mm thick, 10.6 mm wide, and 67.7% in canal occupancy (panel 1 to 6). Spinal cord in the shape of boomerang due to anterior indentation, with signal hyperintensity at C5/6 indicating myelopathy (panel 7 to 10) (Fig. 3.15.3).

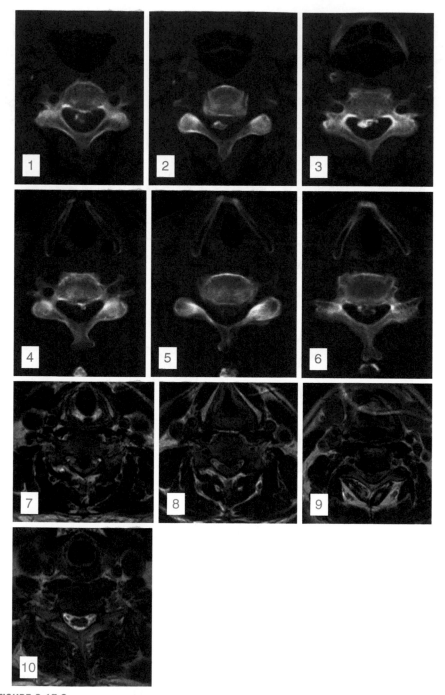

FIGURE 3.15.3

Preoperative axial images of the cervical spine and their reference on the sagittal diagram.

Highlights

This case features spinal cord impingement at C3 to C4 and C5 to C6 due to the anterior OPLL and intervertebral soft tissue. The lesion is hill-shaped at C3 to C4. Intervertebral material protrusion and calcification are present at C5/6, and the OPLL involves C6 as well.

Surgical planning

An anterior approach is a way to go in this case of a hill-shaped K-line (−) OPLL with straightened curvature and protruding disc.

ACDF has a minimal role in decompressing structures posterior to vertebral bodies.

ACCF involves resection of multiple vertebral bodies and the use of long construct, which carries a higher risk of fusion failure and implant-related complications.

The decision was made to antedisplace C3 through C6 via ACAF, a procedure characterized by bone preservation that facilitates fusion.

The C5/6 impingement is readily addressed with C5 and C6 antedisplacement combined with endplate preparation, which obviates the need to remove the protruded disc material at the intervertebral disc (Fig. 3.15.4).

Results

Postoperative function: JOA score was 11, Nurick score: 3, VAS: 0, and NDI: 11 (Fig. 3.15.5).

Restored cervical curvature with Cobb angle of 11.4° from C2 through C7.

(1) Axial CT image at C3 vertebra.
(2) Axial CT image at C3/4 disc space.
(3) Axial CT image at C4 vertebra.
(4) Axial CT image at C5 vertebra.
(5) Axial CT image at C5/6 disc space.
(6) Axial CT image at C6 vertebra.
(7) Axial MRI image at C3/4 disc space.
(8) Axial MRI image at C4/5 disc space.
(9) Axial MRI image at C5/6 disc space.
(10) Axial MRI image at C6/7 disc space.

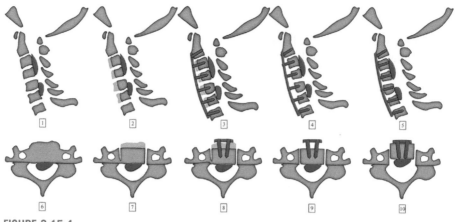

FIGURE 3.15.4

Illustration of the surgical plan on sagittal and axial views.

(1, 6) Illustration of the disease on sagittal and axial views before surgery.

(2, 7) Resection of the anterior part of the vertebral bodies of C3 through C6. A complete trough on the left and a half one on the right at C3 through C6 vertebral bodies.

(3, 8) Titanium plate and vertebra screws placed on C2 to C7.

(4, 9) Completion of the right groove on C3 through C6.

(5, 10) C3 through C6 vertebral bodies antedisplaced with the tightening of screws.

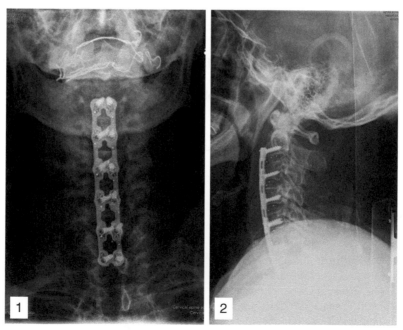

FIGURE 3.15.5

Postoperative X-ray of the cervical spine.

(1) Anteroposterior view.

(2) Lateral view.

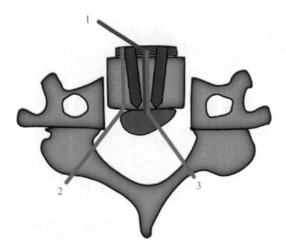

Reference of the sagittal planes

Antedisplaced VOC from C3 to C6 and widened spinal canal shown on postoperative midsagittal CT image (Fig. 3.15.6). Decompressed spinal cord from C3 through C6 surrounded by CSF, shown on postoperative sagittal magnetic resonance imaging (MRI) images (Fig. 3.15.7).

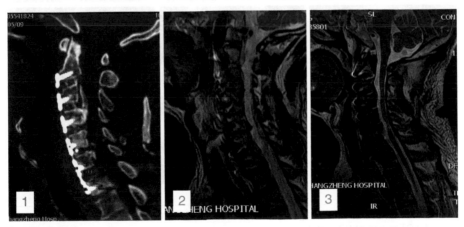

FIGURE 3.15.6

Postoperative sagittal images and their reference on the axial diagram.
(1) Midsagittal CT image.
(2) Right paramedian sagittal MRI image.
(3) Midsagittal MRI image.

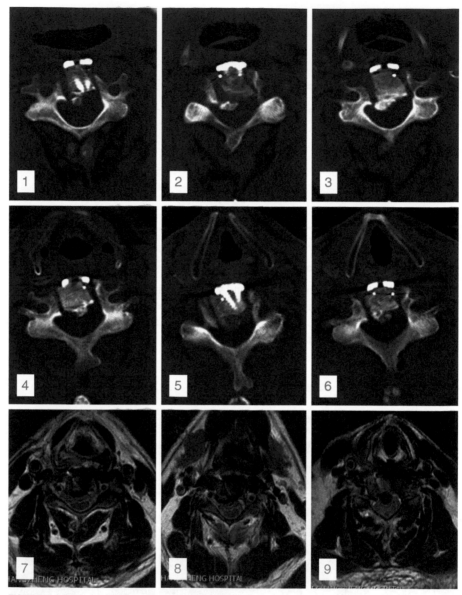

FIGURE 3.15.7

Postoperative axial cervical images and their reference on the sagittal diagram.

(1) Axial CT image at C3 vertebra.

(2) Axial CT image at C3/4 intervertebral space.

(3) Axial CT image at C4 vertebra.

(4) Axial CT image at C5 vertebra.

(5) Axial CT image at C5/6 intervertebral space.

(6) Axial CT image at C6 vertebra.

(7) Axial MRI image at C3/4 disc space.

(8) Axial MRI image at C4/5 disc space.

(9) Axial MRI image at C5/6 disc space.

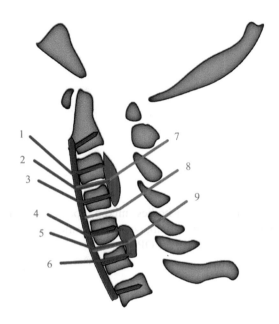

Reference of the axial planes

The VOC dissected from the boney structures on both sides by parasagittal grooves 20.8 mm apart and displaced anteriorly by 4.0 mm on the right and 7.4 mm on the left, shown on postoperative axial CT images. The canal occupancy ratio has decreased to 24.8% at C3/4 in the widened spinal canal. The spinal cord resumes its oval shape with normal CSF around it, as shown on postoperative axial MRI images.

Discussion

Will satisfactory decompression be achieved with antedisplacement of C3, C4, and C6 that skips C5?

Radiological evidence of this case includes established ossification posterior to C6 vertebra, incipient ossification at C5 and C5/6, and bulky disc protrusion at C5/6.

The attempt to skip C5 in ACAF involves undercut decompression of the inferoposterior part of C5 vertebra through the C5/6 disc space.

In general, undercut decompression is easier when performed to the superoposterior border of the caudal segment around the distal portion of the wound but more challenging the other way around due to difficult access. As the C5/6 disc space was prepared in this case, access to and exposure of the posterior part of C5 vertebra was so meager that an undercut decompression was challenging, if not impossible. Thus, the C5 vertebra was included as a part of the VOC.

Case 16: Ossification of posterior longitudinal ligament (OPLL) of cervical spine C2 to C7, of >90% canal occupancy

Index terms

Antedisplacement of four vertebral bodies, mixed-type lesion, wide-based lesion, the thickness of ossification above 9 mm, occupancy ratio above 70%, shelter technique, ACAF + ACDF, and K-line (−) OPLL.

History

Patient: A 57-year-old man.

Chief complaint: Neck pain for 10 years that aggravated with upper extremity numbness and gait instability for one month.

Physical exam: Physical exam was noted for gait disturbance, hypertonic extremities, and decreased superficial sensation of the pulps of the right fingers. Muscle strength was measured at 4/5 on upper limbs and 3/5 on lower limbs. Hyperreflexia for all four extremities, with ankle clonus and bilateral Hoffman and Babinski signs.

Preoperative function: JOA was measured at 9, Nurick score: 3, VAS: 5, and NDI: 21 (Fig. 3.16.1).

Imaging studies

Cobb angle of 16.7° measured from C2 through C7. K-line (−) OPLL from C2 to C5 (Fig. 3.16.2).

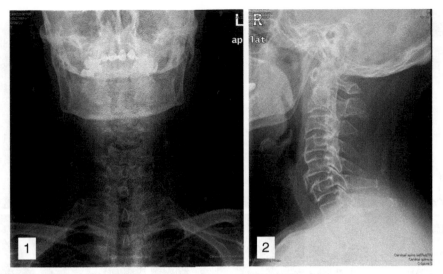

FIGURE 3.16.1

Preoperative X-ray of the cervical spine.
(1) Anteroposterior view.
(2) Lateral view.

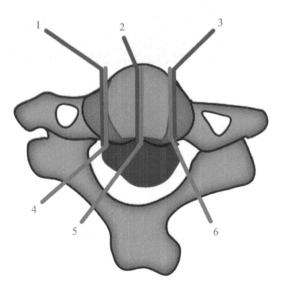

Reference of the sagittal planes

A mixed-type OPLL of C2 to C7, more severe at C3 to C4 and hill-shaped at C3 vertebra (panel 1 to 3). Cervical canal stenosis secondary to OPLL at C3 to C6, C7/

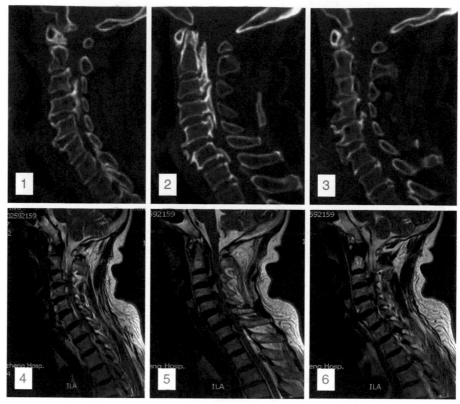

FIGURE 3.16.2

Preoperative sagittal images of the cervical spine and their reference on the axial diagram.

(1) Parasagittal CT at the right uncinate process.
(2) Midsagittal CT.
(3) Parasagittal CT at the left uncinate process.
(4) Parasagittal MRI at the right uncinate process.
(5) Right paramedian sagittal MRI.
(6) Parasagittal MRI at the left uncinate process.

T1 disc herniation, severely impinged, and deformed spinal cord in an "S" curvature (panel 4 to 6) (Fig. 3.16.3).

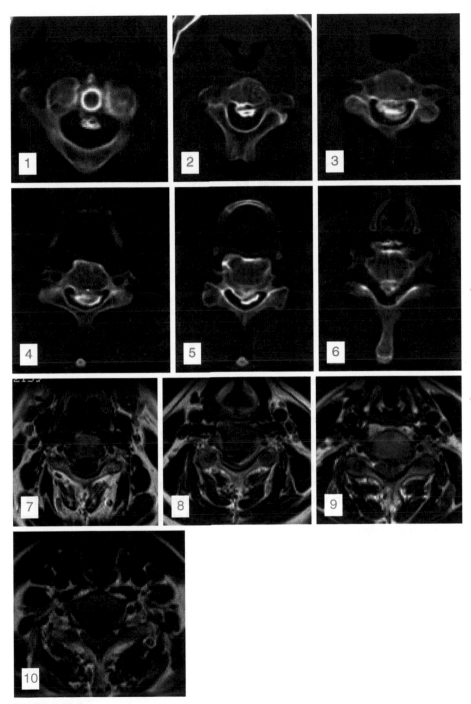

FIGURE 3.16.3

Preoperative axial images of the cervical spine and their reference on the sagittal diagram.

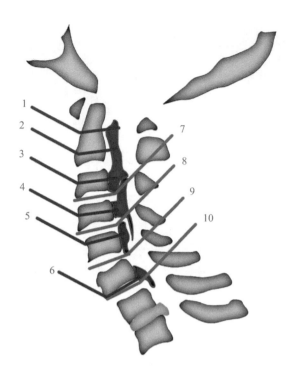

Reference of the axial planes

A large OPLL that encroaches the spinal canal with a wide base at C3 to C4 and C6 instability. The OPLL measures 7.0 mm thick (anteroposterior), 13.2 mm wide (mediolateral), and 50% in canal occupancy at C2; 10.7 mm thick, 16.8 mm wide, and 89.3% in occupancy with a double-layer sign at C3; 9.9 mm thick, 18.1 mm wide, and 92.2% in occupancy at C4; 7.4 mm thick, 14.8 mm wide, and 64.3% in occupancy at C5; and 9.0 mm thick, 12.7 mm wide, and 62.5% in occupancy at C6/7. The anteroposterior dimensions of the vertebral bodies vary between 14.8 and 17.4 mm. The spinal cord is boomerang-shaped at multiple levels due to severe anterior indentation.

(1) Axial CT at C2.
(2) Axial CT at the inferior surface of C2.
(3) Axial CT at C3.
(4) Axial CT at C4.
(5) Axial CT at the superior surface of C5.
(6) Axial CT at C6/7.
(7) Axial MRI at C3/4.
(8) Axial MRI at C4/5.
(9) Axial MRI at C5/6.
(10) Axial MRI at C6/7.

Highlights

This case features a severe mixed-type OPLL of multiple levels with over 90% of canal occupancy and double-layer sign on multiple sections. This case is also complicated with C5/6 instability and C7/T1 disc herniation.

Surgical planning

In this case of severe long-segment OPLL with 90% or higher canal stenosis, any decompression surgery from the anterior or posterior is technically demanding and carries an extremely high risk of injury and complication.

The patient received an ACAF on C3 through C6 with a posteroinferior part of C2 vertebra resected via the shelter technique. An ACDF was performed for C7/T1 disc herniation and neural decompression.

Canal stenosis of 90% or above indicates resection of a large part of the vertebral bodies. Screws purchased to the ossification provide better control of the antedisplacement and construct stability.

Though the OPLL extended its tip high at C2 vertebra, the compressive myelopathy did not go beyond the inferior surface of C2 and C2/3. As such, the posteroinferior part of the C2 vertebra was resected at the impingement-free level to allow for antedisplacement of the rest of the lesion via a shelter procedure (Fig. 3.16.4).

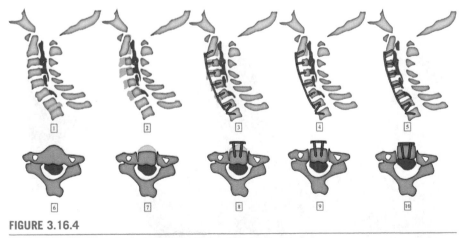

FIGURE 3.16.4

Illustration of the surgical plan on sagittal and axial views.
(1, 6) Illustration of the OPLL on sagittal and axial views before surgery.
(2, 7) Resection of the anterior part of the vertebral bodies of C3 to C6 as well as the posterior part of C2 vertebra. A left groove and a right half-groove with the posterior cortex still intact on C3 to C6.
(3, 8) Titanium plate and screws placed on vertebral bodies from C2 to C7.
(4, 9) Completion of the right groove on C3 through C6.
(5, 10) Antedisplaced C3 through C6 vertebral bodies after screw tightening.

Results

Postoperative function: JOA was scored at 16, Nurick score: 2, VAS: 2, and NDI: 12 (Fig. 3.16.5).

Cobb angle of 25.7° from C2 to C7. Antedisplaced vertebral bodies from C3 through C7 and instrumentation from C2 to T1 where screw length was 14 mm at C2 and C7, and 12 mm at C3 through C6. (Fig. 3.16.6).

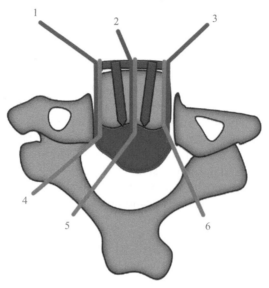

Reference of the sagittal planes

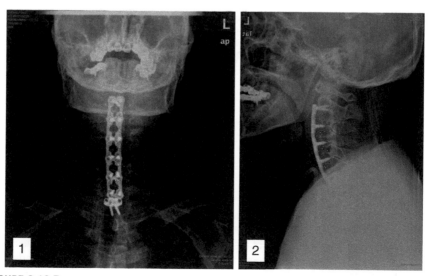

FIGURE 3.16.5

Postoperative cervical X-ray.
(1) Anteroposterior view.
(2) Lateral view.

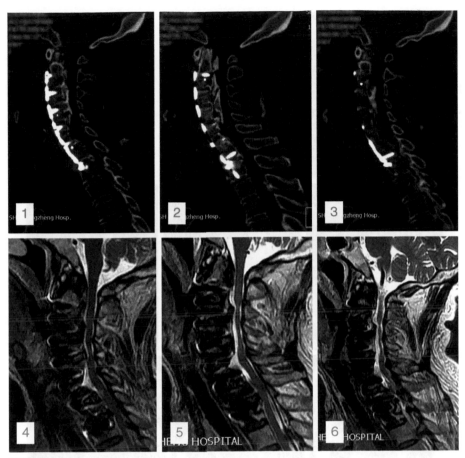

FIGURE 3.16.6

Postoperative sagittal images and their reference on the axial diagram.

(1) Parasagittal CT at the right uncinate process.

(2) Midsagittal CT.

(3) Parasagittal CT at the left intervertebral foramen.

(4) Parasagittal MRI at the right uncinate process.

(5) Midsagittal MRI.

(6) Parasagittal MRI at the left uncinate process.

Ventrally displaced VOC from C2 through C7 and spinal canal of resumed volume (panel 1 to 3). Spinal cord free of compression in natural curvature with residual deformation surrounded by CSF in the cervical spine (panel 4 to 6) (Fig. 3.16.7).

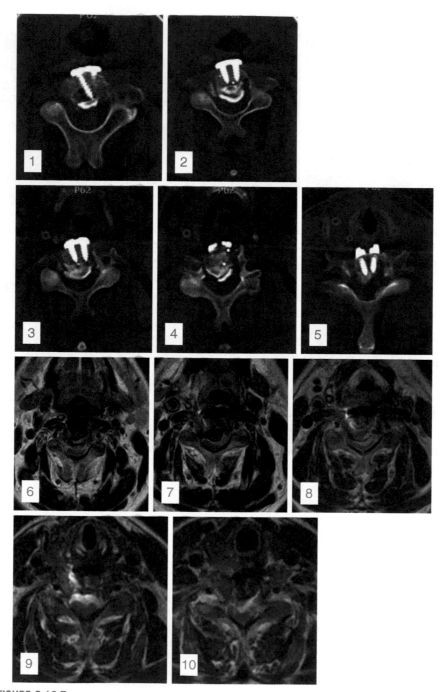

FIGURE 3.16.7

Postoperative axial cervical images and their reference on the sagittal diagram.
(1) Axial CT at the inferior surface of C2.
(2) Axial CT at C3.

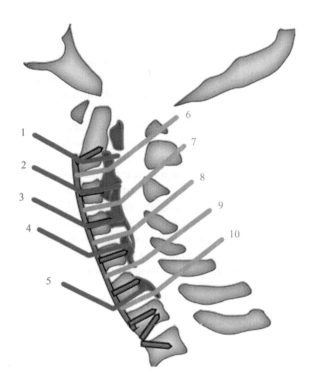

Reference of the axial planes

The vertebral bodies have been dissected with parasagittal cuts on both sides 22.6 mm apart and VOC antedisplaced by 6 mm; canal occupancy has been reduced to 18%, 49%, 45%, and 21% at C2, C3, C4, and C5, respectively (panel 1 to 5). The spinal cord resumes to boomerang shape with normal CSF around it at C3 and C4, levels with the worst impingement (panel 6 to 10).

(3) Axial CT at C4.
(4) Axial CT at the superior surface of C5.
(5) Axial CT at the inferior surface of C6.
(6) Axial MRI at C2/3.
(7) Axial MRI at C3/4.
(8) Axial MRI at C4/5.
(9) Axial MRI at C5/6.
(10) Axial MRI at C6/7.

Discussion

What are the merits of ACAF in OPLL as severe as seen in this case?

The long-segment OPLL in this case extended to the upper cervical spine with canal stenosis of 90% or above complicated with dural ossification and segmental instability.

In such cases, the anterior direct decompression bears surgical challenges and risk of durotomy and neurological deterioration. Only posterior decompression remains a feasible option among conventional techniques.

This patient may benefit little from a posterior decompression procedure and face recurrent myelopathy due to the growing ossification as he was still relatively young.

The ACAF technique averts the iatrogenic risk to the dura mater and the spinal cord, difficulties common to anterior surgeries, as the ossification is kept in situ. Neither does it require titanium mesh and thus it reduces implant-related complications. The antedisplacement of ossification in the ACAF technique results in better decompression, smaller incision, and less tissue disruption than posterior surgeries.

Case 17: Ossification of posterior longitudinal ligament (OPLL) of cervical spine C2 to T1 with Kyphosis

Index terms

Antedisplacement of four vertebral bodies or more, mixed-type OPLL, wide-based OPLL, OPLL extending into the intervertebral foramen, thickness of ossification above 9 mm, canal stenosis between 60% and 70%, shelter technique, cervical kyphosis, K-line (−) OPLL, oblique groove, partial antedisplacement, residual ossification, and inadequate decompression width.

History

Patient: A 45-year-old man.

Chief complaint: Numbness on both hands and gait instability for three months that aggravated over the past two months.

Physical exam: Physical exam was noted for gait disturbance, loss of superficial sensation around the navel, hypertonic upper extremities, numbness of both hands and more severe over the pulps of the middle, fourth, and small fingers. Muscle strength was measured at 3/5 on both upper limbs and 4/5 on both lower limbs. Hyperreflexia on both upper limbs and bilateral Hoffmann signs were noted.

Preoperative function: JOA score was 12, Nurick score: 2, VAS: 0, and NDI: 7.

Imaging studies

A K-line (−) OPLL in a kyphotic cervical spine with Cobb of −16.6° from C2 through C7 (Fig. 3.17.1).

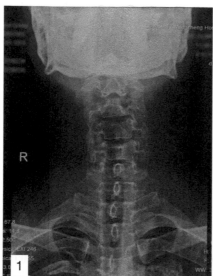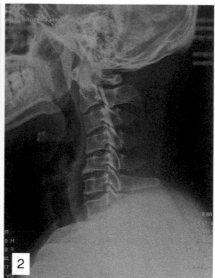

FIGURE 3.17.1

Preoperative X-ray of the cervical spine.
(1) Anteroposterior view.
(2) Lateral view.

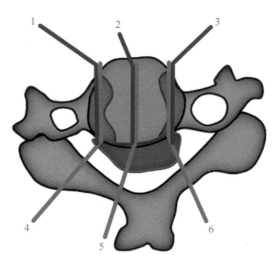

Reference of the sagittal planes

A mixed-type OPLL from C2 to T1 with double layers at C2 and C3/4 and hill shaped at C2/3 and C4 that encroaches the spinal canal (panel 1 to 3) (Fig. 3.17.2). A band-like mass of low signal intensity posterior to the vertebral bodies that occupies

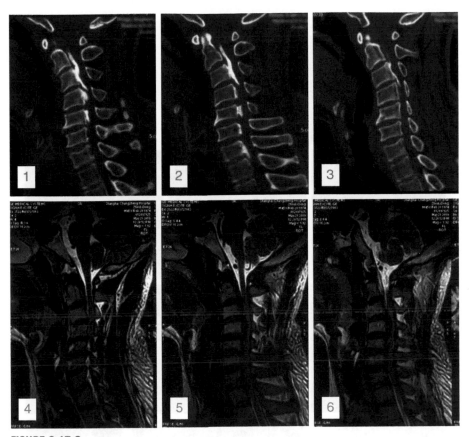

FIGURE 3.17.2

Preoperative sagittal images and their reference on the axial diagram.
(1) Parasagittal CT of the right uncinate process.
(2) Midsagittal CT.
(3) Parasagittal CT of the left uncinate process.
(4) Parasagittal MRI of the right uncinate process.
(5) Midsagittal MRI.
(6) Parasagittal MRI of the left uncinate process.

the spinal canal and compresses the spinal cord, with maximum impingement at C3 and C4, shown on preoperative MR scans; the spinal cord is deformed into an S profile with intramedullary signal hyperintensity suggesting myelopathy (panel 4 to 6) (Fig. 3.17.3).

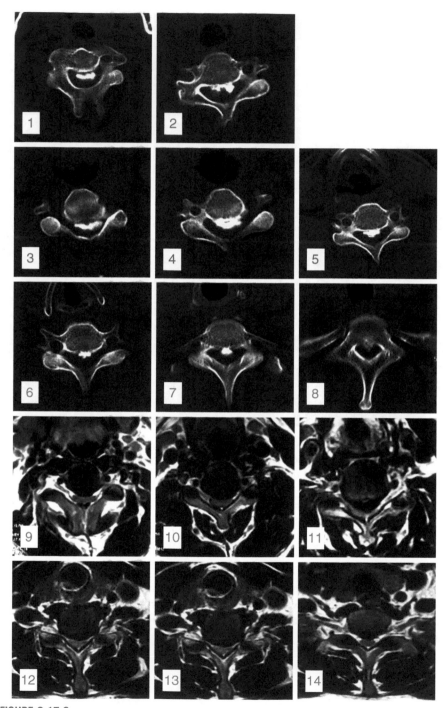

FIGURE 3.17.3

Preoperative axial images of the cervical spine and their reference on the sagittal diagram.

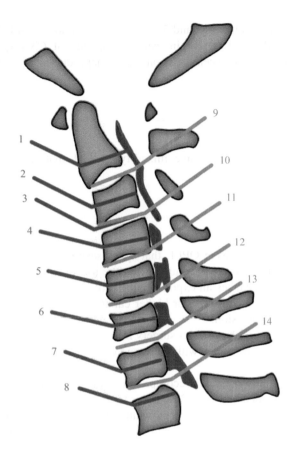

Reference of the axial planes

An OPLL, with a double-layer sign at C3 and C5, that measures 6.4 mm thick (anteroposterior), 14.1 mm wide (mediolateral), and 54.3% in canal occupancy at

(1) Axial CT at the inferior surface of C2.
(2) Axial CT at C3.
(3) Axial CT at C3/4.
(4) Axial CT at C4.
(5) Axial CT at C5.
(6) Axial CT at C6.
(7) Axial CT and C7.
(8) Axial CT and the superior surface of T1.
(9) Axial MRI at C2/3.
(10) Axial MRI at C3/4.
(11) Axial MRI at C4/5.
(12) Axial MRI at C5/6.
(13) Axial MRI at C6/7.
(14) Axial MRI at C7/T1.

C2; 5.1 mm thick, 12.5 mm wide, and 51.5% in canal occupancy at C3; and 9.0 mm thick, 18.8 mm wide, and 69.2% in canal occupancy at C3/4 (panel 1 to 8). Deformed spinal cord in crescent or boomerang shape due to anterior indentation (panel 9 to 14).

Highlights

This case features a severe, extensive, mixed-type OPLL that involves upper levels in a kyphosis cervical spine.

Surgical planning

This case features an extensive OPLL that spans seven levels and reaches C2. If ACCF is performed for direct decompression, the use of extremely long titanium mesh is necessary and carries an exponential risk of a fusion failure.

A K-line (−) OPLL with 60% or higher canal stenosis may not benefit much from posterior decompression.

A staged procedure with posterior surgery followed by segmental decompression for residual impingement comes with increased cost for the patient and higher surgical risk.

A surgery for definitive neural decompression was performed with ACAF of C3 to T1, with shelter procedure for C2, anterior to the tip of the OPLL.

Since the correction of the cervical curvature also provides room for decompression, resection of the anterior bony structure of depth smaller than that of the OPLL was executed (Fig. 3.17.4).

Results

Postoperative function: JOA score was 14, Nurick score: 1, VAS: 0, and NDI: 4.

Restored cervical curvature with Cobb of 10.8° measured from C2 through C7 (Fig. 3.17.5).

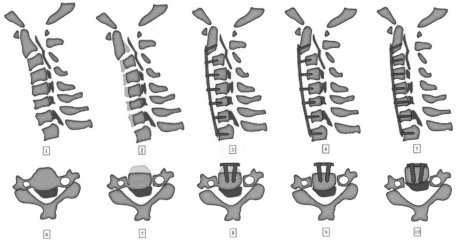

FIGURE 3.17.4

Illustration of the surgical plan on sagittal and axial planes.

(1, 6) Illustration of the OPLL on sagittal and axial views before surgery.

(2, 7) Resection performed to the anterior part of C3 to C7 vertebra and the posterior part of the C2 vertebra. A complete trough is developed on the left vertebral bodies from C3 to C7 while a half one is made on the right side with the posterior bone yet to be dissected.

(3, 8) Plate and screws placed on vertebral bodies from C2 through T1.

(4, 9) The bottom of the right half-groove on C3 through C7 dissected.

(5, 10) Antedisplaced C3 to C7 vertebral bodies as screws were tightened.

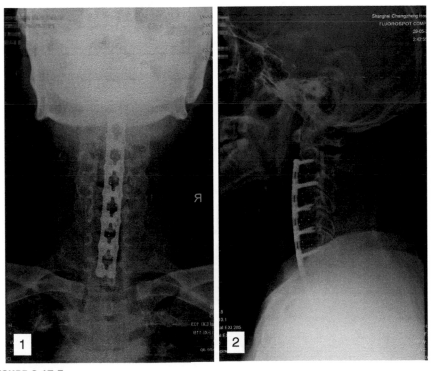

FIGURE 3.17.5

Postoperative cervical spine X-ray.

(1) Anteroposterior view.

(2) Lateral view.

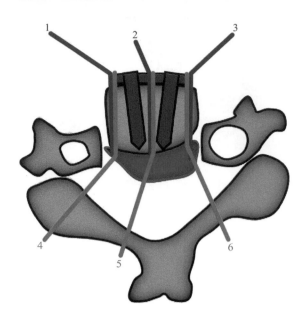

Reference of the sagittal planes

Antedisplaced VOC from C3 to C7 and expanded spinal canal (panel 1 to 3). Spinal cord in resumed curvature surrounded by CS, residual focal CSF obliteration from C2 to C4, and residual compression at C2/3 and C4 (panel 4 to 6).

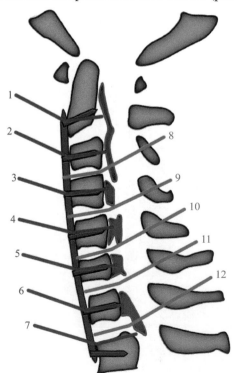

Reference of the axial planes

The vertebral bodies have been dissected with parasagittal cuts on both sides 22.1 mm apart and VOC antedisplaced by 5 mm; canal occupancy has been reduced to 37% at C3/4, the level of maximum compression (panel 1 to 7) (Fig. 3.17.6). The spinal cord at C4 has recovered from crescent shape to boomerang shape with residual indentation; other than C4, the spinal cord is oval and surrounded by CSF (panel 8 to 12) (Fig. 3.17.7).

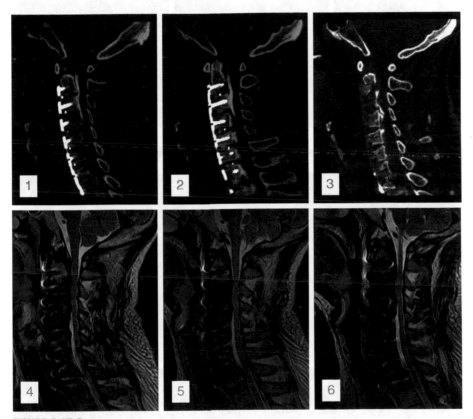

FIGURE 3.17.6

Postoperative sagittal views and their reference on the axial diagram.
(1) Parasagittal CT of the right uncinate process.
(2) Midsagittal CT.
(3) Parasagittal CT of the left uncinate process.
(4) Parasagittal MRI of the right uncinate process.
(5) Midsagittal MRI.
(6) Parasagittal MRI of the left uncinate process.

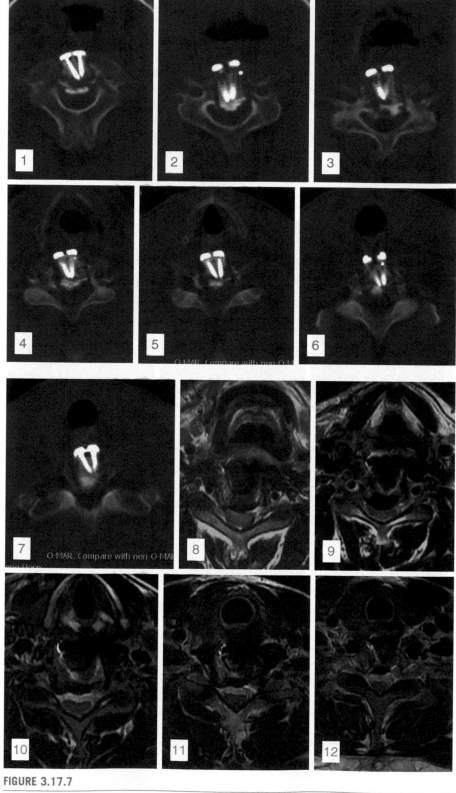

FIGURE 3.17.7

Postoperative axial cervical images and their reference on the sagittal diagram.
(1) Axial CT at the inferior surface of C2.

Discussion

Why did the procedure leave the C2 to C4 partially displaced only?

Decompression was more sufficient at C5 to C7 than at C2 to C4, and CSF obliteration was still present at the latter levels, according to postoperative MRI.

The OPLL was uninterrupted from C2 to C4 and adhered to C3 but not C2 or C4.

Postoperative CT reveals insufficient antedisplacement of C2 to C4 because the volume of resection of anterior C2 was smaller on the right side, causing premature contact between the VOC and the adjacent segments and termination of the displacement.

◀────────────────────────────────────

(2) Axial CT at C3.
(3) Axial CT at C4.
(4) Axial CT at C5.
(5) Axial CT at C6.
(6) Axial CT at C7.
(7) Axial CT at the superior surface of T1.
(8) Axial MRI at C3/4.
(9) Axial MRI at C4/5.
(10) Axial MRI at C5/6.
(11) Axial MRI at C6/7.
(12) Axial MRI at C7/T1.

Case 18: Ossification of posterior longitudinal ligament (OPLL) of cervical spine C2 to T1 with ossification of ligamentum flavum and extension injury

Index terms

Antedisplacement of more than four vertebral bodies, continuous OPLL, wide-based OPLL, OPLL extending into intervertebral foramen, thickness of ossification 7—9 mm, canal occupancy ratio above 70%, shelter technique, history of extension injury, cervical kyphosis, K-line (−) OPLL, and oblique groove.

History

Patient: A 45-year-old man.

Chief complaint: Gait disturbance following a fall five months ago.

Physical exam: Physical exam was noted for gait instability, reduced superficial sensation below the level of sternal angle, and hypertonic extremities. Muscle strength was tested at 4/5 on upper limbs and 3/5 on lower limbs. Brisk tendon reflexes were noted on all four extremities, and Hoffmann and Babinski signs were present bilaterally. Bladder and bowel control was impaired.

Preoperative function: JOA was measured at 9, Nurick score: 4, VAS: 3, and NDI: 24.

Imaging studies

Cobb angle of 3.5° measured from C2 through C7 and K-line (−) OPLL (Fig. 3.18.1).

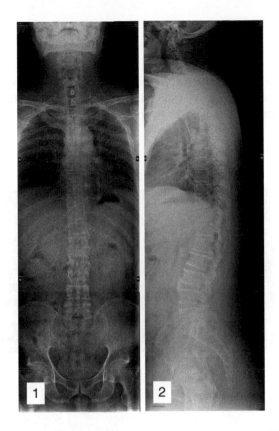

FIGURE 3.18.1

Preoperative X-ray of the whole spine.
(1) Anteroposterior view.
(2) Lateral view.

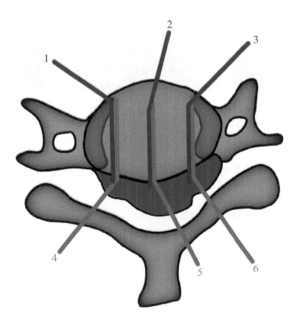

Reference of the sagittal planes

A particularly extensive, continuous flat-type OPLL from C2 to T2 (panel 1 to 3). A hypointense band posterior to vertebral bodies of C2 to T2, effacement of CSF, and S-shaped spinal cord (panel 4 to 6) (Fig. 3.18.2).

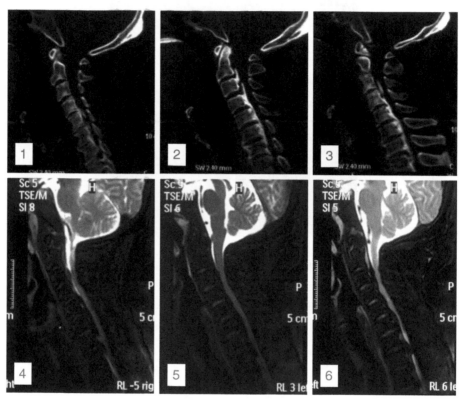

FIGURE 3.18.2

Preoperative sagittal images and their reference on axial diagram.
(1) Parasagittal CT of the right uncinate process.
(2) Midsagittal CT.
(3) Parasagittal CT of the left uncinate process.
(4) Parasagittal MRI of the right uncinate process.
(5) Midsagittal MRI.
(6) Parasagittal MRI of the left uncinate process.

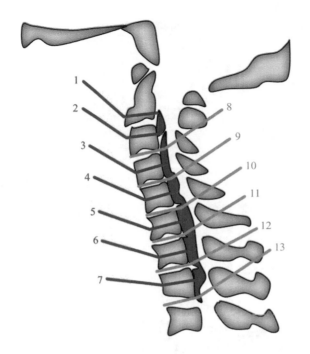

Reference of the axial planes

An extensive wide-based OPLL, more severe from C5 to T1; the lesion measures: 4.2 mm thick, 9.7 mm wide, and 26.8% in canal occupancy at C2; 5.2 mm thick, 14.4 mm wide, and 52% in canal occupancy at C3; 5.5 mm thick, 17.7 mm wide, and 47.4% in canal occupancy at C3/4; 5.4 mm thick, 12.4 mm wide, and 47.8% in canal occupancy at C4; 8.9 mm thick, 19.5 mm wide, and 66.4% in canal occupancy at C4/5; 7.3 mm thick, 19.5 mm wide, and 53.5% in canal occupancy at C5; 10.3 mm thick, 23.0 mm wide, and 68.2% in canal occupancy at C5/6; 8.3 mm thick, 21.2 mm wide, and 62.0% in canal occupancy at C6; 7.3 mm thick, 21.2 mm wide, and 57.5% in canal occupancy at C6/7; 6.7 mm thick, 11.5 mm wide, and 51.5% in canal occupancy at C7; 8.2 mm thick, 17.0 mm wide and 73.2% in canal occupancy at C7/T1; and 6.1 mm thick, 13.9 mm wide, and 49.2% in canal occupancy at T1 (panel 1 to 7). Spinal cord deformation in crescent or boomerang shape with CSF effacement at the levels of severe compression (panel 8 to 13) (Fig. 3.18.3).

Highlights

This case features an extraordinarily extensive, flat-type continuous OPLL from C2 to T1 with a wide base and double-layer sign at C3, shown on preoperative axial CT scans. Canal stenosis is above 70% at the level of maximum compression.

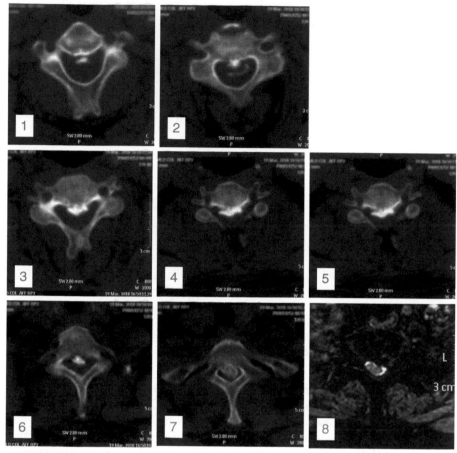

FIGURE 3.18.3

Preoperative axial images of the cervical spine and their reference on the sagittal diagram.
(1) Axial CT at the inferior surface of C2.
(2) Axial CT at C3.
(3) Axial CT at C4.
(4) Axial CT at C5.
(5) Axial CT at C6.
(6) Axial CT at C7.
(7) Axial CT at T1.
(8) Axial MRI at C3/4.
(9) Axial MRI at C4/5.
(10) Axial MRI at C5/6.
(11) Axial MRI at C6/7.
(12) Axial MRI at C7/T1.
(13) Axial MRI at T1/2.

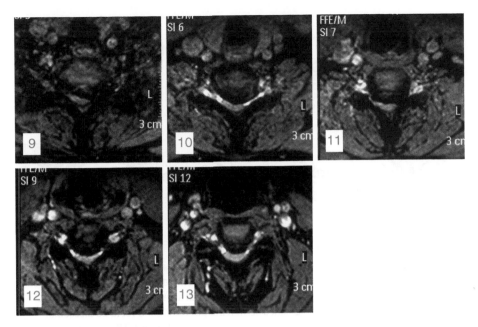

FIGURE 3.18.3 (Continued)

Surgical planning

Among the conventional techniques, indirect decompression through a posterior surgery is the only feasible option for an OPLL that spans eight levels.

However, a posterior surgery carries a significant risk of incomplete decompression due to the K-line (−) lesion and poor cervical curvature. What is more, a posterior surgery does not resolve the risk of recurrent impingement due to ossification progression.

The patient received ACAF for C3 to T1, with the OPLL dissected at C2/3.

Care should be taken to contour the plate properly. Before bony resection of the vertebral bodies, the plate was contoured to fit the anterior cervical cortex.

An undercontoured plate may cause insufficient antedisplacement, whereas an overcontoured one may increase the risk of breakage of the extensive ossification (Fig. 3.18.4).

Results

Postoperative function: JOA score was 7, Nurick score: 4, VAS: 1, and NDI: 23.

Cobb angle restored to 9.4° measured from C2 through C7 and instrumentation from C2 to T2 (Fig. 3.18.5).

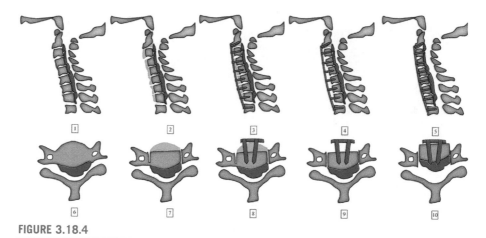

FIGURE 3.18.4

Illustration of the surgical plan on sagittal and axial planes.

(1, 6) Illustration of the OPLL on sagittal and axial views before surgery.

(2, 7) Resection performed to the anterior part of C2 to T1 vertebra and the posteroinferior part of C2 vertebra. A complete trough is developed along the left side of vertebral bodies from C2 to T1 while a half one is made on the right side with the posterior bone yet to be dissected.

(3, 8) Plate and screws placed on vertebral bodies from C2 through T2.

(4, 9) The bottom of the right half-groove on C2 through T1 dissected.

(5, 10) Antedisplaced C2 to T1 vertebral bodies as screws are tightened.

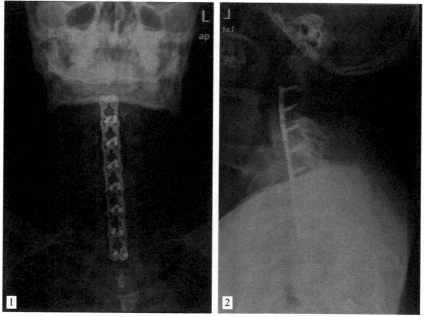

FIGURE 3.18.5

Postoperative cervical spine X-ray.

(1) Anteroposterior view.

(2) Lateral view.

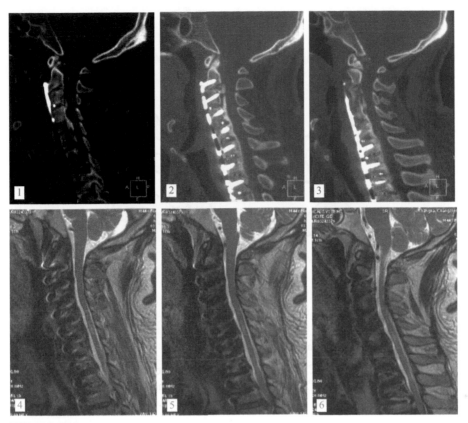

FIGURE 3.18.6

Postoperative sagittal views and their reference on the axial diagram.

(1) Parasagittal CT of the right uncinate process.

(2) Midsagittal CT.

(3) Parasagittal CT of the left uncinate process.

(4) Parasagittal MRI of the right uncinate process.

(5) Midsagittal MRI.

(6) Parasagittal MRI of the left uncinate process.

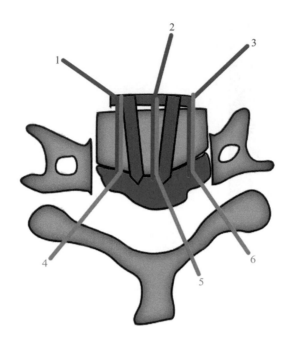

Reference of the sagittal planes

    Ventrally displaced VOC from C3 through T1 and the spinal canal with resumed volume (panel 1 to 3) (Fig. 3.18.6). Spinal cord surrounded by CSF in the cervical spine with restored lordosis (panel 4 to 6) (Fig. 3.18.7).

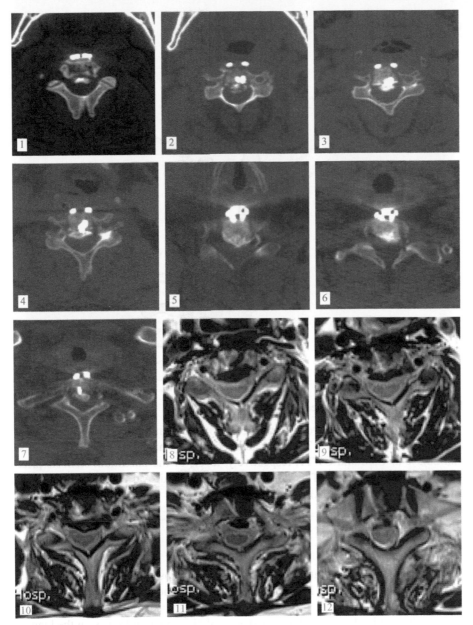

FIGURE 3.18.7

Postoperative axial cervical images and their reference on the sagittal diagram.

(1) Axial CT at the inferior surface of C2.

(2) Axial CT at C3.

(3) Axial CT at C4.

(4) Axial CT at C5.

(5) Axial CT at C6.

(6) Axial CT at C7.

(7) Axial CT at T1.

(8) Axial MRI at C4/5.

(9) Axial MRI at C5/6.

(10) Axial MRI at C6/7.

(11) Axial MRI at C7/T1.

(12) Axial MRI at T1/T2.

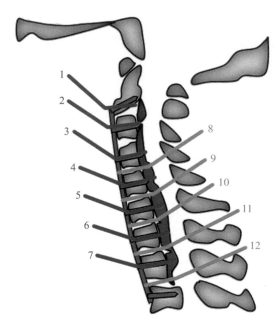

Reference of the axial planes

The vertebral bodies have been dissected with cuts on both sides 21.3 mm apart and VOC antedisplaced by 7.3 mm. Canal occupancy has been reduced to 28.7% and 20.3% at C5/6 and C7/T1, respectively, levels of the maximum stenosis prior to surgery (panel 1 to 7). The spinal cord has resumed oval or triangle shape on cross-section (panel 8 to 12).

Discussion

Why was the cervical curvature not corrected in this case?

This case represents the longest VOC antedisplacement en bloc with the ACAF technique in this book, where the instrumentation spans from the upper cervical spine to the cervicothoracic spine. The degree of plate contour hinges on the length, interruption, and focal weakness of the OPLL.

Loss of segmental motion was present as the continuous OPLL had adhered to the posterior wall of the vertebral bodies.

In extensive-segment OPLL, when the VOC is displaced toward a contoured plate, there is a risk of premature termination of the antedisplacement process since it is difficult to get all the levels to contact the plate.

In such a case, the attempt to maximize the antedisplacement may strip the screws, break the ossification, fails the decompression, and even injure the dura mater and spinal cord.

Therefore, the plate was contoured based on the anterior cortex as the latter was accessible during the surgery.

Case 19: Ossification of posterior longitudinal ligament (OPLL) of cervical spine C2 to C5 and C7 to T1

Index terms

Antedisplacement of more than four vertebral bodies, mixed-type lesion, wide-based lesion, extension into the intervertebral foramen, thickness of ossification above 9 mm, occupancy ratio 60%–70%, K-line (−) disease, and residual ossification.

History

Patient: A 46-year-old man.

Chief complaint: Neck discomfort for three months.

Physical exam: Hypertonicity of the lower extremities. Muscle strength was measured at 4/5 on all extremities. Hyperreflexia was found on both lower limbs, with Hoffmann and Babinski signs bilaterally.

Preoperative function: JOA was measured at 15, Nurick score: 1, VAS: 0, and NDI: 3.

Imaging studies

Cobb angle of 25.3° measured from C2 through C7, Pavlov ratio above 0.75, and a K-line (−) OPLL lesion spanning from C2 to C5 (Fig. 3.19.1).

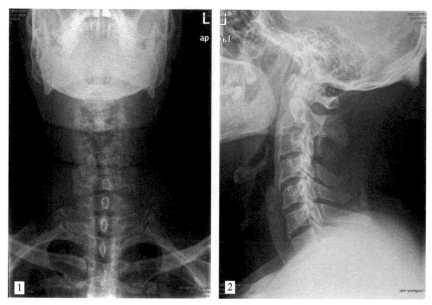

FIGURE 3.19.1

Preoperative X-ray of the cervical spine.
(1) Anteroposterior view.
(2) Lateral view.

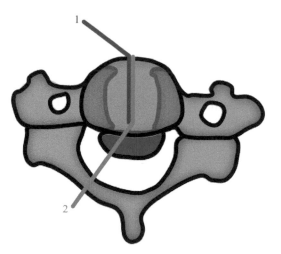

Reference of the sagittal planes

OPLL from C2/3 to C5 and C7 to T1/2, with C6 unaffected (panel 1). Spinal cord impingement at C2/3 to C4/5 and C5/6 to T1/2 (panel 2) (Fig. 3.19.2).

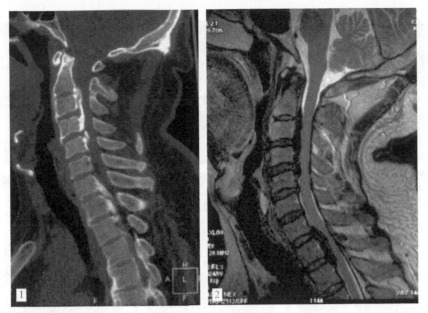

FIGURE 3.19.2

Preoperative sagittal images and their reference on axial diagram.
(1) Midsagittal CT.
(2) Midsagittal MRI.

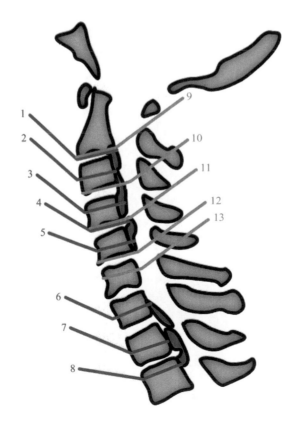

Reference of the axial planes

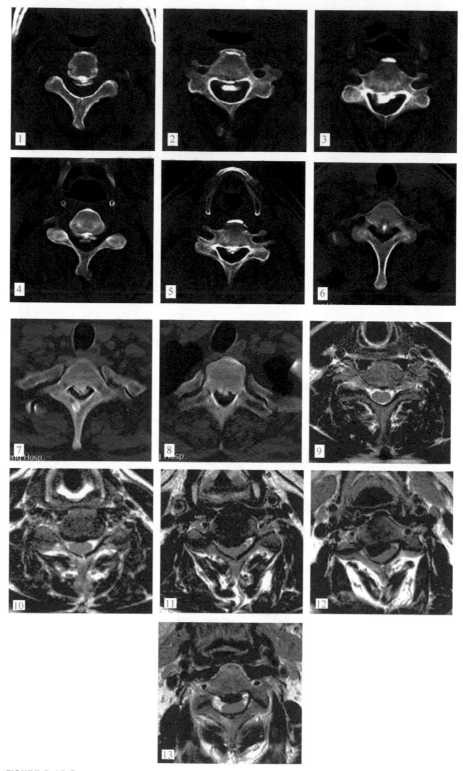

FIGURE 3.19.3

Preoperative axial images of the cervical spine and their reference on the sagittal diagram.

The OPLL measures 5.6 mm thick (anteroposterior), 13.8 mm wide (coronal width), and 44.8% in canal occupancy at C3. At C3/4, it is eccentric to the right and hill-shaped with canal encroachment measuring 7.2 mm thick, 17.7 mm wide, and 61.5% in canal occupancy (Fig. 3.19.3). The lesion is 5.2 mm thick, 10.9 mm wide, and 41.6% in canal occupancy at C4; and 6.4 mm thick, 14.4 mm wide, and 49.2% in canal occupancy at C4/5. It is hill-shaped and measured at 9.6 mm thick, 14.6 mm wide, and 55.2% in canal occupancy at C7/T1; and centered in the spinal canal of 9.6 mm thick, 14.5 mm wide, and 69.9% in canal occupancy at T1 (panel 1 to 8). The spinal cord is impinged at C2/3 to C4/5, with C3/4 and C4/5 being more severe, in the shape of a triangle or boomerang (panel 9 to 13).

Highlights

Overall, the OPLL in this case spans from the upper cervical spine to the thoracic spine skipping C6. As such, the upper part is from C2/3 to C5 while the lower part from C7 to T1/2.

Surgical planning

In extraordinarily long OPLL, extensive decompression is required, and posterior surgeries are often performed conventionally. However, a long incision in the neck results in significant disruption of soft tissues and elevated risk of axial symptoms.

What is more, the extensive posterior decompression should cause a limited posterior shift of the spinal cord in the case of neural palsy. And a posterior surgery with preserved segmental motion comes with the long-term risk of curvature deformities and recurrent neuropathy.

(1) Axial CT at the inferior surface of C2.
(2) Axial CT at C3.
(3) Axial CT at C4.
(4) Axial CT at the inferior surface of C4.
(5) Axial CT at C5.
(6) Axial CT at C7.
(7) Axial CT at T1.
(8) Axial CT at T2.
(9) Axial MRI at the inferior surface of C2.
(10) Axial MRI at the inferior surface of C3.
(11) Axial MRI at the inferior surface of C4.
(12) Axial MRI at the inferior surface of C5.
(13) Axial MRI at C6.

The decision was made to perform ACAF that skips C6 and decompresses the upper and lower parts of the disease, respectively, with antedisplacement of C3 to C5 and C7 to T1.

Tracheal mobilization exercise was prescribed before surgery to reduce the resistance of tracheal retraction during surgery and airway discomfort after surgery.

To enhance exposure, the spine was accessed lateral to the omohyoid for the upper part and medial to the omohyoid for the lower part of the lesion.

Two transverse incisions were made on the neck (Fig. 3.19.4).

Results

Postoperative function: JOA score was 16, Nurick score: 0, VAS: 0, and NDI: 13.

Properly instrumented spine with two plates, one on C2 to C6 and the other on C6 to T2, and antedisplaced C3 to C5 and C7 to T1 (Fig. 3.19.5).

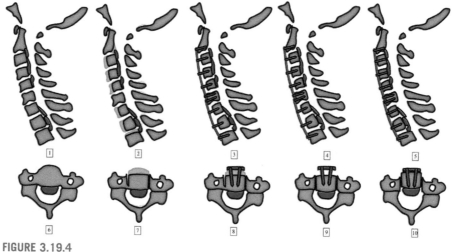

FIGURE 3.19.4

Illustration of the surgical plan on sagittal and axial planes.
(1, 6) Illustration of the OPLL on sagittal and axial views before surgery.
(2, 7) The anterior part of the vertebral bodies of C3, C4, C5, and C7 and the posteroinferior part of the C2 vertebra are partially resected. A complete trough is developed on the left vertebral bodies on C3, C4, C5, C7, and T1 while a half one is made on the right side with the posterior bone yet to be dissected.
(3, 8) Plate and screws placed on vertebral bodies from C2 through T2.
(4, 9) The bottom of the right half-groove on C3, C4, C5, C7, and T1 dissected.
(5, 10) Screws are tightened to hoist the C3 to C5 and C7 to T1 vertebral bodies.

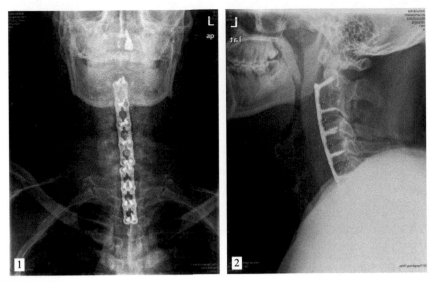

FIGURE 3.19.5

Postoperative cervical spine X-ray.
(1) Anteroposterior view.
(2) Lateral view.

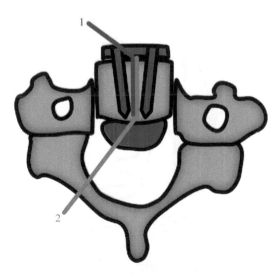

Reference of the sagittal planes

Ventrally displaced vertebral bodies of C3 to C5 and C7 to T1, and expanded spinal canal (panel 1) (Fig. 3.19.6). Spinal cord around normal CSF in unobstructed canal (panel 2) (Fig. 3.19.7).

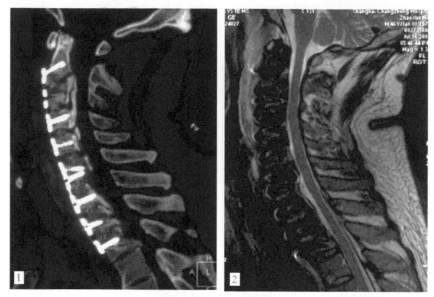

FIGURE 3.19.6

Postoperative sagittal views and their reference on the axial diagram.
(1) Midsagittal CT.
(2) Midsagittal MRI.

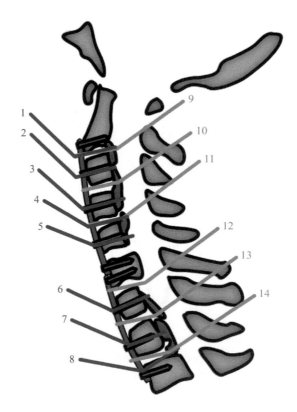

Reference of the axial planes

The vertebral bodies have been dissected with parasagittal cuts on both sides 20.3 and 24.7 mm apart, and VOC antedisplaced by 3 and 8.1 mm at the upper (C3 to C5)

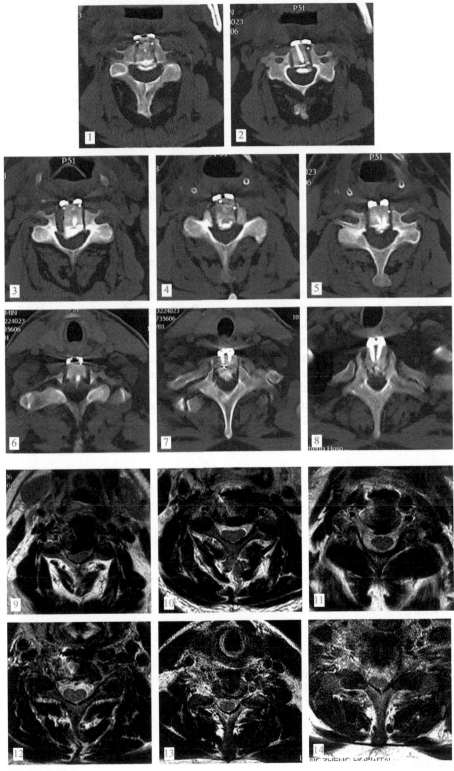

FIGURE 3.19.7

Postoperative axial cervical images and their reference on the sagittal diagram.
(1) Axial CT at C2/3.
(2) Axial CT at C3/4.

and the lower part (C7 to T1), respectively; in the expanded canal, the occupancy has been reduced to 26.0% and 0% at the upper and lower parts, respectively (panel 1 to 8). The spinal cord free of impingement at C3 and T1 (panel 9 to 14).

Discussion

What are the advantages of the dual transverse skin incision over a long craniocaudal one in this case?

The antedisplacement procedure was directed at two blocks: the upper block from C3 to C4 and the lower on from C7 to T1. Overall, the procedure involved the entire cervical spine. This is too challenging to approach the spine with one transverse incision.

If the spine is approached from one longitudinal incision, it would be from the mandible to the clavicle, leaving a long scar after surgery. In addition, as the C6 was not to be antedisplaced, it was not necessary to expose from the upper instrumented level to the lower one.

The use of dual transverse incisions provides adequate visualization while averting cicatricial contracture from an extensive longitudinal wound.

The upper incision, developed on the right side, provided access from C2 to C5 whereas the lower, on the left side, from C7 to T1 to avoid injury to the right recurrent laryngeal nerve around the inferior levels.

(3) Axial CT at C4.
(4) Axial CT at C4/5.
(5) Axial CT at C5.
(6) Axial CT at C7.
(7) Axial CT at T1.
(8) Axial CT at the superior surface of T2.
(9) Axial MRI at C2/3.
(10) Axial MRI at C3/4.
(11) Axial MRI at C4/5.
(12) Axial MRI at C6/7.
(13) Axial MRI at C7/T1.
(14) Axial MRI at T1/2.

Case 20: Ossification of posterior longitudinal ligament (OPLL) of cervical spine C2 to C6

Index terms

Antedisplacement of four vertebral bodies, segmental OPLL, wide-based lesion, the thickness of ossification 5–7 mm, occupancy ratio above 70%, shelter technique, undercut decompression, oblique groove, and inadequate antedisplacement.

History

Patient: A 63-year-old man.

Chief complaint: Numbness of all four limbs for 15 years that aggravated in the past four months.

Physical exam: Physical exam was noted for gait instability, paresthesia below the level of the intermammary line, hypertonicity on all four extremities, pain on both arms and forearms, numbness of hands, and an impaired sense of light touch, pinprick, and temperature on lower limbs. Muscle strength was tested at 3/5 on upper limbs and 4/5 on lower limbs. Brisk tendon reflexes were noted on both lower extremities, and Hoffmann and Babinski signs were present bilaterally.

Preoperative function: JOA was measured at 10, Nurick score: 2, VAS: 0, and NDI: 8.

Imaging studies

Cobb angle of 24.6° measured from C2 through C7, Pavlov ratio of 0.64 at C3, and OPLL spanning from C2 to C6 (Fig. 3.20.1).

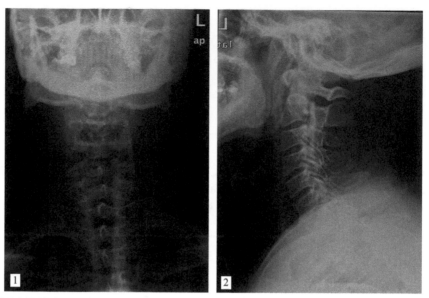

FIGURE 3.20.1

Preoperative X-ray of the cervical spine.
(1) Anteroposterior view.
(2) Lateral view.

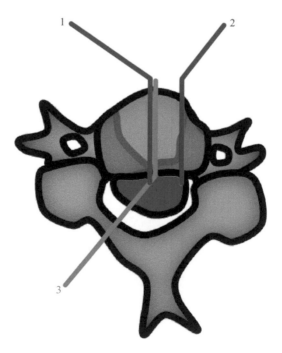

Reference of the sagittal planes

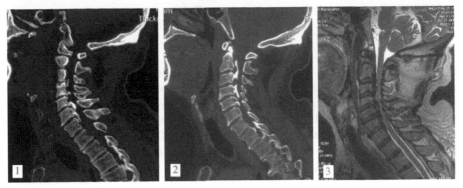

FIGURE 3.20.2

Preoperative sagittal images and their reference on axial diagram.
(1) Midsagittal CT.
(2) Parasagittal CT of the left uncinate process.
(3) Midsagittal MRI.

A segmental OPLL from C2 to C7, more severe from C3 to C6 (panel 1 and 2). Spinal cord compression from C2/3 to C6 with resultant obliteration of the anterior and posterior CSF column at the levels, with the maximum impingement at C3 and C4/5; intramedullary signal hyperintensity at C4 and C5 (panel 3) (Fig. 3.20.2).

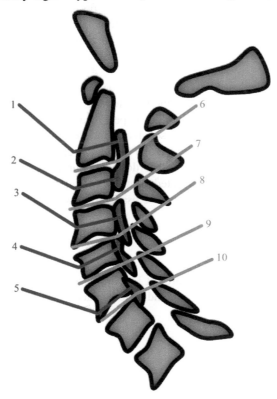

Reference of the axial planes

An OPLL that measures: 4.7 mm thick (anteroposterior), 12.9 mm wide (coronal width), and 36.7% in canal occupancy at C2; 6.7 mm thick, 17.6 mm wide, and 67%

in canal occupancy at C3; 4.7 mm thick, 15.9 mm wide, and 38.8% in canal occupancy at C4; 8.5 mm thick, 15.7 mm wide, and 68.5% in canal occupancy at C5 where the lesion is centered midline with a wide base; 8.1 mm thick, 15.9 mm wide, and 74.3% in canal occupancy at C5/6; and 7.6 mm thick, 11.8 mm wide, and 51.4% in canal occupancy at C6 (panel 1 to 5). The spinal cord in triangular or boomerang shape, and spinal cord signal hyperintensity at C5/6, the level of maximum compression (panel 6 to 10) (Fig. 3.20.3).

Highlights

This case features developmental stenosis of the spinal canal complicated with an extensive OPLL from C2 to C6, resulting in canal occupancy of 70% or higher.

Surgical planning

According to the conventional algorithm, a long-segment K-line (+) OPLL, as seen in this case, will have ample decompression with posterior surgery.

Given the relatively large lordosis, care should be taken to prevent an excessive posterior shift of the spinal cord in the case of neural palsy. However, motion-preserving surgery carries an increased risk of ossification progression and recurrent neuropathy.

The patient received an ACAF procedure for antedisplacement of C3 to C6. Also, the posterior part of C2 and C7 vertebral bodies was undercut.

A longitudinal skin incision was developed to avoid overtensioning the skin edges and excessive retraction to the soft tissue in a long-segment procedure.

The ossification posterior to the C2 and C7 vertebral bodies was undercut.

To accommodate the physiological lordosis, no curvature correction, and thus room for decompression was expected from the plate. Thus, an anterior part of the vertebrae of the same thickness as the ossification was resected (Fig. 3.20.4).

Results

Postoperative function: JOA was scored at 11, Nurick score: 1, VAS: 1, and NDI: 11.

Instrumentation from C2 to C7 and antedisplaced C3 through C6 vertebral bodies (Fig. 3.20.5).

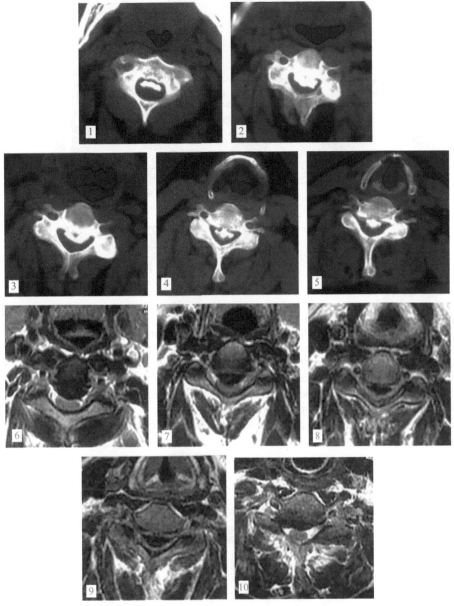

FIGURE 3.20.3

Preoperative axial images of the cervical spine and their reference on the sagittal diagram.
(1) Axial CT at the inferior surface of C2.
(2) Axial CT at C3.
(3) Axial CT at C4.
(4) Axial CT at C5.
(5) Axial CT at C6.
(6) Axial MRI at C2/3.
(7) Axial MRI at C3/4.
(8) Axial MRI at C4/5.
(9) Axial MRI at C5/6.
(10) Axial MRI at C6/7.

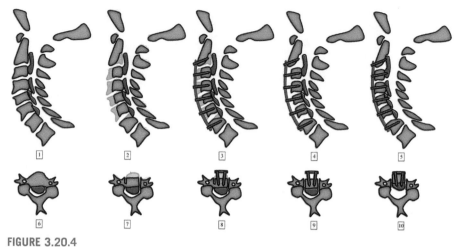

FIGURE 3.20.4

Illustration of the surgical plan on sagittal and axial views.

(1, 6) Illustration of the OPLL on sagittal and axial views before surgery.

(2, 7) Resection of the anterior part of vertebral bodies of C3 through C6, and the posteroinferior part of C2 vertebra; a complete trough on the left and a half one on the right at C3 through C6 vertebral bodies.

(3, 8) Titanium plate and screws placed in vertebral bodies from C2 to C7.

(4, 9) Completion of the right groove on C3 through C6.

(5, 10) Antedisplaced C3 through C6 vertebral bodies after screw tightening.

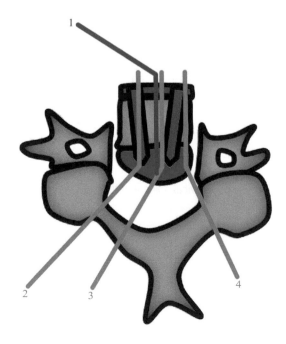

Reference of the sagittal planes

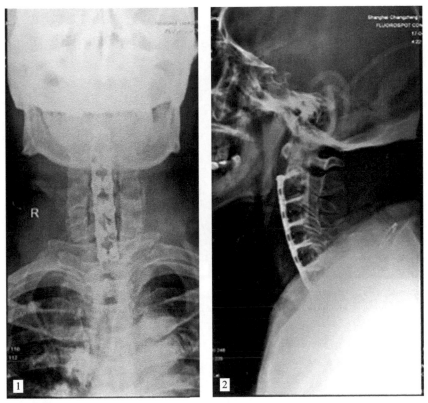

FIGURE 3.20.5

Postoperative X-ray of the cervical spine.
(1) Anteroposterior view.
(2) Lateral view.

Antedisplaced VOC from C3 to C6 and expanded central canal (panel 1) (Fig. 3.20.6). Adequately decompressed spinal cord from C2/3 to C6 surrounded by CSF in the unobstructed spinal canal (panel 2 to 4) (Fig. 3.20.7).

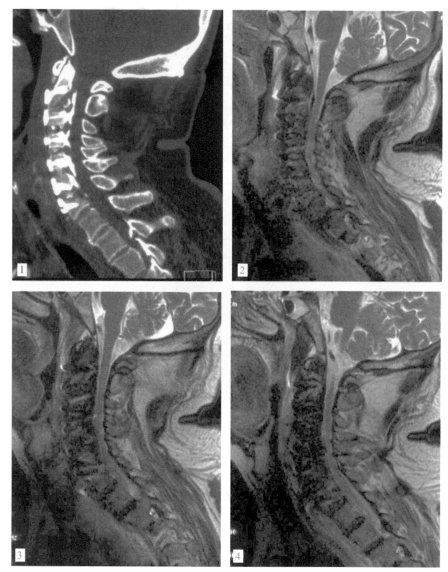

FIGURE 3.20.6

Postoperative sagittal images and their reference on the axial diagram.
(1) Midsagittal CT.
(2) Right parasagittal MRI.
(3) Midsagittal MRI.
(4) Parasagittal MRI of the left uncinate process.

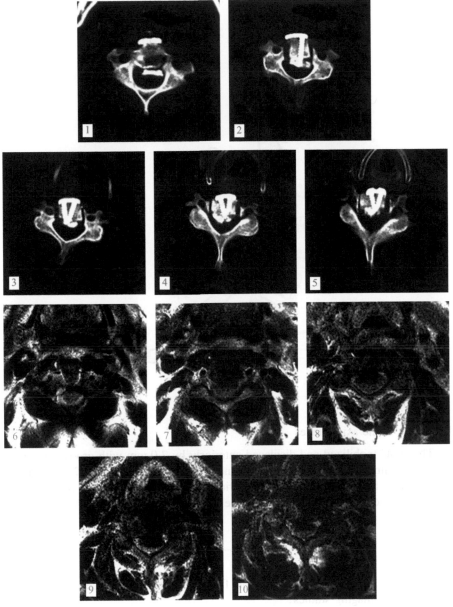

FIGURE 3.20.7

Postoperative axial cervical images and their reference on the sagittal diagram.

(1) Axial CT at the inferior surface of C2.

(2) Axial CT at C3.

(3) Axial CT at C4.

(4) Axial CT at the inferior surface of C5.

(5) Axial CT at the inferior surface of C6.

(6) Axial MRI at C2/3.

(7) Axial MRI at C3/4.

(8) Axial MRI at C4/5.

(9) Axial MRI at C5/6.

(10) Axial MRI at C6/7.

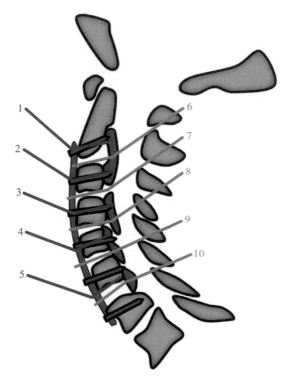

Reference of the axial planes

The VOC mobilized and displaced anteriorly by 7.0 mm with grooves on both sides 23.3 mm apart; expanded spinal canal with occupancy of 47.0% and 34.3% at the levels of maximum impingement prior to surgery (panel 1 to 5). Significantly ameliorated cord compression at C5 (panel 6 to 10).

Discussion

Why were the grooves angulated variably from the parasagittal planes, according to postoperative imaging studies?

The grooves were developed obliquely because of the patient's axially rotated cervical spine.

Preoperative imaging studies, in particular CT and MRI, revealed the cervical spines rotated toward left along the body axis. The spine was further rotated as the patient lay supine.

Therefore, bone-cutting tools directed perpendicular to the floor resulted in oblique grooves on both sides of vertebral bodies.

Despite this obliquity, ample decompression was still obtained in this narrow-based disease. However, we also noted the right groove on C4 almost blew the medial wall of the transverse foramen, with only 1 mm bony septation.

Case 21: Ossification of posterior longitudinal ligament (OPLL) of cervical spine (C2 to C6)

Index terms

Antedisplacement of four vertebral bodies, mixed-type ossification of posterior longitudinal ligament (OPLL), wide-based lesion, the thickness of ossification 5–7 mm, occupancy ratio above 60%–70%, shelter technique, and oblique grooves.

History

Patient: A 45-year-old man.

Chief complaint: Numbness of upper limbs that aggravated over the past 10 days with weakness of all four extremities.

Physical exam: Physical exam was noted for gait instability, paresthesia below the level of the intermammary line, and on upper extremities, hypertonicity on all four extremities, and hyperpathia on the lateral side of the arm and the radial side of the forearm on the right. Muscle strength was tested at 4/5 on the left upper limb, 3/5 on the right upper limb, and 4/5 on lower limbs. Tendon reflexes were brisk on the left upper extremity and lower limbs, but intact on the right upper limb. Hoffmann sign was present bilaterally.

Preoperative function: Japanese Orthopedic Association (JOA) was measured at 11, Nurick score: 3, visual analog scale (VAS): 0, and neck disability index (NDI): 8.

Imaging studies

Cobb angle of 8.8° measured from C2 through C7 and K-line (+) OPLL at the levels of C2 to C5 and C6/7 (Fig. 3.21.1).

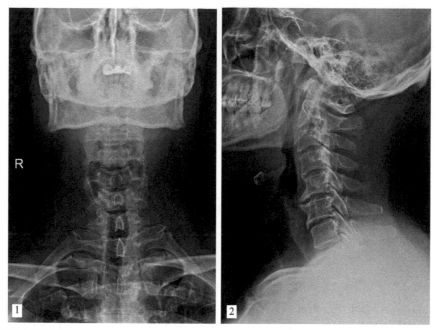

FIGURE 3.21.1

Preoperative X-ray of the cervical spine.
(1) Anteroposterior view.
(2) Lateral view.

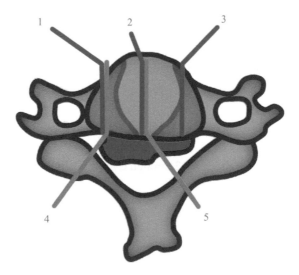

Reference of the sagittal planes

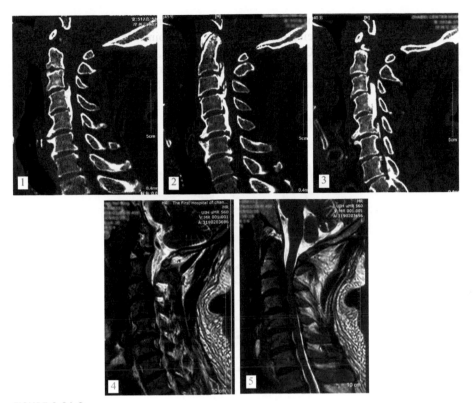

FIGURE 3.21.2

Preoperative sagittal images and their reference on the axial diagram.
(1) Parasagittal CT of the right uncinate process.
(2) Midsagittal CT.
(3) Parasagittal CT of the left uncinate process.
(4) Parasagittal MRI of the right uncinate process.
(5) Midsagittal MRI.

On a sagittal view of computed tomography (CT) scan, a mixed-type OPLL from C2 to C6, with C3 and C4 being the most severe. A hypointense band in the front of the spinal canal from C2 to C6, spinal cord compression, obliteration of the anterior and posterior cerebrospinal fluid (CSF) columns, and intramedullary signal hyperintensity shown on sagittal magnetic resonance imaging (MRI) images (Fig. 3.21.2).

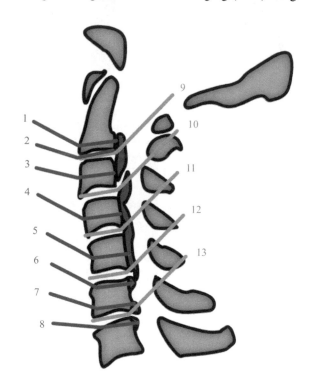

Reference of the axial planes

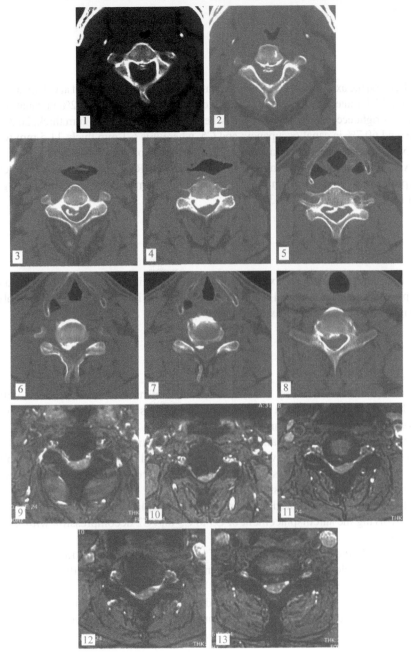

FIGURE 3.21.3

Preoperative axial images of the cervical spine and their reference on the sagittal diagram.

(1) Axial CT at the inferior surface of C2.

(2) Axial CT at C2/3.

(3) Axial CT at C3.

(4) Axial CT at C4.

(5) Axial CT at C5.

(6) Axial CT at C6.IT.

(7) Axial CT at the inferior surface of C6.

(8) Axial CT at C7.

(9) Axial MRI at C2/3.

(10) Axial MRI at C3/4.

Based on the axial view of CT, the ossification is eccentric to the right at C3, measuring 6.1 mm thick (anteroposterior), 17.2 mm wide (mediolateral), and 45.2% in canal occupancy. Its right eccentricity involves C4, where it is wide-based, 6.8 mm thick, 20.3 mm wide, and 60.7% in canal occupancy; and C5, where it is 6.1 mm thick, 11.5 mm wide, and 50% in canal occupancy (and Fig. 3.21.3, panel 1 to 8).

As shown on the axial magnetic resonance (MR) imaging, the spinal cord compression is more severe on the right side with intramedullary hyperintense signal (and Fig. 3.21.3, panel 9 to 13).

Highlights

This case features a severe, extensive, flat-typed, continuous OPLL from C2 to C6 complicated with spinal canal stenosis. The OPLL is right paracentral and involves the right neural foramina. It is wide-based at C4.

Surgical planning

This case is characterized by a K-line (+) OPLL of more than three levels with a double-layer sign. An indirect decompression via a posterior approach offers higher safety with a lower risk of dural tear or cord injury.

Imaging studies also reveal, however, the maximum canal stenosis above 60% and poor cervical curvature, which suggests a limited posterior shift of the spinal cord, incomplete decompression, and possible recurrence of neuropathy due to aggravating curvature and ossification.

The patient received anterior controllable antedisplacement fusion (ACAF) surgery involving the antedisplacement of C3 to C5 and C2 decompression with shelter technique.

Caution should be taken to the levels of a wide-based or paracentral lesion, where the grooves developed off the base of the uncinate process may cut through the ossification and cause residue lesion (Fig. 3.21.4).

Therefore, the surgeon is recommended to start the groove off the base of the uncinate process and deviate laterally as he or she goes deeper to ensure the dissection incorporates the entire ossification (Fig. 3.21.5).

Results

Postoperative function: JOA score was 15, Nurick score: 1, VAS: 0, and NDI: 6.
Cobb angle of 15.3° from C2 to C7 and cervical curvature corrected.

(11) Axial MRI at C4/5.
(12) Axial MRI at C5/6.
(13) Axial MRI at C6/7.

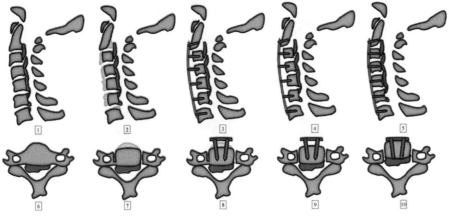

FIGURE 3.21.4

Illustration of the surgical plan on sagittal and axial planes.

(1, 6) Illustration of the OPLL on sagittal and axial views before surgery.

(2, 7) Resection performed to the anterior part of C3 to C6 vertebral bodies and the posterior part of C2 vertebra. A complete trough is developed on the left vertebral bodies from C3 to C6 while a half one is made on the right side with the posterior bone yet to be dissected.

(3, 8) Plate and screws placed on vertebral bodies from C2 through C7.

(4, 9) The bottom of the right half-groove on C3 through C6 dissected.

(5, 10) Antedisplaced C3 to C6 vertebral bodies as screws were tightened.

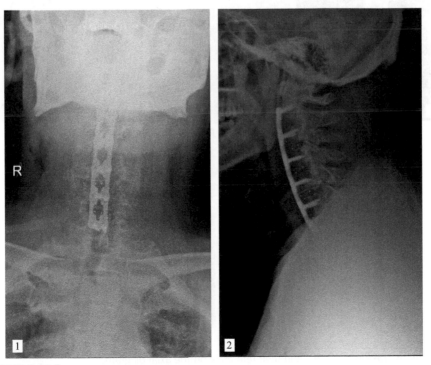

FIGURE 3.21.5

Postoperative cervical spine X-ray.

(1) Anteroposterior view.

(2) Lateral view.

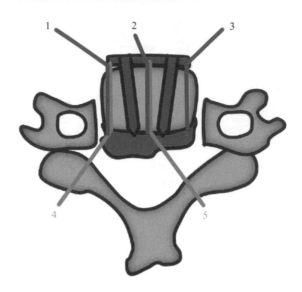

Reference of the sagittal planes

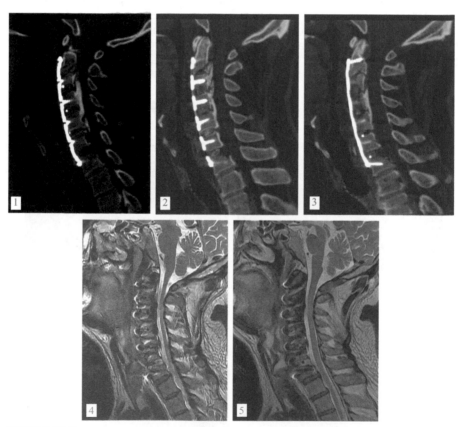

FIGURE 3.21.6

Postoperative sagittal views and their reference on the axial diagram.
(1) Parasagittal CT of the right uncinate process.
(2) Midsagittal CT.
(3) Parasagittal CT of the left uncinate process.
(4) Parasagittal MRI of the right uncinate process.
(5) Midsagittal MRI.

Antedisplaced vertebra-OPLL complex (VOC) from C2 to C6 with anteriorized vertebral bodies from C3 to C6 facilitated by shelter technique, shown on postoperative midsagittal CT image (Fig. 3.21.6, panel 1 to 3). Spinal cord with restored curvature free of indentation and surrounded by CSF shown on postoperative sagittal MRI images (Fig. 3.21.6, panel 4 to 5).

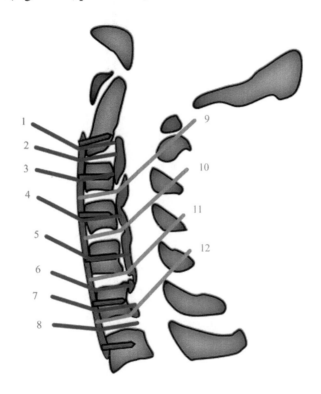

Reference of the axial planes

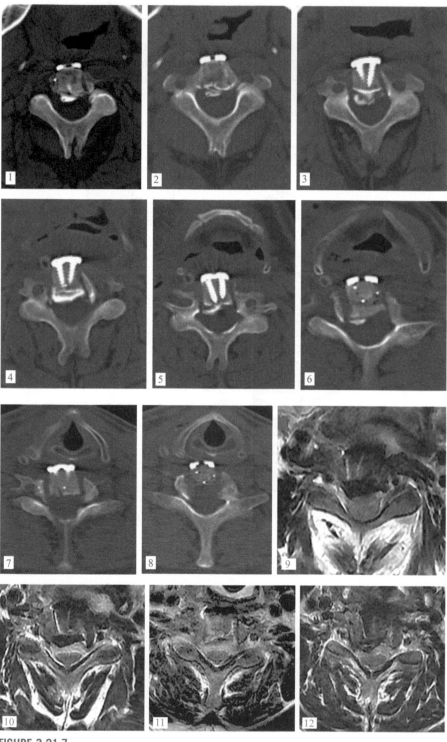

FIGURE 3.21.7

Postoperative axial cervical images and their reference on the sagittal diagram.
(1) Axial CT at the inferior surface of C2.
(2) Axial CT at C2/3.

The VOC has been sufficiently antedisplaced by 5.8 mm with a sagittal right groove and an oblique left groove 21.3 mm apart; canal stenosis at the most severe level improved to 23.2% shown on postoperative axial CT (Fig. 3.21.7, panel 1 to 8).

The spinal cord resumes its oval shape with normal CSF around it, as shown on postoperative axial MRI images (Fig. 3.21.7, panel 9 and 12).

Discussion

Why did the grooves on C3 through C5 deviate toward the left side as the dissection went deeper, shown on postoperative CT images?

The surgeon operated in a position that lures them into deviating the parasagittal cuts toward their opposite side.

Care should be taken to direct the bone groove perpendicular to the floor. The tendency to deviate the cut can be offset by tilting the surgical degree toward the surgeon's side Tables 10–25.

Alternatively, a surgical microscope can be used to maintain visualization perpendicular to the floor.

Proper patient positioning is essential as well to ensure the patient faces upward and avoid rotation of the cervical spine.

◀──────────────────────────────────

(3) Axial CT at C3.
(4) Axial CT at C4.
(5) Axial CT at C5.
(6) Axial CT at the superior surface of C6.
(7) Axial CT at the inferior surface of C6.
(8) Axial CT at the C6/7.
(9) Axial MRI at C3/4.
(10) Axial MRI at C4/5.
(11) Axial MRI at C5/6.
(12) Axial MRI at C6/7.

Case 22: Ossification of posterior longitudinal ligament (OPLL) of cervical spine (At C2 to C3/4 and C4/5 to C5)

Index terms

Antedisplacement of two vertebral bodies, mixed-type OPLL, wide-based OPLL, thickness of ossification 7–9 mm, canal stenosis between 60% and 70%, shelter technique, and cervical kyphosis.

History

Patient: A 50-year-old man.

Chief complaint: Numbness and weakness of the left upper limb for six months and gait instability for one month.

Physical exam: Wheeled in the clinic, the patient was noted for paresthesia below the level of sternal angle on the left flank, decreased perianal sensation, and weak anal wink reflex. Hypertonicity on all four extremities. The decreased superficial sensation on the left forearm and left foot, and atrophic left deltoid. Muscle strength was tested at 4/5 on the other sites of the upper limbs and on lower limbs. Tendon reflexes were not elicited on the left upper arm but brisk on lower extremities. Hoffmann and Babinski signs were present bilaterally.

Preoperative function: JOA was measured at 7, Nurick score: 4, VAS: 0, and NDI: 23.

Imaging studies

Cervical kyphosis with Cobb angle of C2 to C7 is −6.7°, Pavlov ratio is 0.65, bony density is abnormally increased, ossification of anterior longitudinal ligament can be seen in C4 ~ T1, and K-line (−) OPLL at C2 ~ C4 (Fig. 3.22.1).

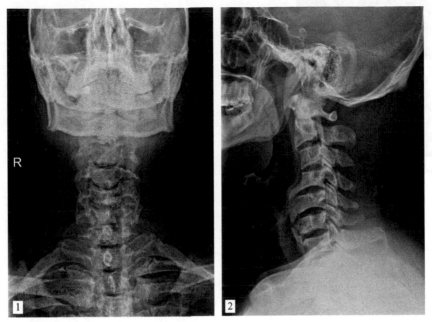

FIGURE 3.22.1

Preoperative X-ray of the cervical spine.
(1) Anteroposterior view.
(2) Lateral view.

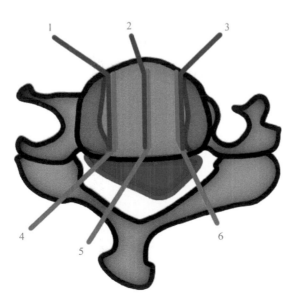

Reference of the sagittal planes

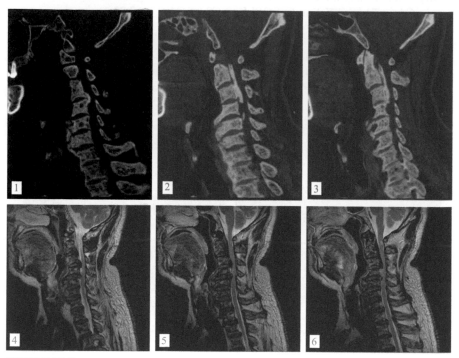

FIGURE 3.22.2

Preoperative sagittal images of the cervical spine and their reference on the axial diagram.

(1) Parasagittal CT of the right uncinate process.

(2) Midsagittal CT.

(3) Parasagittal CT of the left uncinate process.

(4) Parasagittal MRI of the right uncinate process.

(5) Midsagittal MRI.

(6) Parasagittal MRI of the left uncinate process.

According to sagittal CT images, a mixed-type OPLL that involves C2 to C5 and most protuberant at C3 and C3/4 with hill-shaped at C3/4 (Fig. 3.22.2, panel 1 to 3).

A hypodense band posterior to the vertebral bodies that occupies the spinal canal from C2 to C3; disc protrusion at C4/5; spinal cord compression, in particular at C3 and C4/5; intramedullary signal hyperintensity at C2 and C4, suggesting myelopathy shown on sagittal MRI images (Fig. 3.22.2, panel 4 to 6).

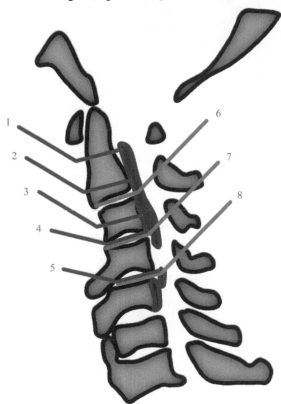

Reference of the axial planes

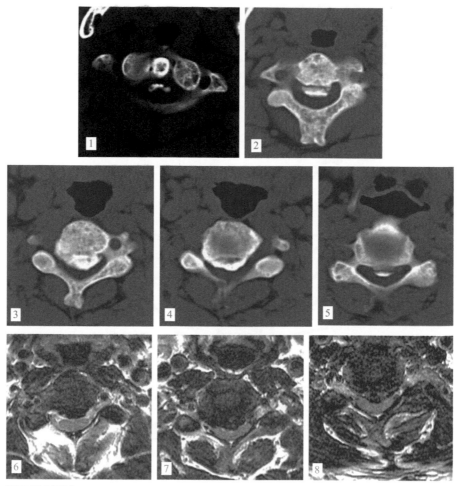

FIGURE 3.22.3

Preoperative axial images of the cervical spine and their reference on the sagittal diagram.

(1) Axial CT at C2.

(2) Axial CT at the inferior surface of C2.

(3) Axial CT at C3.

(4) Axial CT at C3/4.

(5) Axial CT at C4/5.

(6) Axial MRI at C2/3.

(7) Axial MRI at C3/4.

(8) Axial MRI at C4/5.

Preoperative axial CT image: The OPLL measures 6.9 mm thick (anteroposterior), 17.2 mm wide (mediolateral), and 51.5% in OR at C2. At C3, the wide-based OPLL measures 7.9 mm thick, 21.2 mm wide, and 64.8% in canal stenosis. A double-layer sign is present at C3 and C4/5. An ossification of the anterior longitudinal ligament on C4 to T1, with the most thick of 14.1 mm (Fig. 3.22.3, panel 1 to 5).

Preoperative axial MRI image: Cord compression at C2, C3, and C4/5, particularly at the latter two levels where it appears boomerang-shaped due to severe anterior indentation (Fig. 3.22.3, panel 6 to 8).

Highlights

This case features OPLL of C2 to C3/4 and C4/5 to C5, not attached to the C2 vertebra. The double-layer sign at C3 and C3/4 suggests the likelihood of dural ossification. Ossification of the anterior longitudinal ligament from C4 to T1. Cervical kyphosis from C2 to C4. The cancellous bone of increased density and sclerotic bone are shown on preoperative CT images.

Surgical planning

Patients with K-line (−) OPLL in a kyphotic cervical spine will benefit little from posterior decompression. What is more, C2 and C4 bear more cervical motion as compensation to the ossification of the anterior longitudinal ligament from C4 to C7. Therefore, a posterior procedure may leave the ossification to advance, deteriorate the cervical curvature, and subject the patient to recurrent neuropathies.

The involvement of the upper cervical spine makes anterior surgeries too challenging with a higher risk of morbidities. Also, the wide-base and double-layer components of the lesion are associated with increased risk of the residual lesion and durotomy for the anterior cervical corpectomy and fusion (ACCF) procedure (Fig. 3.22.4).

The patient received ACAF for C3 and C4 antedisplacement and shelter procedure for the tip behind C2. During surgery, the ossification anterior to the C4 and C5 was removed to access the vertebral bodies (Fig. 3.22.5).

Results

Postoperative function: JOA score was 10, Nurick score: 3, VAS: 0, and NDI: 19.

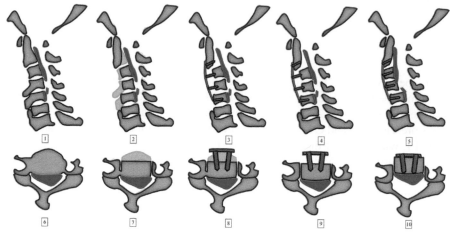

FIGURE 3.22.4

Illustration of the surgical plan on sagittal and axial views.

(1, 6) Illustration of the OPLL on sagittal and axial views before surgery.

(2, 7) Resection of the anterior part of the vertebral bodies of C3 to C6 as well as the posteroinferior part of C2 vertebra. A left groove and a right half-groove with the posterior cortex still intact on C3 and C4.

(3, 8) Titanium plate and screws placed in vertebral bodies from C2 to C5.

(4, 9) Completion of the right groove on C3 through C4.

(5, 10) Antedisplaced C2 through C4 vertebral bodies after screw tightening.

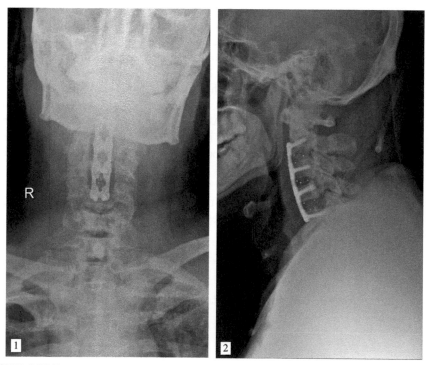

FIGURE 3.22.5

Postoperative cervical X-ray.

(1) Anteroposterior view.

(2) Lateral view.

Restored curvature with Cobb angle of 18.5° from C2 to C7.

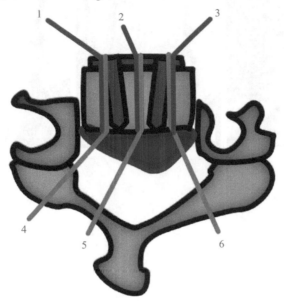

Reference of the sagittal planes

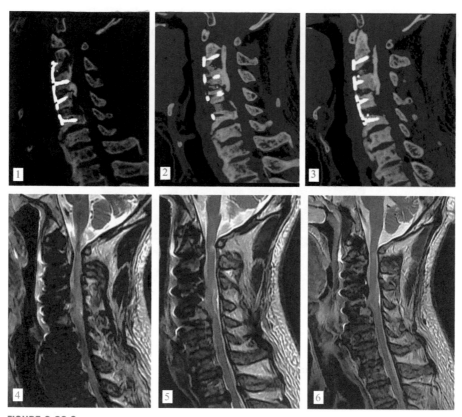

FIGURE 3.22.6

Postoperative sagittal images and their reference on the axial diagram.
(1) Parasagittal CT of the right uncinate process.
(2) Midsagittal CT.
(3) Parasagittal CT of the left uncinate process.
(4) Parasagittal MRI of the right uncinate process.
(5) Midsagittal MRI.
(6) Parasagittal MRI of the left uncinate process.

Improved cervical curvature, ventrally displaced VOC of C3 to C4, expanded spinal canal, and incomplete antedisplacement due to engagement of the OPLL tip at C2 and the vertebra shown on sagittal CT images (Fig. 3.22.6, panel 1 to 3).

Adequate decompression of the spinal cord with normal CSF around it; physiological lordosis restored; the area of signal hyperintensity at C2 and C4 shrunk and attenuated shown on sagittal MRI images (Fig. 3.22.6, panel 4 and 5).

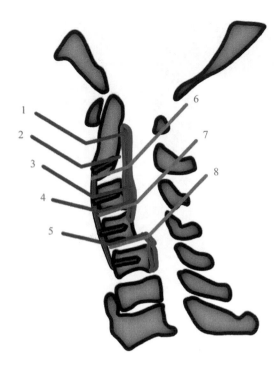

Reference of the axial planes

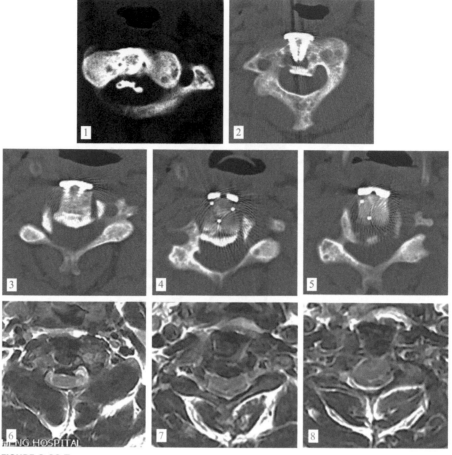

FIGURE 3.22.7

Postoperative axial cervical images and their reference on the sagittal diagram.

(1) Axial CT at C2.

(2) Axial CT at the inferior surface of C2.

(3) Axial CT at C3.

(4) Axial CT at C3/4.

(5) Axial CT at C4/5.

(6) Axial MRI at C2/3.

(7) Axial MRI at C3/4.

(8) Axial MRI at C4/5.

Postoperative axial CT images: The vertebral bodies have been dissected with parasagittal cuts on both sides 21.2 mm apart and VOC antedisplaced by 8.0 mm, and canal occupancy has been reduced to 27.4% at C2 and 0% at C3 (Fig. 3.22.7, panel 1 to 5).

Postoperative axial MR images: The spinal cord resumes oval or triangular shape with normal CSF around it (Fig. 3.22.7, panel 6 to 8).

Discussion

1. Why was the OPLL posterior to C2 inadequately antedisplaced, shown on postoperative images? Is complete decompression achievable with a lesion dissection at C2?

   The incomplete antedisplacement at C2 stemmed from insufficient height and width of the shelter intended for the OPLL's tip. Therefore, the VOC came into contact with the rest of the C2 vertebra.

   For OPLL that extends too proximally, the shelter technique faces a higher challenge, and the dissociation of the OPLL at C2/3 is too risky.

   With the presence of cord compression, evidenced by CSF effacement of C2 and intramedullary signal hyperintensity at C1 on MRI, if C2 compression is not addressed, the dissociated tip of the lesion will slop dorsally as the cervical lordosis comes back, which will result in residual or even worsened cord compression.

2. What was the impact of the dense cancellous bone on the surgery? Conversely, what are the cautions in antedisplacement for osteoporotic bone?

   The increasingly calcified cancellous bone made it difficult to place screws by untapped insertion. Therefore, the bone was prepared with a burr before screw insertion.

   The screw purchase is not compromised in sclerotic cancellous bone, and antedisplacement is usually successful without the risk of screw pull-out.

   In contrast, in elderly patients with decreased bone volume and osteoporosis, the ACAF technique may result in inadequate antedisplacement of the VOC. During the early stage of the antedisplacement, screws are partially inserted in the vertebral bodies. In osteoporotic bone with the thinned anterior cortex of the vertebra, the screw purchase is so compromised that the screw yields to the friction generated by the antedisplacement maneuver. As a result, the displacement effort may fail due to the screw pull-out.

   The use of an instrument for the hoisting maneuver is recommended for prolonged hoisting. At the end of the hoisting maneuver, the screws can be substituted with longer ones or salvage screws that engage the posterior vertebral cortex for better screw purchase.

   In addition, osteoporosis carries a higher risk of iatrogenic injury as visualization is hampered by excessive hemorrhage following decortication.

Case 23: Ossification of posterior longitudinal ligament (OPLL) of cervical spine (At C2 to C5)

Index terms

Antedisplacement of three vertebral bodies, continuous OPLL, thickness of ossification 5—7 mm, canal stenosis between 60% and 70%, shelter technique, and K-line (−) OPLL.

History

Patient: A 66-year-old woman.

Chief complaint: Nuchal pain, numbness of all extremities, and gait instability for two years that aggravated for two months.

Physical exam: Physical exam was noted for gait instability, paresthesia of the neck, decreased superficial sensation on the back below the level of the intermammary line, hypertonicity on all four extremities, and weakened tactile sensation of forearms, calves, and soles bilaterally. Muscle strength was tested at 4/5 on the left upper limb, 3/5 on the right upper limb, and 4/5 on the lower extremities. Brisk tendon reflexes were noted on both lower extremities and ankle, and Babinski sign was present bilaterally.

Preoperative function: JOA was measured at 7, Nurick score: 3, VAS: 3, and NDI: 19.

Imaging studies

Cobb angle of 19.3° measured from C2 through C7, Pavlov ratio of 0.46—0.59 from C3 to C7, and K-line (−) OPLL at C2 to C7 (Fig. 3.23.1).

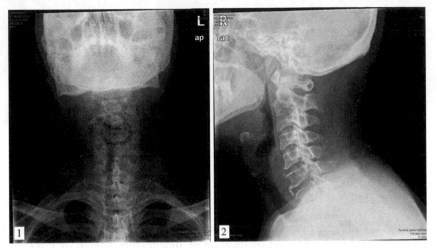

FIGURE 3.23.1

Preoperative X-ray of the cervical spine.
(1) Anteroposterior view.
(2) Lateral view.

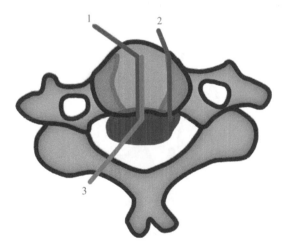

Reference of the sagittal planes

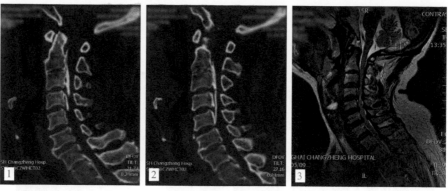

FIGURE 3.23.2

Preoperative sagittal images and their reference on axial diagram.
(1) Midsagittal CT.
(2) Left parasagittal CT.
(3) Midsagittal MRI.

Sagittal CT images, extensive ossification of ligaments characterized by OPLL of C2 to C5 and C7 to T1, and ossification of ligamentum flavum of C7/T1 and T1/2. The continuous OPLL is more severe at C2 to C5 and double-layered at C4 and C5 (Fig. 3.23.2, panel 1 and 2).

Preoperative sagittal MR images: Spinal cord compressed both anteriorly and posteriorly from C3/4 to C6/7 with intramedullary signal hyperintensity at C4/5, indicating myelopathy (Fig. 3.23.2, panel 3).

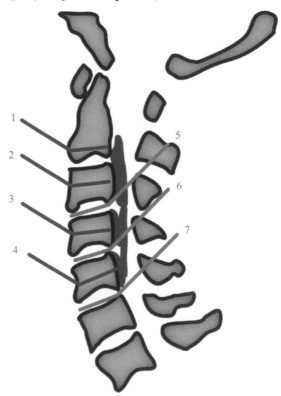

Reference of the axial planes

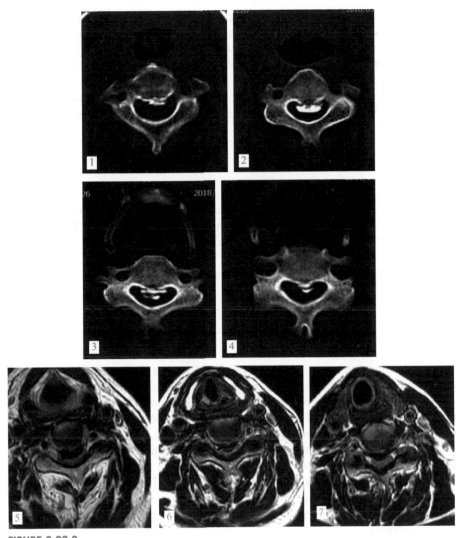

FIGURE 3.23.3

Preoperative axial images of the cervical spine and their reference on the sagittal diagram.
(1) Axial CT at the inferior surface of C2.
(2) Axial CT at C3.
(3) Axial CT at C4.
(4) Axial CT at C5.
(5) Axial MRI at C3/4.
(6) Axial MRI at C4/5.
(7) Axial MRI at C5/6.

The OPLL is flat and centered in the spinal canal with a double-layer sign at C4 and C5. It measures 5.1 mm thick (anteroposterior), 13.7 mm wide (mediolateral), and 54.8% in canal occupancy at C3; and 5.1 mm thick, 12.5 mm wide, and 60% in canal occupancy at C4, shown on postoperative axial CT images (Fig. 3.23.3, panel 1 to 4).

Deformed spinal cord in the shape of boomerang and crescent due to anterior indentation of the hypointense mass in the spinal canal, shown on postoperative axial MR images (Fig. 3.23.3, panel 5 to 7).

Highlights

This case features developmental spinal canal stenosis complicated with extensive and continuous ossification of ligaments, in particular at C2 to C5. The lesion is associated with dural ossification, suggested by a double-layer sign on axial CT, C6/7 disc protrusion, and hypertrophy of ligamentum flavum at C3/4 to C6/7. Due to impingement at C2/3 to C6/7 in the pincer pattern, the spinal cord appears like a string of beads.

Surgical planning

This case features an extensive, K-line (+) OPLL with a double-layer sign. Among the conventional procedures, posterior decompression is an option.

Since the canal stenosis reaches 60% at the most affected level, a significant posterior shift of the spinal cord is needed for adequate decompression, which increases the risk of postoperative neural palsy.

To achieve direct decompression and avoid unintended tension of the neural element due to excessive cord shift, an ACAF from C3 to C5 was performed with anterior cervical discectomy and fusion (ACDF) at C6/7.

Since the correction of the cervical curvature also provides room for decompression, resection was performed to the anterior bony structure of depth smaller than the OPLL thickness.

Results

Postoperative function: JOA score was 15, Nurick score: 0, VAS: 1, and NDI: 10 (Fig. 3.23.4).

Instrumentation from C2 to C7 and antedisplaced C3 to C5 vertebral bodies (Fig. 3.23.5).

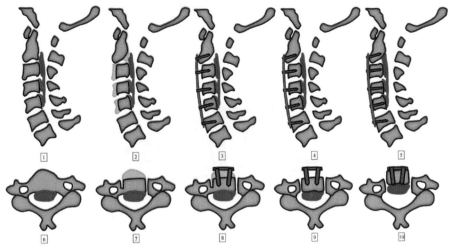

FIGURE 3.23.4

Illustration of the surgical plan on sagittal and axial planes.

(1, 6) Illustration of the OPLL on sagittal and axial views before surgery.

(2, 7) Resection performed to the anterior part of C3 to C5 vertebra and the posteroinferior part of C2 vertebra. A complete trough is developed on the left vertebral bodies from C3 to C5 while a half one is made on the right side with the posterior bone yet to be dissected.

(3, 8) Plate and screws placed on vertebral bodies from C2 through C6.

(4, 9) The bottom of the right half-groove on C3 through C5 dissected.

(5, 10) Antedisplaced C3 to C5 vertebral bodies as screws were tightened.

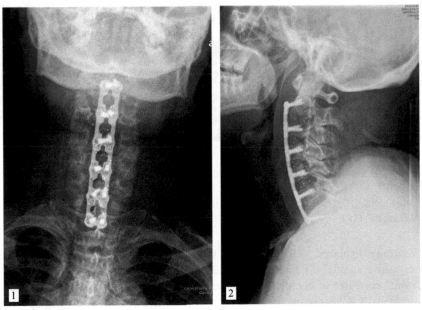

FIGURE 3.23.5

Postoperative cervical spine X-ray.

(1) Anteroposterior view.

(2) Lateral view.

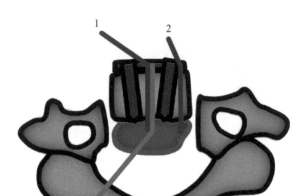

Reference of the sagittal planes

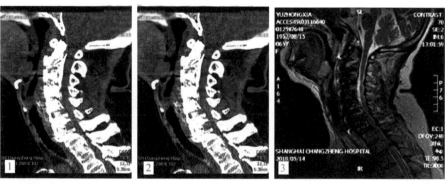

FIGURE 3.23.6

Postoperative sagittal views and their reference on the axial diagram.
(1) Midsagittal CT.
(2) Parasagittal CT of the left uncinate process.
(3) Midsagittal MRI.

Ventrally displaced VOC from C3 to C5, and expanded spinal canal, shown on postoperative sagittal CT images (Fig. 3.23.6, panel 1 and 2).

Spinal cord free of compression in the cervical spine with residual deformation surrounded by CSF columns anteriorly and posteriorly, shown on postoperative sagittal MR image (Fig. 3.23.6, panel 3).

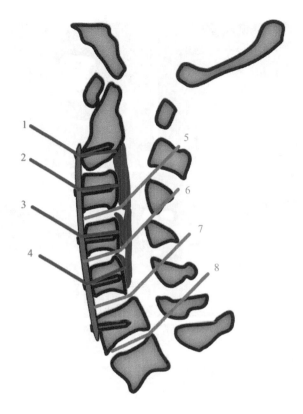

Reference of the axial planes

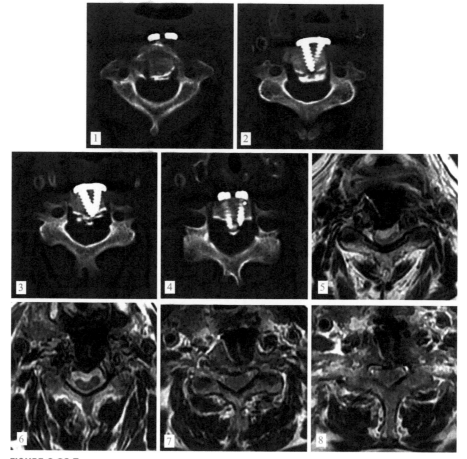

FIGURE 3.23.7

Postoperative axial cervical images and their reference on the sagittal diagram.
(1) Axial CT at the inferior surface of C2.
(2) Axial CT at C3.
(3) Axial CT at C4.
(4) Axial CT at C5.
(5) Axial MRI at C3/4.
(6) Axial MRI at C4/5.
(7) Axial MRI at C5/6.
(8) Axial MRI at C6/7.

The vertebral bodies have been dissected with parasagittal grooves on both sides, medial to the neural foramina, 21 mm apart, and VOC antedisplaced by 5.2 mm; the spinal canal is free of ossification with canal occupancy reduced to 0% at all levels shown on postoperative axial CT images (Fig. 3.23.7, panel 1 to 4).

The unimpinged spinal cord resumes an oval shape with normal CSF around it. It has recovered from crescent shape to boomerang shape at C3/4 and C4/5, levels with the worst impingement before surgery shown on postoperative axial CT images (Fig. 3.23.7, panel 5 to 8).

Discussion

Why was ACDF performed to C6/7 rather than C6 antedisplacement?

Preoperative imaging studies revealed a C6 spared from OPLL with preserved CSF volume around the spinal cord.

The spinal cord was pincered at C5/6 and C6/7 by degenerative disc material ventrally and hypertrophic ligamentum flavum dorsally without evidence of ossification.

In other words, the cord compression was present at disc spaces around C6 but not at C6, and such compression did not stem from ossification components. Therefore, the C6 vertebra was preserved while the C6/7 was decompressed with ACDF.

Case 24: Cervical spinal stenosis and cervical hyperextension injury

---

Index terms

Antedisplacement of three vertebral bodies, segmental OPL, thickness of ossification below 5 mm, canal occupancy ratio below 50%, and history of extension injury.

History

Patient: A 43-year-old man.

Chief complaint: Numbness and weakness of all extremities for six days following a cervical trauma.

Physical exam: Physical exam was noted for the decreased superficial sensation of the left palm and left lower limb. Muscle strength was tested at 3/5 on upper limbs and 4/5 on lower limbs. Brisk tendon reflexes and Babinski signs were present bilaterally.

Preoperative function: JOA was measured at 13, Nurick score: 3, VAS: 0, and NDI: 9.

Imaging studies

Cobb angle of 25.3° measured from C2 through C7; Pavlov ratio of 0.57, 0.50, and 0.53 at C5 to C7, respectively; and a K-line (+) OPLL (Fig. 3.24.1).

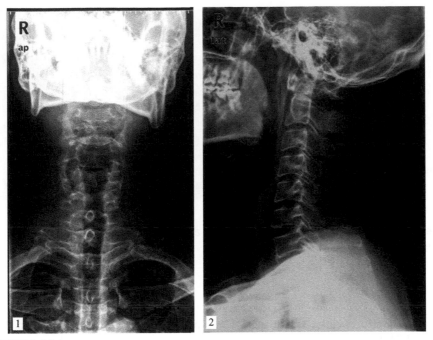

FIGURE 3.24.1

Preoperative X-ray of the cervical spine.
(1) Anteroposterior view.
(2) Lateral view.

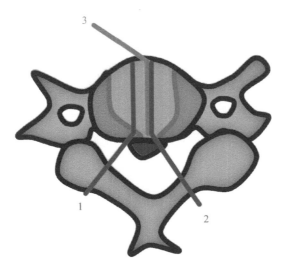

Reference of the sagittal planes

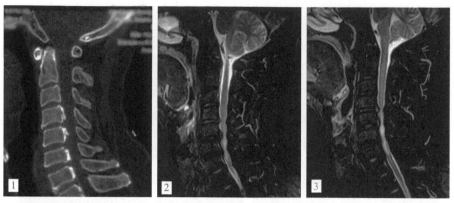

FIGURE 3.24.2

Preoperative sagittal images of the cervical spine and their reference on the axial diagram.

(1) Midsagittal CT.

(2) Right parasagittal CT.

(3) Midsagittal MRI.

Preoperative sagittal CT images: Flat-type segmental OPLL from C4 to T1 (Fig. 3.24.2, panel 1).

Preoperative sagittal MR images: Obliteration of anterior and posterior CSF columns at C4/5 and C7. The cord compression is most severe at C4/5 with pincer pattern indentation; widened intramedullary central canal from C5 to C7 with cysts within the cord (Fig. 3.24.2, panel 2 and 3).

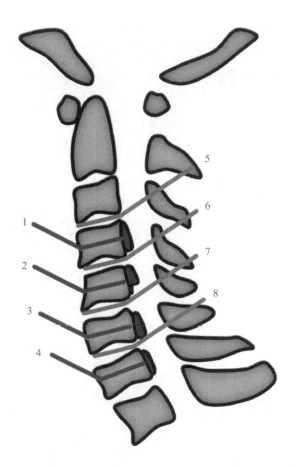

Reference of the axial planes

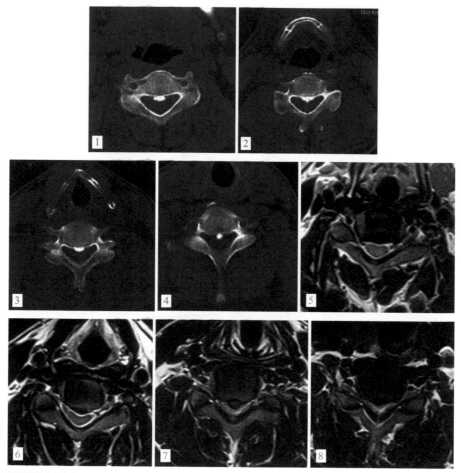

FIGURE 3.24.3

Preoperative axial images of the cervical spine and their reference on the sagittal diagram.

(1) Axial CT at C3/4.
(2) Axial CT at C4/5.
(3) Axial CT at C5/6.
(4) Axial CT at C6/7.
(5) Axial MRI at C4.
(6) Axial MRI at C5.
(7) Axial MRI at C6.
(8) Axial MRI at C7.

A midline-centered and wide-based OPLL, measuring 4.3 mm thick (anteroposterior), 10.2 mm wide (mediolateral), and 42.9% in canal occupancy at the most protuberant level, shown on axial CT images (Fig. 3.24.3, panel 1 to 4).

The spinal cord is crescent- or boomerang-shaped at multiple levels due to severe indentation, shown on axial MR images (Fig. 3.24.3, panel 5 to 8).

Highlights

This case features a hyperextension cervical injury superimposed to developmental spinal canal stenosis from C5 to C7 and stenosis secondary to an extensive OPLL. His diseases were further complicated by disc material protrusion and pincer from the hypertrophic ligamentum flavum. The spinal cord was found with cysts and widened central canal at C5 to C7. The OPLL involves C4 and T1 levels but has not caused cord impingement.

Surgical planning

This case is characterized by an extensive, K-line (+) OPLL in a cervical spine in physiological lordosis. The conventional indirect decompression via a posterior approach provides an option.

But posterior surgeries involve significant muscular disruption and may cause sustained neck pain after surgery. There are also risks for a worsen curvature, progression of ossification, and recurrent neuropathy further down the road.

An ACAF was planned for the patient that antedisplace C5 to C7 levels with stenosis.

Thorough thinking is needed to plan for the instrumented levels. Cord compression was most severe at C5 to C7 and absent at C4 and T1 where the OPLL did not efface the CSF columns. Therefore, the surgery was planned on C4/5 to C7/T1.

Given the preserved physiological lordosis, an anterior part of the vertebrae of the same thickness as the ossification was resected.

Results

Postoperative function: JOA score was 14, Nurick score: 1, VAS: 0, and NDI: 7 (Fig. 3.24.4).

Instrumentation from C4 to T1, and antedisplaced C5 to C7 (Fig. 3.24.5).

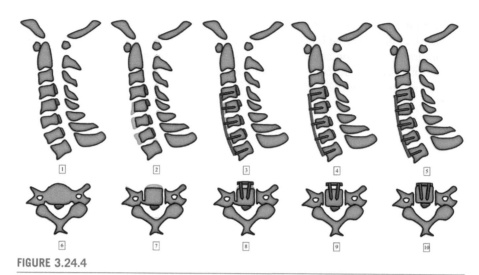

FIGURE 3.24.4

Illustration of the surgical plan on sagittal and axial planes.

(1, 6) Illustration of the OPLL on sagittal and axial views before surgery.

(2, 7) Resection was performed to the anterior part of C5 to C7 vertebra. A complete trough is developed on the left vertebral bodies from C5 to C7 while a half one is made on the right side with the posterior bone yet to be dissected.

(3, 8) Plate and screws placed on vertebral bodies from C4 through T1.

(4, 9) The bottom of the right half-groove on C5 through C7.

(5, 10) Antedisplaced C5 to C7 vertebral bodies as screws were tightened.

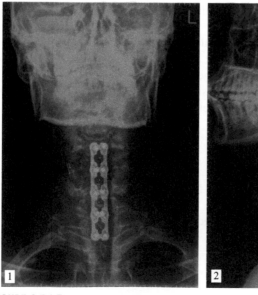
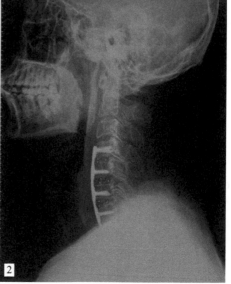

FIGURE 3.24.5

Postoperative cervical spine X-ray.

(1) Anteroposterior view.

(2) Lateral view.

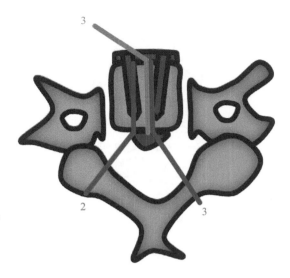

Reference of the sagittal planes

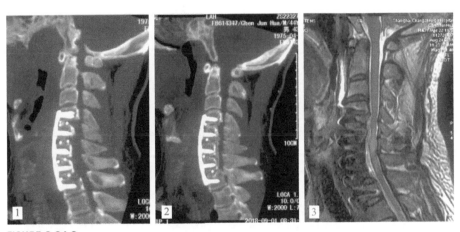

FIGURE 3.24.6

Postoperative sagittal views and their reference on the axial diagram.
(1) Left parasagittal CT.
(2) Midsagittal CT.
(3) Midsagittal MRI.

Postoperative sagittal CT images: VOC of C5, C6, and C7 antedisplaced by 4 mm engaged with the plate, and expanded spinal canal (Fig. 3.24.6, panel 1 and 2).

Postoperative sagittal MR image: The spinal cord free of compression in restored curvature surrounded by anterior and posterior CSF columns, though still with cysts (Fig. 3.24.6, panel 3 and 4).

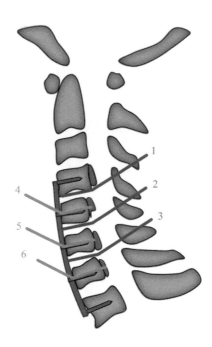

Reference of the axial planes

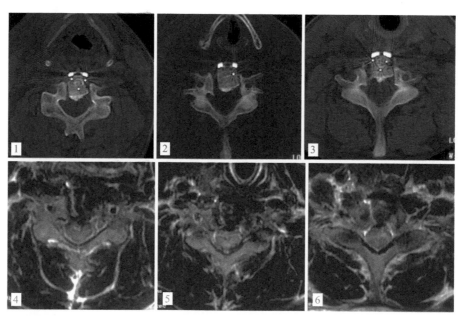

FIGURE 3.24.7

Postoperative axial cervical images and their reference on the sagittal diagram.
(1) Axial CT at C4/5.
(2) Axial CT at C5/6.
(3) Axial CT at C6/7.
(4) Axial MRI at C5.
(5) Axial MRI at C7.
(6) Axial MRI at C7.

Grooves on both sides of the vertebral bodies 17.3 mm apart; spinal stenosis reduced to 0% shown on postoperative axial CT images (Fig. 3.24.7, panel 1 to 5).

The spinal cord, adequately decompressed, resumes oval shape with a widened intramedullary central canal shown on postoperative axial MR images (Fig. 3.24.7, panel 6 to 8).

Discussion

Why were the OPLL at C4 and T1 left out from the antedisplacement?

Preoperative imaging studies revealed a severely compressed spinal cord with effacement of the anterior and posterior CSF columns and widened intramedullary central canal from C5 to C7.

Since the spinal cord at C4 and T1 was still surrounded by CSF ventrally and dorsally with Pavlov ratio above 75%, the OPLL had not impinged the cord yet.

Therefore, C4 and T1 were not antedisplaced for motion preservation.

Case 25: Ossification of posterior longitudinal ligament (OPLL) of Cervical spine (C4 to C6, cervical kyphosis)

Index terms

Antedisplacement of three vertebral bodies, continuous OPLL, wide-based OPLL, thickness of ossification 7–9 mm, canal occupancy ratio above 70%, and cervical kyphosis.

History

Patient: A 47-year-old man.

Chief complaint: Numbness of the upper limbs for one year that aggravated for two months with gait instability.

Physical exam: Physical exam was noted for gait instability, hypertonicity on all four extremities, and impaired tactile sensation on all finger pulps, more severe on the right side. Muscle strength was tested at 3/5 on upper limbs. Brisk tendon reflexes were noted on both upper extremities. Hoffmann and Babinski signs were present bilaterally.

Preoperative function: JOA was measured at 11, Nurick score: 3, VAS: 0, and NDI: 14.

Imaging studies

Cobb angle of $-12.9°$ measured from C2 through C7, spinal canal stenosis, and Pavlov ratio of 68% (Fig. 3.25.1).

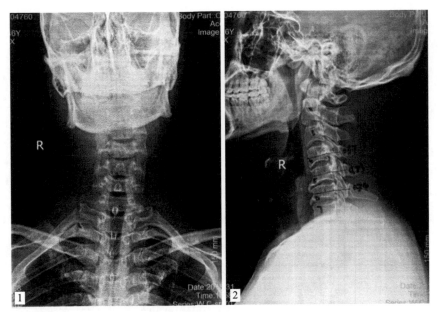

FIGURE 3.25.1

Preoperative X-ray of the cervical spine.
(1) Anteroposterior view.
(2) Lateral view.

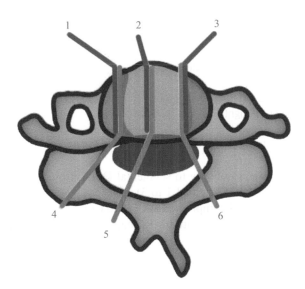

Reference of the sagittal planes

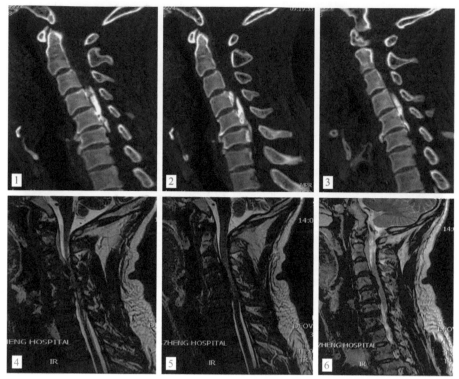

FIGURE 3.25.2

Preoperative sagittal images of the cervical spine and their reference on the axial diagram.

(1) Parasagittal CT of the right uncinate process.
(2) Midsagittal CT.
(3) Parasagittal CT of the left uncinate process.
(4) Parasagittal MRI of the right uncinate process.
(5) Midsagittal MRI.
(6) Parasagittal MRI of the left uncinate process.

Spinal canal stenosis secondary to segmental OPLL from C4 to C6, shown on sagittal CT images (Fig. 3.25.2, panel 1 to 3).

The kyphotic spinal cord compressed at C3/5 to C6/7, and intramedullary signal hyperintensity at C4, shown on sagittal MR images (Fig. 3.25.2, panel 4 to 6).

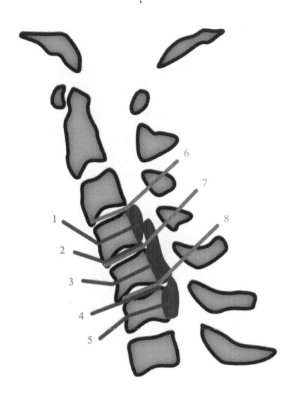

Reference of the axial planes

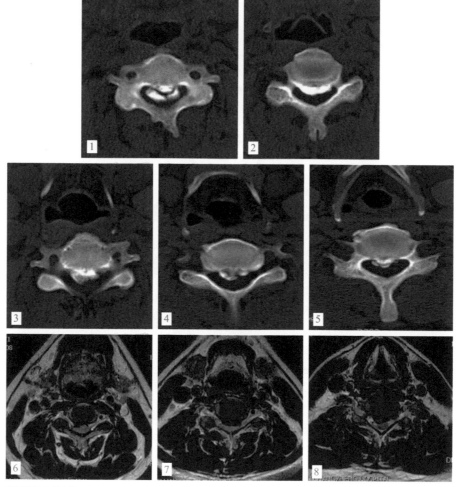

FIGURE 3.25.3

Preoperative axial images of the cervical spine and their reference on the sagittal diagram.
(1) Axial CT at C4.
(2) Axial CT at C4/5.
(3) Axial CT at C5.
(4) Axial CT at C5/6.
(5) Axial CT at C6.
(6) Axial MRI at C3/4.
(7) Axial MRI at C4/5.
(8) Axial MRI at C5/6.

Double-layer sign present at C4 and C5. The OPLL measures 8.7 mm thick (anteroposterior) and 18.4 mm wide (mediolateral), and 72.5% in canal occupancy. At C4/5, it is wide-based and measured at 5.1 mm thick, 20.2 mm wide, and 44.7% canal occupancy; and at C5, it is 8.4 mm thick, 16.6 mm wide, and 62.5% in OR, shown on axial CT images (Fig. 3.25.3, panel 1 to 5).

Deformed spinal cord in crescent or boomerang shape due to anterior indentation and intramedullary signal hyperintensity at C5, shown on axial MR images (Fig. 3.25.3, panel 6 to 8).

Highlights

This case features a kyphotic cervical spine with developmental stenosis superimposed with stenosis secondary to extensive OPLL from C4 to C6. The OPLL is flat and segmental on sagittal views with a double-layer sign on axial views.

Surgical planning

In this case of K-line (−) OPLL with more than 60% of canal stenosis, direct decompression via anterior approach and lordosis reconstruction with plate serve as a conventional option.

Given the wide-based OPLL at C4 and C4/5 and limited decompression width available from a partial corpectomy, there is a risk of insufficient decompression. Also, the use of instrumentation for multiple segments constitutes an increased risk of hardware-related complications.

Given the possible involvement of the dura, suggested by the double-layer sign at C4 and C6, care should be exercised to dissect the ossification off the dura in case of a dural tear or cord injury.

The patient received ACAF with antedisplacement of VOC from C4 to C6.

As the OPLL was wider at C5/6, grooves developed off the base of the uncinate processes may provide inadequate decompression to the right side of the lesion and leave residual lesion around the neural exit foramen. Therefore, it is sensible to lateralize the groove for a thorough decompression (Fig. 3.25.4).

Results

Postoperative function: JOA score was 11, Nurick score: 2, VAS: 0, and NDI: 10.

Improved cervical curvature with a Cobb angle of 11.5° from C2 through C7 (Fig. 3.25.5).

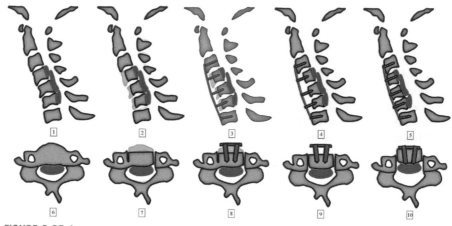

FIGURE 3.25.4

Illustration of the surgical plan on sagittal and axial views.

(1, 6) Illustration of the OPLL on sagittal and axial views before surgery.

(2, 7) Resection of the anterior part of the vertebral bodies of C4 to C6. A left groove and a right half-groove with the posterior cortex still intact on C4 to C6.

(3, 8) Titanium plate and screws placed in vertebral bodies from C3 to C7.

(4, 9) Completion of the right groove on C4 through C6.

(5, 10) Antedisplaced C4 through C6 vertebral bodies after screw tightening.

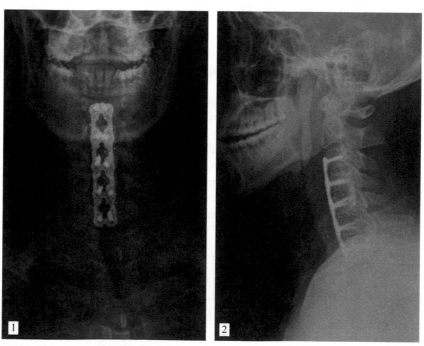

FIGURE 3.25.5

Postoperative cervical X-ray.

(1) Anteroposterior view.

(2) Lateral view.

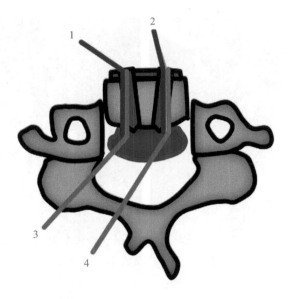

Reference of the sagittal planes

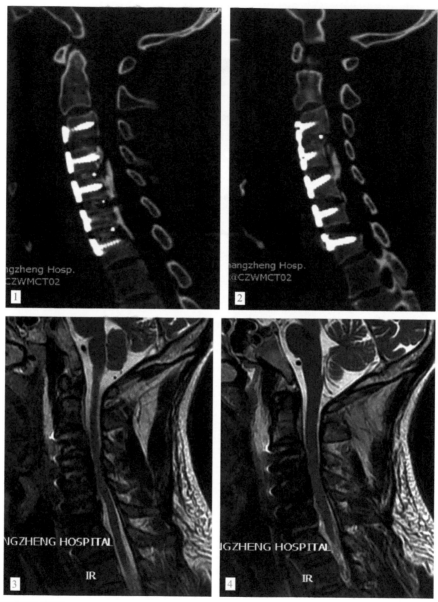

FIGURE 3.25.6

Postoperative sagittal images and their reference on the axial diagram.
(1) Right parasagittal CT.
(2) Left parasagittal CT.
(3) Right parasagittal MRI.
(4) Left parasagittal MRI.

Cervical lordosis restored. Antedisplaced VOC from C4 to C6 and widened spinal canal, shown on postoperative sagittal CT images (Fig. 3.25.6, panel 1 and 2).

Spinal cord free of compression in lordotic curvature surrounded by CSF shown on postoperative sagittal MR images (Fig. 3.25.6, panel 3 and 4).

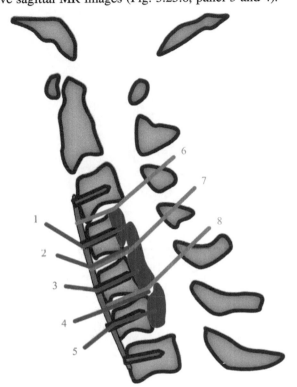

Reference of the axial planes

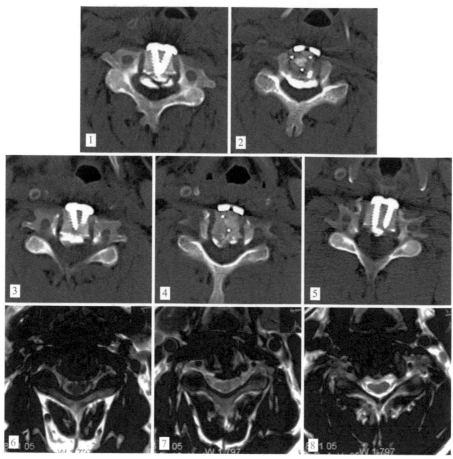

FIGURE 3.25.7

Postoperative axial cervical images and their reference on the sagittal diagram.

(1) Axial CT at C4.
(2) Axial CT at C4/5.
(3) Axial CT at C5.
(4) Axial CT at C5/6.
(5) Axial CT at C6.
(6) Axial MRI at C2/3.
(7) Axial MRI at C3/4.
(8) Axial MRI at C4/5.

Postoperative crossing CT images: The vertebral bodies of C4 to C6 have been dissected with parasagittal cuts on both sides 22.4 mm apart and the VOC antedisplaced by 4 mm; canal occupancy has been reduced to 38.9% and 30% at C4 and C5, respectively (Fig. 3.25.7, panel 1 to 5).

The spinal cord resumes to oval or triangular shape, shown on postoperative crossing MR image (Fig. 3.25.7, panel 6 and 8).

Discussion

When the resection of the vertebra measures only half the thickness of the ossification, does it cause insufficient decompression at C4 to C5, the levels of more severe ossification? How can we avoid this problem?

The OPLL in this case measured 8.7 and 5.1 mm at the thickest and thinnest levels, respectively. Resection of the anterior vertebra referenced off the maximum thickness of the lesion will result in excessive antedisplacement of levels where the ossification was less severe. Therefore, the anterior resection shall measure thinner than the maximum thickness of the ossification.

In this patient with cervical kyphosis, the surgery involves not only decompression but also curvature restoration through a prebent plate. As the cervical spine comes back into lordosis, it creates extra room for the antedisplacement of the ossification. Taking this advantage can preserve the bony structure and achieve better intervertebral fusion.

On postoperative CT review, the anterior part of the vertebral bodies had been removed by 4 mm, half the maximum thickness of the ossification.

Though the spinal cord had been mobilized off the compression and the C6 vertebra, the level of minimal disease, had not been overly displaced, there was residual effacement of CSF at C4 to C5, levels of more severe disease.

Such a problem caused by variable thickness across the lesion shall be avoided with meticulously planned depths of resection from the anterior vertebral bodies.

Case 26: Ossification of posterior longitudinal ligament (OPLL) of cervical spine (At C2 to C4)

Index terms

Antedisplacement of two vertebral bodies, continuous OPLL, wide-based lesion, thickness of ossification 5—7 mm, occupancy ratio below 50%, shelter technique, and insufficient antedisplacement.

History

Patient: A 53-year-old man.

Chief complaint: Nuchal discomfort for 10 years that worsened with gait instability for five years.

Physical exam: Physical exam was noted for gait instability, paresthesia (painful) on both shoulders, hypertonicity on all four extremities, and impaired tactile sensation on the plantar side of both feet. Muscle strength was tested at 4/5 on the upper limbs and 4/5 on lower limbs. Tendon reflexes were brisk on all four extremities. Hoffmann and Babinski signs were present bilaterally.

Preoperative function: JOA was measured at 15, Nurick score: 1, VAS: 0, and NDI: 0.

Imaging studies

Straightened cervical spine with Cobb angle of 5.1° from C2 through C7, and K-line (+) OPLL from C2 to C4 (Fig. 3.26.1).

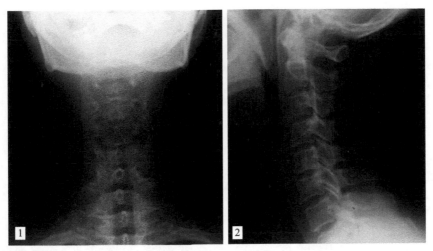

FIGURE 3.26.1

Preoperative X-ray of the cervical spine.

(1) Anteroposterior view.

(2) Lateral view.

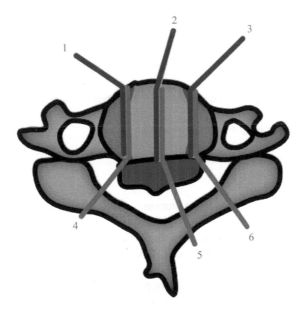

Reference of the sagittal planes

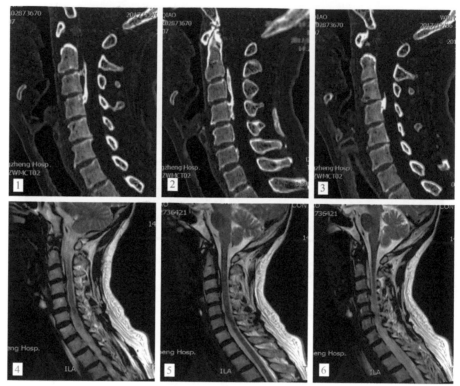

FIGURE 3.26.2

Preoperative sagittal images of the cervical spine and their reference on the axial diagram.

(1) Parasagittal CT of the right uncinate process.
(2) Midsagittal CT.
(3) Parasagittal CT of the left uncinate process.
(4) Parasagittal MRI of the right uncinate process.
(5) Midsagittal MRI.
(6) Parasagittal MRI of the left uncinate process.

Preoperative sagittal CT images: A flat-type continuous OPLL from C2 to C4 with the ossified mass attached to C4 vertebral bodies but not C2 or C3 (Fig. 3.26.2, panel 1 to 3).

Preoperative sagittal MR images: A hypointense band in the front of the spinal canal from C2 to C4 that causes anterior indentation of the spinal cord and obliteration of the anterior and posterior CSF columns (Fig. 3.26.2, panel 4 to 6).

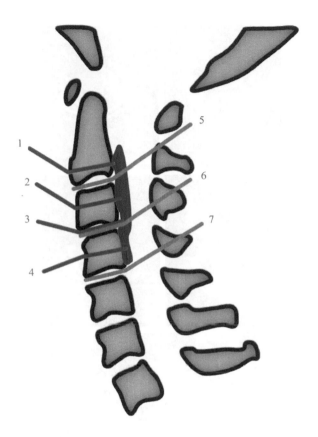

Reference of the axial planes

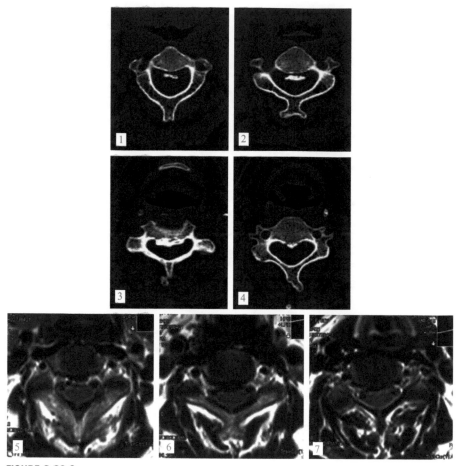

FIGURE 3.26.3

Preoperative axial images of the cervical spine and their reference on the sagittal diagram.

(1) Axial CT at the inferior surface of C2.
(2) Axial CT at C3.
(3) Axial CT at C3/4.
(4) Axial CT at C4.
(5) Axial MRI at C2/3.
(6) Axial MRI at C3/4.
(7) Axial MRI at C4/5.

The OPLL is smaller at C2 and C3; it measures 5.6 mm thick (anteroposterior), 10.8 mm wide (mediolateral), and 38.1% in canal occupancy; gaps between the lesion and vertebral bodies are present; at C3/4, the lesion is wider and measured 5.2 mm thick, 16.3 mm wide, and 40.6% in OR, shown on axial CT images (Fig. 3.26.3, panel 1 to 4).

Compressed spinal cord due to anterior indentation of the hypointense mass in the front of the spinal canal, and effacement of the surrounding CSF, shown on axial MR images (Fig. 3.26.3, panel 5 to 7),

Highlights

This case features spinal canal stenosis secondary to a flat-type continuous OPLL from C2 to C4, centered at midline, and not attached to vertebral bodies. It has a broader base at C3/4.

Surgical planning

In this case of K-line (+) OPLL that spans three levels and extends to the upper cervical spine, indirect decompression via a posterior approach is a conventional option.

Given the poor cervical curvature and the ventral-based compression on the spinal cord, indicated by the lesion and the posterior CSF column on preoperative MRI scans, a posterior surgery may lead to inadequate decompression.

Another option is an anterior surgery with ACCF on C3 and C4 and undercutting the posterior part of C2 vertebra. At C3/4 where the lesion is wider, after grooves are developed on the vertebral bodies according to the ACCF technique, further decompression to the residual lesion lateral to the grooves is needed, which comes with the risk of injury and insufficient clearance.

The patient received ACAF for antedisplacement of C3 and C4 and a shelter procedure for the posterior part of the C2 vertebra.

Since extra room in the spinal canal is obtained from curvature correction, the anterior resection shall measure thinner than the OPLL thickness.

At C3/4, the OPLL spans 15.9 mm on the coronal plane, wider than the distance between the uncinate processes on both sides, 15.5 mm. Therefore, the grooves were developed off the anterior base of the uncinate processes, followed by palpation of the lateral edge of the lesion with a neural hook and properly expand the grooves toward the edge of the lesion (Fig. 3.26.4).

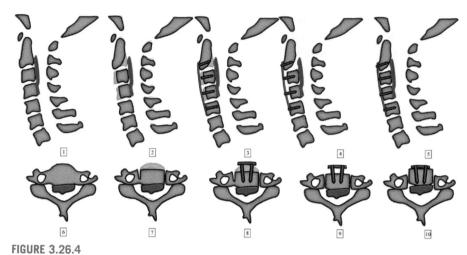

FIGURE 3.26.4

Illustration of the surgical plan on sagittal and axial planes.

(1, 6) Illustration of the OPLL on sagittal and axial views before surgery.

(2, 7) Resection performed to the anterior part of C3 to C4 vertebral bodies and the posterior part of the C2 vertebra. A complete trough is developed on the left vertebral bodies from C3 to C4 while a half one is made on the right side with the posterior bone yet to be dissected.

(3, 8) Plate and screws placed on vertebral bodies from C2 through C5.

(4, 9) The bottom of the right half-groove on C3 through C6 dissected.

(5, 10) Antedisplaced C3 to C4 vertebral bodies as screws were tightened.

Results

Postoperative function: JOA score was 15, Nurick score: 0, VAS: 0, and NDI: 5.

Improved cervical curvature with a Cobb angle of 17° from C2 through C7 (Fig. 3.26.5).

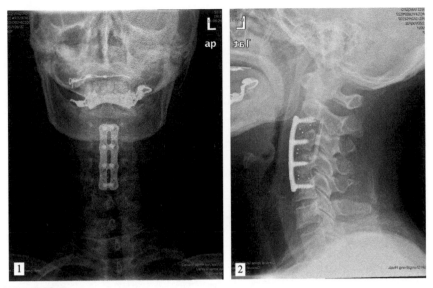

FIGURE 3.26.5

Postoperative cervical spine X-ray.
(1) Anteroposterior view.
(2) Lateral view.

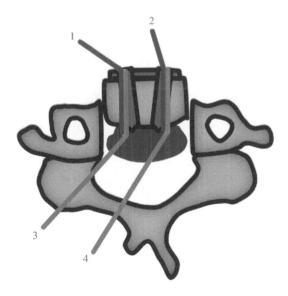

Reference of the sagittal planes

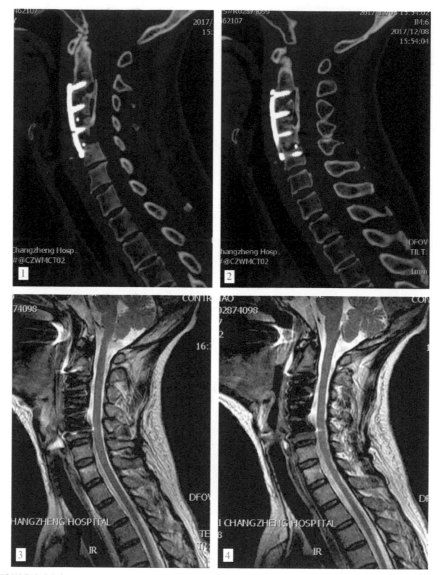

FIGURE 3.26.6

Postoperative sagittal views and their reference on the axial diagram.
(1) Parasagittal CT of the right uncinate process.
(2) Midsagittal CT.
(3) Parasagittal CT of the left uncinate process.
(4) Parasagittal MRI of the right uncinate process.
(5) Midsagittal MRI.
(6) Parasagittal MRI of the left uncinate process.

Antedisplaced VOC from C3 to C4 with the posteroinferior part of the C2 vertebra resected shown on postoperative sagittal CT images (Fig. 3.26.6, panel 1 and 2).

Expanded spinal canal with restored anterior and posterior CSF columns shown on postoperative sagittal MR images (Fig. 3.26.6, panel 3 and 4).

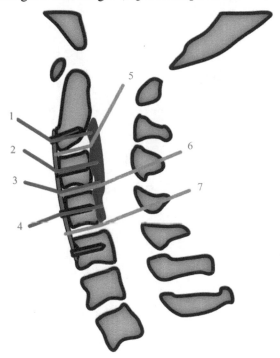

Reference of the axial planes

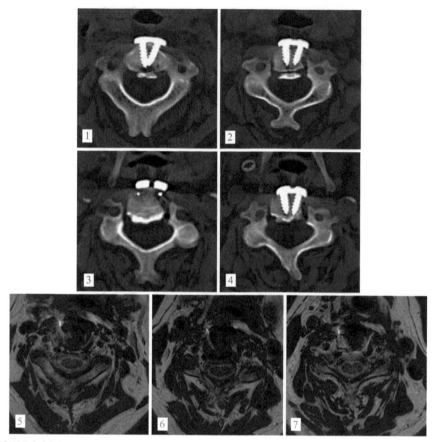

FIGURE 3.26.7

Postoperative axial cervical images and their reference on the sagittal diagram.

(1) Axial CT at the inferior surface of C2.

(2) Axial CT at C3.

(3) Axial CT at C3/4.

(4) Axial CT at C4.

(5) Axial MRI at C2/3.

(6) Axial MRI at C3/4.

(7) Axial MRI at C4/5.

The vertebral bodies of C2 to C4 have been dissected with parasagittal cuts on both sides 21.8 mm apart and the VOC antedisplaced by 5.4 mm, and canal occupancy has been reduced to 0%, shown on postoperative axial CT images (Fig. 3.26.7, panel 1 to 4).

The spinal cord, cleared of compression, resumes its oval shape at C2/3 to C4/5, shown on postoperative axial MR images (Fig. 3.26.7, panel 5 to 7).

Discussion

In this case with mild-to-moderate cord compression, indicated from preoperative imaging studies, how much antedisplacement was needed in the ACAF technique?

This patient was symptomatic, though, with a mild ossification. In the spinal cord with mild compression, antedisplacement of a small distance is enough for an adequate decompression and symptom resolution.

To account for the progression of ossification down the road, the anterior cervical column was resected by the thickness consistent with that of the lesion, which reduced canal stenosis to 0%.

Case 27: Ossification of posterior longitudinal ligament (OPLL) of cervical spine (At C4 to C5)

Index terms

Antedisplacement of two vertebral bodies, continuous OPLL, wide-based OPLL, thickness of ossification 5–7 mm, canal stenosis between 50% and 60%, and shelter technique.

History

Patient: A 64-year-old man.

Chief complaint: Pain, numbness, and weakness of all four extremities for two years that aggravated with gait instability for one month.

Physical exam: Physical exam was noted for gait instability, hypertonicity on all four extremities, impaired tactile sensation on all finger pulps, and paresthesia (painful) on lower limbs. Muscle strength was tested at 4/5 on upper limbs. Brisk tendon reflexes were noted on both upper extremities. Hoffmann sign was present bilaterally.

Preoperative function: JOA was measured at 12, Nurick score: 1, VAS: 3, and NDI: 14.

Imaging studies

Cobb angle of 14.8° from C2 through C7, Pavlov ratio above 0.75, and OPLL of C4 through C5 (Fig. 3.27.1).

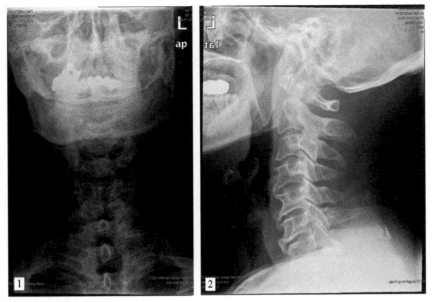

FIGURE 3.27.1

Preoperative X-ray of the cervical spine.
(1) Anteroposterior view.
(2) Lateral view.

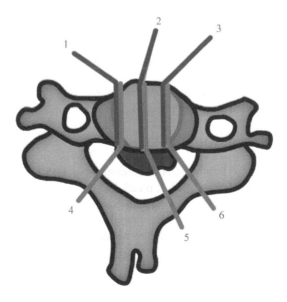

Reference of the sagittal planes

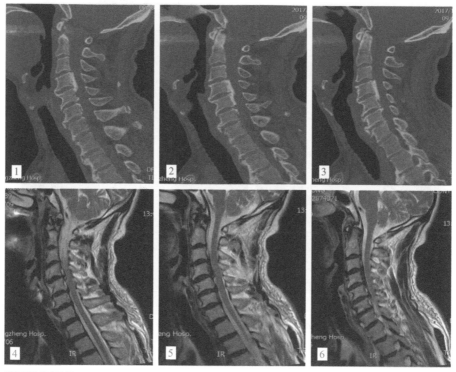

FIGURE 3.27.2

Preoperative sagittal images of the cervical spine and their reference on the axial diagram.

(1) Parasagittal CT of the right uncinate process.
(2) Midsagittal CT.
(3) Parasagittal CT of the left uncinate process.
(4) Parasagittal MRI of the right uncinate process.
(5) Midsagittal MRI.
(6) Parasagittal MRI of the left uncinate process.

Preoperative sagittal CT images: A continuous-type OPLL from C4 to C5 that featured peak-type at C4/5 (Fig. 3.27.2, panel 1 to 3).

Preoperative sagittal MR images: A hypointense band in the front of the spinal canal from C4 to C5 protuberant into the spinal canal, and obliteration of the anterior and posterior CSF columns at C5/6 due to the herniated disc (Fig. 3.27.2, panel 4 to 6).

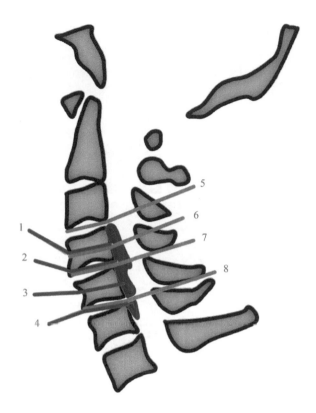

Reference of the axial planes

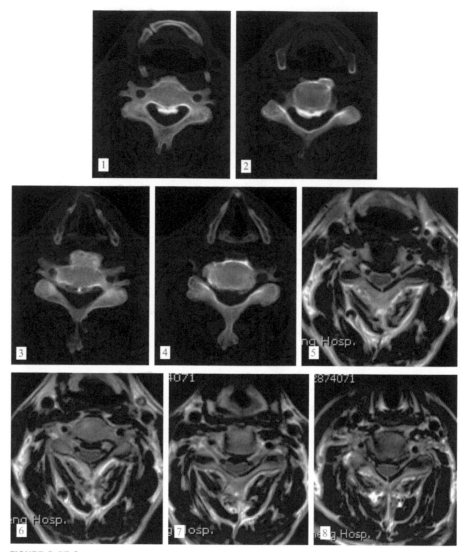

FIGURE 3.27.3

Preoperative axial images of the cervical spine and their reference on the sagittal diagram.

(1) Axial CT at C4.
(2) Axial CT at C4/5.
(3) Axial CT at C5.
(4) Axial CT at C5/6.
(5) Axial MRI at C3/4.
(6) Axial MRI at C4.
(7) Axial MRI at C4/5.
(8) Axial MRI at C5/6.

Preoperative axial CT images: At C4, it is narrow-based and measured at 4.0 mm thick (anteroposterior), 13.7 mm wide (mediolateral), and 33.9% in OR; and at C5, it becomes wide-based and measures 6.0 mm thick, 18.2 mm wide, and 50% in OR (Fig. 3.27.3, panel 1 to 4).

Preoperative axial MR images: Due to anterior indentation of a hypointense mass, the spinal cord featured triangular-type and diminished CSF (Fig. 3.27.3, panel 5 to 8).

Highlights

This case features a short-segment continuous OPLL of C4 to C5, most severe at C4/5.

Surgical planning

In this short-segment continuous OPLL without imagery evidence of dural involvement, a direct decompression via ACCF constitutes a low-risk option.

The wide-based component at C4/5 creates a challenge in the ACCF technique as an adequate decompression shall involve the lesion lateral to the bone cut.

The patient received ACAF surgery for antedisplacement of C4 and C5. With preserved cervical lordosis, minimal decompression can be gained from curvature correction. Therefore, the bone at the front of the vertebra with the same thickness as the ossification was resected (Fig. 3.27.4).

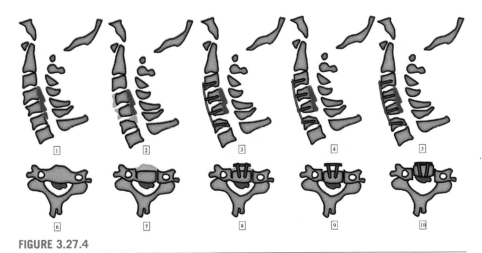

FIGURE 3.27.4

Illustration of the surgical plan on sagittal and axial planes.

(1, 6) Illustration of the OPLL on sagittal and axial views before surgery.

(2, 7) Resection performed to the anterior part of C4 and C5 vertebral bodies and the posterosuperior part of C6 vertebra. A complete trough is developed on the left vertebral bodies from C4 to C5 while a half one is made on the right side with the posterior bone yet to be dissected.

(3, 8) Plate and screws placed on vertebral bodies from C3 through C6.

(4, 9) The bottom of the right half-groove on C4 and C5 dissected.

(5, 10) Antedisplaced C4 and C5 vertebral bodies as screws were tightened.

Results

Postoperative function: JOA score was 17, Nurick score: 0, VAS: 0, and NDI: 3.

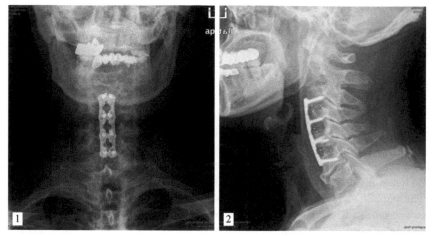

FIGURE 3.27.5

Postoperative cervical spine X-ray.
(1) Anteroposterior view.
(2) Lateral view.

Instrumentation from C3 to C6, and antedisplaced C4 and C5 vertebral bodies (Fig. 3.27.5).

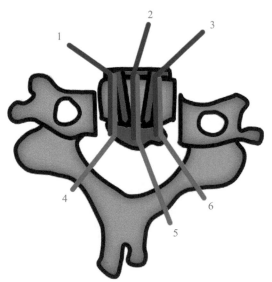

Reference of the sagittal planes

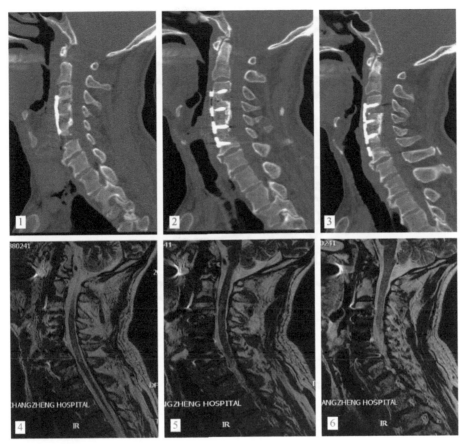

FIGURE 3.27.6

Postoperative sagittal views and their reference on the axial diagram.

(1) Parasagittal CT of the right uncinate process.

(2) Midsagittal CT.

(3) Parasagittal CT of the left uncinate process.

(4) Parasagittal MRI of the right uncinate process.

(5) Midsagittal MRI.

(6) Parasagittal MRI of the left uncinate process.

VOC of C4 and C5 antedisplaced by 3.5 and 6.0 mm, respectively, shown on postoperative sagittal CT images (Fig. 3.27.6, panel 1 to 3).

Expanded spinal canal with anterior and posterior CSF columns restored, shown on postoperative sagittal MR images (Fig. 3.27.6, panel 4 to 6).

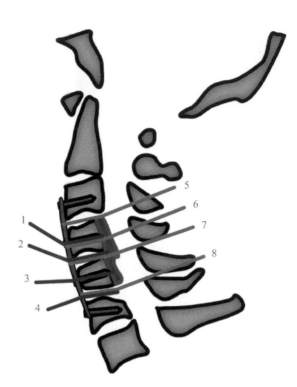

Reference of the axial planes

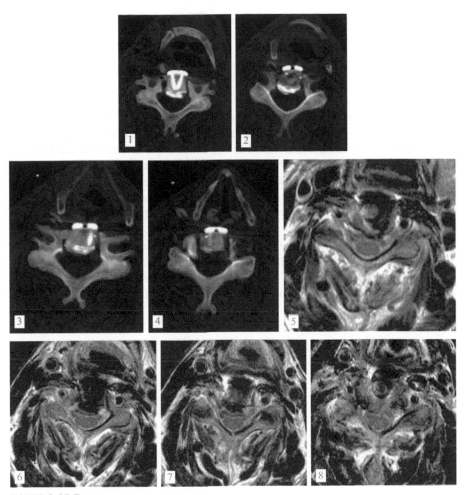

FIGURE 3.27.7

Postoperative axial cervical images and their reference on the sagittal diagram.

(1) Axial CT at C4.

(2) Axial CT at C4/5.

(3) Axial CT at C5.

(4) Axial CT at C5/6.

(5) Axial MRI at C3/4.

(6) Axial MRI at C4.

(7) Axial MRI at C4/5.

(8) Axial MRI at C5/6.

Postoperative axial CT images: Bony grooves on both sides of the vertebral bodies 21.8 mm apart; spinal stenosis reduced to 26% and 0% at C4 and C5, respectively (Fig. 3.27.7, panel 1 to 4).

Postoperative axial MR images: The spinal cord is decompressed adequately and resumes to oval shape (Fig. 3.27.7, panel 5 to 8).

Discussion

There seems to be excessive CSF posterior to the C5 vertebra after surgery. Does excessive antedisplacement of the vertebra cause it? How can this be avoided?

On postoperative images, the VOC has been ventrally displaced more at C5 than at C4, which results in overantedisplacement of C5 and excessive room for CSF.

This was caused by the excessive resection of the anterior part of the vertebra. Though the thickness of resection was consistent with that of the ossification, the decompression was amplified by the prebent plate, and the C5 vertebra ended up overly displaced.

When the decompression is expectable from curvature correction, the resected part of the anterior vertebra needs to be thinner than the OPLL.

An inappropriate distance of antedisplacement can be avoided with software-assisted preoperative planning that addresses the volume of resection on the anterior vertebral bodies, the extent of plate contouring, and the distance of antedisplacement.

Case 28: Ossification of posterior longitudinal ligament (OPLL) of cervical spine (At C2 to C4)

Index terms

Antedisplacement of two vertebral bodies, continuous OPL, wide-based OPLL, thickness of ossification 5—7 mm, canal occupancy ratio below 50%, and shelter technique.

History

Patient: A 54-year-old man.

Chief complaint: Discomfort of the neck and shoulders for 10 years that aggravated with weakness of extremities for two months.

Physical exam: Physical exam was noted for paresthesia on the neck and shoulders, and hypertonicity on all four extremities. Muscle strength was tested at 4/5 on all the extremities. Tendon reflexes were brisk on the triceps brachii and knees bilaterally. Hoffmann and Babinski signs were present bilaterally.

Preoperative function: JOA score was 14, Nurick score: 2, VAS: 4, and NDI: 17.

Imaging studies

Straightened cervical spine with Cobb angle of 16.5° from C2 through C7, and Pavlov ratio of 70%, a K-line (+) OPLL of C2 through C4 (Fig. 3.28.1).

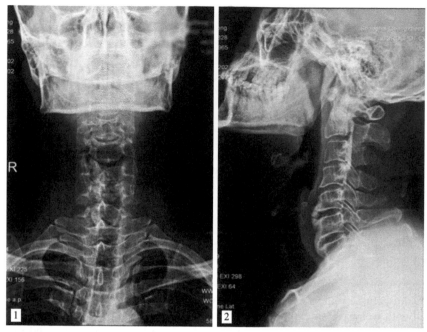

FIGURE 3.28.1

Preoperative X-ray of the cervical spine.
(1) Anteroposterior view.
(2) Lateral view.

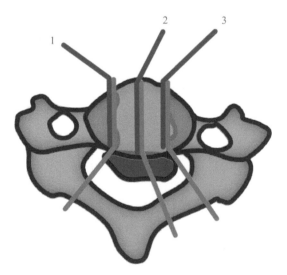

Reference of the sagittal planes

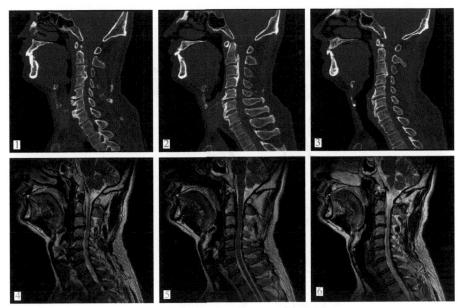

FIGURE 3.28.2

Preoperative sagittal images of the cervical spine and their reference on the axial diagram.
(1) Parasagittal CT of the right uncinate process.
(2) Midsagittal CT.
(3) Parasagittal CT of the left uncinate process.
(4) Parasagittal MRI of the right uncinate process.
(5) Midsagittal MRI.
(6) Parasagittal MRI of the left uncinate process.

Flat-type continuous OPLL from C2 to C4 shown on preoperative sagittal CT image (Fig. 3.28.2, panel 1 to 3).

A hypointense band in the front of the spinal canal, compressed spinal cord in the kyphotic cervical spine, and obliteration of the anterior and posterior CSF columns shown on preoperative sagittal MR image (Fig. 3.28.2, panel 4 to 6).

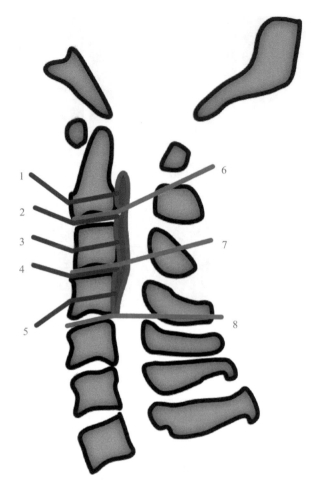

Reference of the axial planes

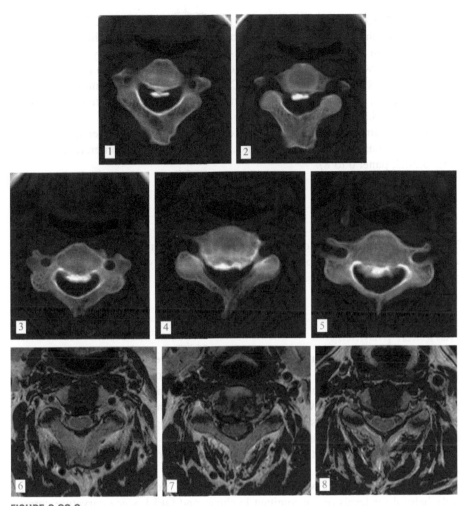

FIGURE 3.28.3

Preoperative axial images of the cervical spine and their reference on the sagittal diagram.

(1) Axial CT at the inferior surface of C2.
(2) Axial CT at C2/3.
(3) Axial CT at C3.
(4) Axial CT at C3/4.
(5) Axial CT at C4.
(6) Axial MRI at C2/3.
(7) Axial MRI at C3/4.
(8) Axial MRI at C4/5.

Axial CT images: The OPLL features narrow-based at C2 and C2/3, with separation between the lesion and the C2 vertebra. It measures: 5.2 mm thick (anteroposterior), 11.1 mm wide (mediolateral), and 46.8% in canal occupancy at C2; 4.0 mm thick, 14.4 mm wide, and 33.9% in canal occupancy at C3; 6.6 mm thick, 18.8 mm wide, and 42.6% in canal occupancy at C3/4 where the lesion is midline-centered and wide-based; and 5.4 mm thick, 16.5 mm wide, and 47.8% in canal occupancy at C4 (Fig. 3.28.3, panel 1 to 5).

Axial MR images: Deformed spinal cord due to anterior indentation from a hypointense mass in the front of the spinal canal and obliteration of CSF (Fig. 3.28.3, panel 6 to 8).

Highlights

This case features developmental cervical canal stenosis and kyphosis from C2 to C4 complicated with OPLL from C2 to C4, which is flat-type on sagittal views and wide-based at C3/4.

Surgical planning

In this K-line (+) continuous OPLL that spans three levels and extends into the upper cervical spine, indirect decompression via a posterior procedure is an option.

However, a posterior procedure may lead to incomplete decompression in a straightened cervical spine with kyphosis at C2 to C4. Though preserving segmental motions, laminoplasty does not cease the kyphosis progression, which may cause recurrent compression further down the road.

An ACAF procedure with antedisplacement of C3 and C4 and a shelter technique for the posteroinferior part of C2 were planned.

Physiological lordosis was to be corrected with a prebent plate. This is particularly helpful for levels of concomitant kyphosis and OPLL since curvature correction will bring about extra room for compression clearance. As such, the anterior resection of the vertebral bodies measures thinner than that of the ossification (Fig. 3.28.4).

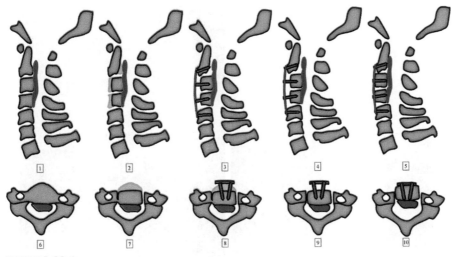

FIGURE 3.28.4

Illustration of the surgical plan on sagittal and axial planes.

(1, 6) Illustration of the OPLL on sagittal and axial views before surgery.

(2, 7) Resection performed to the anterior part of C3 and C4 vertebral bodies. A complete trough on the left vertebral bodies of C3 and C4 while a half one on the right side with the posterior bone yet to be dissected.

(3, 8) Plate and screws placed on vertebral bodies from C2 through C5.

(4, 9) The bottom of the right half-groove on C3 through C6 dissected.

(5, 10) Antedisplaced C3 and C4 vertebral bodies as screws were tightened.

Results

Postoperative function: JOA score was 16, Nurick score: 0, VAS: 0, and NDI: 3.
    Instrumentation from C2 to C5 and antedisplaced C3 to C4 (Fig. 3.28.5).

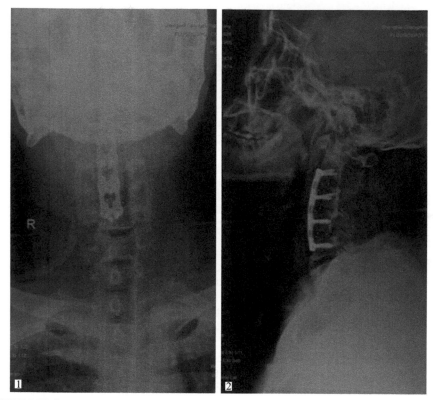

FIGURE 3.28.5

Postoperative cervical spine X-ray.
(1) Anteroposterior view.
(2) Lateral view.

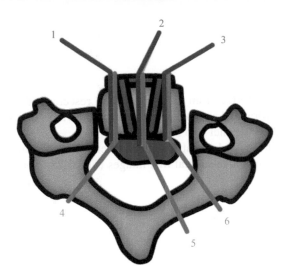

Reference of the sagittal planes

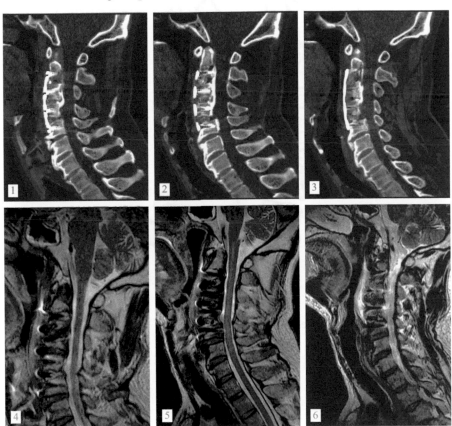

FIGURE 3.28.6

Postoperative sagittal views and their reference on the axial diagram.
(1) Right parasagittal CT.
(2) Midsagittal CT.
(3) Left parasagittal CT.
(4) Right parasagittal MRI.
(5) Midsagittal MRI.
(6) Left parasagittal MRI.

Ventrally displaced VOC from C2 to C4, partial resection of the posteroinferior part of the C2 vertebra, and expanded spinal canal shown on postoperative sagittal CT images (Fig. 3.28.6, panel 1 to 3).

Spinal cord with restored curvature free of indentation and surrounded by ample CSF shown on postoperative sagittal MR images (Fig. 3.28.6, panel 4 to 6).

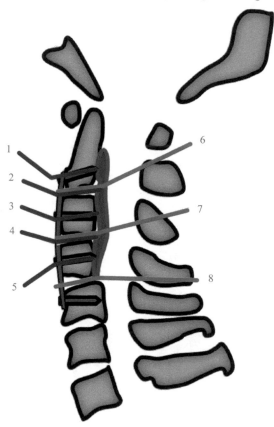

Reference of the axial planes

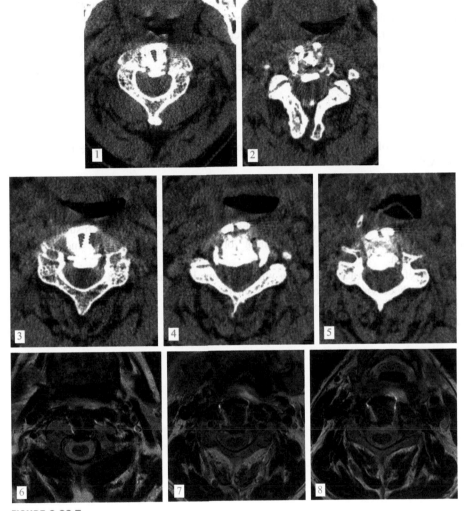

FIGURE 3.28.7

Postoperative axial cervical images and their reference on the sagittal diagram.
(1) Axial CT at C3.
(2) Axial CT at C2/3.
(3) Axial CT at C3.
(4) Axial CT at C3/4.
(5) Axial CT at C4.
(6) Axial MRI at C2/3.
(7) Axial MRI at C3/4.
(8) Axial MRI at C4/5.

As shown on postoperative axial CT image, the VOC has been sufficiently ante-displaced by 4.5 mm with sagittal grooves 22.3 mm apart; canal stenosis reduced to 18.4% and 14.9% at C2 and C3/4, respectively (Fig. 3.28.7, panel 1 to 5).

As shown on postoperative axial MR image, the spinal cord recovers to an oval shape surrounded CSF (Fig. 3.28.7, panel 6 to 8).

Discussion

In this case of OPLL in a spine with focal kyphosis, how to restore lordosis via ACAF?

In cases with cervical kyphosis, the use of a contoured plate in the ACAF technique restores curvature and provides more room for vertebra antedisplacement.

However, if surgeons contour the plate only with experience and visual judgment, they run the risk of over- or underbending the plate, which will result in excessive or insufficient antedisplacement of the vertebral bodies and residual compression.

Therefore, curvature planning with software is recommended in ACAF for patients with cervical kyphosis. Based on the accurate calculation from software, the surgeon removes the exact amount of bone needed and contours the plate with a curvature gauge.

Case 29: Cervical spinal stenosis, ossification of posterior longitudinal ligament (OPLL) of cervical spine (At C5 to C6)

Index terms

Antedisplacement of two vertebral bodies, segmental OPLL, wide-based lesion, the thickness of ossification above 9 mm, and occupancy ratio above 60%—70%.

History

Patient: A 54-year-old man.

Chief complaint: Discomfort of the neck and shoulders for 10 years that aggravated with weakness of extremities for two months.

Physical exam: Physical exam was noted for gait instability and hypertonicity on all four extremities. Muscle strength was tested at 4/5 on the upper limbs and 4/5 on lower limbs. Tendon reflexes were brisk on the triceps brachii and knee bilaterally. Hoffmann and Babinski signs were present bilaterally.

Preoperative function: JOA was measured at 10, Nurick score: 3, VAS: 3, and NDI: 16.

Imaging studies

Cobb angle of 20.2° from C2 through C7, Pavlov ratio 65%, and OPLL from C5 to C6 (Fig. 3.29.1).

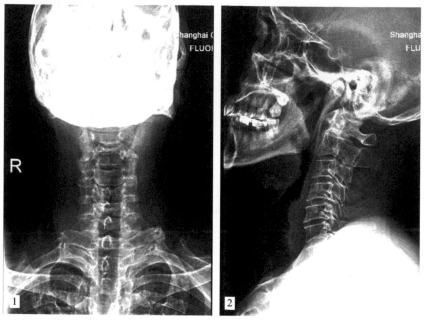

FIGURE 3.29.1

Preoperative X-ray of the cervical spine.
(1) Anteroposterior view.
(2) Lateral view.

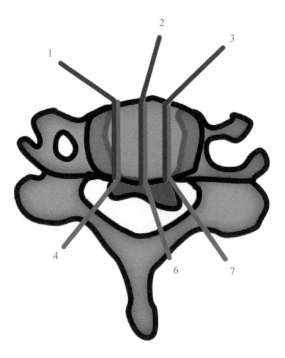

Reference of the sagittal planes

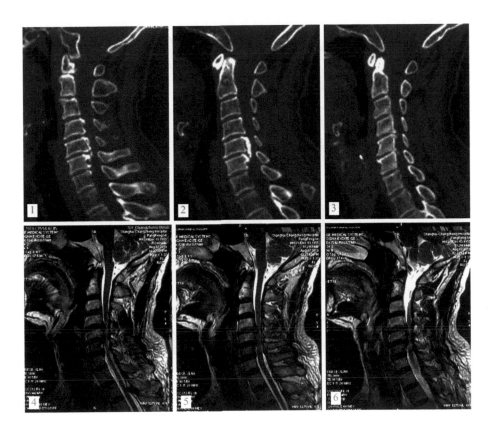

FIGURE 3.29.2

Preoperative sagittal images and their reference on axial diagram.
(1) Right parasagittal CT.
(2) Midsagittal CT.
(3) Left parasagittal CT.
(4) Right parasagittal MRI.
(5) Midsagittal MRI.
(6) Left parasagittal MRI.

According to preoperative CT sagittal images, a flat-type segmental OPLL from C5 to C6 (Fig. 3.29.2, panel 1 to 3). Spinal cord compression from C4/5 to C5/6 at the levels of the vertebra and intervertebral space, shown on postoperative sagittal MR images (Fig. 3.29.2, panel 4 to 6).

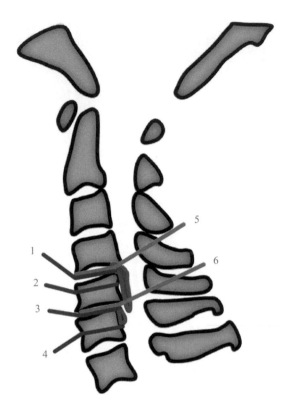

Reference of the axial planes

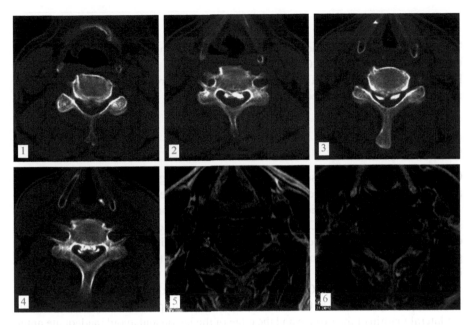

FIGURE 3.29.3

Preoperative axial images of the cervical spine and their reference on the sagittal diagram.
(1) Axial CT at C4/5.
(2) Axial CT at C5.
(3) Axial CT at C5/6.
(4) Axial CT at C6.
(5) Axial MRI at C4/5.
(6) Axial MRI at C5/6.

Based on axial CT images, the OPLL is mushroom-shaped and wide-based at C5 to C6 and with a double-layer sign at C5/6 and C6. It measures 7.4 mm thick (anteroposterior), 13.6 mm wide (mediolateral), and 61.7% in canal occupancy at C4/5; 5.3 mm thick, 9.1 mm wide at the base, 14.9 mm at the widest part, and 54.6% in canal occupancy at C5; 5.3 mm thick, 18.5 mm wide, and 51% in canal occupancy at C5/6; 5.3 mm thick, 10.3 mm wide at the base, 16.4 mm at the widest part, and 46.5% in canal occupancy at C6 (Fig. 3.29.3, panel 1 to 4).

Based on axial MR images, spinal cord in the shape of boomerang due to anterior indentation, with signal hyperintensity indicating myelopathy (panel 5 to 6).

Highlights

This case features developmental spinal canal stenosis complicated with OPLL from C5 to C6. This flat-typed OPLL mainly involves C5 while extending less than halfway across the height of C6. It is wide-based, mushroom-shaped, and protuberant at C5 and double-layered at C6.

Surgical planning

Conventionally, such short-segment OPLL can be managed with ACCF of C5 alone and undercutting of the superoposterior part of C6 vertebra.

Because this OPLL is wider than the typical decompression width achieved in a subtotal corpectomy, an ACCF may lead to incomplete decompression. As such, care should be taken to decompress the residual lesions lateral to the sagittal grooves. Also, the attempt to directly resect lesion from the ossified dura may result in durotomy.

The patient received ACAF with antedisplacement of C5 and C6. With this mushroom-shaped lesion at C5, care should be taken to probe the relations between the lateral margin of the groove and the edge of the lesion and avoid inadequate antedisplacement of the VOC (see the Discussion part below) (Fig. 3.29.4).

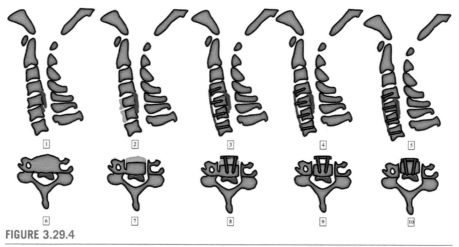

FIGURE 3.29.4

Illustration of the surgical plan on sagittal and axial planes.
(1, 6) Illustration of the OPLL on sagittal and axial views before surgery.
(2, 7) Resection performed to the anterior part of C5 to C6 vertebra. A complete trough is developed on the left vertebral bodies from C5 to C6 while a half one is made on the right side with the posterior bone yet to be dissected.
(3, 8) Plate and screws placed on vertebral bodies from C4 through C7.
(4, 9) The bottom of the right half-groove on C5 through C6 dissected.
(5, 10) Antedisplaced C5 to C6 vertebral bodies as screws were tightened.

Results

Postoperative function: JOA score was 15, Nurick score: 1, VAS: 1, and NDI: 5.

Instrumentation from C4 to C7 and antedisplaced C5 and C6 vertebral bodies (Fig. 3.29.5).

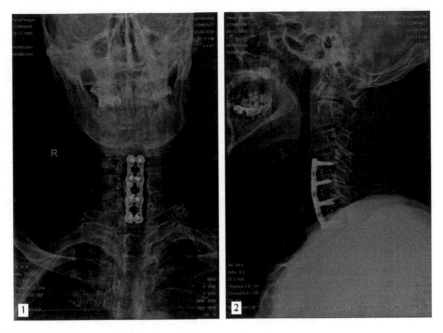

FIGURE 3.29.5

Postoperative cervical spine X-ray.
(1) Anteroposterior view.
(2) Lateral view.

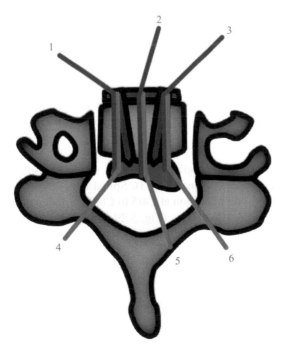

Reference of the sagittal planes

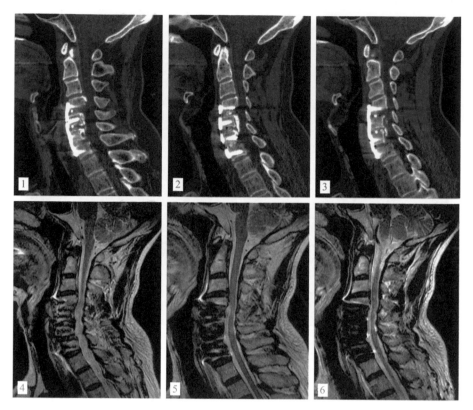

FIGURE 3.29.6

Postoperative sagittal views and their reference on the axial diagram.
(1) Right parasagittal CT.
(2) Midsagittal CT.
(3) Left parasagittal CT.
(4) Right parasagittal MRI.
(5) Midsagittal MRI.
(6) Left parasagittal MRI.

As shown on postoperative sagittal CT images, ventrally displaced VOC from C5 to C6 by 6 mm (Fig. 3.29.6, panel 1 to 3). Spinal cord in lordotic curvature surrounded by CSF free of compression at C4/5 to C6/7 but indented at C5/6, as shown on postoperative sagittal MR images (Fig. 3.29.6, panel 4 to 6).

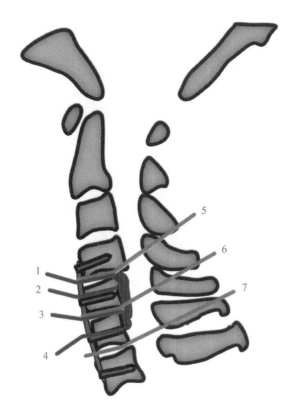

Reference of the axial planes

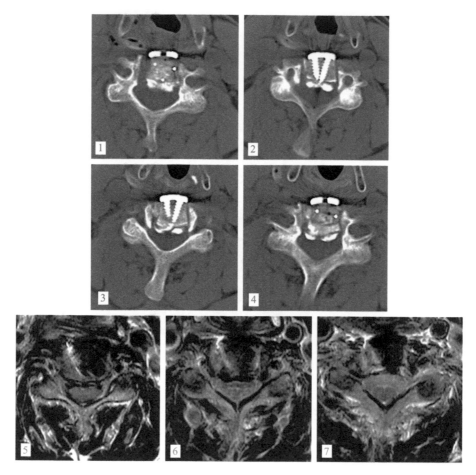

FIGURE 3.29.7

Postoperative axial cervical images and their reference on the sagittal diagram.
(1) Axial CT at C3/4.
(2) Axial CT at C4.
(3) Axial CT at C4/5.
(4) Axial CT at C5.
(5) Axial MRI at C3/4.
(6) Axial MRI at C4/5.
(7) Axial MRI at C5/6.

As shown on postoperative axial CT images, the vertebral bodies have been dissected with parasagittal cuts on both sides off the base of uncinate processes 21.8 mm apart, and the canal occupancy reduced to 20% (Fig. 3.29.7, panel 1 to 4).

As shown on postoperative axial MR images, the spinal cord has recovered to an oval and triangular shape, surrounded by an ample amount of CSF (Fig. 3.29.7, panel 5 to 7).

Discussion

Given the absence of imagery evidence for cord compression at C6/7, is it possible to antedisplace C5 alone while undercutting the posterosuperior part of the C6 vertebra?

First, the ossification dorsal to C5 was loosely connected to that at C6, leaving a gap posterior to C5/6. Thus, the antedisplacement of C5 alone may risk incomplete antedisplacement of the ossification at C6.

Second, given that the ossification at the posterosuperior level of C6 was markedly thick and spanned about half the vertebral height, the undercutting of the posterosuperior of the C6 vertebra may result in minimal endplate area and fusion failure.

Indeed, radiological evidence of OPLL was present at the posterosuperior level of C6 and its posteroinferior level. Along with the MRI evidence of moderate effacement of CSF at C6, these signs suggested a risk of ossification progression and recurrent myelopathy if C6 is to be undercut instead of antedisplaced.

Therefore, the C6 was also displaced ventrally.

Case 30: Ossification of posterior longitudinal ligament (OPLL) of cervical spine (At C2 to C4)

Index terms

Antedisplacement of two vertebral bodies, continuous OPL, the thickness of ossification 5—7 mm, canal occupancy ratio 50%—60%, shelter technique, and inadequate antedisplacement.

History

Patient: A 56-year-old woman.

Chief complaint: Numbness and weakness of the lower limbs for four months aggravated over the past two months.

Physical exam: Physical exam was noted for gait instability and impaired tactile sensation on the lower extremities. Muscle strength was tested at 4/5 on the lower limbs. Brisk tendon reflexes were noted on the right biceps and triceps brachii, the left triceps brachii and brachioradialis, and the knees. Babinski sign was present bilaterally.

Preoperative function: JOA was measured at 10, Nurick score: 3, VAS: 3, and NDI: 18.

Imaging studies

A lordotic cervical spine with a Cobb angle of 14.5° from C2 through C7 and K-line (+) OPLL (Fig. 3.30.1).

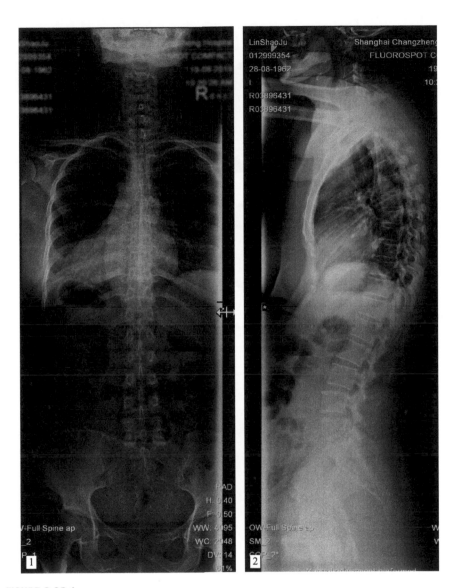

FIGURE 3.30.1

Preoperative whole-spine X-ray.
(1) Anteroposterior view.
(2) Lateral view.

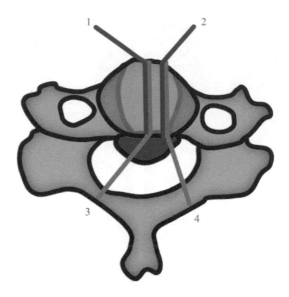

Reference of the sagittal planes

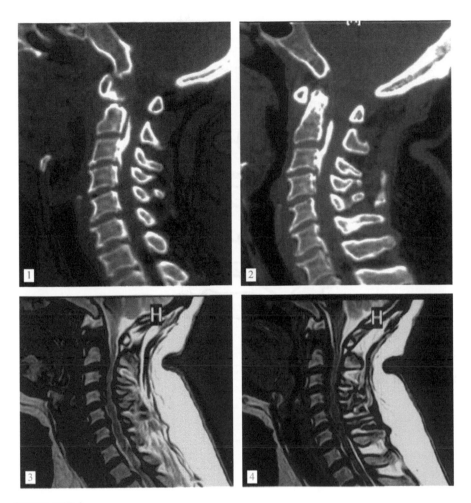

FIGURE 3.30.2

Preoperative sagittal images and their reference on axial diagram.
(1) Midsagittal CT.
(2) Left parasagittal CT.
(3) Midsagittal MRI.
(4) Left parasagittal MRI.

As shown on sagittal CT images, a multisegment cervical OPLL that is most severe at C2 to C4 and features continuous- and flat-type (Fig. 3.30.2, panel 1 and 2).

As shown on sagittal MR images, an impinged spinal cord due to the anterior indentation of a hypointense mass in the anterior of the spinal canal from C2 to C4 (panel 3 and 4).

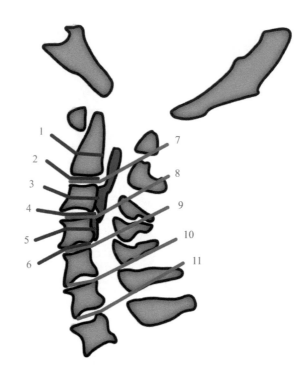

Reference of the axial planes

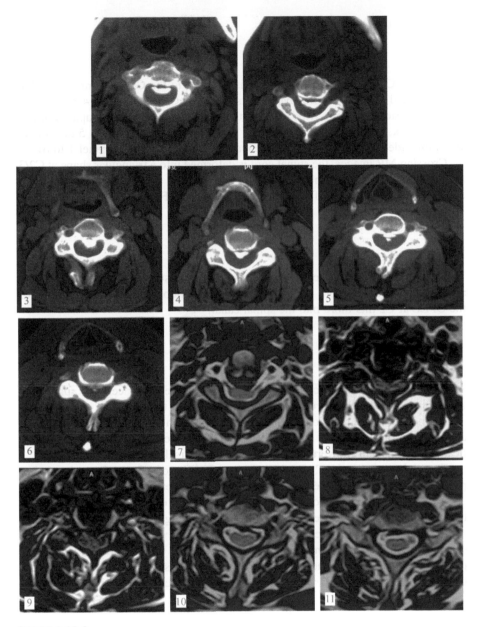

FIGURE 3.30.3

Preoperative axial images of the cervical spine and their reference on the sagittal diagram.
(1) Axial CT at C2.
(2) Axial CT at C2/3.
(3) Axial CT at C3.
(4) Axial CT at C3/4.
(5) Axial CT at C4.
(6) Axial CT at C4/5.
(7) Axial MRI at C2/3.
(8) Axial MRI at C3/4.
(9) Axial MRI at C4/5.
(10) Axial MRI at C5/6.
(11) Axial MRI at C6/7.

Crossing CT images, the ossification is attached to the C3 vertebra but not the upper cervical spine. A double-layer sign is present at C4. It measures: 4.8 mm thick (anteroposterior), 13.3 mm wide (mediolateral), and 40% in canal occupancy at C2; 4.7 mm thick, 9.7 mm wide, and 46.5% in canal occupancy at C3; 5 mm thick, 10.1 mm wide, and 51.5% in canal occupancy at C4 (Fig. 3.30.3, panel 1 to 6).

Crossing MR images, the spinal cord is deformed into a triangular shape at C2/3 to C4/5 with CSF effacement; a hypointense mass in the spinal canal has not caused cord compression or CSF effacement at C5/6 to C6/7 (Fig. 3.30.3, panel 7 to 11).

Highlights

This case features a multilevel continuous OPLL, most severe at C2 to C4. It is attached to the C3 vertebra but not the C2 or C4 vertebral bodies. Also, the tip of the OPLL at C2 tilts more into the spinal canal.

Surgical planning

A conventional anterior decompression surgery for the upper cervical spine may lead to incomplete decompression and complication in this case.

An indirect decompression via the posterior approach provides a less challenging and risky option but runs the risk of incomplete decompression at C2, where the ossification extends half the vertebral height and tilts dorsally.

The patient received ACAF with antedisplacement of C3 and C4 and a shelter procedure that undercuts the posterior part of the C2 vertebra.

A relatively large resection was performed to the posterior part of the C2 vertebra because the ossification extended half the vertebral height and tilted dorsally.

Thus, fusion was augmented with autologous bone grafting in the C2/3 interspace and compression maneuver on the screws at the top and bottom levels. For proper antedisplacement, the initial screw insertion was done on the levels caudal to C2, whereas those for C2 were inserted only after antedisplacement (Fig. 3.30.4).

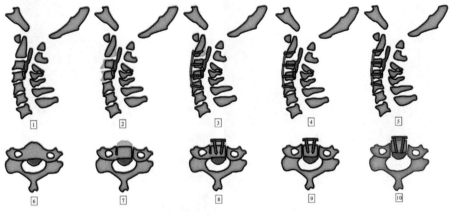

FIGURE 3.30.4

Illustration of the surgical plan on sagittal and axial views.
(1, 6) Illustration of the OPLL on sagittal and axial views before surgery.
(2, 7) Resection performed to the anterior part of C3 to C4 vertebral bodies and the posterior part of the C2 vertebra. A complete trough is developed on the left vertebral bodies from C3 to C4 while a half one is made on the right side with the posterior bone yet to be dissected.
(3, 8) Plate and screws placed on vertebral bodies from C2 through C5.
(4, 9) The bottom of the right half-groove on C3 through C4 dissected.
(5, 10) Antedisplaced C3 and C4 vertebral bodies as screws were tightened.

Results

Postoperative function: JOA score was 13, Nurick score: 0, VAS: 1, and NDI: 5.

Instrumentation from C2 to C5, and antedisplaced C3 to C4 vertebral bodies (Fig. 3.30.5).

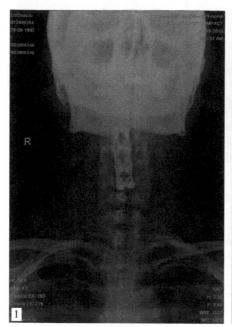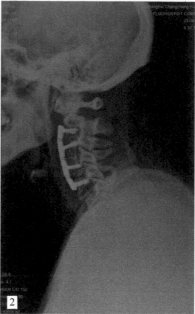

FIGURE 3.30.5

Postoperative cervical X-ray.
(1) Anteroposterior view.
(2) Lateral view.

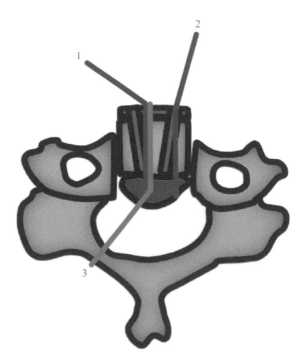

Reference of the sagittal planes

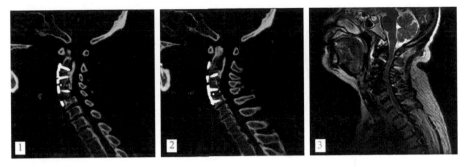

FIGURE 3.30.6

Postoperative sagittal images and their reference on the axial diagram.
(1) Midsagittal CT.
(2) Left parasagittal CT.
(3) Midsagittal MRI.

Ventrally displaced VOC from C3 to C4 with posterior partially corpectomy of C2, and expanded spinal canal shown on postoperative midsagittal CT images (Fig. 3.30.6, panel 1 and 2).

Adequate decompression of the spinal cord with normal CSF around it shown on postoperative midsagittal MR image (Fig. 3.30.6, pane 3).

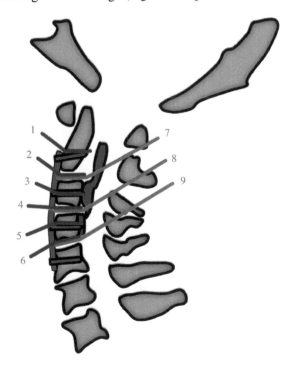

Reference of the axial planes

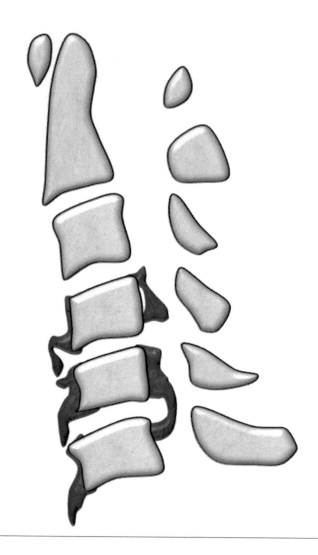

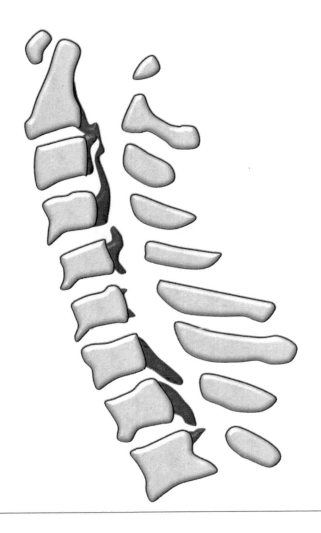

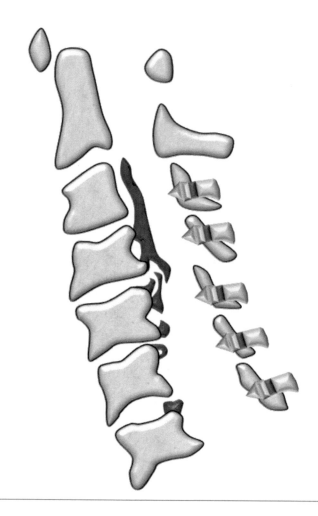

As shown on axial CT images, the posterior part of the C2 vertebra has been resected with shelter technique; vertebral bodies have been dissected with parasagittal cuts on both sides 14.1 mm apart at C2 and 18.4 mm apart at C3 and C4; VOC antedisplaced by 3.6 mm and canal occupancy reduced to 22.4% at C3, where partial antedisplacement is obtained; and VOC antedisplaced by 4.7 mm and canal occupancy reduced to 0% at C4 (Fig. 3.30.7, panel 1 to 6).

As shown on postoperative axial MR image, the spinal cord resumes to oval shape with normal CSF around it (Fig. 3.30.7, panel 7 to 9).

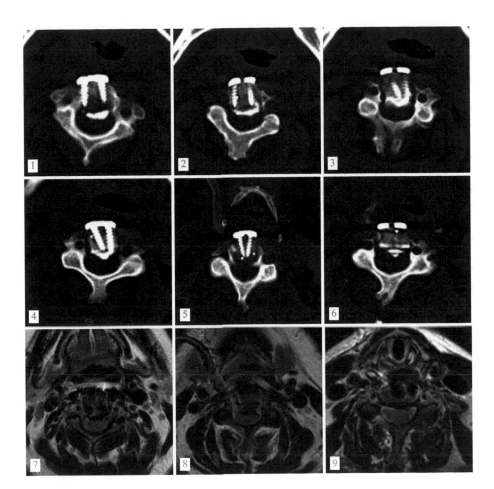

FIGURE 3.30.7

Postoperative axial cervical images and their reference on the sagittal diagram.
(1) Axial CT at the inferior surface of C2.
(2) Axial CT at C2/3.
(3) Axial CT at C3.
(4) Axial CT at C3/4.
(5) Axial CT at C4.
(6) Axial CT at C4/5.
(7) Axial MRI at C2/3.
(8) Axial MRI at C3/4.
(9) Axial MRI at C4/5.

Discussion

What are the causes of insufficient antedisplacement of C2 and C3, according to postoperative imagery studies?

The insufficient antedisplacement involving both C2 and C3 found its cause in the insufficient antedisplacement of the C3 vertebra. Given that the ossification was continuous from C2 to C3, the initial plan was to displace C2 and C3 together ventrally by antedisplacing C3. It turned out that C3 was not sufficiently hoisted, which resulted in residual compression of the two levels.

Oblique bone cuts, osteoporosis, and engaging screws are common causes of insufficient antedisplacement. However, it was distinctively caused by grafting material at C2/3 dislodged to the ventral side of C3.

Autologous bone grafting in C2/3 interspace was planned based on the significant resection of the posterior part of C2 vertebra.

Placed between at C2/3 between markedly reduced contact areas, some grafting material dislodged into the ventral side of C3 during the antedisplacement maneuver and block the migration of C3. Therefore, residual compression is present at C2.

Case 31: Ossification of anterior longitudinal ligament and ossification of posterior longitudinal ligament (OPLL) of cervical spine (At C2 to C7)

Index terms

Antedisplacement of four vertebral bodies, mixed-type ossification of the posterior longitudinal ligament (OPLL), thickness of ossification 7−9 mm, and occupancy ratio between 60% and 70%.

History

Patient: A 73-year-old man.

Chief complaint: Numbness and weakness of the four extremities for four months with aggravation of one month.

Physical exam: Physical exam was noted for gait instability and numbness of both palms and feet. Muscle strength was tested at 4/5 on the upper limbs and 4/5 on lower limbs. Tendon reflexes were brisk on all four extremities. Hoffmann and Babinski signs were present bilaterally.

Preoperative function: Japanese Orthopedic Association (JOA) score was 11, Nurick score: 1, visual analog scale (VAS): 0, and neck disability index (NDI): 8.

Imaging studies

Cobb angle of 14.3° from C2 through C7, Pavlov above 75%, and K-line (−) OPLL (Fig. 3.31.1).

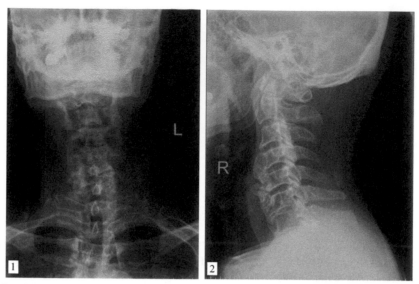

FIGURE 3.31.1

Preoperative X-ray of the cervical spine.
(1) Anteroposterior view.
(2) Lateral view.

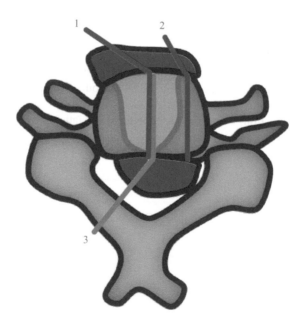

Reference of the sagittal planes

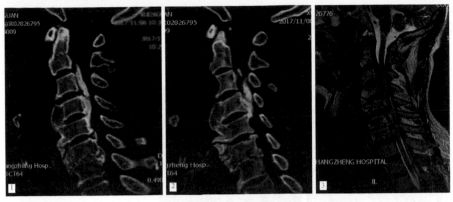

FIGURE 3.31.2

Preoperative sagittal images of the cervical spine and their reference on the axial diagram.
(1) Midsagittal CT.
(2) Left parasagittal CT.
(3) Midsagittal MRI.

A mixed-type OPLL from C2/3 to C6/7, most severe at C4, and ossification of the anterior longitudinal ligament (OALL) from C4 to C6 shown on sagittal computed tomography (CT) images (Fig. 3.31.2, panel 1 and 2).

A straightened spinal cord impinged at C3 to C4, C5/6, and C6/7 with cerebrospinal fluid (CSF) effacement; intramedullary hyperintensity at C6/7 shown on sagittal magnetic resonance (MR) images (Fig. 3.31.2, panel 3).

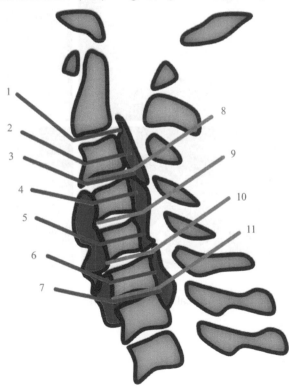

Reference of the axial planes

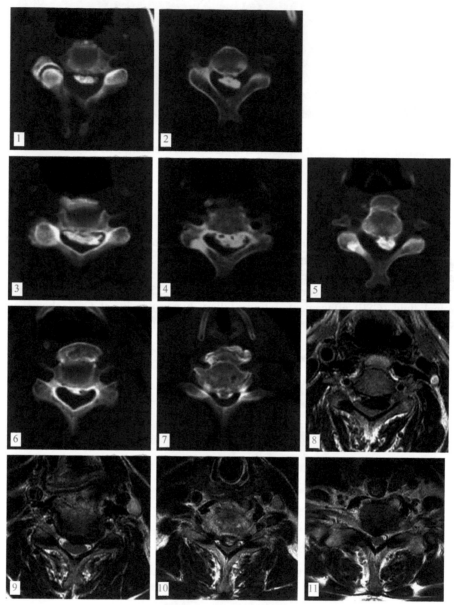

FIGURE 3.31.3

Preoperative axial images of the cervical spine and their reference on the sagittal diagram.
(1) Axial CT of C2/3.
(2) Axial CT of C3.
(3) Axial CT of C3/4.

Reference of the axial planes

According to axial CT images, the OPLL measures:9.0 mm thick (anteroposterior), 14.4 mm wide (mediolateral), and 75.0% in canal occupancy at C3 where it is midline-centered and wide-based; 8.0 mm thick, 19.4 mm wide, and 62.0% in canal occupancy at C3/4; 9.0 mm thick, 22.9 mm wide, and 72% in canal occupancy at C4; 7.5 mm thick, 16.9 mm wide, and 54% in canal occupancy at C4/5; 5.0 mm thick, 3.4 mm wide, and 43.4% in canal occupancy at C6 where it is centered and narrow-based; and 8.0 mm thick, 31.7 mm wide, and 57.1% in canal occupancy at C6/7 (Fig. 3.11.3, panel 1 to 7).

According to axial MR images, a boomerang-shaped spinal cord due to indentation indicating myelopathy (Fig. 3.31.3, Figs. 8—11).

Highlights

This case features severe and extensive ectopic calcification composed of OPLL from C2/3 to C6/7 and OALL from C4 to C6/7. The wide-based OPLL has caused canal stenosis of above 60%.

Surgical planning

This case features a K-line (−), four-level OPLL that is peak-shaped at some levels in a straightened cervical spine with canal occupancy above 60%. These characters are relevant to the risk of incomplete decompression in conventional posterior surgery.

Its bulkiness suggests the risks and challenges in the anterior cervical corpectomy and fusion (ACCF) procedure and the possibility of fusion-associated complications.

The patient received anterior controllable antedisplacement fusion (ACAF) with antedisplacement from C3 to C6 for spinal cord decompression.

The bulk of OALL was to be addressed during surgery, where it would be resected from C4 to C7 referenced off the anterior wall of C3 that was spared

(4) Axial CT of C4.
(5) Axial CT of C5.
(6) Axial CT of C6.
(7) Axial CT of C6/7.
(8) Axial MRI of C3/4.
(9) Axial MRI of C4/5.
(10) Axial MRI of C5/6.
(11) Axial MRI of C6/7.

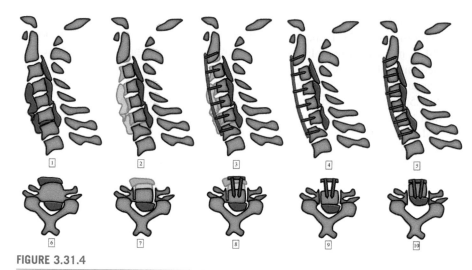

FIGURE 3.31.4

Illustration of the surgical plan on sagittal and axial planes.
(1, 6) Illustration of the OPLL on sagittal and axial views before surgery.
(2, 7) Resection performed to the OALL from C4 to C6, the anterior part of C3 to C6 vertebral bodies, and the posteroinferior margin of the C2 vertebra. A complete trough is developed on the left vertebral bodies from C3 to C6 while a half one is made on the right side with the posterior bone yet to be dissected.
(3, 8) Plate and screws placed on vertebral bodies from C2 through C7.
(4, 9) The bottom of the right half-groove on C3 through C6 dissected.
(5, 10) Antedisplaced C3 to C6 vertebral bodies as screws were tightened.

from the OALL. Fluoroscopy was used during surgery to validate the adequate resection of the ossification ventral to the vertebral bodies.

Given the significant thickness of OPLL, lordosis correction was utilized to gain extra room for decompression and preserve bone (Fig. 3.31.4).

Results

Postoperative function: JOA score was 15, Nurick score: 0, VAS: 0, and NDI: 4.

Antedisplaced C3 to C6 vertebral bodies, instrumentation placed from C2 to C7 with 12 mm screws used at C2–C6 (Fig. 3.31.5).

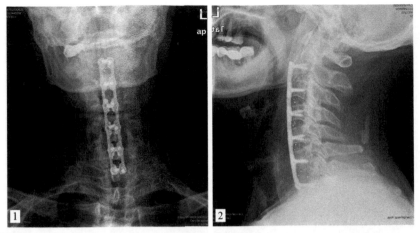

FIGURE 3.31.5

Postoperative cervical spine X-ray.
(1) Anteroposterior view.
(2) Lateral view.

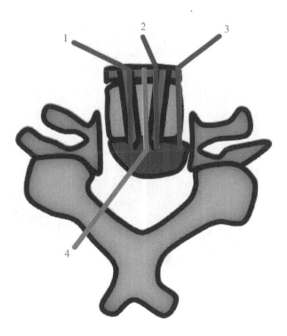

Reference of the sagittal planes

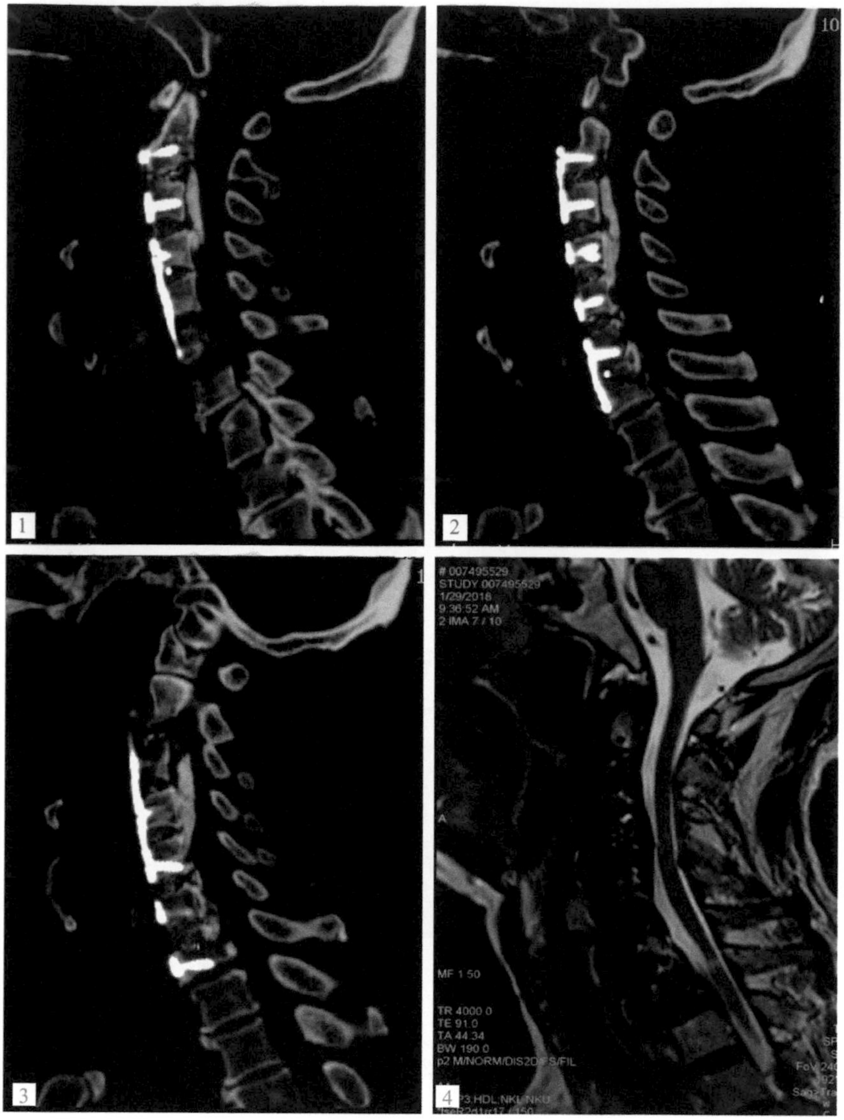

FIGURE 3.31.6

Postoperative sagittal views and their reference on the axial diagram.
(1) Right parasagittal CT.
(2) Left parasagittal CT.
(3) Parasagittal CT of the left uncinate process.
(4) Midsagittal MRI.

Postoperative sagittal views of CT images: Ventrally displaced vertebrae-OPLL complex (VOC) from C3 to C6, expanded spinal canal, and OALL from C4 to C6 resected (Fig. 3.31.6, panel 1 to 3). Postoperative sagittal views of MR image: Spinal cord in lordotic curvature surrounded by CSF free of compression at C3 to C6/7 (Fig. 3.31.6, panel 4).

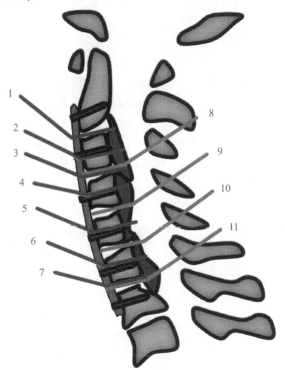

Reference of the axial planes

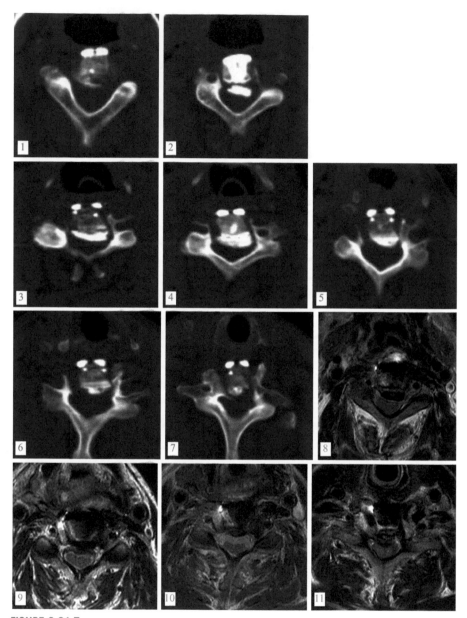

FIGURE 3.31.7

Postoperative axial cervical images and their reference on the sagittal diagram.
(1) Axial CT of C2/3.
(2) Axial CT of C3.
(3) Axial CT of C3/4.
(4) Axial CT of C4.

The vertebral bodies have been dissected with parasagittal cuts on both sides 23.9 mm apart and antedisplaced by 6.1 mm; after the spinal canal expansion, the canal occupancy reduced to 29.0% and 19.3% at C3 and C6/7, respectively, as shown on axial cervical CT scan (Fig. 3.31.7, panel 1 to 7).

The spinal cord has resumed the oval shape surround by an ample amount of CSF at C3 and C6, as shown on axial cervical MR images (Fig. 3.31.7, panel 8 to 11).

Discussion

How can excessive or inadequate antedisplacement be avoided in cases with bulky anterior osteophytes or OALL?

In planning an ACAF, the large ectopic ossification ventral to vertebral bodies affects the assessment of bone volume to be resected.

The anterior ossification ventral to the vertebral bodies is resected before that of the vertebral bodies referenced from the thickness of OPLL. Otherwise, overly or inadequate resection of the anterior vertebral bodies leads to overly or insufficient antedisplacement, respectively.

In the case presented here, both excessive and inadequate OALL resection was present across the entire lesion, resulting in insufficient antedisplacement at C3/4 to C4, where the OPLL was most severe overly displaced C5, which was less affected by the OPLL.

Therefore, in such a case, distinguishing the margin between OALL and the inherent structure of vertebral bodies is crucial but challenging in a severely degenerated cervical spine.

To achieve this objective, the fluoroscopy can be utilized during surgery. Alternatively, the proper margin is indicated by the gaps between the two components, if there is any.

(5) Axial CT of C5.
(6) Axial CT of C6.
(7) Axial CT of C6/7.
(8) Axial MRI of C3/4.
(9) Axial MRI of C4/5.
(10) Axial MRI of C5/6.
(11) Axial MRI of C6/7.

Case 32: Ossification of posterior longitudinal ligament (OPLL) of cervical spine (At C2 to C6)

Index terms

Antedisplacement of three vertebral bodies, segmental OPLL, the thickness of ossification 5–7 mm, canal stenosis below 50%, shelter technique, K-line (−) disease, and inadequate antedisplacement.

History

Patient: A 48-year-old man.

Chief complaint: Numbness and pain of the extremities and gait instability for three years.

Physical exam: Physical exam was noted for gait disturbance, decreased sensation in the perineal and perianal areas, hypertonicity on all four extremities, hyperalgesia of the upper limbs, and decreased sensation on the lower extremities, in particular the anterior thigh. Muscle strength was tested at 3/5 on both hands and 4/5 for the rest of the system. Brisk tendon reflexes were elicited on the lower extremities. Hoffmann and Babinski signs were present bilaterally.

Preoperative function: JOA score was 12, Nurick score: 2, VAS: 0, and NDI: 8.

Imaging studies

Cobb angle of 6.0° in a straightened cervical spine, Pavlov ratio 55%, and a K-line (−) OPLL (Fig. 3.32.1).

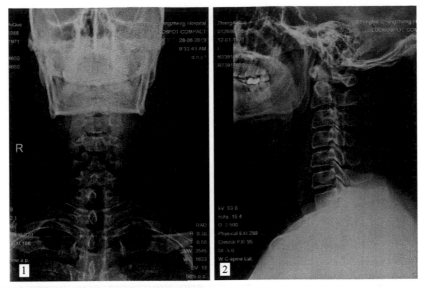

FIGURE 3.32.1

Preoperative X-ray of the cervical spine.
(1) Anteroposterior view.
(2) Lateral view.

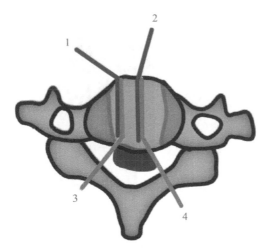

Reference of the sagittal planes

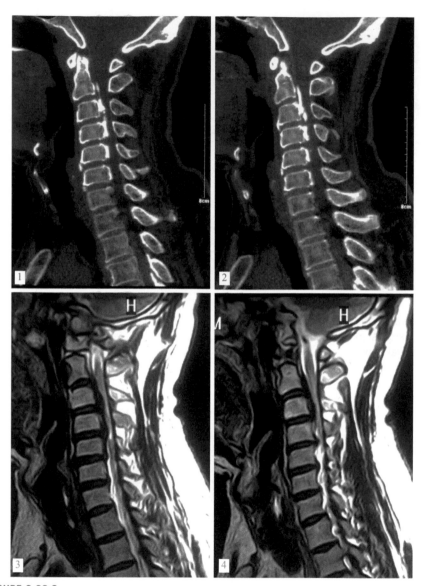

FIGURE 3.32.2

Preoperative sagittal images of the cervical spine and their reference on the axial diagram.

(1) Parasagittal CT of the right uncinate process.

(2) Midsagittal CT.

(3) Parasagittal MRI of the right uncinate process.

(4) Midsagittal MRI.

A segment-type OPLL from C2 to C6 shown on sagittal CT images (Fig. 3.32.2, panel 1 and 2).

Cervical kyphosis and a hypointense band in the front of the spinal canal from C2 to C5/6 protuberant into the spinal canal and spinal cord impingement generated by the OPLL and herniated disc materials. Intramedullary hyperintensity at C3/4 and C4/5 suggests myelopathy, as shown on sagittal MR images (Fig. 3.27.2, panel 4 to 6).

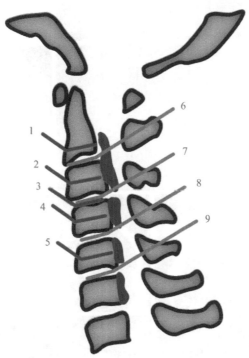

Reference of the axial planes

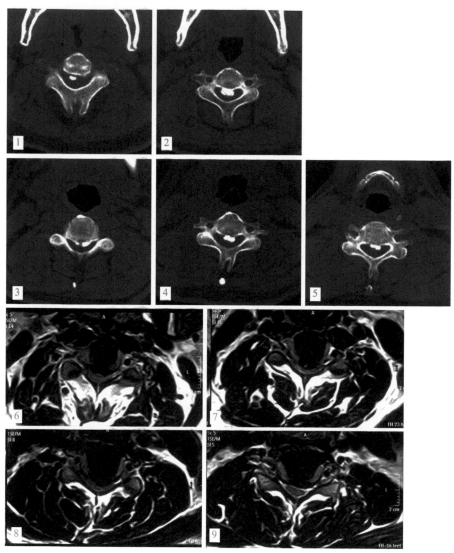

FIGURE 3.32.3

Preoperative axial images of the cervical spine and their reference on the sagittal diagram.
(1) Axial CT of the inferior surface of C2.
(2) Axial CT of C3.
(3) Axial CT of C3/4.
(4) Axial CT of C4.
(5) Axial CT of C5.
(6) Axial MRI of C2/3.
(7) Axial MRI of C3/4.
(8) Axial MRI of C4/5.
(9) Axial MRI of C5/6.

Axial CT images: This narrow-based OPLL measures 5 mm thick (anteroposterior), 13 mm wide (mediolateral), and 41.7% in canal occupancy at C3; 6.0 mm thick, 10 mm wide, and 50% in canal occupancy at C4; and 4 mm thick, 10 mm wide, and 36.4% in canal occupancy at C5 (Fig. 3.32.3, panel 1 to 5).

Axial MR images: Boomerang- or crescent-shaped spinal cord due to anterior indentation and effacement of CSF (Fig. 3.32.3, panel 6 to 9).

Highlights

This case features a straightened cervical spine, developmental stenosis of the spinal canal, a segmental OPLL from C2 to C6 that impinges the spinal cord from C2 to C5, poor spinal cord curvature, and intramedullary hyperintensity at multiple levels.

Surgical planning

In long-segment K-line (+) OPLL as in this case, a posterior surgery achieves adequate decompression among the conventional strategies.

However, in the cervical spine with poor curvature, the posterior indirect decompression may precipitate curvature worsening and recurrent neuropathy.

The muscular disruption caused by posterior exposure may also leave the patient with sustained pain over the neck and shoulders.

This patient received ACAF with antedisplacement of C3 to C5 and a shelter procedure for C2 decompression.

In a straightened cervical spine, as the curvature correction provides extra room for decompression, the anterior resection shall measure thinner than the thickness of the ossification (Fig. 3.32.4).

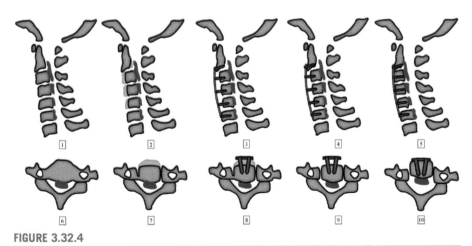

FIGURE 3.32.4

Illustration of the surgical plan on sagittal and axial planes.
(1, 6) Illustration of the OPLL on sagittal and axial views before surgery.
(2, 7) Resection performed to the anterior part of C3 to C5 vertebral bodies. A complete trough is developed on the left vertebral bodies from C3 to C5 while a half one is made on the right side with the posterior bone yet to be dissected.
(3, 8) Plate and screws placed on vertebral bodies from C2 through C6.
(4, 9) The bottom of the right half-groove on C3 through C5 dissected.
(5, 10) Antedisplaced C3 to C5 vertebral bodies as screws were tightened.

Results

Postoperative function: JOA score was 17, Nurick score: 0, VAS: 0, and NDI: 4.

Lordotic cervical spine, Cobb angle of 15.6° from C2 to C7, instrumentation from C2 to C7, and antedisplaced C3 to C5 vertebral bodies (Fig. 3.32.5).

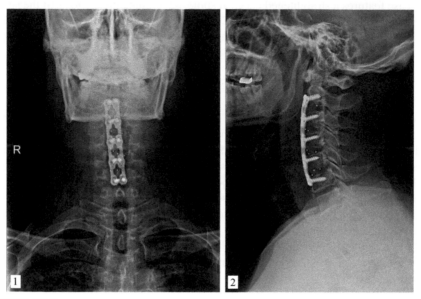

FIGURE 3.32.5

Postoperative cervical spine X-ray.
(1) Anteroposterior view.
(2) Lateral view.

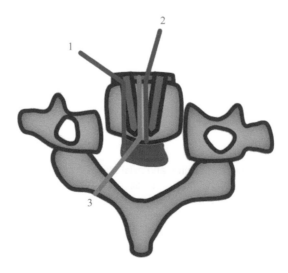

Reference of the sagittal planes

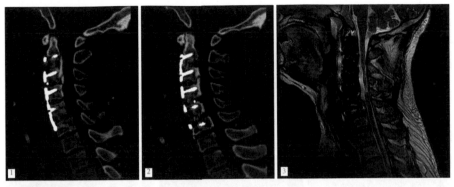

FIGURE 3.32.6

Postoperative sagittal views and their reference on the axial diagram.
(1) Right parasagittal CT.
(2) Midsagittal CT.
(3) Midsagittal MRI.

Ventrally displaced VOC from C2 to C5, and partial resection of the posterior rim of C2 vertebra shown on postoperative midsagittal CT image (Fig. 3.32.6, panel 1 and 2).

Straightened spinal cord free of compression and surrounded by CSF, with ill-defined intramedullary hyperintensity shown on postoperative midsagittal MR image (Fig. 3.32.6, panel 3).

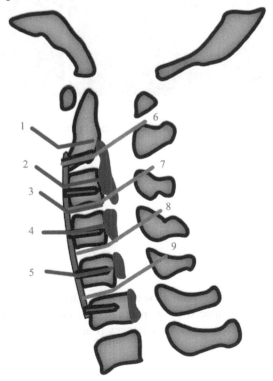

Reference of the axial planes

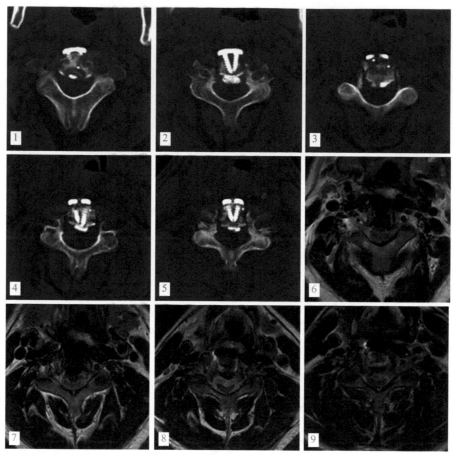

FIGURE 3.32.7

Postoperative axial cervical images and their reference on the sagittal diagram.
(1) Axial CT of C2.
(2) Axial CT of C3.
(3) Axial CT of C3/4.
(4) Axial CT of C4.
(5) Axial CT of C5.
(6) Axial MRI of C2/3.
(7) Axial MRI of C3/4.
(8) Axial MRI of C4/5.
(9) Axial MRI of C5/6.

The vertebral bodies have been dissected with parasagittal cuts on both sides 22 mm apart and antedisplaced by 3 mm, and the canal occupancy reduced to 0% as shown on postoperative axial CT images (Fig. 3.32.7, panel 1 to 5).

It has recovered to an oval and triangular shape, surrounded by an ample amount of CSF as shown on postoperative axial MR images (Fig. 3.32.7, panel 6 to 9).

Discussion

Why was the C3 inadequately antedisplaced? Though adequate decompression was achieved with ACAF, the spinal cord morphology did not recover immediately. What were the causes, and how long does it take to recover the normal shape?

The spinal cord is subject to a slow and gradual change in morphology in slowly progressing diseases such as OPLL. It is asymptomatic due to the robust compensatory capacity until advanced disease.

The development of symptoms signals that the compensatory capacity runs out and neurological deterioration will set in anytime upon unintended compression, particularly the iatrogenic one. That is why ACCF is often risky in such diseases.

In contrast, ACAF provides a safer option as it achieves controlled antedisplacement without the need for ossification resection. Even with sufficient decompression via ACAF, the spinal cord does not resume its original shape immediately.

Case 33: Ossification of posterior longitudinal ligament (OPLL) of cervical spine (At C3 to C6)

Index terms

Antedisplacement of three vertebral bodies, mixed-type OPL, narrow-based disease, thickness of ossification 8.7 mm, and canal occupancy 66%.

History

Patient: A 54-year-old woman.

Chief complaint: Numbness of both hands and gait disturbance for six months.

Physical exam: Physical exam was noted for gait instability, limited range of cervical motion, impaired tactile, pinprick, and temperature sensation on all the fingertips, and clumsiness of both hands. Muscle strength was tested at 4/5 on the upper arms and hands, lower limbs, and dorsal and plantar flexes bilaterally. Normal anal wink. Hypertonicity and brisk tendon reflexes were noted on all four extremities. Hoffmann sign was present bilaterally.

Preoperative function: JOA score was 13, Nurick score: 1, VAS: 0, and NDI: 8.

Imaging studies

A lordotic cervical spine with Cobb angle of 14.6° from C2 through C7; Pavlov ratio of 61%, 63%, 66%, and 57% at C3, C4, C5, and C6, respectively; and K-line (−) OPLL from C3 to C5 (Fig. 3.33.1).

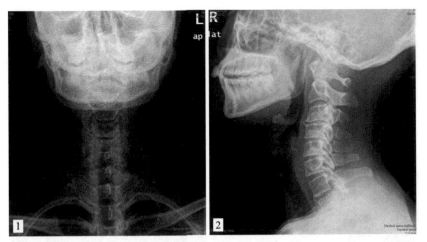

FIGURE 3.33.1

Preoperative X-ray of the cervical spine.
(1) Anteroposterior view.
(2) Lateral view.

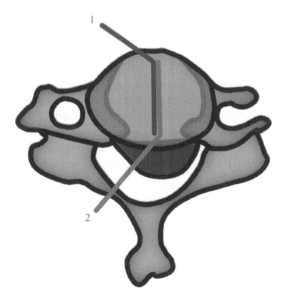

Reference of the sagittal planes

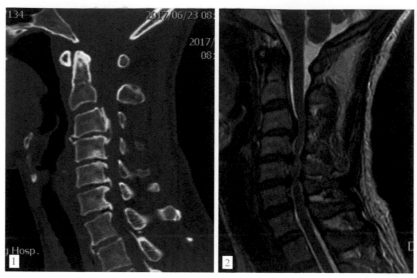

FIGURE 3.33.2

Preoperative sagittal images and their reference on axial diagram.
(1) Midsagittal CT.
(2) Midsagittal MRI.

Based on sagittal CT images: Extensive ossification that involves the posterior longitudinal ligament and ligamentum flavum of the cervicothoracic region, with OPLL being more severe; multisegmental circumscribed OPLL from C3 to C7, most severe at C3/4 (Fig. 3.33.2, panel 1).

Based on sagittal MR images: A kyphotic spinal cord compressed at C3 to C5/6, in particular at the interspace levels; hypertrophic ligamentum flavum at C4/5 to C5/6 (Fig. 3.33.2, panel 2).

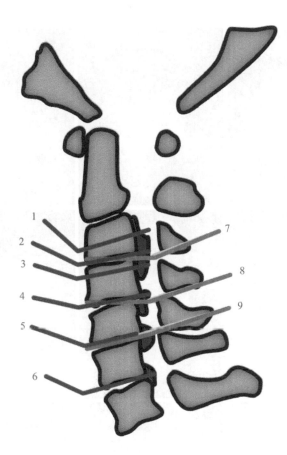

Reference of the axial planes

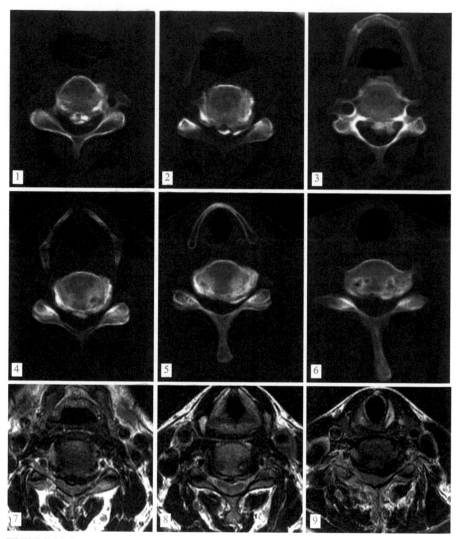

FIGURE 3.33.3

Preoperative axial images of the cervical spine and their reference on the sagittal diagram.

(1) Axial CT of C3.

(2) Axial CT of C3/4.

(3) Axial CT of the superior surface of C4.

(4) Axial CT of C4/5.

(5) Axial CT of C5/6.

(6) Axial CT of C6/7.

(7) Axial MRI of C3/4.

(8) Axial MRI of C4/5.

(9) Axial MRI of C5/6.

The OPLL is eccentric to the left, wide-based, and larger at C2 to C3; it extends to the neural exit foramina at C3/4 and C5/6, with a double-layer sign at C3/4 as shown on axial CT images (Fig. 3.33.3, panel 1 to 6).

Pincer-pattern spinal cord impingement and intramedullary signal hyperintensity at C4/5; spinal cord deformed into boomerang and crescent shape with CSF efface-ment as shown on axial MR images (Fig. 3.33.3, panel 7 to 9).

Highlights

This case features circumscribed OPLL that involves C3 to C6 at the interspaces complicated with severe disc degeneration. Wide-based and left paracentral, the ossification extends to neural exit foramen at some levels.

Surgical planning

In this K-line (−), multifocal circumscribed OPLL that causes over 60% of canal stenosis, an anterior surgery is a preferred conventional strategy.

The decompression at C3 is beyond the strength of anterior cervical discectomy and fusion (ACDF). Also, in patients with severe disc degeneration, interspace decompres-sion is technically challenging in addition to the possible incomplete decompression.

ACCF bears the risk of incomplete decompression in wide-based disease and fusion-related complication due to the use of a long construct.

Among the conventional procedures, ACCF can be used on C3 and C4 where the ossification is more severe, and ACDF for C5/6 with less severe disease.

The patient received ACAF with antedisplacement of C3 to C5 and undercutting of the superior edge of C6.

Given the preserved physiological lordosis, room of decompression generated by curvature correction is less likely and an anterior part of the vertebrae of the same thickness as the ossification was resected.

At the levels of OPLL with severe disc degeneration, the interspace was prepared just enough to accept the cage instead of more aggressively (Fig. 3.33.4).

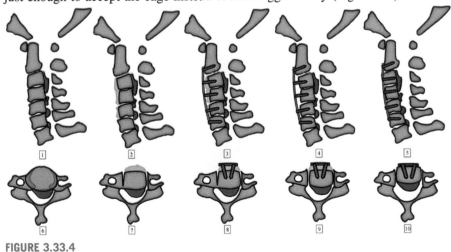

FIGURE 3.33.4

Illustration of the surgical plan on sagittal and axial views.
(1, 6) Illustration of the OPLL on sagittal and axial views before surgery.
(2, 7) Resection of the anterior part of the vertebral bodies of C3 to C6. A left groove and a right half-groove with the posterior cortex still intact on C3 to C6.
(3, 8) Titanium plate and screws placed in vertebral bodies from C2 to C7.
(4, 9) Completion of the right groove on C3 through C6.
(5, 10) Antedisplaced C3 to C6 vertebral bodies as screws were tightened.

Results

Postoperative function: JOA score was 14, Nurick score: 1, VAS: 0, and NDI: 3.

Instrumentation from C2 to C6 and antedisplaced C3 to C5; 16 mm screws in C2 and C6 while 12 mm ones in C3 to C5 (Fig. 3.33.5).

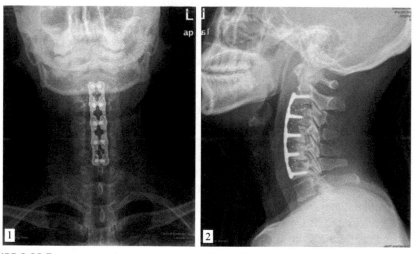

FIGURE 3.33.5

Postoperative cervical X-ray.
(1) Anteroposterior view.
(2) Lateral view.

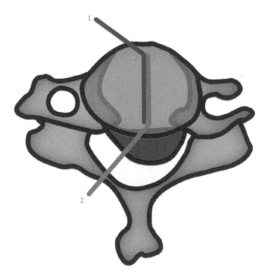

Reference of the sagittal planes

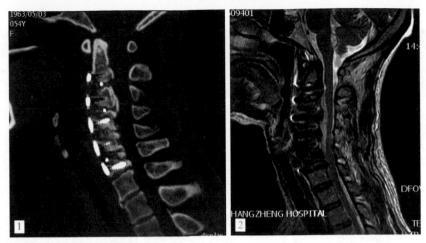

FIGURE 3.33.6

Postoperative sagittal images and their reference on the axial diagram.
(1) Midsagittal CT.
(2) Midsagittal MRI.

Antedisplaced VOC of C3 to C5, debulked posterior rim of C6, and expanded spinal canal shown on sagittal CT image (Fig. 3.33.6, panel 1).

Postoperative sagittal MR image: Spinal cord with partially restored curvature free of indentation and surrounded by CSF (Fig. 3.33.6, panel 2).

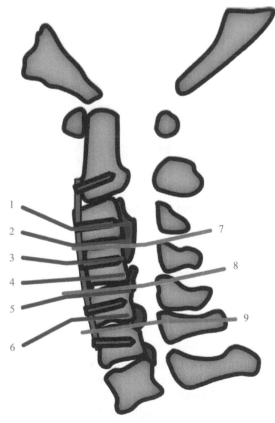

Reference of the axial planes

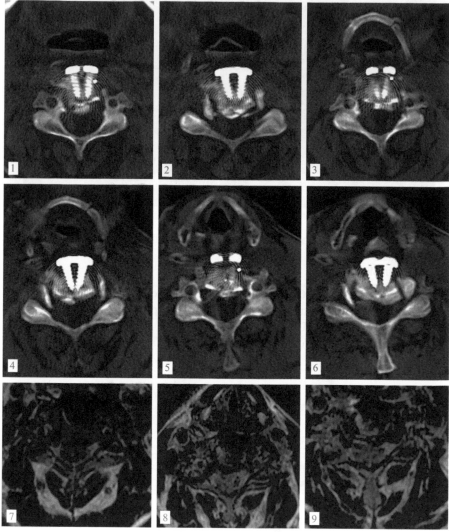

FIGURE 3.33.7

Postoperative axial cervical images and their reference on the sagittal diagram.

(1) Axial CT of C3.

(2) Axial CT of C3/4.

(3) Axial CT of C4.

(4) Axial CT of the inferior surface of C4.

(5) Axial CT of C4/5.

(6). Axial CT of the inferior surface of C5.

(7) Axial MRI of C3/4.

(8) Axial MRI of C4/5.

(9) Axial MRI of C5/6.

Based on postoperative axial CT images, the VOC has been sufficiently antedisplaced by 4.6 mm with sagittal bone cuts 23 mm apart; canal stenosis reduced to 0%; the grooves deviated laterally with the left groove through the pedicle (Fig. 3.33.7, panel 1 to 6). As shown on sagittal CT images, the spinal cord resumes to triangular or boomerang shape with normal CSF around it (Fig. 3.33.7, panel 7 to 9).

Discussion

What are the cautions in addressing severely degenerated disc spaces, as seen at C3/4, C4/5, and C5/6 in this case?

Interspace preparation constitutes an essential step in ACAF aiming for a parallel disc space by disc material removal, endplate preparation on both sides, and resection of anular epiphysis.

Our retrospective analysis revealed that interspace height of less than 4 mm is a negative factor for antedisplacement. This is because a narrow disc space accepts the smallest cage with difficulty and increases resistance during antedisplacement.

The partial removal of endplates with a burr is recommended in cases with severe intervertebral degeneration and stenosis to reduce this resistance and match the disc space to the cage to be used.

Case 34: Cervical spinal stenosis and ossification of posterior longitudinal ligament (At C2 to C7)

Index terms

Antedisplacement of multiple vertebral bodies, multilevel circumscribed OPLL, wide-based lesion, thickness of ossification 6.6 mm, canal stenosis 58%, shelter technique, and K-line (−) OPLL.

History

Patient: A 59-year-old man.

Chief complaint: Pain and numbness of the neck and shoulders for five years with aggravation and gait disturbance for six months.

Physical exam: Physical exam was noted for gait instability; limited range of cervical motion; impaired tactile, pinprick, and temperature sensation on all the extremities, the trunk, and perineal area. Muscle strength was tested at 4/5 on bilateral deltoid, biceps and triceps brachii, wrist flexion and extension, hand grips, iliopsoas, quadriceps femoris, biceps femoris, semitendinosus, semimembranosus, anterior tibialis, triceps surae, and dorsal and plantar flexion. Intact anal wink. Brisk tendon reflexes on knee and ankle bilaterally.

Preoperative function: JOA score was 9, Nurick score: 3, VAS: 4, and NDI: 21.

Imaging studies

A kyphotic deformed cervical spine with C2−C7 Cobb angle of −2.6°; Pavlov ratio of 61%, 63%, 66%, and 57% at C3, C4, C5, and C6, respectively; and a K-line (−) OPLL from C3 to C5 (Fig. 3.34.1).

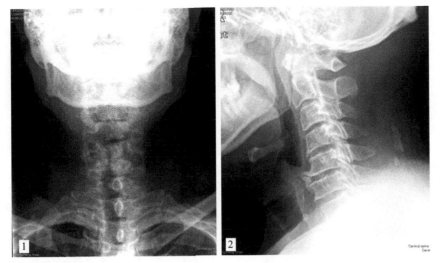

FIGURE 3.34.1

Preoperative X-ray of the cervical spine.

(1) Anteroposterior view.

(2) Lateral view.

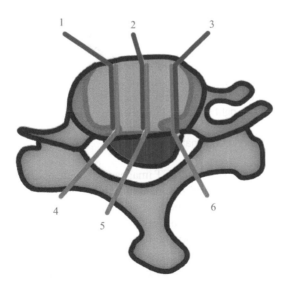

Reference of the sagittal planes

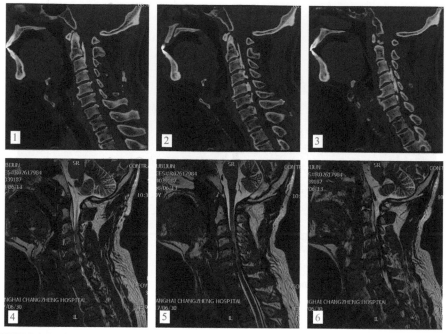

FIGURE 3.34.2

Preoperative sagittal images of the cervical spine and their reference on the axial diagram.
(1) Parasagittal CT of the right uncinate process.
(2) Midsagittal CT.
(3) Parasagittal CT of the left uncinate process.
(4) Parasagittal MRI of the right uncinate process.
(5) Midsagittal MRI.
(6) Parasagittal MRI of the left uncinate process.

As shown on preoperative sagittal CT images, extensive ossification that involves the cervical posterior longitudinal ligament and ligamentum flavum of the cervicothoracic region, with OPLL being more severe; multisegmental noncontinuous circumscribed OPLL from C3 to C7, most severe at C3/4 (Fig. 3.34.2, panel 1 to 3). As shown on sagittal MR images, a kyphotic spinal cord compressed at C3 to C5/6, particularly at the interspace levels; hypertrophic ligamentum flavum at C4/5 to C5/6; pincer-pattern spinal cord impingement and intramedullary signal hyperintensity at C4/5 (Fig. 3.34.2, panel 4 to 6).

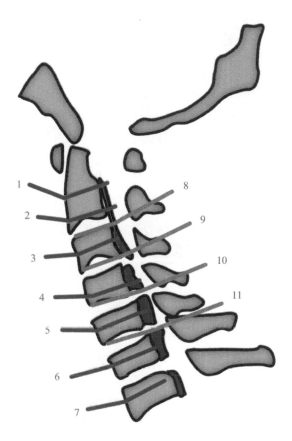

Reference of the axial planes

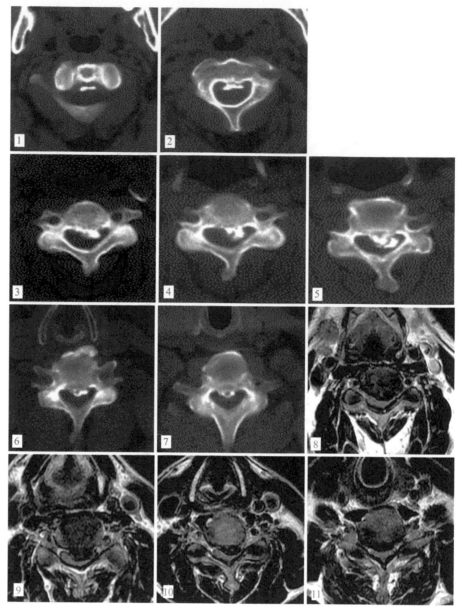

FIGURE 3.34.3

Preoperative axial images of the cervical spine and their reference on the sagittal diagram.

(1) Axial CT of C1.

(2) Axial CT of the inferior surface of C2.

(3) Axial CT of C3.

(4) Axial CT of the inferior surface of C4.

(5) Axial CT of C5.

(6) Axial CT of C6.

(7) Axial CT of C7.

(8) Axial MRI of C2/3.

(9) Axial MRI of C3/4.

(10) Axial MRI of C4/5.

(11) Axial MRI of C5/6.

Based on axial CT image, the OPLL is eccentric to the left, wide-based, and larger at C2 to C3; it extends to the neural exit foramina at C3/4 and C5/6. The OPLL measures 6.5 mm thick (anteroposterior), 10.3 mm wide (mediolateral), and 55% in canal occupancy at C3; 5.6 mm thick, 14.9 mm wide, and 63% in canal occupancy at C3/4 where a double-layer sign is present; and 6.5 mm thick, 18.2 mm wide, and 55% in canal occupancy at C4 (Fig. 3.34.3, panel 1 to 7).

Spinal cord deformed into boomerang and crescent shape with CSF effacement shown on postoperative axial MR image (Fig. 3.34.3, panel 8 to 11).

Highlights

This case features a kyphotic cervical spine, developmental stenosis of the spinal canal, a long mixed-type OPLL from C2 to C7, most severe at C5 where it is eccentric to the left and double-layered.

Surgical planning

This case features a long and K-line (−) OPLL with preoperative imagery evidence of dural ossification. An indirect decompression via a posterior approach may result in a residual complication, whereas a direct compression via ACCF, involving the use of a cylindrical titanium mesh, may risk dural injury, CSF leak, and fusion failure.

The patient received ACAF with antedisplacement of C3 through C6. The OPLL was dissected at C2/3 and left unresected at C2.

As the curvature correction amplifies decompression in a kyphotic cervical spine, the anterior resection shall measure thinner than the ossification thickness (Fig. 3.34.4).

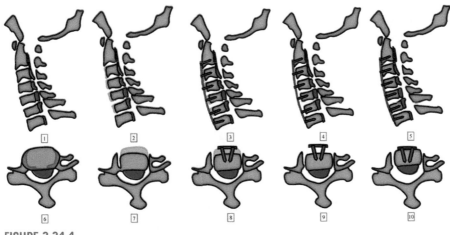

FIGURE 3.34.4

Illustration of the surgical plan on sagittal and axial planes.
(1, 6) Illustration of the OPLL on sagittal and axial views before surgery.
(2, 7) OPLL of C2 to C3 dissected at the interspace level, resection performed to the anterior part of C3 to C6 vertebral bodies, a complete trough developed on the left vertebral bodies from C3 to C6 while a half one is made on the right side with the posterior bone yet to be dissected.
(3, 8) Plate and screws placed on vertebral bodies from C2 through C7.
(4, 9) The bottom of the right half-groove on C3 through C6 dissected.
(5, 10) Antedisplaced C3 to C6 vertebral bodies as screws were tightened.

Results

Postoperative function: JOA score was 16, Nurick score: 1, VAS: 0, and NDI: 5.

Instrumentation from C2 to C6, screws of 16 mm used at C2 and C6, and ones of 12 mm used at C3 to C5 (Fig. 3.34.5).

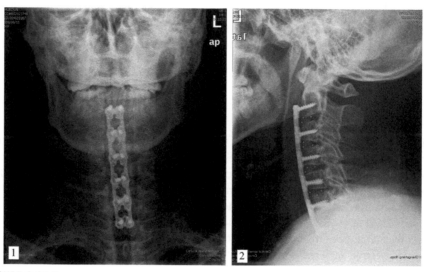

FIGURE 3.34.5

Postoperative cervical spine X-ray.
(1) Anteroposterior view.
(2) Lateral view.

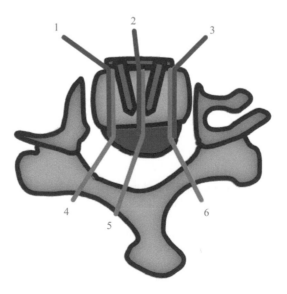

Reference of the sagittal planes

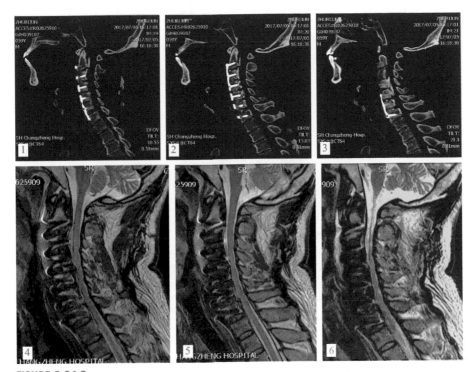

FIGURE 3.34.6

Postoperative sagittal views and their reference on the axial diagram.

(1) Parasagittal CT of the right uncinate process.
(2) Midsagittal CT.
(3) Parasagittal CT of the left uncinate process.
(4) Parasagittal MRI of the right uncinate process.
(5) Midsagittal MRI.
(6) Parasagittal MRI of the left uncinate process.

Ventrally displaced VOC from C3 to C6, expanded spinal canal, and OPLL of C2 to C3 dissected at C2/3, shown on sagittal CT images (Fig. 3.34.6, panel 1 to 3).

Lordotic spinal cord free of compression and surrounded by CSF, shown on sagittal MR images (Fig. 3.34.6, panel 4 to 6).

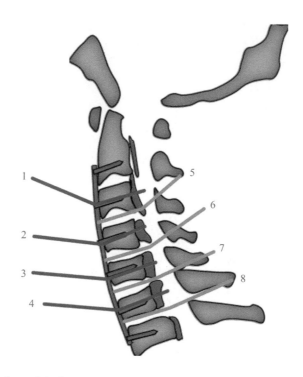

Reference of the axial planes

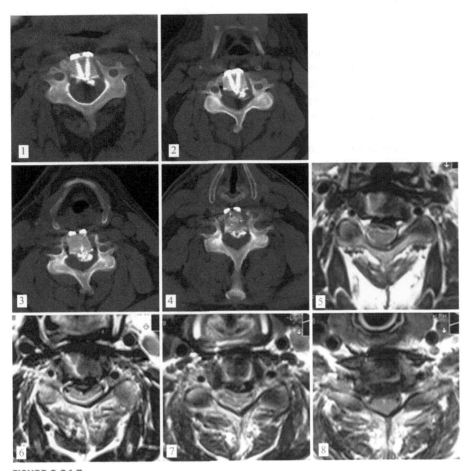

FIGURE 3.34.7

Postoperative axial cervical images and their reference on the sagittal diagram.

(1) Axial CT of C1.

(2) Axial CT of the inferior surface of C2.

(3) Axial CT of C3.

(4) Axial CT of C4.

(5) Axial CT of C5.

(6) Axial CT of C6.

(7) Axial CT of C7.

(8) Axial MRI of C2/3.

(9) Axial MRI of C3/4.

(10) Axial MRI of C4/5.

(11) Axial MRI of C5/6.

As shown on postoperative axial CT imaging, the vertebral bodies have been dissected with parasagittal cuts on both sides 23.1 mm apart and antedisplaced by 5.1 mm, and the canal occupancy reduced to 26.7% at C4 (Fig. 3.34.7, panel 1 to 7).

As shown on postoperative axial MR imaging, it has recovered to an oval and triangular shape, surrounded by an ample amount of CSF (Fig. 3.34.7, panel 8 to 11).

Discussion

What are the considerations for the dissection at C2/3?

The OPLL extended cephalad beyond the margin between C1 and C2.

If the proximal tip of the OPLL is decompressed via a shelter procedure, a significant amount of the C2 vertebra will be resected from posterior, leaving the endplate less than 10 mm long sagittally. This may result in diminished areas for bone grafts and screw purchase.

Also, preoperative magnetic resonance imaging (MRI) suggested that the thin lesion at C2/3 and C2 had not caused neuropathy or CSF effacement.

Therefore, the ossification was dissected at C2/3, and the C2 lesion was not ventrally displaced.

Case 35: Cervical spinal stenosis and ossification of posterior longitudinal ligament (At C3 to C7)

Index terms

Antedisplacement of three vertebral bodies, continuous OPLL, narrow-based OPLL, the thickness of ossification 8.7 mm, and canal occupancy 58%.

History

Patient: A 59-year-old man.

Chief complaint: Pain and numbness of the neck and shoulders for five years with aggravation and gait disturbance for six months.

Physical exam: Physical exam was noted for gait instability; limited range of cervical motion; impaired tactile, pinprick, and temperature sensation on all the extremities, the trunk and perineal area. Muscle strength was tested at 4/5 on bilateral deltoid, biceps and triceps brachii, wrist flexion and extension, hand grips, iliopsoas, quadriceps femoris, biceps femoris, semitendinosus, semimembranosus, anterior tibialis, triceps surae, and dorsal and plantar flexion. Intact anal wink. Brisk tendon reflexes on knee and ankle bilaterally.

Preoperative function: JOA score was 4, Nurick score: 5, VAS: 1, and NDI: 31.

Imaging studies

Pavlov of C5, C6, and C7 measured 59%, 53%, and 60% (Fig. 3.35.1).

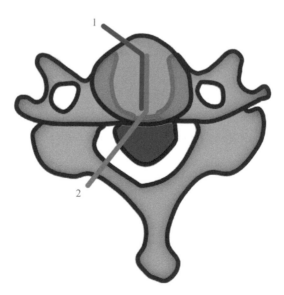

FIGURE 3.35.1

Preoperative bending X-ray.
(1) Hyperflexion view.
(2) Hyperextension view.

Reference of the sagittal planes

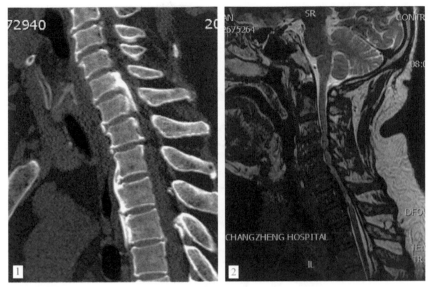

FIGURE 3.35.2

Preoperative sagittal images of the cervical spine and their reference on the axial diagram.
(1) Midsagittal CT.
(2) Midsagittal MRI.

A continuous-type OPLL from C6 to C7 shown on midsagittal CT image (Fig. 3.35.2, panel 1).

As shown on postoperative midsagittal MR image, a spinal cord impinged at C3/4 to T1, in particular at interspace levels from C3/4 to C5/6; cord impingement at C6 to the superior surface of T1 due to the hypointense indentation in the front of the spinal canal; and intramedullary signal hyperintensity at C7/T1 (Fig. 3.35.2, panel 2).

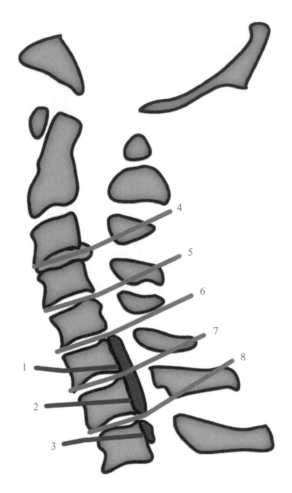

Reference of the axial planes

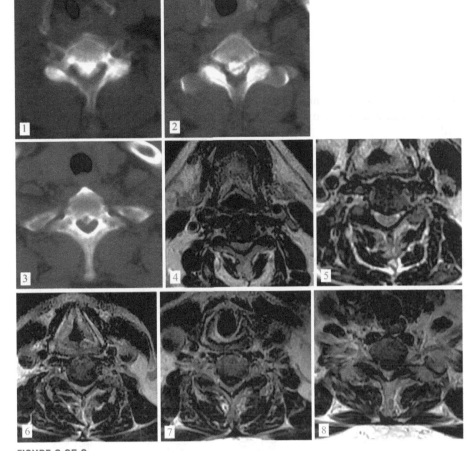

FIGURE 3.35.3

Preoperative axial images of the cervical spine and their reference on the sagittal diagram.

(1) Axial CT of C6.

(2) Axial CT of C7.

(3) Axial CT of the superior surface of T1.

(4) Axial MRI of C4/5.

(5) Axial MRI of C5/6.

(6) Axial MRI of C6/7.

(7) Axial MRI of C7/T1.

As shown on postoperative axial CT imaging, this wide-based OPLL measures: 8.7 mm thick (anteroposterior), 15.1 mm wide (mediolateral), and 58% in canal occupancy at C6; 8.3 mm thick, 16.1 mm wide, and 45% in canal occupancy at C7 where it is double-layered; and 5.2 mm thick, 8.9 mm wide, and 40% in canal occupancy at T1 (Fig. 3.35.3, panel 1 to 3).

As shown on postoperative axial MR imaging, a boomerang- or crescent-shaped spinal cord due to indentation from C3/4 to C7/T1, in particular at C5/6 to C7/T1; and intramedullary snake-eyes sign at C5/6 and hyperintensity at C7/T1 (Fig. 3.35.3, Figs. 4–8).

Highlights

This case features developmental spinal canal stenosis with continuous OPLL from C6 to T1 complicated with cord impingement by herniated disc material.

Surgical planning

In OPLL that involves the initiation of the thoracic kyphosis, spinal canal expansion alone may cause incomplete decompression and limited posterior shift of the spinal cord.

Conventionally, direct decompression via an anterior surgery is feasible with care exercised in locating the incision properly and protecting the thyroid during surgery.

The patient received ACAF with antedisplacement of C5 to C7, and undercutting of the ossification along the superior edge of T1. The protruded C3/4 disc material was managed with ACDF.

As the surgery involved extensive levels, one transverse incision alone may not provide enough access. Thus, dual transverse incisions of the same side or one longitudinal incision is preferred.

Given the location of the cervicothoracic junction, room of decompression generated by curvature correction is less likely, and an anterior part of the vertebrae of the same thickness as the ossification was resected (Fig. 3.35.4).

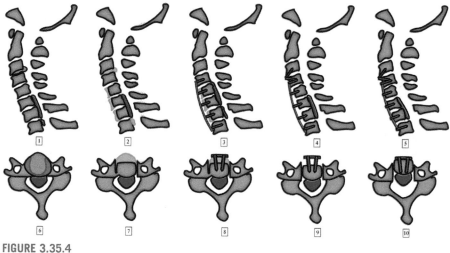

FIGURE 3.35.4

Illustration of the surgical plan on sagittal and axial planes.

(1, 6) Illustration of the OPLL on sagittal and axial views before surgery.

(2, 7) Resection of the anterior part of the vertebral bodies of C5 to C7, the posteroinferior rim of C7 vertebra, and C3/4 intervertebral disc; a left groove and a right half-groove with the posterior cortex still intact on C6 and C7.

(3, 8) Titanium plate and screws inserted in vertebral bodies from C4 to T1.

(4, 9) Completion of the right groove on C6 and C7, and placement of a cage in C3/4 and instrumentation.

(5, 10) Antedisplaced C6 and C7 vertebral bodies as screws were tightened.

Results

Postoperative function: JOA score was 5, Nurick score: 4, VAS: 0, and NDI: 25.

Cobb angle of 22.0° from C2 to C7, antedisplaced VOC from C5 to C7, and instrumentation with 16 mm screws in C4 and T1, and 12 mm ones in C5 to C7 (Fig. 3.35.5).

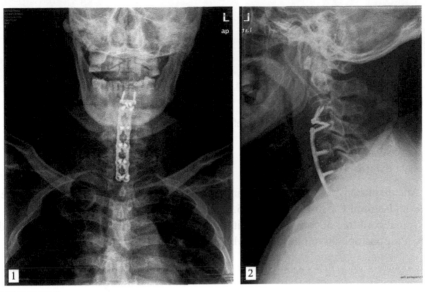

FIGURE 3.35.5

Postoperative cervical X-ray.
(1) Anteroposterior view.
(2) Lateral view.

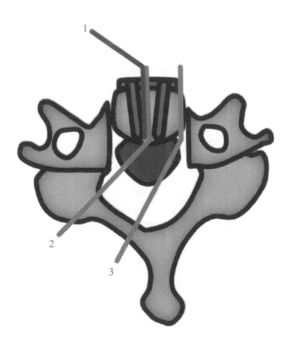

Reference of the sagittal planes

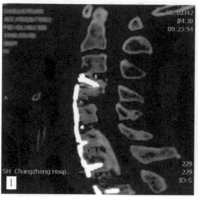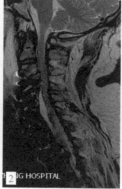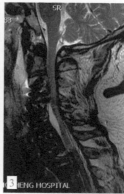

FIGURE 3.35.6

Postoperative sagittal images and their reference on the axial diagram.
(1) Midsagittal CT.
(2) Midsagittal MRI.
(3) Right parasagittal MRI.

Antedisplaced VOC of C5 to C7 and expanded spinal canal shown on postoperative midsagittal CT image (Fig. 3.35.6, panel 1).

Spinal cord free of compression with an ample amount of CSF on the ventral side shown on postoperative midsagittal MR image (Fig. 3.35.6, panel 2 and 3).

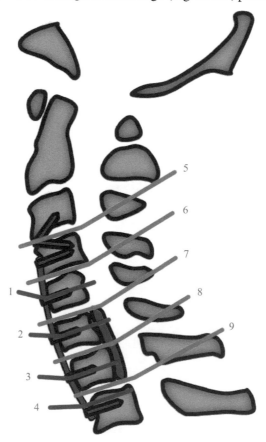

Reference of the axial planes

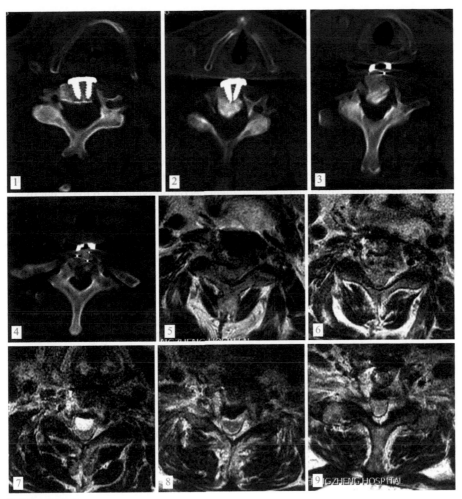

FIGURE 3.35.7

Postoperative axial cervical images and their reference on the sagittal diagram.

(1) Axial CT of C5.

(2) Axial CT of C6.

(3) Axial CT of C7.

(4) Axial CT of the superior surface of T1.

(5) Axial MRI of C3/4.

(6) Axial MRI of C4/5.

(7) Axial MRI of C5/6.

(8) Axial MRI of C6/7.

(9) Axial MRI of C6/T1.

The VOC has been antedisplaced by 7 mm with bone cuts 23.9 mm apart and deviated toward the left; canal stenosis reduced to 20% at T1 and 0 at C6 and C7; and the left groove at C7 through the pedicle, shown on postoperative axial CT image (Fig. 3.35.7, panel 1 to 4).

The spinal cord free of compression resumes to a triangular or oval shape with normal CSF around it, shown on postoperative axial MR image (Fig. 3.35.7, panel 5 to 9).

Discussion

What are the causes of the excessive ventral CSF volume at C5, shown on MRI?

This case was developmental stenosis of the spinal canal from C5 to C7 complicated with OPLL from C6 to C7, according to preoperative imaging studies. The anterior part of vertebral bodies was resected by the thickness of the OPLL calculated before surgery, which achieved excellent decompression at C6 to C7 but over-displacement of C5.

Indeed, the depth of resection of the anterior vertebral bodies should be calculated individually on levels involved in and spared of OPLL. This calculation is based on the thickness of OPLL and the plate contour at the levels with OPLL. In contrast, the calculation at the levels spared from OPLL should aim for Pavlov above 75% in the expanded spinal canal.

Resection performed on the levels spared from OPLL by the thickness of the OPLL results in over-resection and excessive antedisplacement.

An excessively resected vertebra increases the risk of screw engagement with the posterior vertebral cortex and reduces the surface area available for interspace fusion.

What is more, overly antedisplaced vertebral bodies tether the nerve roots on both sides and cause palsy, in particular when severe adhesion is present between the dura mater and the posterior vertebral cortex.

Therefore, anterior resection should be tailored to each level in cases where the thickness of OPLL varies among the levels, or the OPLL is complicated with developmental spinal canal stenosis.

Case 36: Ossification of posterior longitudinal ligament (OPLL) of cervical spine (At C5 to T1)

Index terms

Antedisplacement of two vertebral bodies, segmental OPLL, narrow-based OPLL, thickness of ossification 6.1   mm, and occupancy ratio 45%.

History

Patient: A 55-year-old man.

Chief complaint: Numbness of the right hand for five years with aggravation and numbness of the right sole for six months.

Physical exam: The patient walked with a steady gait. Muscle strength was tested at 4+/5 on the deltoid, biceps and triceps brachii, wrist flexion and extension, hand grips, iliopsoas, quadriceps femoris, biceps femoris, semitendinosus, semimembranosus, anterior tibialis, triceps surae, and dorsal and plantar flexion on the right side. Brisk tendon reflexes on the biceps and triceps brachii, brachioradialis, knees, and ankles bilaterally. Hoffmann sign was documented on the left side.

Preoperative function: JOA score was 15, Nurick score: 1, VAS: 3, and NDI: 9.

Imaging studies

A lordotic cervical spine with Cobb angle of 26.5° from C2 through C7 with Pavlov ratio of above 75%. And OPLL noticed at C5 and C6 (Fig. 3.36.1).

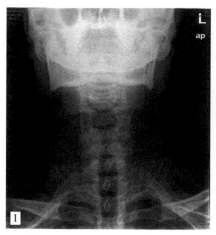
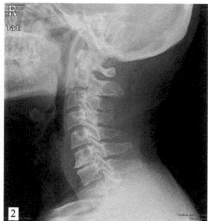

FIGURE 3.36.1

Preoperative X-ray of the cervical spine.
(1) Anteroposterior view.
(2) Lateral view.

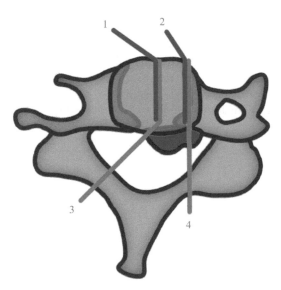

Reference of the sagittal planes

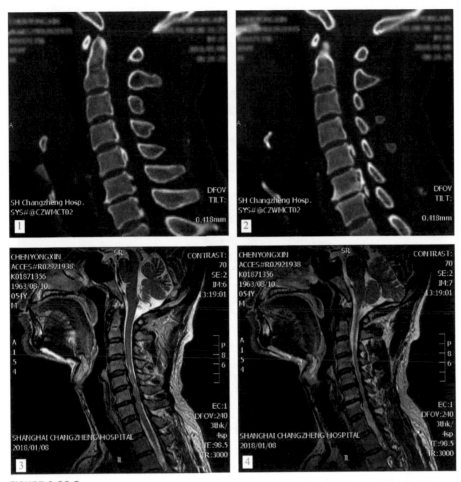

FIGURE 3.36.2

Preoperative sagittal images of the cervical spine and their reference on the axial diagram.

(1) Midsagittal CT.
(2) Parasagittal CT of the left uncinate process.
(3) Midsagittal MRI.
(4) Parasagittal MRI of the left uncinate process.

A segment-type OPLL from C5 to C6/7 shown on sagittal CT image (Fig. 3.36.2, panel 1 and 2).

Spinal canal stenosis from C4/5 to C6/7; spinal cord compression from C4/5 to C6/7, more severe at interspace levels; CSF effacement; and intramedullary signal hyperintensity at C4/5 and C5/6 shown on sagittal MR image (Fig. 3.36.2, panel 3 and 4).

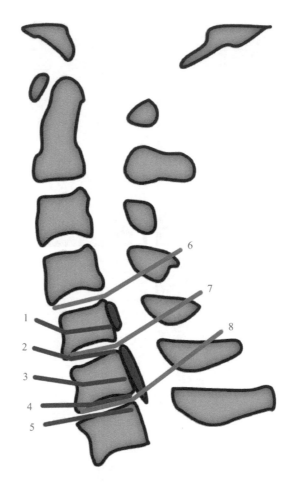

Reference of the axial planes

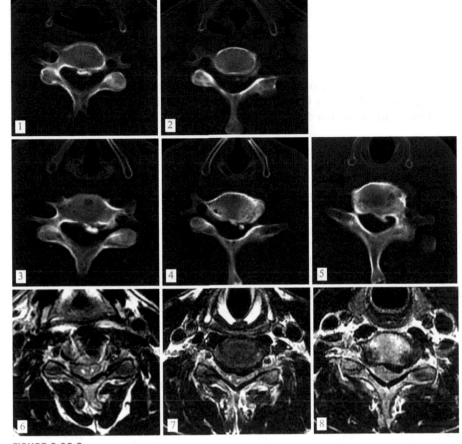

FIGURE 3.36.3

Preoperative axial images of the cervical spine and their reference on the sagittal diagram.

(1) Axial CT of C5.

(2) Axial CT of C5/6.

(3) Axial CT of C6.

(4) Axial CT of C6/7.

(5) Axial CT of the superior surface of C7.

(6) Axial MRI of C4/5.

(7) Axial MRI of C5/6.

(8) Axial MRI of C6/7.

Based on axial CT image, the OPLL is eccentric to the left and narrow-based. It measures 3.8 mm thick (anteroposterior), 10.2 mm wide (mediolateral), and 31% in canal occupancy at C5; 4.2 mm thick, 7.5 mm wide, and 40% in canal occupancy at C5/6; 5.9 mm thick, 9.4 mm wide, and 45% in canal occupancy at C6; 5.1 mm thick, 6.1 mm wide, and 43% in canal occupancy at C6/7; and 5.8 mm thick, 10.4 mm wide, and 40% in canal occupancy at C7 (Fig. 3.36.3, panel 1 to 5).

Based on axial MR image, spinal cord deformed into a boomerang and triangular shape at C5/6 to C6/7, and intramedullary snake-eyes sign at C4/5 and C5/6 (Fig. 3.36.3, panel 6 to 8).

Highlights

This case features developmental stenosis of the spinal canal complicated with flat-type segmental OPLL from C5 to C7, a short-segment disease. The OPLL is eccentric to the right and narrow-based.

Surgical planning

A short-segment OPLL can be managed with anterior decompression. Given the left eccentricity of the OPLL and the extension into the left neural exit foramen at C5/6, care should be taken to further decompress the residual lesion within the spinal canal after vertebra preparation.

An ACAF with antedisplacement of C5 and C6 was planned for this case.

For the lesion at C6/7, the plan was to displace it anteriorly into the interspace by removing the superior endplate of C7 and the inferior endplate of C6.

Given the preserved physiological lordosis, an anterior part of the vertebrae of the same thickness as the ossification was resected (Fig. 3.36.4).

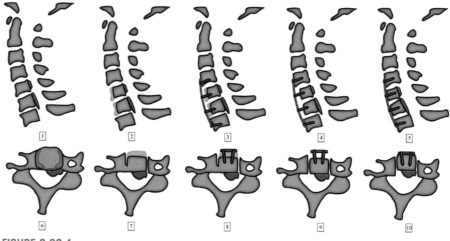

FIGURE 3.36.4

Illustration of the surgical plan on sagittal and axial planes.
(1, 6) Illustration of the OPLL on sagittal and axial views before surgery.
(2, 7) Resection performed to the anterior part of C5 to C6 vertebral bodies and the posteroinferior rim of C2 vertebra, a complete trough developed on the left vertebral bodies from C5 to C6 while a half one on the right side with the posterior bone yet to be dissected.
(3, 8) Plate and screws placed on vertebral bodies from C4 through C7.
(4, 9) The bottom of the right half-groove on C5 through C6 dissected.
(5, 10) Antedisplaced C5 to C6 vertebral bodies as screws were tightened.

Results

Postoperative function: JOA score was 15, Nurick score: 0, VAS: 0, and NDI: 0.

Instrumentation from C4 to C7 and antedisplaced C5 to C6; the screw in C5 has gone through the posterior vertebral cortex and into the spinal canal (Fig. 3.36.5).

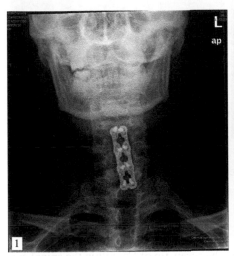
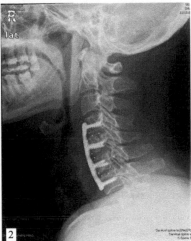

FIGURE 3.36.5

Postoperative cervical spine X-ray.

(1) Anteroposterior view.

(2) Lateral view.

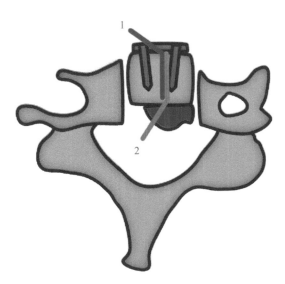

Reference of the sagittal planes

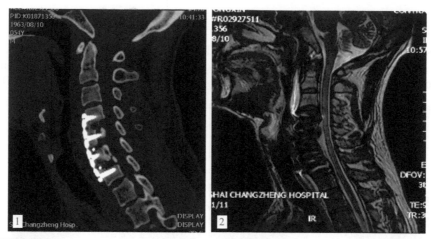

FIGURE 3.36.6

Postoperative sagittal views and their reference on the axial diagram.
(1) Midsagittal CT.
(2) Midsagittal MRI.

Antedisplaced VOC of C5 to C6, with the screw tip of C5 within the spinal canal, shown on postoperative midsagittal CT image (Fig. 3.36.6, panel 1).

Spinal cord free of compression in restored curvature and surrounded by CSF, the intramedullary hyperintensity diminished, shown on postoperative midsagittal MR image (Fig. 3.36.6, panel 2).

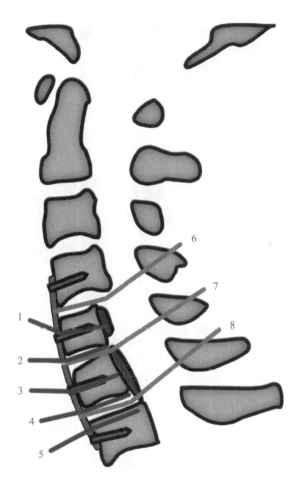

Reference of the axial planes

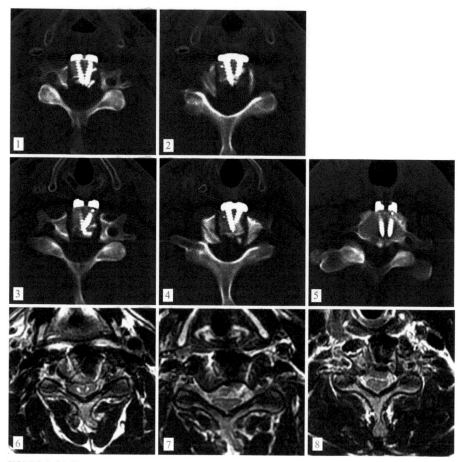

FIGURE 3.36.7

Postoperative axial cervical images and their reference on the sagittal diagram.
(1) Axial CT of C5.
(2) Axial CT of C5/6.
(3) Axial CT of C6.
(4) Axial CT of C6/7.
(5) Axial CT of the superior surface of C7.
(6) Axial MRI of C4/5.
(7) Axial MRI of C5/6.
(8) Axial MRI of C6/7.

Based on postoperative axial CT images, the VOC has been antedisplaced by 7.8 mm at C5 and 3.4 mm at C6 with sagittal bone cuts 21.9 mm apart, and canal stenosis reduced to 0% (Fig. 3.36.7, panel 1 to 5). The cord has recovered to an oval shape, surrounded by an ample amount of CSF, shown on postoperative axial MR images (Fig. 3.36.7, panel 6 to 8).

Discussion

Does the C5 screw engagement into the ossification counteract the antedisplacement or cause complications?

The postoperative imaging studies indicated the spinal cord surrounded by CSF, excessively antedisplaced C5, and the C5 screw went through the posterior vertebral cortex. This resulted in diminished migration of the ossification.

When the anterior part of C5 vertebra was significantly resected, the screw went through the posterior vertebral cortex and engaged in the ossification. The ossification was just loosely attached to the vertebra, and the antedisplacement maneuver did not adequately involve the ossification and left it behind.

In relatively small lesions, as seen in this case, the insufficiently displaced ossification at C5 did not affect the magnitude of decompression. But this may happen to lesions of larger size. Therefore, in lesions loosely attached to the vertebra, surgeons are recommended against purchasing the screw in the ossification in case of limited antedisplacement of the VOC.

Case 37: Ossification of posterior longitudinal ligament (OPLL) of cervical spine (At C2 to C4)

Index terms

Antedisplacement of two vertebral bodies, continuous OPLL, wide-based OPLL, and K-line (−) OPLL.

History

Patient: A 42-year-old man.

Chief complaint: Nuchal pain and numbness and weakness of all four extremities for three months.

Physical exam: Physical exam was noted for gait disturbance; reduced physiological curvature of the spine; an impaired sense of light touch, pinprick, temperature, vibration, and position; and impaired fine movements. Muscle strength was tested at 4/5 on the upper limbs and 4-/5 on the lower limbs. Brisk tendon reflexes on knees and ankles bilaterally. Hoffmann was positive on the left side.

Preoperative function: JOA score was 12, Nurick score: 1, VAS: 2, and NDI: 9.

Imaging studies

OPLL from C2 to C4, and Pavlov ratio above 75% across the whole cervical spine (Fig. 3.37.1).

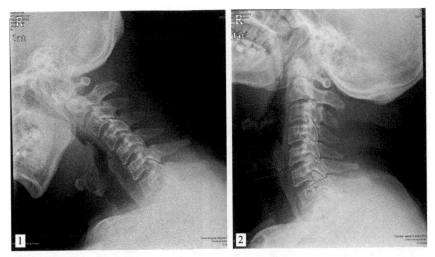

FIGURE 3.37.1

Preoperative bending X-ray.
(1) Hyperflexion view.
(2) Hyperextension view

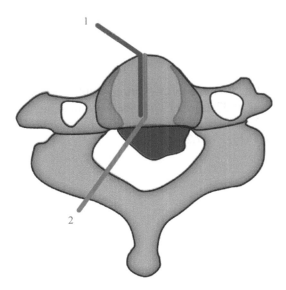

Reference of the sagittal planes

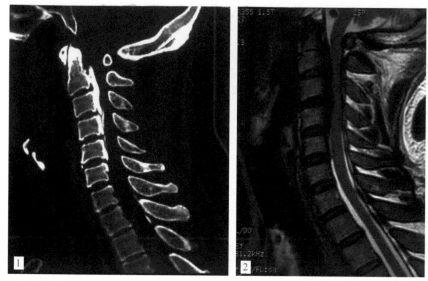

FIGURE 3.37.2

Preoperative sagittal images of the cervical spine and their reference on the axial diagram.
(1) Midsagittal CT.
(2) Midsagittal MRI.

A continuous OPLL from C2 to C4, with a double-layer sign at C4 shown on sagittal CT image (Fig. 3.37.2, panel 1). Spinal cord in straightened curvature and compressed from C2 to C4/5 due to the anterior hypointense indentation shown on sagittal MR image (Fig. 3.37.2, panel 2).

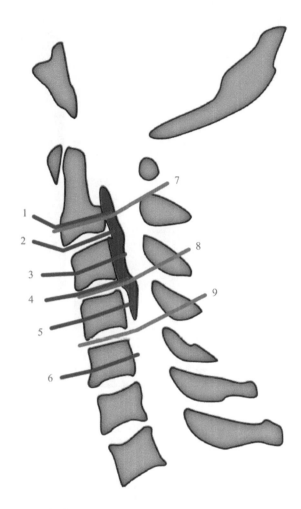

Reference of the axial planes

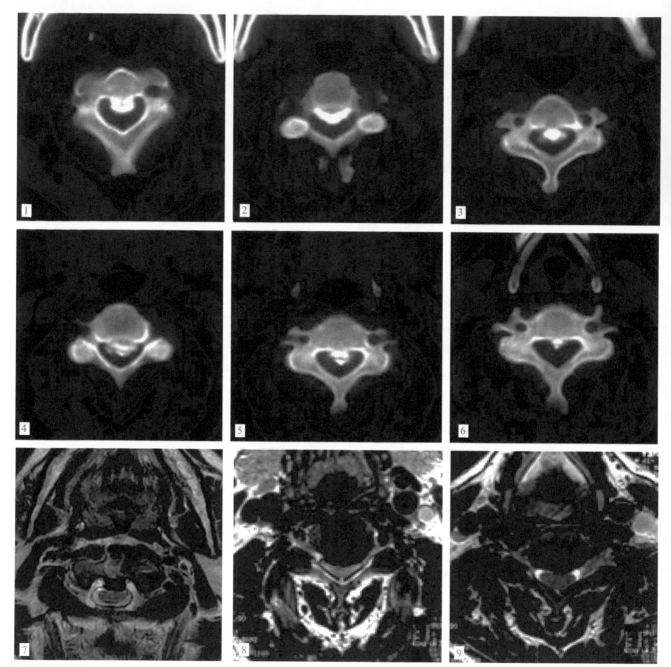

FIGURE 3.37.3

Preoperative axial images of the cervical spine and their reference on the sagittal diagram.

(1) Axial CT of C2.
(2) Axial CT of C2/3.
(3) Axial CT of C3.
(4) Axial CT of C3/4.
(5) Axial CT of C4.
(6) Axial CT of C5.
(7) Axial MRI of the inferior surface of C2.
(8) Axial MRI of C3/4.
(9) Axial MRI of C4/5.

Shown on postoperative axial CT images, the OPLL is found at C2 to C5 on axial images, with C2 to C4 being more severe and wide-based at interspace levels. This OPLL measures:7 mm thick (anteroposterior), 11.9 mm wide (mediolateral), and 38.9% in canal occupancy at C2; 5.2 mm thick, 20.3 mm wide, and 36.9% in canal occupancy at C2/3; 5.1 mm thick, 11.4 mm wide, and 34.2% in canal occupancy at C3; 5.1 mm thick, 15.3 mm wide, and 38.3% in canal occupancy at C3/4; and 7.2 mm thick, 11.8 mm wide, and 48.6% in canal occupancy at C4 (Fig. 3.37.3, panel 1 to 6).

Shown on postoperative axial MR images, a boomerang-shaped or triangular spinal cord due to indentation and intramedullary signal hyperintensity at C3/4 (Fig. 3.37.3, Figs. 7—9).

Highlights

This case features a centered continuous OPLL from C2 to C4 that extends high up the C2 vertebra. It is wide-based at C2/3 and double-layered at C2, C3/4, and C4.

Surgical planning

For continuous OPLL that extends into the upper cervical spine, an anterior decompression bears an increased risk of complications and surgical challenges. Posterior surgeries yield insufficient decompression due to the K-line (−) disease and lead to curvature deterioration and ossification progression.

An ACAF with antedisplacement of C3 and C4 and curvature correction via a properly contoured plate was planned for this case.

The OPLL had a significant extension in the upper cervical spine, more than half the height of the C2 vertebra, a shelter procedure may result in leaving the tip of the ossification in the canal and residual compression.

The dissection of the OPLL at C2/3 did not seem to work either given the ossification presence in the interspace level. The dissection maneuver may exert direct insult to the spinal cord. Even if it is safely dissected, the antedisplacement may create a step across the upper cervical spine and cause spinal cord impingement.

Therefore, the posteroinferior part of C2 vertebra was to be resected, followed by dissection of the OPLL at the level spared from cord impingement. The VOC will then be ready for antedisplacement.

In a kyphotic cervical spine, as the curvature correction provides extra room for decompression, the anterior resection shall measure thinner than the thickness of the ossification (Fig. 3.37.4).

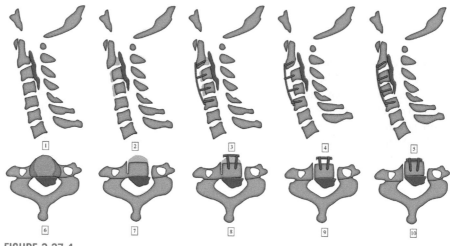

FIGURE 3.37.4

Illustration of the surgical plan on sagittal and axial planes.

(1, 6) Illustration of the OPLL on sagittal and axial views before surgery.

(2, 7) Resection performed to the anterior part of C3 and C4 vertebral bodies; a complete trough developed on the left vertebral bodies of C3 and C4 while a half one on the right side with the posterior bone yet to be dissected.

(3, 8) Plate and screws placed on vertebral bodies from C2 through C5.

(4, 9) The bottom of the right half-groove on C3 and C4 dissected.

(5, 10) Antedisplaced C3 and C4 vertebral bodies as screws were tightened.

Results

Postoperative function: JOA score was 17, Nurick score: 0, VAS: 0, and NDI: 0.

Cobb angle of 12.5° from C2 to C7, antedisplaced C3 to C5 vertebral bodies, and instrumentation except for the left screw in C3 (Fig. 3.37.5).

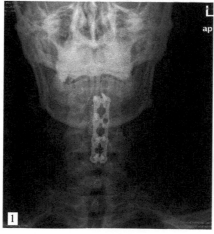
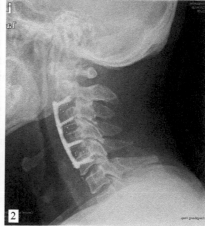

FIGURE 3.37.5

Postoperative cervical spine X-ray.

(1) Anteroposterior view.

(2) Lateral view.

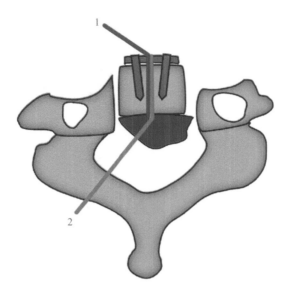

Reference of the sagittal planes

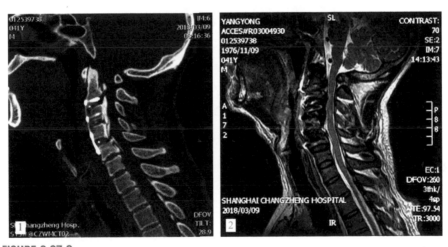

FIGURE 3.37.6

Postoperative sagittal views and their reference on the axial diagram.
(1) Midsagittal CT.
(2) Midsagittal MRI.

Ventrally displaced VOC and OPLL dissected at C2/3 shown on postoperative midsagittal CT image (Fig. 3.37.6, panel 1).

Lordotic spinal cord free of compression and surrounded by CSF shown on postoperative midsagittal MR image (Fig. 3.37.6, panel 2).

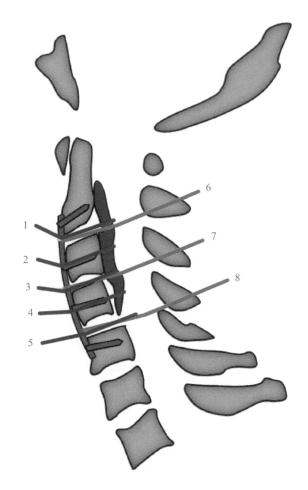

Reference of the axial planes

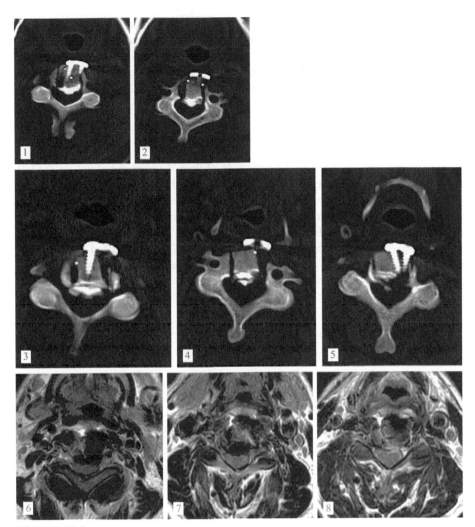

FIGURE 3.37.7

Postoperative axial cervical images and their reference on the sagittal diagram.

(1) Axial CT of C2/3.
(2) Axial CT of C3.
(3) Axial CT of C3/4.
(4) Axial CT of C4.
(5) Axial CT of C4/5.
(6) Axial MRI of C2/3.
(7) Axial MRI of C3/4.
(8) Axial MRI of C4/5.

As shown on postoperative axial CT images, the vertebral bodies have been dissected with parasagittal cuts on both sides 19.6 mm apart and antedisplaced by 4.2 mm, and the canal occupancy reduced to 21.4% (Fig. 3.37.7, panel 1 to 5). As shown on postoperative axial MR images, the spinal cord has recovered to an oval shape, surrounded by an ample amount of CSF (Fig. 3.37.7, panel 6 to 8).

Discussion

The screw was only inserted to the right side of the C4 vertebra but not on the left side. What were the barriers, and how can we avoid them?

Since the initial right groove on the C4 vertebra was medial to the OPLL's edge, it was lateralized later. Second, this right groove was oblique and resulted in a narrower decompression width on C3.

Third, given the left eccentric plate, when the VOC was hoisted via the right screw in C4, it resulted in a deviation of the C4 vertebra to the right side, and its left side was no longer accessible for screw insertion.

Case 38: Ossification of posterior longitudinal ligament (OPLL) of cervical spine (At C2 to C4)

Index terms

Antedisplacement of two vertebral bodies, mixed-type OPLL, wide-based disease, shelter technique, thickness of ossification 6 mm, and canal occupancy 57%.

History

Patient: A 54-year-old man.

Chief complaint: Numbness and pain on the upper extremities for one year with aggravation and gait disturbance for three months.

Physical exam: Physical exam was noted for gait instability, reduced cervical lordosis, and a limited range of cervical motion. Muscle strength was tested at 4+/5 on bilateral deltoid, biceps and triceps brachii; 4/5 on wrist flexion and extension, hand grips; 5-/5 on iliopsoas, quadriceps femoris, biceps femoris, semitendinosus, semimembranosus, and anterior tibialis on both sides, triceps surae, dorsal and plantar flexion on both sides. Brisk tendon reflexes on bilateral biceps and triceps brachii, radiobrachialis, knee, and ankle bilaterally.

Preoperative function: JOA score was 11, Nurick score: 1, VAS: 3, and NDI: 4.

Imaging studies

A straightened cervical spine with a Cobb angle of 13.4° from C2 through C7; Pavlov ratio above 75%, and a K-line (−) OPLL of C2 through C4 (Fig. 3.38.1).

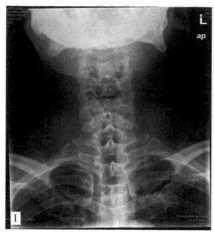
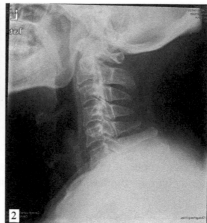

FIGURE 3.38.1

Preoperative X-ray of the cervical spine.
(1) Anteroposterior view.
(2) Lateral view.

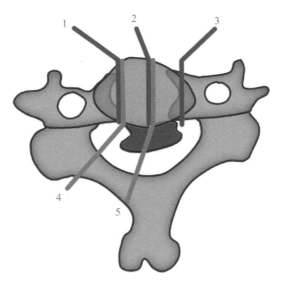

Reference of the sagittal planes

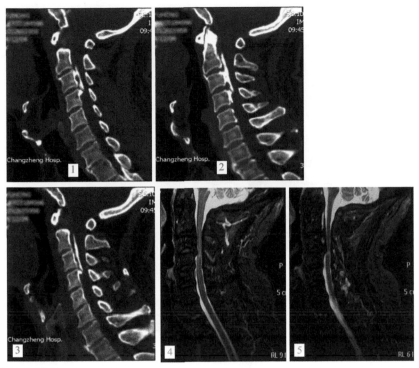

FIGURE 3.38.2

Preoperative sagittal images of the cervical spine and their reference on the axial diagram.

(1) Right parasagittal CT.
(2) Midsagittal CT.
(3) Left parasagittal CT.
(4) Midsagittal MRI.
(5) Left parasagittal MRI.

Preoperative sagittal CT images: OPLL from C2 to C4 with gaps from the C2 vertebra (Fig. 3.38.2, panel 1 to 3). Preoperative sagittal MR images: spinal cord compression from C2 to C4, more severe at C3/4 with intramedullary signal hyper-intensity suggesting myelopathy (Fig. 3.38.2, panel 4 and 5).

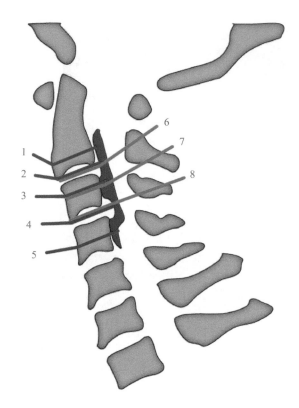

Reference of the axial planes

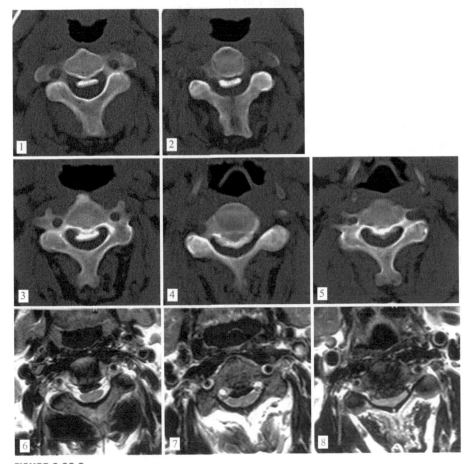

FIGURE 3.38.3

Preoperative axial images of the cervical spine and their reference on the sagittal diagram.
(1) Axial CT of C2.
(2) Axial CT of C2/3.
(3) Axial CT of C3.
(4) Axial CT of C3/4.
(5) Axial CT of C4.
(6) Axial MRI of C2/3.
(7) Axial MRI of C3/4.
(8) Axial MRI of C4/5.

Based on preoperative axial CT images, the OPLL is wide-based and larger at C4/5. It measures:4.5 mm thick (anteroposterior), 14.3 mm wide (mediolateral), and 35% in canal occupancy at C2; 5.1 mm thick, 14.8 mm wide, and 54% in canal occupancy at C2/3; 6 mm thick, 15.1 mm wide, and 49% in canal occupancy at

C3 where double-layer sign is present; 5.5 mm thick, 20.3 mm wide, and 57% in canal occupancy at C3/4; and 3.1 mm thick, 10.5 mm wide, and 27.4% in canal occupancy at C4 (Fig. 3.38.3, panel 1 to 5).

Based on preoperative axial MR images, compressed spinal cord in the shape of triangle or boomerang at C2 to C3/4 with ill-defined intramedullary hyperintensity (Fig. 3.38.3, Figs. 6—8).

Highlights

This case features mixed-type OPLL from C2 to C4 that is wide-based at C3/4 and double-layered at C3.

Surgical planning

In three-segment K-line (+) OPLL that extends into the upper cervical spine, as in this case, indirect decompression via a posterior surgery achieves adequate decompression among the conventional strategies.

An ACAF with antedisplacement of C3 to C4 with shelter technique on C2 was planned for this patient.

As the curvature correction amplifies the decompression, the anterior resection shall measure thinner than the OPLL thickness (Fig. 3.38.4).

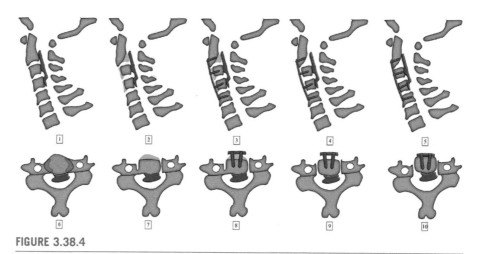

FIGURE 3.38.4

Illustration of the surgical plan on sagittal and axial planes.

(1, 6) Illustration of the OPLL on sagittal and axial views before surgery.

(2, 7) Resection performed to the anterior part of C3 to C4 vertebral bodies and the posteroinferior part of C2 vertebra; a complete trough developed on the left vertebral bodies from C3 to C4 while a half one made on the right side with the posterior bone yet to be dissected.

(3, 8) Plate and screws placed on vertebral bodies from C2 through C5.

(4, 9) The bottom of the right half-groove on C3 and C4 dissected.

(5, 10) Antedisplaced C3 and C4 vertebral bodies as screws were tightened.

Results

Postoperative function: JOA score was 13, Nurick score: 1, VAS: 2, and NDI: 8.

Instrumentation from C2 to C5, and antedisplaced C3 to C4 vertebral bodies (Fig. 3.38.5).

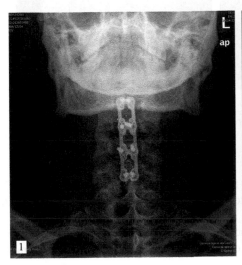
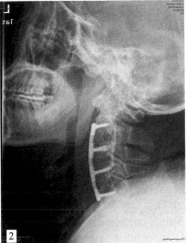

FIGURE 3.38.5

Postoperative cervical spine X-ray.
(1) Anteroposterior view.
(2) Lateral view.

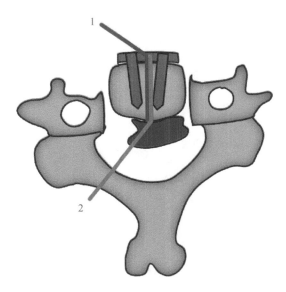

Reference of the sagittal planes

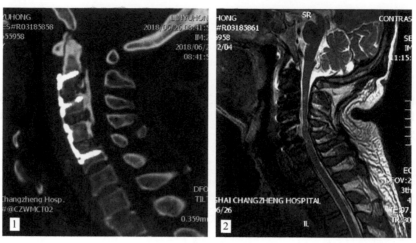

FIGURE 3.38.6

Postoperative sagittal views and their reference on the axial diagram.
(1) Midsagittal CT.
(2) Midsagittal MRI.

Ventrally displaced VOC from C3 to C4, and decompression of the level of C2 via a shelter technique shown on postoperative midsagittal CT image (Fig. 3.38.6, panel 1).

Spinal cord free of compression and surrounded by CSF, with residual compression associated curvature shown on postoperative midsagittal MR image (Fig. 3.38.6, panel 2).

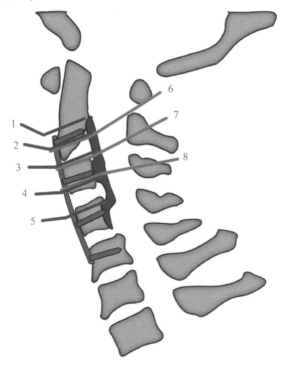

Reference of the axial planes

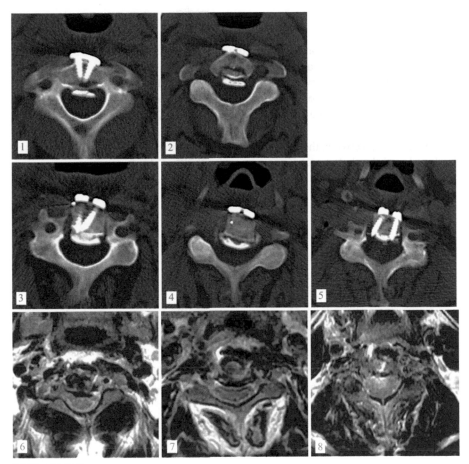

FIGURE 3.38.7

Postoperative axial cervical images and their reference on the sagittal diagram.

(1) Axial CT of C1.

(2) Axial CT of C2.

(3) Axial CT of C2/3.

(4) Axial CT of C3.

(5) Axial CT of the superior surface of C4.

(6) Axial MRI of C2.

(7) Axial MRI of C2/3.

(8) Axial MRI of C3.

The vertebral bodies have been dissected with parasagittal cuts on both sides 14.4 mm apart at C2 and 20.5 mm apart at C3 to C4, and antedisplaced by 4.3 mm, and the canal occupancy reduced to 19% as shown on postoperative axial CT image (Fig. 3.38.7, panel 1 to 5).

It has recovered to an oval and triangular shape, surrounded by an ample amount of CSF as shown on postoperative axial CT image (Fig. 3.38.7, panel 6 to 8).

Discussion

Can adequate decompression be achieved with antedisplacement of C3? What were the reasons for a two-level antedisplacement?

According to preoperative imaging studies, the OPLL was adhered to the C3 vertebra but not C2 or C4 vertebra, where gaps existed between them. As the lesion involved less than half of the vertebral height at C2 and C4, their posterior part could be undercut.

Given the gap between the lesion and the C4 vertebra, both C3 and C4 were antedisplaced, and the shelter technique was performed to C2 only.

Case 39: Cervical spinal stenosis and ossification of posterior longitudinal ligament (At C4 to C5)

Index terms

Antedisplacement of two vertebral bodies.

History

Patient: A 53-year-old man.

Chief complaint: Numbness of the right lower limb for four months with aggravation and numbness and weakness of both hands for one month.

Physical exam: Physical exam was noted for gait instability, straightened cervical spine, limited range of cervical motion, and impaired fine movements. Muscle strength was tested at 4+/5 on bilateral deltoid, biceps and triceps brachii, wrist flexion and extension, hand grips, iliopsoas, quadriceps femoris, biceps femoris, semitendinosus, semimembranosus, anterior tibialis, triceps surae, and dorsal and plantar flexion. Brisk tendon reflexes were noted on the knee and ankle bilaterally. The patient reported pain on the right upon straight leg raise (SLR) and dorsiflexion trigger. Hoffmann sign was positive on the left side.

Preoperative function: JOA score was 10, Nurick score: 3, VAS: 1, and NDI: 13.

Imaging studies

A straightened cervical spine with Cobb angle of 7.1° from C2 through C7; Pavlov ratio of 68% at C4, and K-line (+) OPLL posterior to C5 and C6 (Fig. 3.39.1).

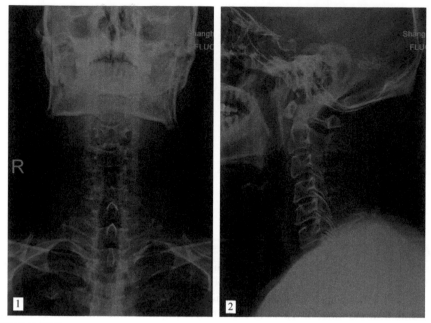

FIGURE 3.39.1

Preoperative X-ray of the cervical spine.
(1) Anteroposterior view.
(2) Lateral view.

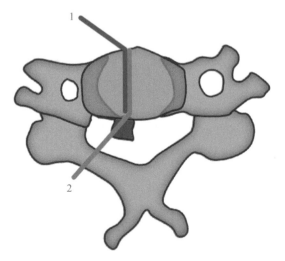

Reference of the sagittal planes

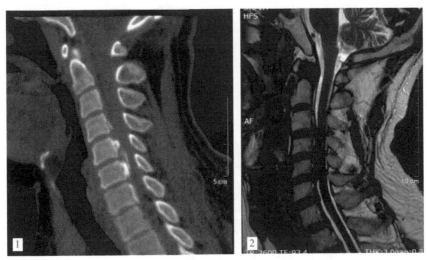

FIGURE 3.39.2

Preoperative sagittal images of the cervical spine and their reference on the axial diagram.
(1) Midsagittal CT.
(2) Midsagittal MRI.

A flat-type and small OPLL posterior to the C5 vertebra shown on midsagittal CT image (Fig. 3.39.2, panel 1).

A straightened spinal cord compressed at C4 to C5/6, in particular at C5/6 shown on midsagittal CT image (Fig. 3.39.2, panel 2).

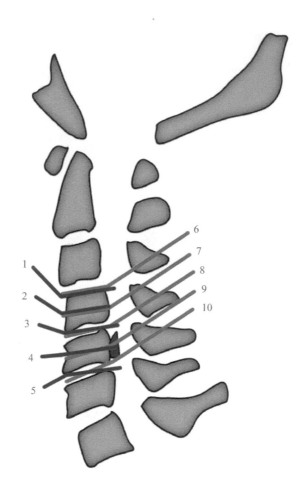

Reference of the axial planes

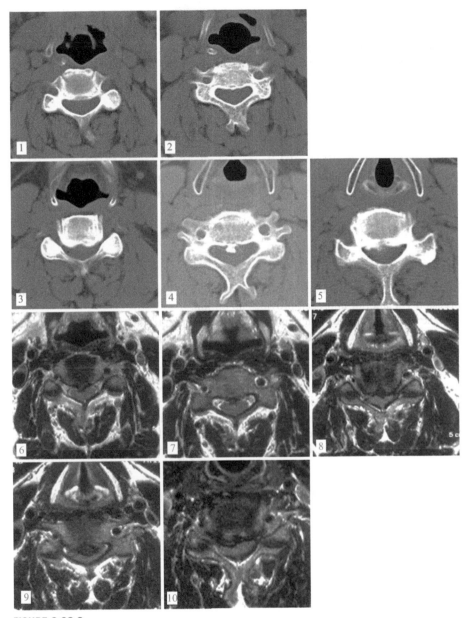

FIGURE 3.39.3

Preoperative axial images of the cervical spine and their reference on the sagittal diagram.
(1) Axial CT of C3/4.
(2) Axial CT of C4.
(3) Axial CT of C4/5.

Based on preoperative axial CT images, the ossification measures 4 mm thick (anteroposterior), 6 mm wide (mediolateral), and 36.4% in canal occupancy at C5 (Fig. 3.39.3, panel 1 to 5). Based on preoperative axial MR images, spinal cord deformed into boomerang and crescent shape, in particular at C4/5 to C5/6 (Fig. 3.39.3, panel 6 to 10).

Highlights

This case features developmental stenosis of the spinal canal at C4 to C5 complicated with a flat-type single-segment OPLL at C5 and intervertebral disc herniation at C3/4 to C5/6. Spinal cord compression was more prominent at the interspace levels.

Surgical planning

In cases with concomitant disc herniation and short-segment OPLL, a direct decompression via anterior approach provides an option.

The ACDF technique can manage compression due to interspace herniation but not ossification posterior to the C5 vertebra. An alternative among the conventional strategies is ACCF with C4 and C5 corpectomy that decompresses the spinal canal and removes the impinging interspace material.

An ACAF with antedisplacement of C4 and C5 was planned for this case with developmental canal stenosis superimposed with OPLL and secondary stenosis.

As the curvature correction via contoured plate provides extra decompression in a straightened cervical spine, the anterior resection shall measure thinner than the OPLL thickness (Fig. 3.39.4).

---

(4) Axial CT of C5.
(5) Axial CT of C5/6.
(6) Axial MRI of C3/4.
(7) Axial MRI of C4.
(8) Axial MRI of C4/5.
(9) Axial MRI of C5.
(10) Axial MRI of C5/6.

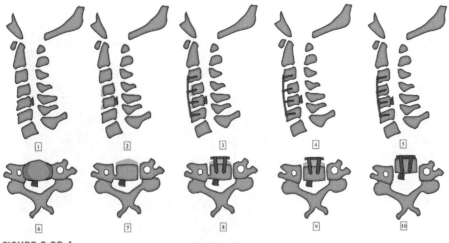

FIGURE 3.39.4

Illustration of the surgical plan on sagittal and axial planes.

(1, 6) Illustration of the OPLL on sagittal and axial views before surgery.

(2, 7) Resection performed to the anterior part of C4 to C5 vertebral bodies, a complete trough developed on the left vertebral bodies from C4 to C5 while a half one is made on the right side with the posterior bone yet to be dissected.

(3, 8) Plate and screws placed on vertebral bodies from C3 through C6.

(4, 9) The bottom of the right half-groove on C4 through C5 dissected.

(5, 10) Antedisplaced C4 to C5 vertebral bodies as screws were tightened.

Results

Postoperative function: JOA score was 15, Nurick score: 1, VAS: 1, and NDI: 7.

Improved curvature of cervical spine with a Cobb angle of 22.3° from C2 to C7, and antedisplaced C4 to C5 vertebral bodies (Fig. 3.39.5).

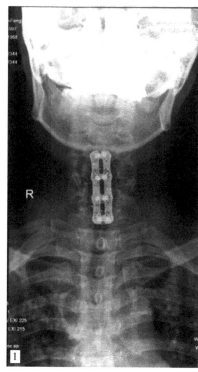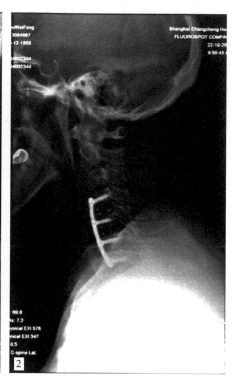

FIGURE 3.39.5

Postoperative cervical spine X-ray.
(1) Anteroposterior view.
(2) Lateral view.

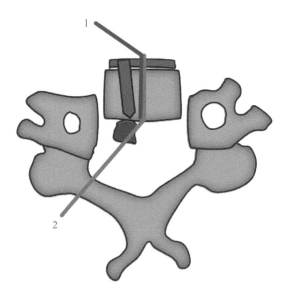

Reference of the sagittal planes

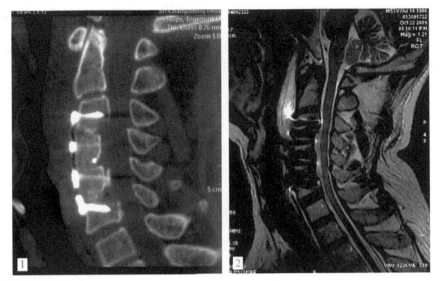

FIGURE 3.39.6

Postoperative sagittal cervical images and their reference on the axial diagram.

(1) Midsagittal CT.

(2) Midsagittal MRI.

Antedisplaced C4 to C5 vertebral bodies and expanded spinal canal shown on postoperative midsagittal CT image (Fig. 3.39.6, panel 1).

Lordotic spinal cord free of compression and surrounded by CSF shown on postoperative midsagittal MR image (Fig. 3.39.6, panel 2).

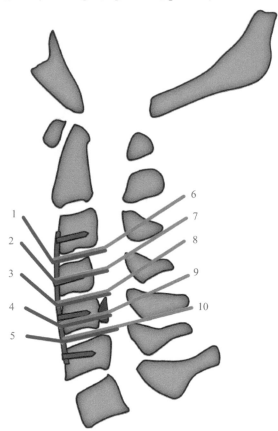

Reference of the axial planes

The vertebral bodies have been dissected with parasagittal cuts on both sides 24 mm apart and antedisplaced by 7 mm, and the canal occupancy reduced to 0%, as shown on postoperative axial CT images (Fig. 3.39.7, panel 1 to 5).

It has recovered to an oval shape, surrounded by an ample amount of CSF, as shown on postoperative axial MR images (Fig. 3.39.7, panel 6 to 10).

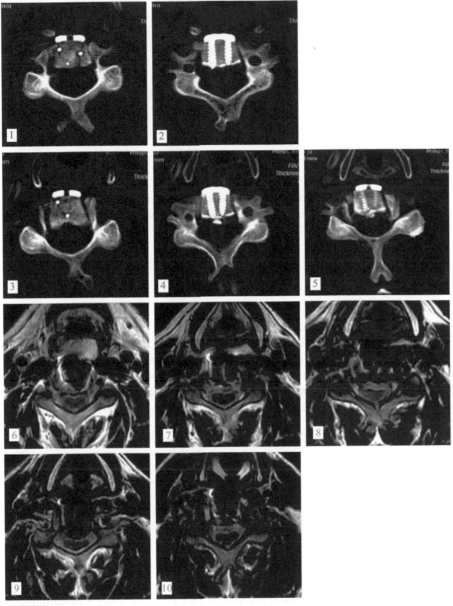

FIGURE 3.39.7

Postoperative axial cervical images and their reference on the sagittal diagram.

(1) Axial CT of C3/4.
(2) Axial CT of C4.
(3) Axial CT of C4/5.
(4) Axial CT of C5.
(5) Axial CT of C5/6.
(6) Axial MRI of C3/4.
(7) Axial MRI of C4.
(8) Axial MRI of C4/5.
(9) Axial MRI of C5.
(10) Axial MRI of C5/6.

Case 40: Cervical trauma and ossification of posterior longitudinal ligament (OPLL) (At C3 to C5)

Index terms

Antedisplacement of one vertebra, continuous OPLL, wide-based disease, C6 ~ C7 interspinous cerclage, undercutting, the thickness of ossification 6 mm, and canal occupancy of 55%.

History

Patient: A 53-year-old man.

Chief complaint: Numbness of the extremities for 18 months and weakness of limbs and gait instability for two months.

Physical exam: Physical exam was noted for gait disturbance, decreased sense of pinprick and temperature on the right hand and right lower limb, and hypertonic upper limbs. Muscle strength was tested at 4/5 on both upper limbs. Hyperreflexia of bilateral biceps brachii, brachioradialis, and both lower limbs. Hoffmann sign was present on both sides.

Preoperative function: JOA score was 8, Nurick score: 3, VAS: 0, and NDI: 12.

Imaging studies

Highlights

This case features a short-segment continuous OPLL from C3 to C5 superimposed with C6 and C7 interspinous cerclage due to trauma-related segmental instability. The OPLL is adhered to the C4 vertebra but not C3 or C5.

Surgical planning

Conventionally, a short-segment OPLL in a straightened cervical spine can be managed with ACCF for direct cord decompression and curvature restoration.

A straightened cervical spine with Cobb angle of 4.2° from C2 through C7; Pavlov ratio of 57%, 62%, and 67% at C3, C4, and C5, respectively; a K-line (+) OPLL at C3—C4; and posterior instrumentation between C6 and C7 (Fig. 3.40.1).

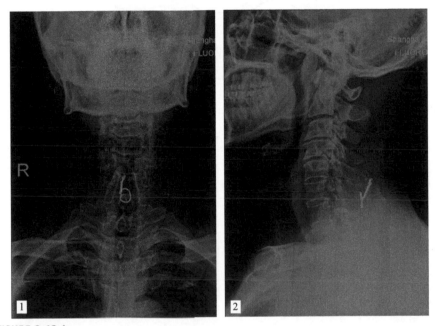

FIGURE 3.40.1

Preoperative X-ray of the cervical spine.
(1) Anteroposterior view.
(2) Lateral view.

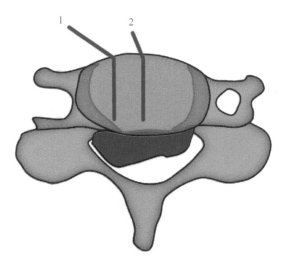

Reference of the sagittal planes

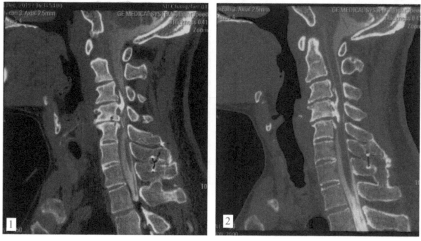

FIGURE 3.40.2

Preoperative sagittal images of the cervical spine and their reference on the axial diagram.

(1) Right parasagittal CT.

(2) Midsagittal CT.

Preoperative CT: A continuous OPLL from C3 to C5. The OPLL adheres to the C4 vertebra and extends caudally and cephalad without attachment on C3 or C5 vertebral bodies (Fig. 3.40.2, panel 1 and 2).

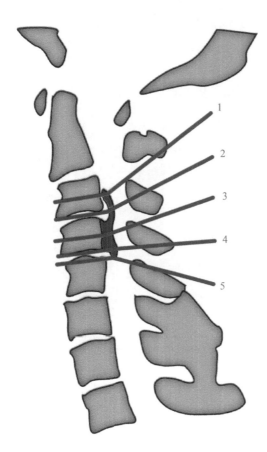

Reference of the axial planes

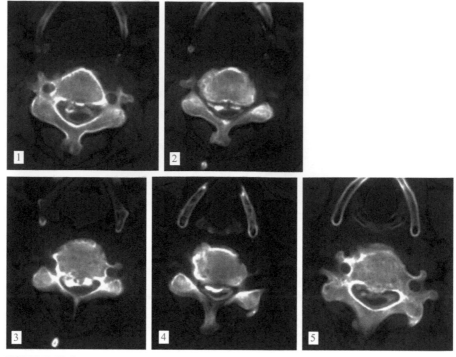

FIGURE 3.40.3

Preoperative axial images of the cervical spine and their reference on the sagittal diagram.
(1) Axial CT of C3.
(2) Axial CT of C3/4.
(3) Axial CT of C4.
(4) Axial CT of C4/5.
(5) Axial CT of the superior surface of C5.

The OPLL is wide-based at C3/5 to C4. It measures 5 mm thick (anteroposterior), 15.8 mm wide (mediolateral), and 55.6% in canal occupancy at C3; 4 mm thick, 18.2 mm wide, and 47% in canal occupancy at C3/4; 6 mm thick, 17.9 mm wide, and 55% in canal occupancy at C4; 3 mm thick, 15 mm wide, and 32% in canal occupancy at C4/5; and 2.7 mm thick, 6.3 mm wide, and 30% in canal occupancy at C5 (Fig. 3.40.3, panel 1 to 5) (Fig. 3.40.4).

In considering the resection levels, given that the OPLL involves half the C3 vertebral height but less than that at C5, the resection should involve at least C3 and C4.

Decompression of the residual lesion lateral to the bone cuts may be needed in an ACCF procedure because of the wide-based component at C3 to C3/4.

An ACAF with C4 antedisplacement and undercutting of the posterior part of C3 and C5 vertebral bodies were planned for this patient.

For the prolapsed disc space at C3/4 and C4/5 documented on preoperative imaging studies, during intervertebral preparation, the inferior endplate of C3 and the superior endplate of C5 were removed for enhanced visualization.

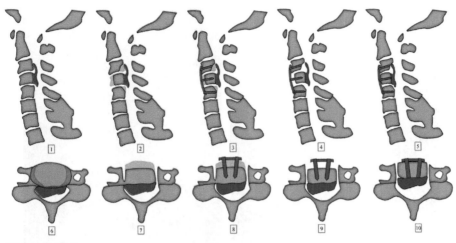

FIGURE 3.40.4

Illustration of the surgical plan on sagittal and axial planes.

(1, 6) Illustration of the OPLL on sagittal and axial views before surgery.

(2, 7) Resection performed to the anterior part of C4 vertebra, the posteroinferior part of C3 vertebra, and the posterosuperior part of C5 vertebra; a complete trough developed on the left of the C4 vertebra while a half one on the right side with the posterior bone yet to be dissected.

(3, 8) Plate and screws placed on vertebral bodies from C3 through C4.

(4, 9) The bottom of the right half-groove on C4 dissected.

(5, 10) Antedisplaced C4 vertebra as screws were tightened.

Results

Postoperative function: JOA score was 8, Nurick score: 3, VAS: 3, and NDI: 15.

Discussion

What are the values of ACAF in this case?

This case features a continuous OPLL adhered to C4 but not C3 or C5. The OPLL had extended to these two levels by less than half the vertebral height with gaps with the vertebra.

If ACCF, one of the conventional options, is performed, C4 corpectomy alone may not yield decompression at C3 and C5, in particular for C3. To obtain thorough decompression, the ACCF should involve more than C4 alone.

In contrast, decompression posterior to C3 and C5 vertebral bodies can be obtained via undercutting in the ACAF technique. In other words, the antedisplacement of C4 alone provides decompression of the two adjacent levels as well, and ACAF allows for better motion preservation.

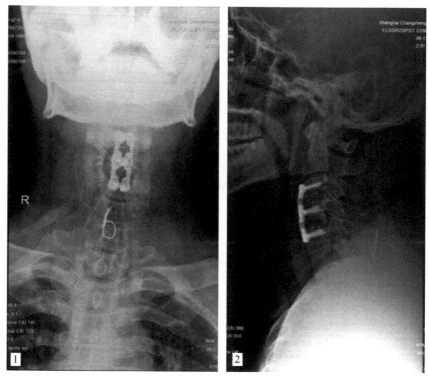

FIGURE 3.40.5

Postoperative cervical spine X-ray.
(1) Anteroposterior view.
(2) Lateral view.

Improved cervical curvature, Cobb angle of 14.9° from C2 to C7, antedisplaced C4 vertebra, and instrumentation from C3 to C5 (Fig. 3.40.5).

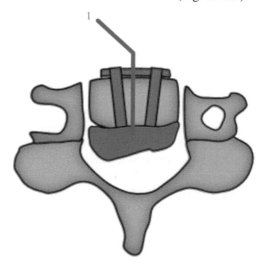

Reference of the sagittal planes

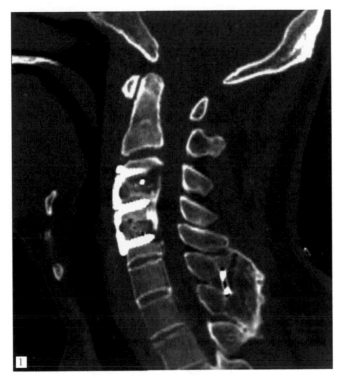

FIGURE 3.40.6

Postoperative sagittal cervical images and their reference on the axial diagram.
(1) Midsagittal CT.

Ventrally displaced VOC of C4, undercutting posterior part of C3 and C5 vertebral bodies, and expanded spinal canal shown on postoperative midsagittal CT image (Fig. 3.40.6, panel 1).

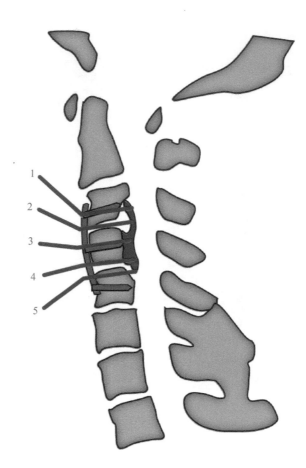

Reference of the axial planes

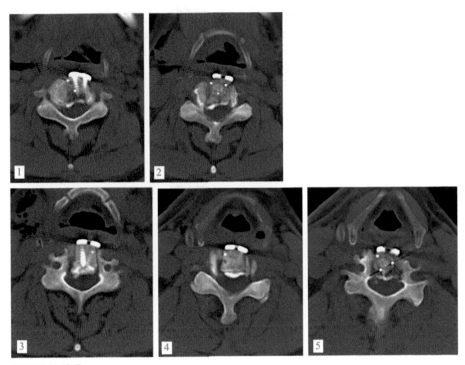

FIGURE 3.40.7

Postoperative axial cervical images and their reference on the sagittal diagram.
(1) Axial CT of C3.
(2) Axial CT of C3/4.
(3) Axial CT of C4.
(4) Axial CT of C4/5.
(5) Axial CT of the superior surface of C5.

The vertebral bodies have been dissected with parasagittal cuts on both sides 21 mm apart and antedisplaced by 5 mm, and the canal occupancy reduced to 20.3% at C3 as shown on postoperative axial CT image (Fig. 3.40.7, panel 1 to 5).

Discussion

For such cases with spinal canal stenosis, how ACAF is compared with ACCF?

In this case, the spinal canal stenosis had a predominant developmental component with little contribution from the OPLL.

In developmental stenosis, both ACCF and ACAF achieve decompression via expanding the anterior room of the spinal canal. In ACCF, specifically, given the absent anterior wall of the spinal canal, there is a restriction on the width between the bone cuts on both sides in case of an excessive anterior shift of the spinal cord.

In contrast, the anterior wall of the spinal canal is preserved in ACAF, serving as a barrier for the anterior shift of the spinal cord. Also, the bilateral bone cuts can be wider apart, facilitating a thorough decompression.

Since more bone stock is preserved in ACAF than ACCF, a fusion-related complication occurs less often in ACAF.

Case 41: Ossification of posterior longitudinal ligament (OPLL) of cervical spine (At C3 to C5)

Index terms

Antedisplacement of two vertebra, continuous ossification of the posterior longitudinal ligament (OPLL), wide-based disease, undercutting, the thickness of ossification 7–9 mm, and canal occupancy of 50%–60%.

History

Patient: A 55-year-old woman.

Chief complaint: Weakness of all the extremities for eight months.

Physical exam: Physical exam was noted for gait instability; impaired tactile sensation on the trunk; hypermyotonia of four extremities. Muscle strength was tested at 4-/5 on upper limbs and 4/5 on lower limbs; tendon hyperreflexia and bilateral Hoffmann sign (+).

Preoperative function: Japanese Orthopedic Association (JOA) score was 6, Nurick score: 4, visual analog scale (VAS): 0, and neck disability index (NDI): 25.

Imaging studies

A straightened cervical spine with Cobb angle of 5.4° from C2 through C7; a K-line (+) OPLL spanning from C3 to C5 (Fig. 3.41.1).

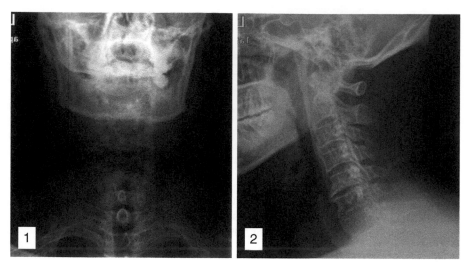

FIGURE 3.41.1

Preoperative cervical X-ray.
(1) Anteroposterior image.
(2) Lateral image.

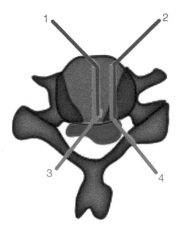

Location maps of the sagittal planes

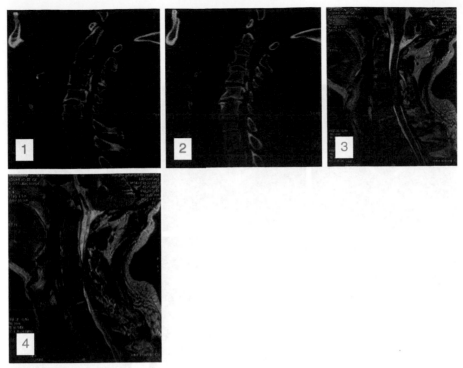

FIGURE 3.41.2

Preoperative sagittal images and their location maps on axial diagram.
(1) Midsagittal CT.
(2) Left parasagittal CT.
(3) Midsagittal MRI.
(4) Left parasagittal MRI.

Shown on sagittal computerized tomography (CT) images, a continuous-type OPLL from C3 to C5 that most serious at the level of C4/5 (Fig. 3.41.2, panel 1 and 2).

Shown on sagittal magnetic resonance (MR) images, the spinal cord was compressed at C3/4 ~ C5/6, with the curvature straight. The compression was focused on the C3/4 and C4/5 intervertebral spaces, and the intramedullary signal changes were seen at the corresponding segments (Fig. 3.41.2, panel 3 and 4).

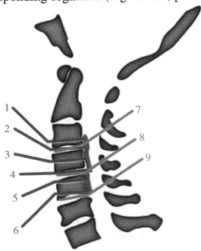

Location maps of the axial planes

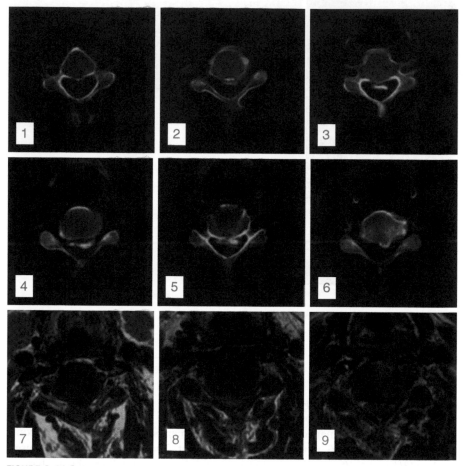

FIGURE 3.41.3

Preoperative axial images of the cervical spine and their location maps on the sagittal diagram.

(1) Axial CT of C3.
(2) Axial CT of C3/4.
(3) Axial CT of C4.
(4) Axial CT of C4/5.
(5) Axial CT of the superior part of C5.
(6) Axial CT of the inferior part of C5.
(7) Axial MRI of C3/4.
(8) Axial MRI of C4/5.
(9) Axial MRI of C5/6.

Shown on axial **CT** images, the ossified mass featured wide-based at C4/5 and measured 4.5 mm thick (anteroposterior), 13.9 mm wide (mediolateral), and 34.9% in canal occupancy at C3/4 with double-layer sign present; 8 mm thick, 20.9 mm wide, and 57.6% in canal occupancy at C4/5 (Fig. 3.41.3, panel 1 to 6).

The axial preoperative MRI: Spinal cord was compressed and deformed with intramedullary signal changes at C4/5; at C3/4, the cord was not completely compressed, and cerebrospinal fluid (CSF) signals were still visible around the spinal cord (Fig. 3.41.3, panel 7 to 9).

Highlights

This case features short-level continuous-type OPLL from C3 to C5 and wide-based lesion at C4/5 with double-layer sign at C3/4 and C5.

Surgical planning

This case features a K-line (+), short-level OPLL in a straightened cervical spine, which is suited for anterior decompression. However, the ossified mass charactered wide base and the existence of double-layer sign. These characters are relevant to the risk of incomplete decompression and dural injury.

The patient received anterior controllable antedisplacement fusion (ACAF) with antedisplacement from C4 to C5 for spinal cord decompression.

Given the impaired curvature of OPLL, lordosis correction was utilized to gain extra room for decompression and preserve bone (Fig. 3.41.4).

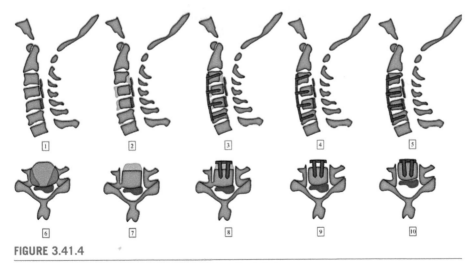

FIGURE 3.41.4

Illustration of the surgical plan on sagittal and axial planes.
(1, 6) Illustration of the ossification on sagittal and axial views before surgery.
(2, 7) Resection performed to the anterior part of C4 to C5 vertebral bodies and posterior inferior part of C3, a complete groove developed on the left vertebral bodies from C4 to C5 while a half one is made on the right side with the posterior cortical bone yet to be dissected.
(3, 8) Plate and screws placed on vertebral bodies from C3 through C6.
(4, 9) The bottom of the right half-groove on C4 through C5 dissected.
(5, 10) Antedisplaced C4 to C5 vertebral bodies as screws were tightened.

Results

Postoperative functional score: JOA score was 12, Nurick score: 3, VAS: 0, and NDI: 23.

Corrected cervical curvature, Cobb angle of 24.4° from C2 to C7, instrumentation from C3 to C6, and antedisplaced C4 to C5 (Fig. 3.41.5).

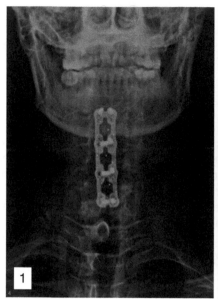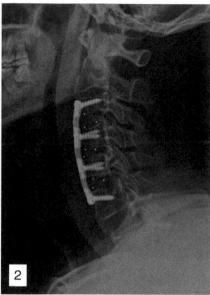

FIGURE 3.41.5

Postoperative cervical X-ray.
(1) Anteroposterior image.
(2) Lateral image.

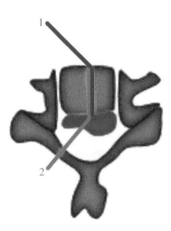

Location maps of the sagittal planes

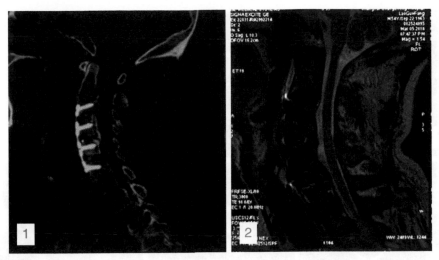

FIGURE 3.41.6

Postoperative sagittal images and their location maps on axial diagram.
(1) Midsagittal CT.
(2) Midsagittal MRI.

Ventrally displaced vertebral-OPLL complex (VOC) from C4 to C5 with the spinal canal enlarged shown on postoperative midsagittal CT image (Fig. 3.41.6, panel 1).

Satisfactory decompression of spinal cord, recovery of spinal cord curvature, and anterior and posterior CSF band shown on postoperative midsagittal MR image (Fig. 3.41.6, panel 2).

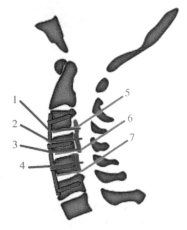

Location maps of the axial planes

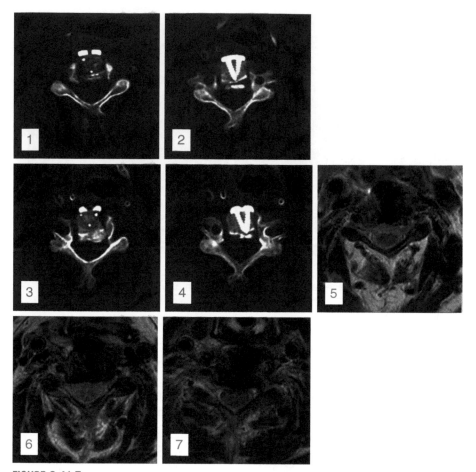

FIGURE 3.41.7

Postoperative axial images of the cervical spine and their location maps on the sagittal diagram.

(1) Axial CT of C3/4.
(2) Axial CT of C4.
(3) Axial CT of C4/5.
(4) Axial CT of C5.
(5) Axial MRI of C3/4.
(6) Axial MRI of C4/5.
(7) Axial MRI of C5/6.

As shown on postoperative axial CT images, the VOCs have been dissected with parasagittal grooves on both sides, 21.4 mm apart, and antedisplaced by 6.8 mm. The OR reduced to 0% (Fig. 3.41.7, panel 1 to 4). The spinal cord resumes its oval shape with normal CSF around it, as shown on postoperative axial MRI images (Fig. 3.41.7, panel 5 to 7).

Discussion

How to choose antedisplaced segments?

This case is the first application of undercutting technique in ACAF. As the involved segment in this patient was short, the main compression was located at C4–C5 without compression behind the C3/4 intervertebral space. We made the following preoperative planning for the operation.

Antedisplaced C4 and C5 and dissected the ossified mass at C3/4 intervertebral space. There are few segments involved in operation, but transecting ossification needs to separate between ossification and dura, which increases the risk of operation. Although hosting C3–C5 vertebrae decompressed all ossified segments completely, there was no compression behind C3, so the operative segment was too long. We utilized the undercutting technique. The VOC at the level of C4 and C5 was dissociated with the posterior lower edge of C3 resected, so the ossified mass at level of C3/4 moved forward together. In this way, the leakage of CSF caused by transverse ossification can be avoided, and the cervical motion also preserved.

Case 42: Ossification of posterior longitudinal ligament (OPLL) of cervical spine (At C3 to C5)

Index terms

Circumscribed (localized) OPLL.

History

Patient: A 49-year-old man.

Chief complaint: Weakness of all the extremities and numbness of the upper limbs for six months that aggravated over the past 20 days.

Physical exam: Physical exam was noted for gait instability; straightened cervical spine; mildly limited range of cervical motion; impaired tactile and pinprick sensation on the hands and lower extremities, worse in the left; an impaired sense of temperature over the right extremity and the right trunk below the costal arch; and reduced fine movements. Muscle strength was tested at 4/5 on bilateral deltoid, biceps and triceps brachii, wrist flexion and extension, hand grips, iliopsoas, quadriceps femoris, biceps femoris, semitendinosus, semimembranosus, anterior tibialis, triceps surae, and dorsal and plantar flexion. Hyperreflexic radiobrachialis was documented.

Preoperative function: JOA score was 12, Nurick score: 3, VAS: 0, and NDI: 13.

Imaging studies

A lordotic cervical spine with Cobb angle of 9.2° from C2 through C7; Pavlov ratio above 75%; and a K-line (+) OPLL from C3 to C5 (Fig. 3.42.1).

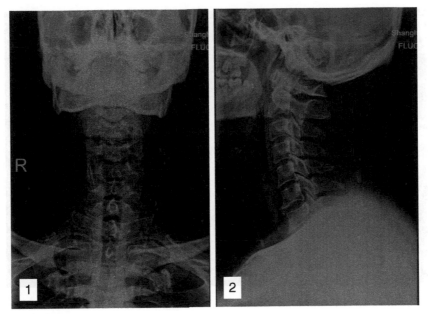

FIGURE 3.42.1

Preoperative X-ray of the cervical spine.
(1) Anteroposterior view.
(2) Lateral view.

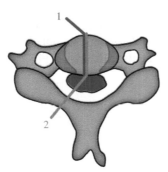

Reference of the sagittal planes

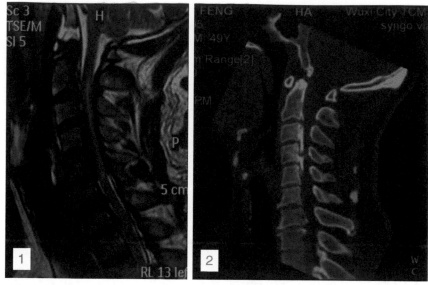

FIGURE 3.42.2

Preoperative sagittal images and their reference on axial diagram.
(1) Midsagittal CT.
(2) Midsagittal MRI.

A flat- and mixed-type OPLL from C3 to C5 shown on postoperative midsagittal CT image (Fig. 3.42.2, panel 1).

Compression at C2/3 to C5/6 along the straightened spinal cord due to anterior hypointense indentation, and widened intramedullary central canal from C2 to C5/6 shown on postoperative midsagittal MR image (Fig. 3.42.2, panel 2) (Fig. 3.42.3).

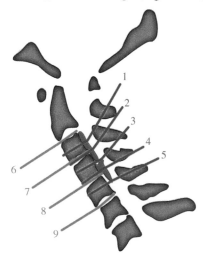

Reference of the axial planes

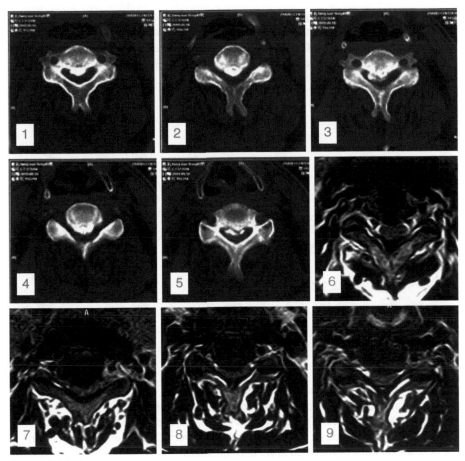

FIGURE 3.42.3

Preoperative axial images of the cervical spine and their reference on the sagittal diagram.

(1) Axial CT of C3.
(2) Axial CT of C3/4.
(3) Axial CT of C4.
(4) Axial CT of C4/5.
(5) Axial CT of C5.
(6) Axial MRI of C2/3.
(7) Axial MRI of C3/4.
(8) Axial MRI of C4/5.
(9) Axial MRI of C5/6.

Shown on axial CT images, the OPLL, narrow-based and double-layered at C4 and C5, measures: 5 mm thick (anteroposterior), 13 mm wide (mediolateral), and 40% in canal occupancy at C3; 6 mm thick, 15 mm wide, and 66.7% in canal occupancy at C4; and 5 mm thick, 15 mm wide, and 45.5% in canal occupancy at C5 (Fig. 3.42.4, panel 1 to 5).

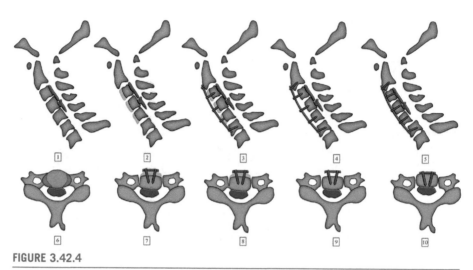

FIGURE 3.42.4

Illustration of the surgical plan on sagittal and axial planes.
(1, 6) Illustration of the OPLL on sagittal and axial views before surgery.
(2, 7) Resection performed to the anterior part of C3, C4, and C5 vertebral bodies; a complete trough developed on the left vertebral bodies from C3 to C5 while a half one on the right side with the posterior bone yet to be dissected.
(3, 8) Plate and screws placed on vertebral bodies from C2 through C6.
(4, 9) The bottom of the right half-groove on C3, C4, and C5 dissected.
(5, 10) Antedisplaced C3, C4, and C5 vertebral bodies as screws were tightened.

Shown on axial MR images, a triangular or boomerang-shaped spinal cord due to indentation from C2/3 to C5/6 with intramedullary signal hyperintensity (Fig. 3.42.4, panel 6 to 10).

Highlights

This case features extensive ectopic ossification that involves the posterior longitudinal ligament from C3 to C5 and ligamentum flavum from T1/2 to T2/3, with OPLL of C3 to C5 being more compressive on the spinal cord. This OPLL is continuous and flat, with a double-layer sign at C5 and C6. Ectasia of the intramedullary central canal from C2 to C5/6 is documented.

Surgical planning

For a K-line (+) OPLL that spans three vertebral bodies, indirect decompression via a posterior procedure is an option. On the other hand, a posterior procedure comes with the risk of incomplete decompression as spinal canal stenosis had reached 60%.

An ACAF with antedisplacement of C3 to C5 was planned for this patient, where C5 was included in the antedisplacement since the OPLL had extended beyond half of the vertebra height.

Given the preserved physiological lordosis, room of decompression generated by curvature correction is less likely and an anterior part of the vertebrae of the same thickness as the ossification was resected.

Results

Postoperative function: JOA score was 15, Nurick score: 1, VAS: 0, and NDI: 116.

Corrected cervical curvature, Cobb angle of 16.8° from C2 to C7, instrumentation placed from C3 to C7, and antedisplaced C4 to C6 vertebral bodies (Fig. 3.42.5).

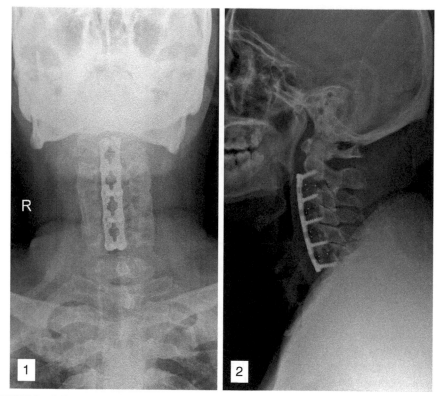

FIGURE 3.42.5

Postoperative cervical spine X-ray.
(1) Anteroposterior view.
(2) Lateral view.

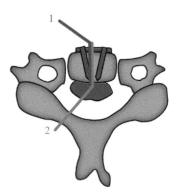

Reference of the sagittal planes

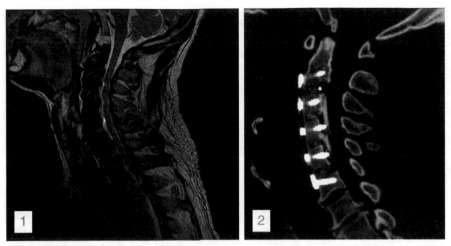

FIGURE 3.42.6

Postoperative sagittal views and their reference on the axial diagram.
(1) Midsagittal CT.
(2) Midsagittal MRI.

Ventrally displaced VOC from C3 to C5, and screw going through the posterior vertebral wall, shown on sagittal CT image (Fig. 3.42.6, panel 2).

Lordotic spinal cord free of compression and surrounded by CSF, and the ectasia of the intramedullary central canal reduced, shown on sagittal MR images (Fig. 3.42.6, panel 2).

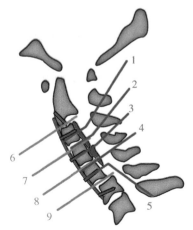

Reference of the axial planes

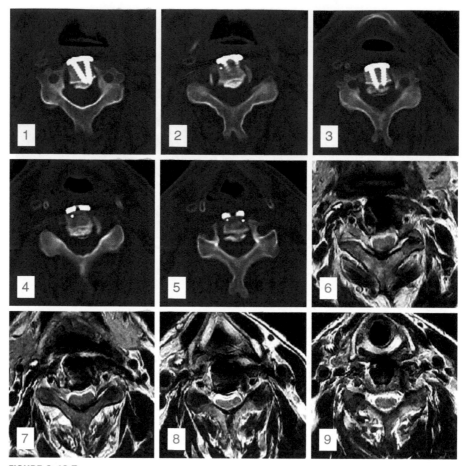

FIGURE 3.42.7

Postoperative axial cervical images and their reference on the sagittal diagram.
(1) Axial CT of C3.
(2) Axial CT of C3/4.
(3) Axial CT of C4.
(4) Axial CT of C4/5.
(5) Axial CT of C5.
(6) Axial MRI of C2/3.
(7) Axial MRI of C3/4.
(8) Axial MRI of C4/5.
(9) Axial MRI of C5/6.

The vertebral bodies have been dissected with parasagittal cuts on both sides 22 mm apart and antedisplaced by 5 mm, and the canal occupancy reduced to 20% at C4 where the ossification had been most severe before surgery shown on postoperative axial CT images (Fig. 3.42.7, panel 1 to 5).

It has recovered to an oval shape surrounded by an ample amount of CSF shown on postoperative midsagittal MR images (Fig. 3.42.7, panel 6 to 9).

Discussion

Screw going through the posterior wall of the vertebra may block the displacement of the VOC. How can we avoid this?

Postoperative CT images revealed that screws in C4 and C5 through the posterior wall of vertebral bodies and engaged with the ossification, gaps between the ossification and C4 and C5 increased from baseline and microfracture of the OPLL at C5.

Vertebral bodies not attached to the OPLL are usually overcut anteriorly. As such, the use of 14 mm or 16 mm screws easily results in posterior cortex penetration, and the screw tips block the further migration of the ossification, leading to incomplete VOC displacement.

What is worse, patients with a stenosed spinal canal may end up with dural tears. To avoid this adverse outcome, screw lengths are selected based on those in the upper and lower instrumented vertebrae after the VOC has contacted the plate.

Case 43: Cervical canal stenosis, history of cervical surgery

Index terms

Antedisplacement of three vertebral bodies, wide-based OPLL, canal occupancy ratio 50%—60%, status post-anterior cervical corpectomy and fusion (ACCF), and previous anterior surgery.

History

Patient: A 48-year-old man.

Chief complaint: Pain and numbness of the right upper limb for six months and status postanterior cervical surgery.

Physical exam: The patient walked with a steady gait. Other findings included a limited range of cervical motion; tenderness and pain on percussion on the spinous processes, interspinous space, and paraspinal areas across the cervical spine; impaired sense of light touch, pinprick, and temperature on the radial side of the forearm and the small finger of the right side. Muscle strength was tested at 4/5 on deltoid, biceps and triceps brachii, wrist flexion and extension, and hand grips on the right side.

Preoperative function: JOA score was 14, Nurick score: 1, VAS: 3, and NDI: 12.

Imaging studies

History of subtotal corpectomy and fusion of C6; lordotic cervical spine with Cobb angle of 18.8° from C2 through C7; segmental kyphosis from C5 to C7 with Cobb angle of −5.6°; partially pulled out the screw noticed at C7 level with gaps formed between the anterior wall of vertebral bodies and the plate (Fig. 3.43.1).

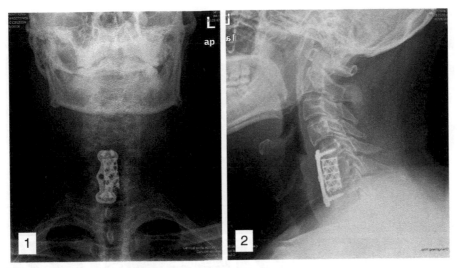

FIGURE 3.43.1

Preoperative X-ray of the cervical spine.
(1) Anteroposterior view.
(2) Lateral view.

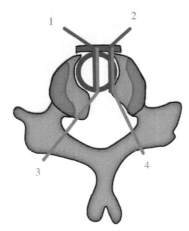

Reference of the sagittal planes

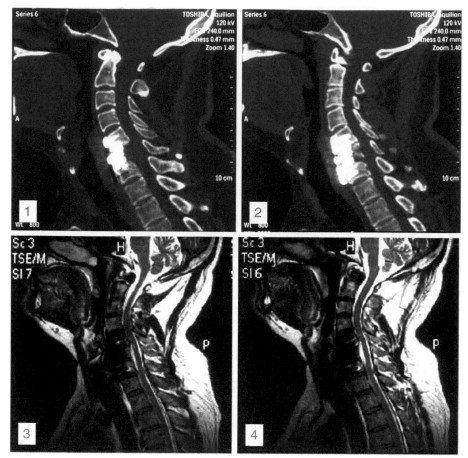

FIGURE 3.43.2

Preoperative sagittal images of the cervical spine and their reference on the axial diagram.

(1) Midsagittal CT.
(2) Left paramedian sagittal CT image.
(3) Midsagittal MRI.
(4) Left paramedian sagittal MRI image.

Shown on sagittal CT images, subtotal corpectomy of C6 performed accompanied with subsided mesh and dorsally displaced C5 vertebra (Fig. 3.43.2, panel 1 and 2). Shown on sagittal MR images, spinal cord featured the shape of "S," dorsally displaced C5 that violates the spinal canal, and compressed spinal cord (Fig. 3.43.2, panel 3 and 4).

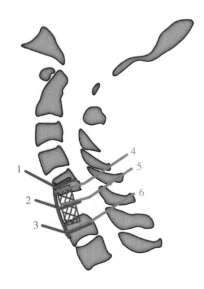

Reference of the axial planes

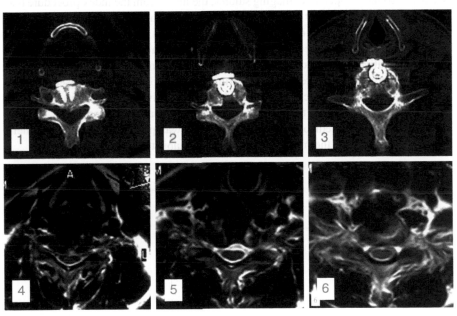

FIGURE 3.43.3

Preoperative axial images of the cervical spine and their reference on the sagittal diagram.

(1) Axial CT of C5.
(2) Axial CT of C6.
(3) Axial CT of C7.
(4) Axial MRI of C5.
(5) Axial MRI of C6.
(6) Axial MRI of C7.

Subtotal corpectomy has been performed on C6 where the width of resection is 12 mm, shown on axial CT images (Fig. 3.43.3, panel 1 to 3).

The spinal cord deformed into a triangular shape at C5, dots of intramedullary signal hyperintensity, and CSF effacement, shown on axial MR images (Fig. 3.43.3, panel 4 to 6).

Highlights

The patient had received ACCF for C6 due to "cervical myelopathy." The assessment performed in this admission revealed subsided mesh, posteriorly displaced and rotated C5 vertebra that violates the spinal canal, and neurological deficit due to cord compression.

Surgical planning

According to the preoperative imaging studies, the mesh from the index procedure had been well fused and difficult to remove. In conventional anterior revision surgery, the resection involves the bone on both sides of the vertebra and adjacent levels. Therefore, a reconstruction may come with the risk of fusion-related complications.

An alternative from the conventional procedures is indirect decompression via a posterior approach with screw-based instrumentation. Given the increased lordosis above C5, however, laminectomy may lead to an excessive posterior shift of the spinal cord, undue tension on the nerve roots, and nerve palsy development.

An ACAF with antedisplacement of C5 to C7 was planned for this case where screws are engaged in the mesh to provide extra stability (Fig. 3.43.4).

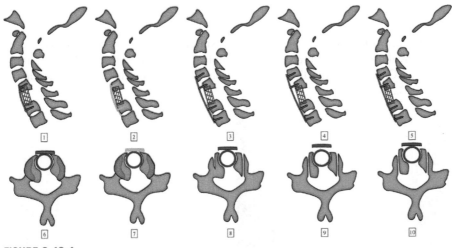

FIGURE 3.43.4

Illustration of the surgical plan on sagittal and axial planes.

(1, 6) Illustration of the OPLL on sagittal and axial views before surgery.

(2, 7) Removing the titanium plate and screw from the previous operation. Resection performed to the anterior part of C5 and C7 vertebral bodies, a complete trough developed on the left vertebral bodies from C5 to C7 while a half one on the right side with the posterior bone yet to be dissected.

(3, 8) Plate and screws placed on vertebral bodies from C3 through T1.

(4, 9) The bottom of the right half-groove on C5 through C7 dissected.

(5, 10) Antedisplaced C5 to C7 vertebral bodies as screws were tightened.

Results

Postoperative function: JOA score was 16, Nurick score: 1, VAS: 2, and NDI: 9.

Cervical spine in restored curvature, Cobb angle of 21.7° from C2 to C7, ante-displaced C5 to C7 within the titanium mesh, and well-positioned instrumentation (Fig. 3.43.5).

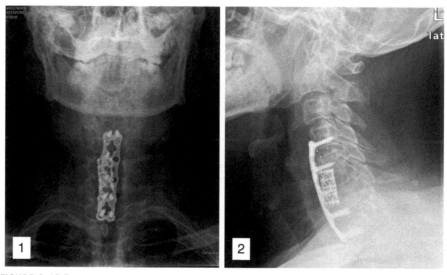

FIGURE 3.43.5

Postoperative cervical spine X-ray.
(1) Anteroposterior view.
(2) Lateral view.

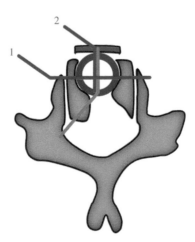

Reference of the sagittal planes

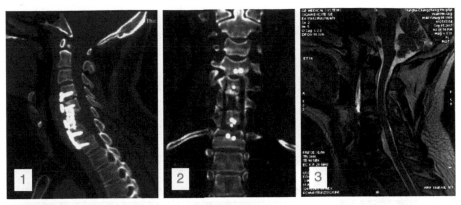

FIGURE 3.43.6

Postoperative sagittal and coronal views and their reference on the axial diagram.
(1) Midsagittal CT.
(2) Coronal CT.
(3) Midsagittal MRI.

Postoperative sagittal CT: Antedisplaced VOC from C5 to C7 and widened spinal canal shown on postoperative midsagittal CT image. Postoperative coronal CT showed that the decompressed width of ACCF was 14 mm and the width of ACAF was 20.4 mm (Fig. 3.43.6, panel 1 and 2).

Postoperative sagittal MRI: Spinal cord free of compression in restored lordosis (Fig. 3.43.6, panel 3).

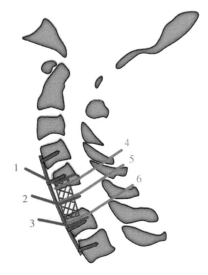

Reference of the axial planes

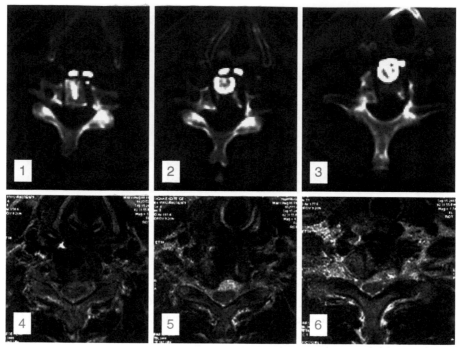

FIGURE 3.43.7

Postoperative axial cervical images and their reference on the sagittal diagram.
(1) Axial CT of C5.
(2) Axial CT of C6.
(3) Axial CT of C7.
(4) Axial MRI of C5.
(5) Axial MRI of C6.
(6) Axial MRI of C7.

Antedisplaced VOC of C5 to C7 by 4 mm by bilateral bony grooves of 20.8 mm. But left-deviated bone cuts on C6 and C7 shown on postoperative axial CT images (Fig. 3.43.7, panel 1 to 3).

At C5, in particular, the unimpinged spinal cord surrounded by CSF shown on postoperative axial MR images (Fig. 3.43.7, panel 4 to 6).

Discussion

What are the cautions during antedisplacement of the mesh in ACAF?

Screws are engaged in the mesh only through its openings. Therefore, little freedom existed for the position and angle of screw insertion, and a second screw may not be possible. Therefore, only one screw was used in the mesh for the antedisplacement.

Second, if two screws were inserted upon the completion of antedisplacement, they might converge and engage. Therefore, only one definitive screw was used on the mesh.

The relation between the mesh and the screw to be used was evaluated, in particular for a mesh with tight openings. If the screw does not seem to fit in the openings, the mesh is trimmed to allow for screw insertion.

Case 44: Cervical canal stenosis, history of cervical surgery

Index terms

Antedisplacement of two vertebral bodies, segmental OPLL, and history of anterior cervical surgery.

History

Patient: A 50-year-old man.

Chief complaint: Status postanterior cervical surgery, numbness and weakness of all the extremities, and tightness and stiffness of the trunk for one year.

Physical exam: Physical exam was noted for gait instability, reduced cervical lordosis, and a limited range of cervical motion. Muscle strength was tested at 3/5 on bilateral deltoid, biceps and triceps brachii; 3/5 on wrist flexion and extension, hand grips; 4/5 on iliopsoas, quadriceps femoris, biceps femoris, semitendinosus, semimembranosus, and anterior tibialis on both sides, triceps surae, dorsal and plantar flexion on both sides. Symmetrical brisk tendon reflexes were noted on bilateral biceps and triceps brachii, radiobrachialis, knee, and ankle. Hoffmann and Babinski signs were elicited on both sides.

Preoperative function: JOA score was 12, Nurick score: 2, VAS: 0, and NDI: 6.

Imaging studies

Instrumentation from C4 to C7 and Pavlov ratio of 69%, 70%, and 68% from C4 to C6 (Fig. 3.44.1).

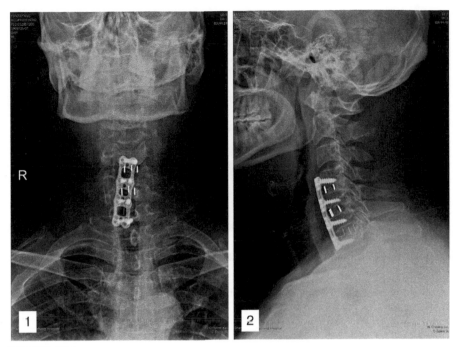

FIGURE 3.44.1

Preoperative X-ray of the cervical spine.
(1) Anteroposterior view.
(2) Lateral view.

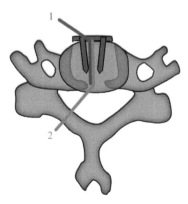

Reference of the sagittal planes

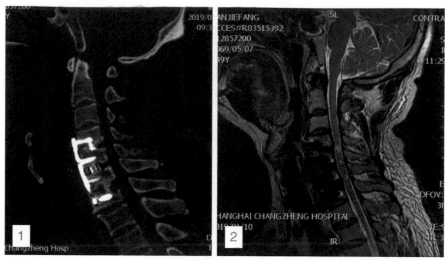

FIGURE 3.44.2

Postoperative sagittal and coronal views and their reference on the axial diagram.
(1) Midsagittal CT.
(2) Coronal CT.

Segment-type OPLL from C5 to C6 shown on midsagittal CT image (Fig. 3.44.2, panel 1).

Straightened cervical spine, CSF partial effacement from C4 to C6/7, spinal cord compression at C4 and C6/7, and patchy intramedullary signal hyperintensity from C4/5 to C6/7 shown on midsagittal MR image (Fig. 3.44.2, panel 2).

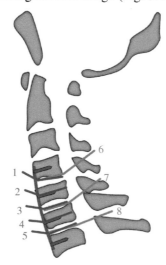

Reference of the axial planes

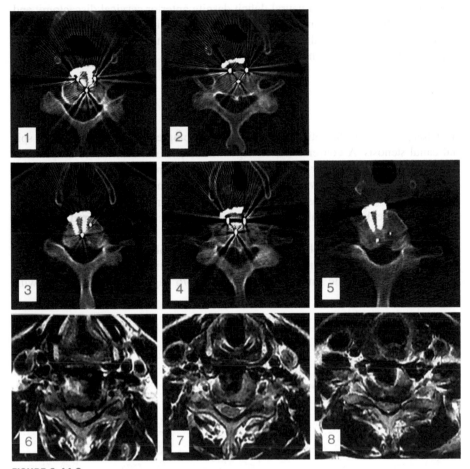

FIGURE 3.44.3

Preoperative axial images of the cervical spine and their reference on the sagittal diagram.

(1) Axial CT of C4/5.
(2) Axial CT of C5.
(3) Axial CT of C5/6.
(4) Axial CT of C6.
(5) Axial CT of C6/7.
(6) Axial MRI of C4/5.
(7) Axial MRI of C5/6.
(8) Axial MRI of C6/7.

Based on axial CT images, this ossified mass measures:2.3 mm thick (anteroposterior), 16.4 mm wide (mediolateral), and 17.3% in canal occupancy at C5; and 4.7 mm thick, 18.8 mm wide, and 32% in canal occupancy at C6 (Fig. 3.44.3, panel 1 to 5). Based on axial MR images, the compressed spinal cord at interspace levels from C4/5 to C6/7, more severe at C4/5 and C6/7 where the cord is a triangle with intramedullary hyperintensity (Fig. 3.44.3, Figs. 6 to 8).

Highlights

This case features persistent neural deficit despite anterior cervical discectomy and fusion (ACDF) of C4, C5, and C6/7 for the prior diagnosis of "cervical myelopathy." Developmental stenosis of the spinal canal and incomplete decompression of the stenosed levels are noted on imaging studies.

Surgical planning

In status post-ACDF, the patient needed further decompression of the levels with spinal canal stenosis. A conventional strategy was to perform indirect decompression through the posterior, further expanding the spinal canal in this lordotic cervical spine.

Alternatively, an ACAF with antedisplacement of C5 and C6, the maximum stenosis levels, offers a ventral expansion of the spinal canal and in situ cord decompression.

To facilitate the antedisplacement of C5 and C6, the cages in C4/5 and C6/7 need to be first removed.

The C5/6 cage left in place may contact with the plate prematurely and cause incomplete antedisplacement. Therefore, during resection of the anterior part of the vertebral bodies, the anterior border of the C5/6 cage should be reduced with a burr (Fig. 3.44.4).

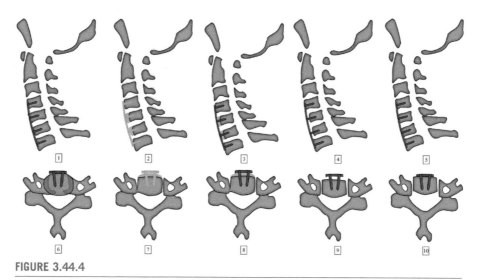

FIGURE 3.44.4

Illustration of the surgical plan on sagittal and axial planes.
(1, 6) Illustration of the OPLL on sagittal and axial views before surgery.
(2, 7) Removal of the plate and screws from the index procedure, resection of the anterior part of C5 to C6 vertebral bodies, a complete trough developed on the left vertebral bodies from C5 to C6 while a half one on the right side with the posterior bone yet to be dissected.
(3, 8) Plate and screws placed on vertebral bodies from C4 through C7.
(4, 9) The bottom of the right half-groove on C5 and C6 dissected.
(5, 10) Antedisplaced C5 and C6 vertebral bodies as screws were tightened.

Results

Postoperative function: JOA score was 14, Nurick score: 1, VAS: 0, and NDI: 4.

Antedisplaced C5 and C6 vertebral bodies, and new cages in C4/5 and C6/7 disc spaces (Fig. 3.44.5).

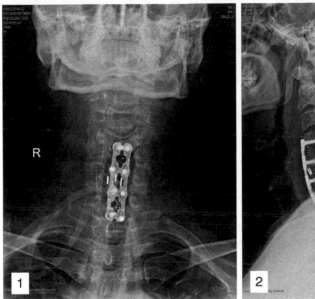
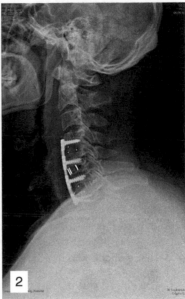

FIGURE 3.44.5

Postoperative cervical spine X-ray.
(1) Anteroposterior view.
(2) Lateral view.

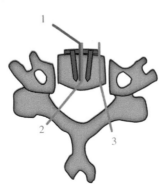

Reference of the sagittal planes

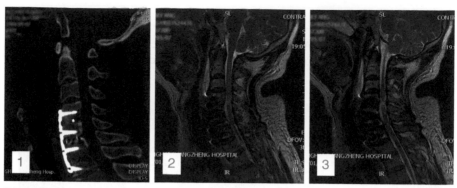

FIGURE 3.44.6

Postoperative sagittal views and their reference on the axial diagram.
(1) Midsagittal CT.
(2) Midsagittal MRI.
(3) Parasagittal MRI of the left uncinate process.

Antedisplaced C5 and C6 and expanded spinal canal shown on postoperative midsagittal CT image (Fig. 3.44.6, panel 1).

Spinal cord free of compression and surrounded by CSF, with residual intramedullary signal hyperintensity shown on postoperative sagittal MR images (Fig. 3.44.6, panel 2 and 3).

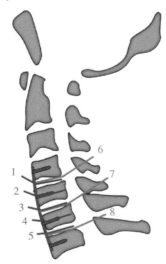

Reference of the axial planes

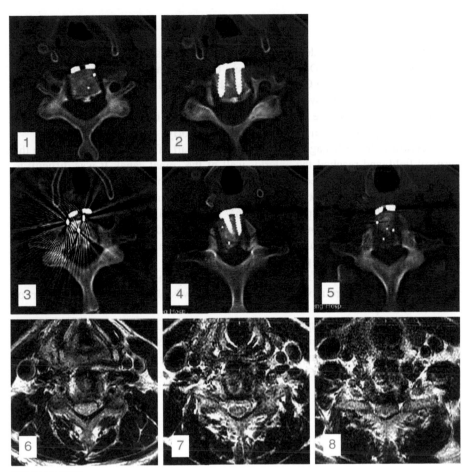

FIGURE 3.44.7

Postoperative axial cervical images and their reference on the sagittal diagram.

(1) Axial CT of C4/5.
(2) Axial CT of C5.
(3) Axial CT of C5/6.
(4) Axial CT of C6.
(5) Axial MRI of C6/7.
(6) Axial MRI of C4/5.
(7) Axial MRI of C5/6.
(8) Axial MRI of C6/7.

The vertebral bodies have been dissected with parasagittal cuts on both sides 23.5 mm apart and antedisplaced by 4.8 mm, reducing canal occupancy to 0% shown on postoperative axial CT images (Fig. 3.44.7, panel 1 to 5).

It has recovered to an oval shape, surrounded by an ample amount of CSF shown on postoperative midsagittal MR images (Fig. 3.44.7, panel 6 to 8).

Discussion

The C6/7 cage from the index ACDF is still seen on postoperative imaging results. Why was it left in place? Does it become a barrier to the antedisplacement?

To antedisplace C5 and C6 in this case, the C4/5 and C6/7 cages from the index surgery needed to be removed.

The C4/5 cage could be safely removed as it sat on the anterior part of the disc space, relatively away from the dura mater posteriorly.

In contrast, the C6/7 cage sat on the posterior part of the disc space, deep in the surgical field, and reached the anterior wall of the spinal canal. It was difficult to develop a safe plane between the cage and the dura mater. The index C6/7 cage was partially left in situ in case of a high-risk maneuver on the dura mater.

We found the posterior part of the C6/7 cage was tightly fused to the adjacent vertebral bodies and disallowed attempts of dissection during the revision surgery. To avoid iatrogenic trauma to the dura mater and the spinal cord, the posterior half of the cage was left in place.

The cage was dissected from the inferior surface of the C6 vertebra with burr and nerve hook. To obtain reliable fusion, a new cage was placed in the anterior part of the C6/7 disc space.

The insufficient antedisplacement of C6, suggested by imaging studies, was attributable to two constraining elements: first, the excessive friction between the index cage and the inferior surface of C6, and second, the residual osteophytes along the posterior border of the C6 vertebra blocked its antedisplacement.

Case 45: Ossification of posterior longitudinal ligament (OPLL) of cervical spine (At C2 to C4), history of cervical surgery.

Index terms

Continuous OPLL, wide-based disease, the thickness of ossification 7–9 mm, canal stenosis above 70%, ACAF performed with ACCF, status postposterior cervical surgery, and K-line (−) OPLL.

History

Patient: A 65-year-old woman.

Chief complaint: Status postcervical surgery received four years ago and gait disturbance for six months.

Physical exam: Physical exam was noted for gait disturbance, impaired tactile sensation on the palm and back of the hands, and the soles. Muscle strength was tested at 3/5 on the left deltoid and 4-/5 on the lower limbs. Hoffmann and Babinski signs were positive on both sides.

Preoperative function: JOA score was 9, Nurick score: 5, VAS: 5, and NDI: 15.

Imaging studies

A straightened cervical spine with a C2–C7 Cobb angle of 8.1° and K-line (−) OPLL at C2 to C4 (Fig. 3.45.1).

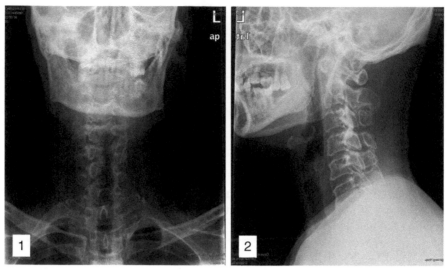

FIGURE 3.45.1

Preoperative X-ray of the cervical spine.
(1) Anteroposterior view.
(2) Lateral view.

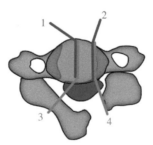

Reference of the sagittal planes

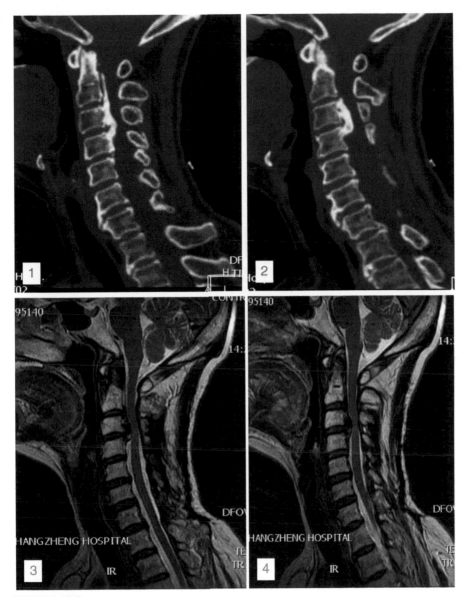

FIGURE 3.45.2

Preoperative sagittal images of the cervical spine and their reference on the axial diagram.
(1) Right parasagittal CT.
(2) Parasagittal CT of the left uncinate process.
(3) Midsagittal MRI.
(4) Parasagittal MRI of the left uncinate process.

Preoperative sagittal CT images: A continuous OPLL from C2 to C4; eccentric to the left, it peaks and violates the spinal canal at C3/4 (Fig. 3.45.2, panel 1 and 2).

Preoperative sagittal MRI images: Spinal cord compression at C3 and C3/4 due to anterior indentation of mixed-signal intensity; and kyphotic spinal cord at the compression levels (Fig. 3.45.2, panel 3 and 4).

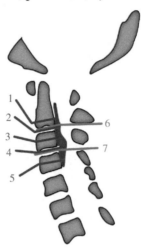

Reference of the axial planes

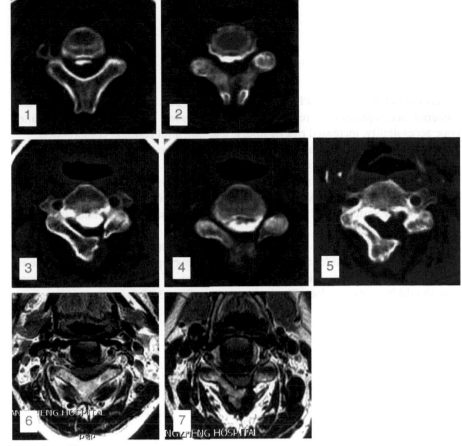

FIGURE 3.45.3

Preoperative axial images of the cervical spine and their reference on the sagittal diagram.

(1) Axial CT of the inferior surface of C2.

(2) Axial CT of C2/3.

(3) Axial CT of C3.

(4) Axial CT of C3/4.

(5) Axial CT of C4.

(6) Axial MRI of C2/3.

(7) Axial MRI of C3/4.

Based on axial CT images, laminoplasty from C3 to C7 was performed with the door opened on the left side. The OPLL is narrow-based and centered at C2 and C4, whereas wide-based and left paracentral at C2/3 to C3/4. It measures: 5.5 mm thick (anteroposterior) and 15.6 mm wide (mediolateral) at C3; 8.9 mm thick and 20.3 mm wide at C3/4; and 7.2 mm thick and 18.6 mm wide at C4 (Fig. 3.45.3, panel 1 to 5).

Based on axial MR images, compressed spinal cord in the shape of a triangle or even boomerang (Fig. 3.45.3, panel 6 and 7).

Highlights

This case features a continuous OPLL from C2 to C4, most severe at C3/4 and wide-based at C2/3 to C3/4, in a straightened cervical spine. She received a prior surgery of posterior subtotal laminectomy, which provided insufficient door opening and thus insufficient decompression at C3 and C4, levels of maximum cord compression. Spinal cord rotation was also noted.

Surgical planning

In this case of K-line (−) OPLL in the straightened cervical spine with status post-posterior decompression, a revision surgery performed posterior would encounter poor accessibility, increased risk of injury, and potential residual compression.

Such risk of residual compression is not fully addressed with conventional anterior procedures due to the wide-base component at C2/3 to C3/4. The extension into the upper cervical spine carries extra challenges for conventional anterior surgery.

An ACAF with antedisplacement of the C3 vertebra and resection of the upper half of the C4 vertebra was planned to expand the spinal canal without sacrificing the C4/5 disc space.

Notice was also given to C3, where the ossification reached the intervertebral foramina on the right side, and the bone groove developed off the anterior base of the uncinate process may leave out lateral residues of the lesion. Thus, the bone cuts should be expanded laterally during surgery (Fig. 3.45.4).

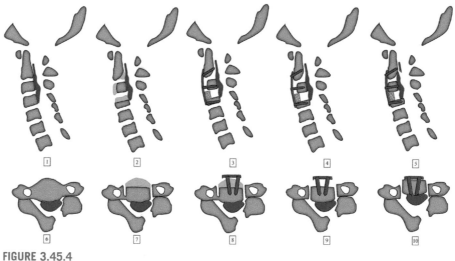

FIGURE 3.45.4

Illustration of the surgical plan on sagittal and axial planes.

(1, 6) Illustration of the OPLL on sagittal and axial views before surgery.

(2, 7) Resection performed to the anterior part of C3, the posteroinferior part of the C2 vertebra, and the superior half of the C4 vertebra; a complete trough developed along the left vertebra of C3 while a half one on the right side with the posterior bone yet to be dissected.

(3, 8) A mesh in place between C3 and C4, and plate and screws inserted on vertebral bodies from C2 through C4.

(4, 9) The bottom of the right half-groove on C3 dissected.

(5, 10) Antedisplaced C3 vertebra as screws were tightened.

Results

Postoperative function: JOA score was 17, Nurick score: 0, VAS: 0, and NDI: 0.

Improved cervical curvature, and a Cobb angle of 21.5° from C2 to C7 (Fig. 3.45.5).

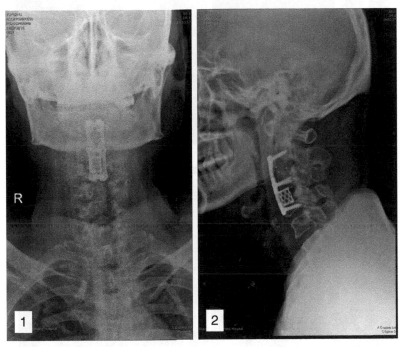

FIGURE 3.45.5

Postoperative cervical spine X-ray.
(1) Anteroposterior view.
(2) Lateral view.

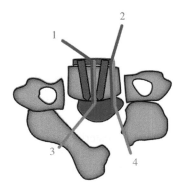

Reference of the sagittal planes

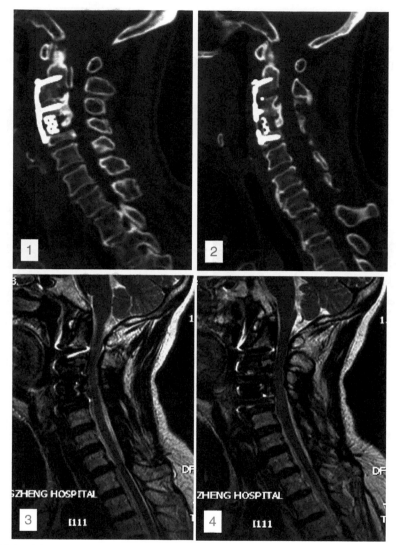

FIGURE 3.45.6

Postoperative sagittal views and their reference on the axial diagram.
(1) Midsagittal CT.
(2) Parasagittal CT of the left uncinate process.
(3) Midsagittal MRI.
(4) Parasagittal MRI of the left uncinate process.

Partial resection performed to the posterior part of C2 vertebra; OPLL dissected at C2 level; C4 vertebra partially substituted with a mesh; ventral displacement of VOC by 6.2 mm, composed of C3 to C4 and the partial ossification posterior to C2; and expanded spinal canal shown on postoperative midsagittal CT image (Fig. 3.45.6, panel 1 and 2).

Lordotic spinal cord free of compression and surrounded by CSF shown on post-operative midsagittal MR image (Fig. 3.45.6, panel 3 and 4).

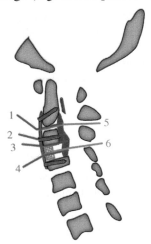

Reference of the axial planes

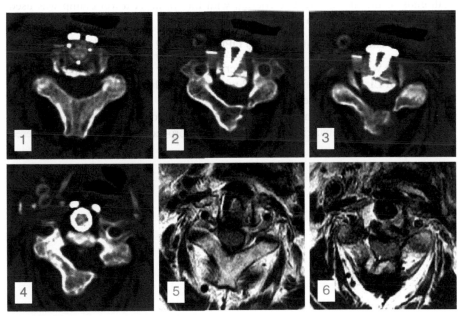

FIGURE 3.45.7

Postoperative axial cervical images and their reference on the sagittal diagram.
(1) Axial CT of C2/3.
(2) Axial CT of C3.
(3) Axial CT of the inferior surface of C3.
(4) Axial CT of C3/4.
(5) Axial MRI of C2/3.
(6) Axial MRI of C3/4.

The vertebral bodies have been dissected with parasagittal cuts on both sides 20.3 mm apart at C2 and C3 and 21.9 mm at C4 shown on postoperative axial CT image (Fig. 3.45.7, panel 1 to 4).

The spinal cord has recovered to an oval shape surrounded by an ample amount of CSF, suggesting excellent decompression shown on postoperative axial MR image (Fig. 3.45.7, panel 5 and 6).

Discussion

1. What was the decision-making process for substituting the superior half of C4 vertebra with a mesh instead of antedisplacement of C4?

With the absence of MRI evidence of disc degeneration at C4/5, we preferred to preserve this motion segment, avoid C4 antedisplacement, and resect the only the superior part of C4 vertebra instead. This partial corpectomy left a void too large for any cage, so a mesh was inserted.

A mesh of proper height was used to avoid the unintended distraction of the disc space. The antedisplacement maneuver was facilitated by placing gauze pads on both ends of the mesh to reduce friction with the mesh. A towel clamp was used to facilitate mesh migration when there was difficult or insufficient migration.

2. Does the shelter technique apply to OPLL at the C2 and C4?

This case was treated prior to the description of the shelter technique.

As the OPLL extended high up to C2 with a thin tip that had not caused impingement, it was dissected at the interspace level.

Since CSF leak was encountered during ossification dissection, a drain was placed through the lumbar cistern at the end of the procedure. The patient recovered two weeks later.

Case 46: Ossification of posterior longitudinal ligament (OPLL) of cervical spine (At C3 to T1), history of cervical surgery

Index terms

Antedisplacement of three vertebral bodies, mixed-type OPLL, the thickness of ossification above 9 mm, canal occupancy ratio 60%–70%, undercutting decompression, and status postposterior cervical surgery.

History

Patient: A 60-year-old man.

Chief complaint: Numbness of both hands, and impaired ambulation for three years with one-year aggravation, presented five years after a posterior cervical surgery.

Physical exam: Physical exam was noted for gait instability, impaired tactile sensation of palms, and hypertonicity on all the extremities. Muscle strength was tested at 4/5 on both hands and lower limbs. Tendon reflexes were brisk on the lower extremities. Hoffmann and Babinski signs were present bilaterally.

Preoperative function: JOA score was 5, Nurick score: 5, VAS: 8, and NDI: 23.

Imaging studies

Devoid laminae and posterior elements from C3 to C6 and Cobb angle of 17.7° from C2 through C7 (Fig. 3.46.1).

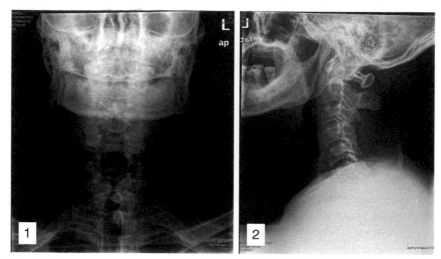

FIGURE 3.46.1

Preoperative X-ray of the cervical spine.
(1) Anteroposterior view.
(2) Lateral view.

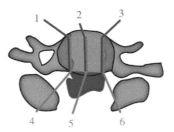

Reference of the sagittal planes

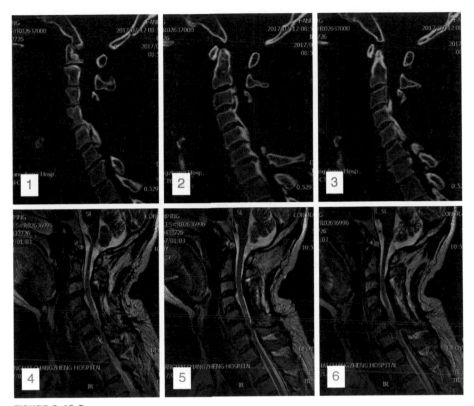

FIGURE 3.46.2

Preoperative sagittal images of the cervical spine and their reference on the axial diagram.
(1) Sagittal CT at the right uncinate process.
(2) Midsagittal CT.
(3) Sagittal CT at the left uncinate process.
(4) Sagittal MRI at the right uncinate process.
(5) Midsagittal MRI.
(6) Sagittal MRI at the left uncinate process.

Preoperative sagittal CT images: A mixed-type OPLL from C3 to T1, status of postposterior cervical surgery with devoid inferior lamina of C3, superior lamina of C6 and C4 and C5 posterior elements (Fig. 3.46.2, panel 1 to 3).

Preoperative sagittal MR images: Hypointense mass posterior to C3 to T1 vertebral bodies, residual compression from the previous posterior surgery, spinal cord compression at C5/6 to C6/7, pincer-pattern impingement of the spinal cord at C6/7, and intramedullary signal hyperintensity and partial CSF effacement of the ventral side at C5/6 (Fig. 3.46.2, panel 4 to 6).

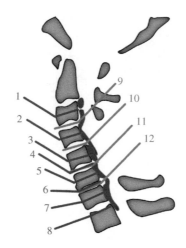

Reference of the axial planes

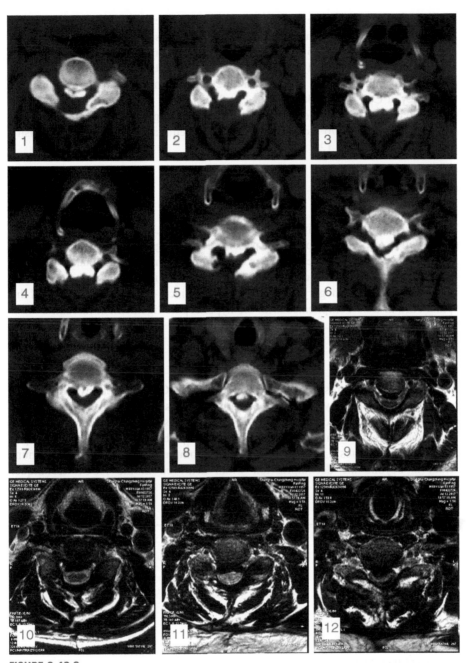

FIGURE 3.46.3

Preoperative axial images of the cervical spine and their reference on the sagittal diagram.

Based on axial CT images, the devoid posterior element dorsal to the spinal canal from C3 to C6 is evident on axial images. The OPLL is mushroom-shaped and violates the spinal canal at C5 and C5/6. It measures: 8.5 mm thick (anteroposterior), 13.2 mm wide (mediolateral) at the stem, and 19.1 mm at the maximum width at C5/6 where it is narrow-based; and 9.0 mm thick, 14.3 mm wide, and 65.2% in canal occupancy at C6/7 (Fig. 3.46.3, panel 1 to 8).

Based on axial CT images, a triangle and boomerang-shaped spinal cord due to indentation from C5/6 to C6/7 with intramedullary signal hyperintensity (Fig. 3.46.3, Figs. 9 to 12).

Highlights

This case features an extensive, flat, and mixed-type OPLL with a mushroom-shaped cross-section at C5/6. The patient experienced neurological improvement after the index surgery, which included resection of the inferior rim of C3 lamina, the superior rim of C6 lamina, and C4 and C5 laminae. Neural deficit recurred five years later and became progressive. Imagery evidence suggested pincer-pattern compression of the spinal cord at C6/7 complicated with the hypertrophic ligamentum flavum.

Surgical planning

The posterior decompression can be extended with a C6 laminectomy. However, a posterior procedure may lead to poor surgical access and recurrent myelopathy due to progressive kyphosis, ossification growth, and scaring down the road.

A conventional alternative is ACCF for C5 to C7. The mushroom-shaped component at C5 constitutes a risk for incomplete decompression because its maximum width is beyond the decompression width achieved in the ACCF technique.

(1) Axial CT of C3.
(2) Axial CT of C4.
(3) Axial CT of C5.
(4) Axial CT of C5/6.
(5) Axial CT of C6.
(6) Axial CT of C6/7.
(7) Axial CT of C7.
(8) Axial CT of C7/T1.
(9) Axial MRI of C3/4.
(10) Axial MRI of C4/5.
(11) Axial MRI of C5/6.
(12) Axial MRI of C6/7.

Meanwhile, the use of multisegmental instrumentation comes with an increased risk of failure.

An ACAF with antedisplacement for C5 to C7, levels with residual compression, with undercutting decompression of the posterior rim of the T1 vertebra was planned for this patient.

The mushroom-shaped lesion at C5 and C5/6 merits extra attention. Measuring 19.1 mm wide, it was wider than the distance between the uncinate processes on both sides 17.4 mm apart. The ossification was 3.7 mm from the right vertebral artery and 6.4 mm from the left one at the level of maximal width. When palpating with a neural hook, the surgeon should differentiate between the edge of the base of the ossification verse its edge at the maximal width (Fig. 3.46.4).

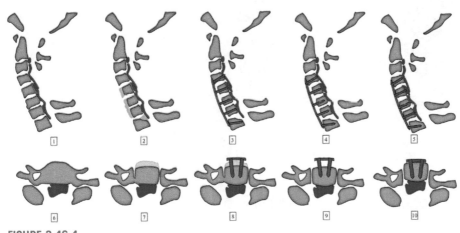

FIGURE 3.46.4

Illustration of the surgical plan on sagittal and axial planes.

(1, 6) Illustration of the OPLL on sagittal and axial views before surgery.

(2, 7) Resection performed to the anterior part of C5 to C7 vertebral bodies and the posterosuperior rim of the T1 vertebra; a complete trough developed on the left vertebral bodies from C5 to C7 while a half one on the right side with the posterior bone yet to be dissected.

(3, 8) Plate and screws placed on vertebral bodies from C4 through T1.

(4, 9) The bottom of the right half-groove on C5 through C7 dissected.

(5, 10) Antedisplaced C5 to C7 vertebral bodies as screws were tightened.

Results

Postoperative function: JOA score was 12, Nurick score: 1, VAS: 2, and NDI: 7.

Instrumentation from C4 to T1 and antedisplaced C5 to C7 vertebral bodies (Fig. 3.46.5).

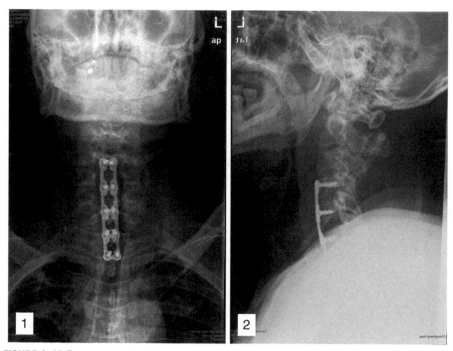

FIGURE 3.46.5

Postoperative cervical spine X-ray.
(1) Anteroposterior view.
(2) Lateral view.

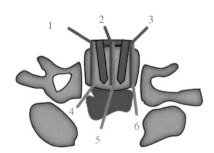

Reference of the sagittal planes

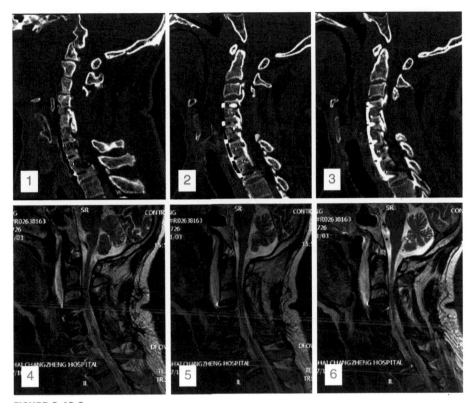

FIGURE 3.46.6

Postoperative sagittal views and their reference on the axial diagram.
(1) Sagittal CT of the right uncinate process.
(2) Midsagittal CT.
(3) Sagittal CT of the left uncinate process.
(4) Sagittal MRI at the right uncinate process.
(5) Midsagittal MRI.
(6) Sagittal MRI at the left uncinate process.

Ventrally displaced VOC from C5 to C7 and expanded spinal canal shown on postoperative sagittal CT images (Fig. 3.46.6, panel 1 to 3).

Spinal cord in lordotic curvature surrounded by CSF free of compression at C6 to C7 shown on postoperative sagittal CT images (Fig. 3.46.6, panel 4 to 6; Fig. 3.46.7, panel 8 to 11).

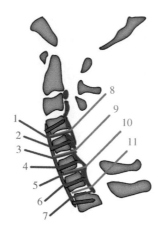

Reference of the axial planes

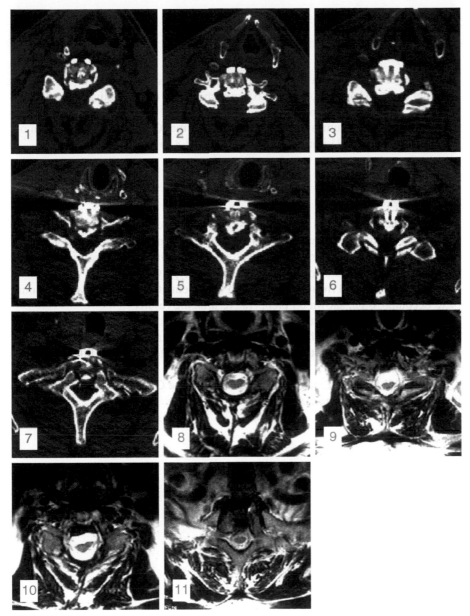

FIGURE 3.46.7

Postoperative axial cervical images and their reference on the sagittal diagram.

(1) Axial CT of C4/5.

(2) Axial CT of C5.

(3) Axial CT of C5/6.

(4) Axial CT of C6.

(5) Axial CT of C6/7.

(6) Axial CT of C7.

(7) Axial CT of T1.

(8) Axial MRI of C4/5.

(9) Axial MRI of C5/6.

(10) Axial MRI of C6/7.

(11) Axial MRI of C7/T1.

The vertebral bodies have been dissected with parasagittal cuts on both sides 20.8 mm apart and antedisplaced by 6.2 mm shown on postoperative axial CT images (Fig. 3.46.7, panel 1 to 7).

The spinal cord resumes its oval shape with normal CSF around it, as shown on postoperative axial MRI images (Fig. 3.46.7, panel 8 to 11).

Discussion

What was the rationale behind the decision of the levels of decompression? Is it possible to exclude C7 from the antedisplacement complex?

This case features recurrent neuropathy after sustained relief from a posterior decompression procedure for an extensive, mixed-type OPLL.

The OPLL spanned from C3 to T1, with C6/7 being the primary level of incomplete decompression, shown on preoperative imaging results.

The location of the most severe cord compression at C6/7 and the compression contributor of OPLL were the bases for C7 antedisplacement. With a gap present at the C6/7, undercutting of the superior rim of C7 vertebra offers little room for antedisplacement.

As the OPLL was not readily dissected at C5/6, the C5 vertebra was included in the antedisplacement complex.

Case 47: Ossification of posterior longitudinal ligament (OPLL) of cervical spine (At C4 to C6), history of cervical surgery

Index terms

Antedisplacement of three vertebral bodies, segmental OPLL, wide-based OPLL, thickness of ossification 7—9 mm, canal stenosis 60% to 70%, and status postposterior cervical surgery.

History

Patient: A 70-year-old woman.

Chief complaint: Weakness and numbness of the left extremities aggravated for nine months, presented nine months after cervical spine surgery.

Physical exam: The patient was wheeled in with hypertonicity of all the extremities. Muscle strength was tested at 3/5 on the left upper limb, 1/5 on the left hand, 4/5 on the right upper limb, and 3/5 on the lower limbs. Brisk tendon reflexes were elicited on all four extremities with ankle clonus. Hoffmann and Babinski signs were present bilaterally.

Preoperative function: JOA score was 8, Nurick score: 5, VAS: 3, and NDI: 24.

Imaging studies

Devoid laminae and posterior elements on C3 to C5, lateral mass screws placed on the right side of C3 to C7, and C2—C7 Cobb angle of 8.1° in a straightened cervical spine (Fig. 3.47.1).

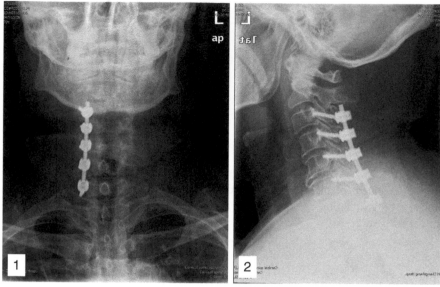

FIGURE 3.47.1

Preoperative X-ray of the cervical spine.
(1) Anteroposterior view.
(2) Lateral view.

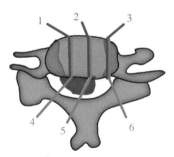

Reference of the sagittal planes

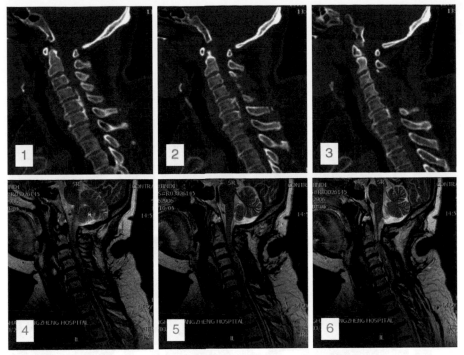

FIGURE 3.47.2

Preoperative sagittal images of the cervical spine and their reference on the axial diagram.

(1) Sagittal CT at the right uncinate process.
(2) Midsagittal CT.
(3) Sagittal CT at the left uncinate process.
(4) Sagittal MRI at the right uncinate process.
(5) Midsagittal MRI.
(6) Sagittal MRI at the left uncinate process.

A segment-type OPLL on C4 to C6 and C6. Status postleft hemilaminectomy and posterior instrumentation and fusion, unresolved poor curvature of the cervical spine, and expanded spinal canal on the left side shown on sagittal CT images (Fig. 3.47.2, panel 1 to 3; and Fig. 3.47.3, panel 1 to 5).

Resumed posterior CSF column from C3 to C6, the insufficient posterior shift of the spinal cord, C4/5 disc protrusion, and pincer-pattern impingement of the spinal cord at C6/7 shown on sagittal MR images (Fig. 3.47.2, panel 4 to 6).

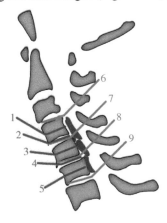

Reference of the axial planes

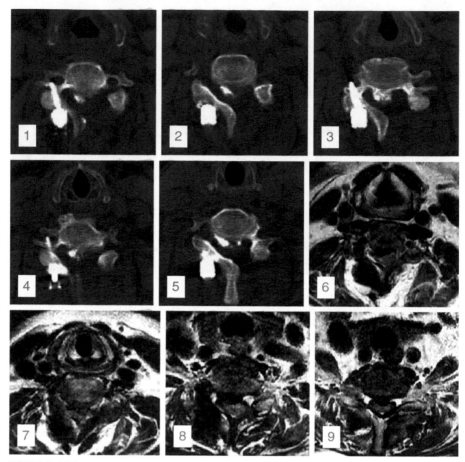

FIGURE 3.47.3

Preoperative axial images of the cervical spine and their reference on the sagittal diagram.

(1) Axial CT of C4.
(2) Axial CT of C4/5.
(3) Axial CT of C5.
(4) Axial CT of C5/6.
(5) Axial CT of C7.
(6) Axial MRI of C3/4.
(7) Axial MRI of C4/5.
(8) Axial MRI of C5/6.
(9) Axial MRI of C6/7.

Based on preoperative axial CT images, a midline-centered narrow-based OPLL at C4–C6 and more prominent on the right side, left hemilaminectomy, and posterior instrumentation and fusion was performed. The ossified mass measures: at C4 7.3 mm thick, 14.7 mm wide, 7.3 mm thick, 11 mm wide at C5 and 4.7 mm thick, 14.1 mm wide at C5.

Based on preoperative axial MR images, residual spinal cord compression and spinal cord rotated toward the laminectomy side (Fig. 3.47.3, panel 6 to 9).

Highlights

This case features a flat-type, wide-based segmental OPLL from C4 to C6 in a cervical spine treated with hemilaminectomy and lateral instrumentation via a posterior approach. With the unresolved neural deficit, the patient sustained recurrent and deteriorating neuropathy.

Surgical planning

Among the conventional options, ACCF from C4 to C6 is feasible. As the posterior part of the spinal canal expanded due to compensation following the prior surgery, the risk of iatrogenic cord injury during ossification resection becomes less likely.

It is worth noted that the risk of residual compression is high at C6 where the wide-based ossification may span wider than the decompression width achieved by subtotal corpectomy.

Another conventional option is to expand the decompression with laminectomies via a posterior approach. However, the surgical dissection of scars and adhesion around the dura mater developed after the index surgery is challenging and time-consuming, let alone the risk of dural tear.

An ACAF with antedisplacement of C4 to C6 was planned on this case. Given the prior posterior fusion, room of decompression generated by curvature correction was less likely, and an anterior part of the vertebrae of the same thickness as the ossification was resected (Fig. 3.47.4).

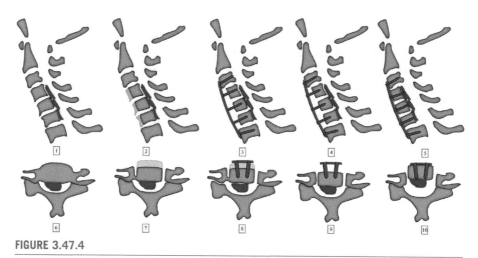

FIGURE 3.47.4

Illustration of the surgical plan on sagittal and axial planes.

(1, 6) Illustration of the OPLL on sagittal and axial views before surgery.

(2, 7) Resection of the anterior part of the vertebral bodies of C4, C5, and C6; a left groove and a right half-groove with the posterior cortex still intact on C4, C5, and C6.

(3, 8) Titanium plate and screws placed in vertebral bodies from C3 to C7.

(4, 9) Completion of the right groove on C4, C5, and C6.

(5, 10) Antedisplaced C4, C5, and C6 vertebral bodies as screws were tightened.

Results

Postoperative function: JOA score was 9, Nurick score: 4, VAS: 2, and NDI: 23.

Cobb angle of 12.5° from C2 to C7 and restored cervical curvature (Fig. 3.47.5).

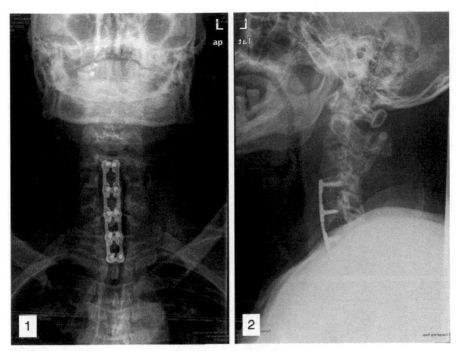

FIGURE 3.47.5

Postoperative cervical X-ray.
(1) Anteroposterior view.
(2) Lateral view.

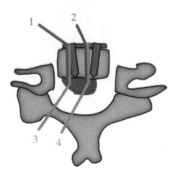

Reference of the sagittal planes

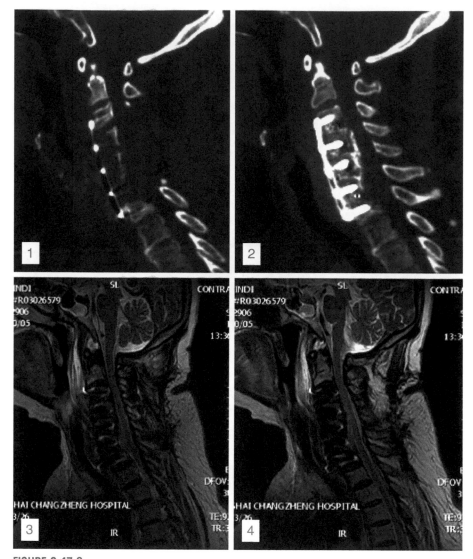

FIGURE 3.47.6

Postoperative sagittal images and their reference on the axial diagram.
(1) Sagittal CT at the right uncinate process.
(2) Midsagittal CT.
(3) Sagittal MRI at the right uncinate process.
(4) Midsagittal MRI.

Postoperative CT images: Antedisplaced VOC of C4 to C6 and expanded spinal canal with tight contact between the vertebral bodies and the titanium plate (Fig. 3.47.6, panel 1 and 2).

Sagittal MR images: Spinal cord free of compression between the anterior and posterior columns of CSF (Fig. 3.47.6, panel 3 and 4).

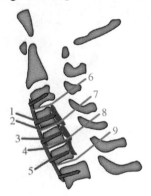

Reference of the axial planes

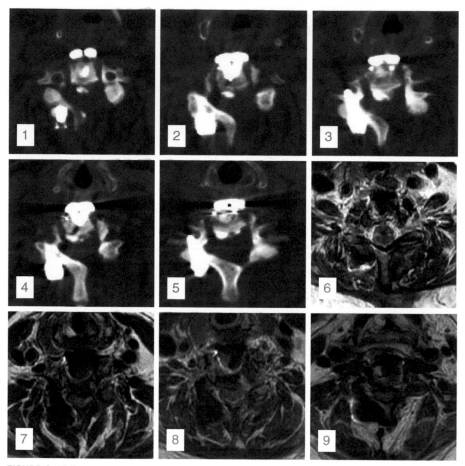

FIGURE 3.47.7

Postoperative axial cervical images and their reference on the sagittal diagram.
(1) Axial CT of C4.
(2) Axial CT of C4/5.
(3) Axial CT of C5.
(4) Axial CT of C5/6.
(5) Axial CT of C6.
(6) Axial MRI of C3/4.
(7) Axial MRI of C4/5.
(8) Axial MRI of C5/6.
(9) Axial MRI of C6/7.

Based on axial CT images, the bony grooves are parasagittal and 22.5 mm apart, and the VOC advanced by 6.3 mm on the left and 5.5 mm on the right (Fig. 3.47.7, panel 1 to 5).

Based on axial MR images, the spinal cord free of compression resumes a triangular or oval shape with normal CSF around it (Fig. 3.47.7, panel 6 to 9).

Discussion

During revision surgery in status postdecompression and fusion via a posterior approach, what are the criteria for a properly contoured plate?

In this case of unresolved cervical curvature following a posterior fusion and instrumentation, a revision surgery via anterior approach yields limited curvature restoration.

Similarly, since the use of positioning pillow had little role in curvature correction, the head was properly supported to maintain the pliability of the trachea and esophagus to allow for easy mobilization during surgery.

The plate was contoured according to the degree of cervical overextension calculated before surgery. With the posterior instrumentation in place, the attempt to restore curvature with an excessively contoured plate produces local lordosis of the antedisplaced levels rather than a global curvature.

In situ decompression and spinal cord derotation achieved via ACAF technique:

The ACAF procedure resolved the rotation of the spinal cord and the secondary neural palsy due to nerve root tethering. The derotation effect is evident from the comparison of postoperative axial MR images from the two surgeries. After the index procedure, the ventral side of the spinal cord rotated toward the laminectomy side at some disc levels. After the revision surgery with ACAF, the rotation was resolved.

After ACAF, more room is gained in the ventral side of the spinal cord so that the spinal cord restores its typical curvature and gets decompression in situ as it is no longer in the posteriorly shifted position from the previous posterior decompression surgery.

Case 48: Ossification of posterior longitudinal ligament (OPLL) of cervical spine (At C3 to C6), history of cervical surgery

Index terms

Antedisplacement of three vertebral bodies, mixed-type OPLL, wide-based disease, and status postposterior cervical surgery.

History

Patient: A 61-year-old man.

Chief complaint: Numbness and weakness of all extremities for two years, presented eight months after cervical surgery.

Physical exam: Physical exam was noted for gait disturbance and numbness on the right trunk below the neck and the perineal areas. The numbness did not resolve after prior surgery, and the patient reported new-onset numbness of the left trunk below the neck. The four extremities were identified with hypertonic muscles and impaired superficial sensation. Muscle strength was tested at 4/5 on upper limbs and 3/5 on lower limbs. Hoffmann and Babinski signs were present bilaterally.

Preoperative function: JOA score was 11, Nurick score: 2, VAS: 3, and NDI: 18.

Imaging studies

OPLL of C3 through C5, laminoplasty performed at C3–C7 and Cobb angle of 10.9° from C2 to C7 (Fig. 3.48.1).

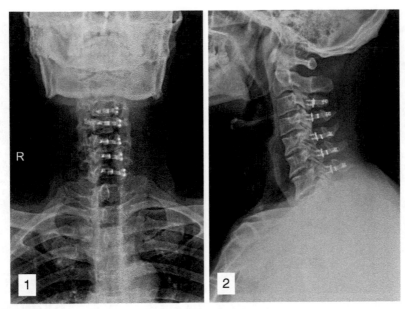

FIGURE 3.48.1

Preoperative X-ray of the cervical spine.
(1) Anteroposterior view.
(2) Lateral view.

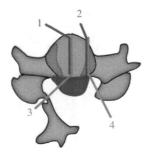

Reference of the sagittal planes

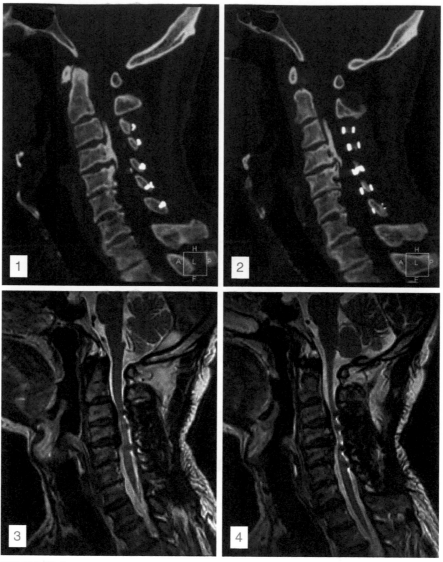

FIGURE 3.48.2

Preoperative sagittal images of the cervical spine and their reference on the axial diagram.

(1) Midsagittal CT.

(2) Sagittal CT at the left uncinate process.

(3) Midsagittal MRI.

(4) Sagittal MRI at the left uncinate process.

Preoperative sagittal CT images: A mixed-type OPLL from C3 to C5, which peaks and violates the spinal canal at C4/5 (Fig. 3.48.2, panel 1 and 2).

Preoperative sagittal MR images: A spinal cord significantly impinged in poor curvature, appearing boomerang-shaped at C4/5 due to indentation (Fig. 3.48.2, panel 2, 3, and 4).

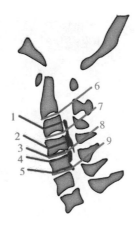

Reference of the axial planes

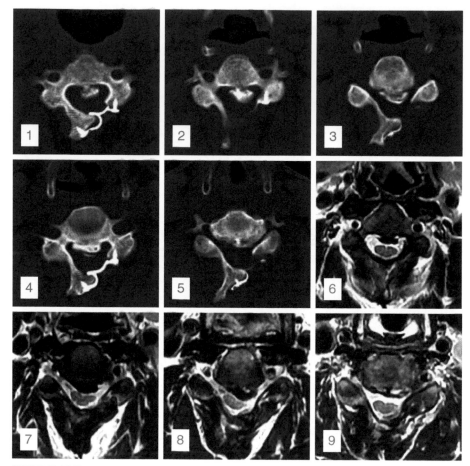

FIGURE 3.48.3

Preoperative axial images of the cervical spine and their reference on the sagittal diagram.

(1) Axial CT of C3.

(2) Axial CT of C4.

(3) Axial CT of C4/5.

(4) Axial CT of the superior surface of C5.

(5) Axial CT of the inferior surface of C5.

(6) Axial MRI of C2/3.

(7) Axial MRI of C3/4.

(8) Axial MRI of C4/5.

(9) Axial MRI of C5/6.

Based on axial CT images, this OPLL measures: 7 mm thick (anteroposterior), 10 mm wide (mediolateral), and 49% in canal occupancy at C3 where a double-layer sign is present; 6.1 mm thick, 13.6 mm wide, and 35% in canal occupancy at C4; 7.6 mm thick, 17.0 mm wide, and 52.4% in canal occupancy at C4/5 where the lesion is wide-based and double-layered; 6.1 mm thick, 16.7 mm wide, and 39% in canal occupancy at the superior surface of C5; and 5.1 mm thick, 18.5 mm wide, and 29% in canal occupancy at the inferior surface of C5 (Fig. 3.48.3, panel 1 to 5).

Based on axial MR images, following the before posterior decompression, the spinal cord shifts posteriorly in partially restored curvature and CSF columns. The spinal cord rotates under the sustained anterior indentation (Fig. 3.48.3, panel 6 to 9).

Highlights

This case features a mixed-type OPLL from C3 to C5. The patient had received a posterior single-door laminoplasty, which yield little long-term functional improvement. The spinal canal was insufficiently expanded after the index surgery, which resulted in residual compression and the sustained anterior indentation on the spinal cord.

Surgical planning

Given the poor cervical curvature, a second posterior surgery may generate an inadequate posterior shift of the spinal cord and residual compression.

In contrast, an ACAF was still feasible to further decompress C3 to C4/5. If partial resection was performed only on C3 and C4 and the disease posterior to the C5 vertebra left not addressed, a step might develop at C4/5 that impinged the spinal cord.

An alternative was ACCF for C3 to C5, but the use of a longer construct would bear a higher risk of hardware-associated complications.

The patient received an ACAF with antedisplacement of C3 to C5, which provided adequate decompression without the risk of iatrogenic injury and fusion-associated complications (Fig. 3.48.4).

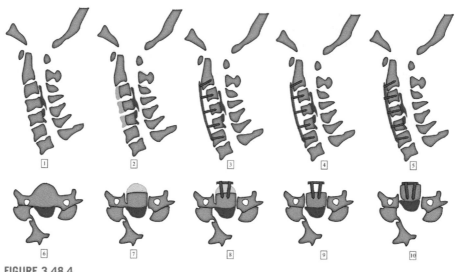

FIGURE 3.48.4

Illustration of the surgical plan on sagittal and axial planes.

(1, 6) Illustration of the OPLL on sagittal and axial views before surgery.

(2, 7) Resection of the anterior part of the vertebral bodies of C3 to C5, a left groove, and a right half-groove with the posterior cortex still intact on C3 to C5.

(3, 8) Titanium plate and screws placed in vertebral bodies from C2 to C6.

(4, 9) Completion of the right groove on C3 to C5.

(5, 10) Antedisplaced C3 to C5 vertebral bodies as screws were tightened.

Results

Postoperative function: JOA score was 11, Nurick score: 1, VAS: 2, and NDI: 12.

Antedisplaced VOC from C3 to C5 and restored cervical curvature and Cobb angle of 20.5° from C2 to C7 (Fig. 3.48.5).

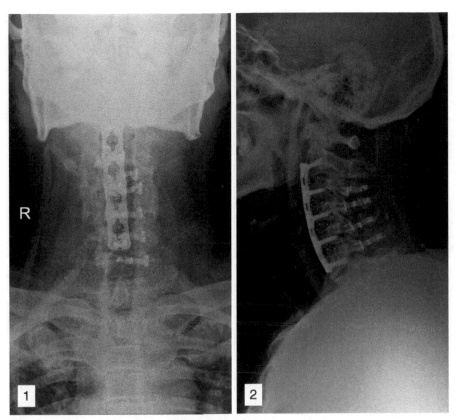

FIGURE 3.48.5

Postoperative cervical X-ray.
(1) Anteroposterior view.
(2) Lateral view.

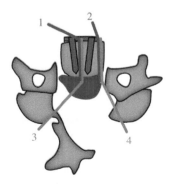

Reference of the sagittal planes

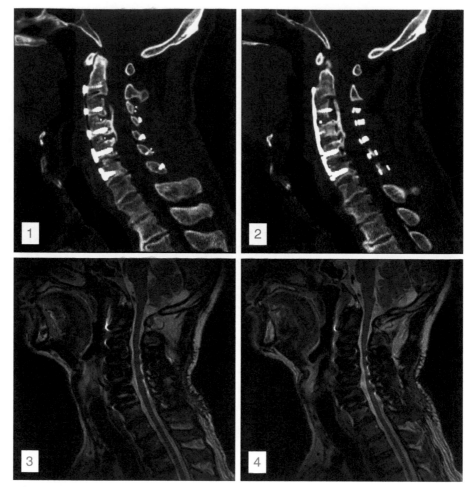

FIGURE 3.48.6

Postoperative sagittal images and their reference on the axial diagram.
(1) Midsagittal CT.
(2) Sagittal CT at the left uncinate process.
(3) Midsagittal MRI.
(4) Sagittal MRI at the left uncinate process.

Antedisplaced VOC from C3 to C5 and widened spinal canal shown on postoperative midsagittal CT image, shown on postoperative sagittal CT images (Fig. 3.48.6, panel 1 and 2).

Spinal cord free of compression with ample amount of CSF on the ventral and dorsal side shown on postoperative sagittal CT images (Fig. 3.48.6, panel 3 and 4).

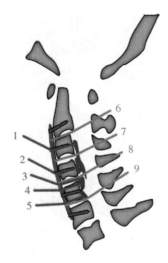

Reference of the axial planes

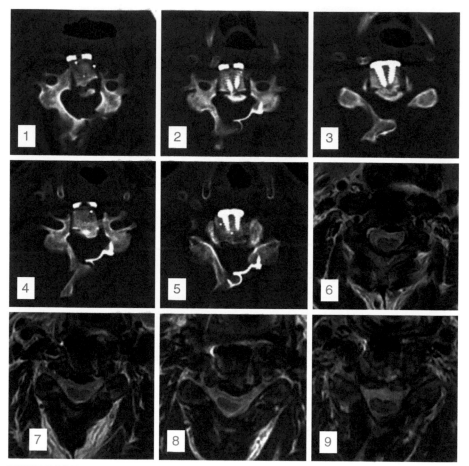

FIGURE 3.48.7

Postoperative axial cervical images and their reference on the sagittal diagram.
(1) Axial CT of C3.
(2) Axial CT of C4.
(3) Axial CT of C4/5.
(4) Axial CT of the superior surface of C5.
(5) Axial CT of the inferior surface of C5.
(6) Axial MRI of C2/3.
(7) Axial MRI of C3/4.
(8) Axial MRI of C4/5.
(9) Axial MRI of C5/6.

VOC ventrally displaced by 4.8 mm, further expanded spinal canal, and canal stenosis reduced to 27.4% and 24.2% shown on postoperative axial CT images (Fig. 3.48.7, panel 1 to 5).

The derotated spinal cord resumes to an oval shape shown on postoperative axial MR images (Fig. 3.48.7, panel 6 to 9).

Discussion

Since the spinal cord compression was most severe at C3 and C4, according to preoperative MRI, was C5 antedisplacement required?

Preoperative MRI suggested C3 to C4 as the levels of decompression in the revision surgery. Though the OPLL extended to C5, the spinal cord of this level still had regular anterior and posterior CSF columns.

In a straightened cervical spine, the antedisplacement of C3 and C4 allowed the spinal cord to adapt to the restored cervical curvature. As such, the spinal cord would contact with the ossification dorsal to the C5 vertebra. The dissection of the lesion at C4/5 did not seem to be a good strategy as it was continuous and bulky at this level.

What is more, using C5 as the lower instrumented level may accelerate the degeneration of C5/6, which is already presented with severe degenerative changes.

Therefore, antedisplacement of three levels, namely C3, C4, and C5, was performed.

Case 49: Ossification of posterior longitudinal ligament (OPLL) of cervical spine (At C3 to C6), history of cervical surgery, cervical hyperextension injury

Index terms

Antedisplacement of three vertebral bodies, mixed-type OPLL, the thickness of ossification above 9 mm, undercut decompression, hyperextension injury, and status postposterior cervical surgery.

History

Patient: A 56-year-old man.

Chief complaint: Numbness and weakness of all the extremities for six months presented one year after anterior cervical surgery.

Past history: The patient sustained a cervical trauma incident one year ago and developed numbness, pain, and weakness of the four extremities, with the upper limbs more severe than the lower limbs. Muscle strength was tested at 3/5 on the lower limbs and 2/5 on the upper limbs. He received a posterior single-door laminoplasty and started to feel improvement in muscle strength, 3/5 upper limbs and 4/5 on lower limbs. However, the numbness of the trunk and extremities resolved little. Four months after the surgery, neural deficit worsened, with muscle strength reduced to 2/5 and increased numbness on the lower limbs.

Physical exam: The patient was brought in on a stretcher with the complaint of numbness and tightness on the trunk. On examination, hypertonicity of all the extremities was present. Sense of light touch, pinprick, and temperature was impaired on the upper extremities. Impaired tactile sensation and hyperalgesia were documented in the lower extremities. Muscle strength was tested at 3/5 on the upper limbs and 2/5 on the lower limbs. Hyperreflexia was present in all the extremities. Hoffmann and Babinski signs were positive on both sides.

Preoperative function: JOA score was at 5, Nurick score: 4, VAS: 4, and NDI: 28.

Imaging studies

Straightened cervical spine with a Cobb angle of 3.8°, OPLL of C2 through C6 (Fig. 3.49.1).

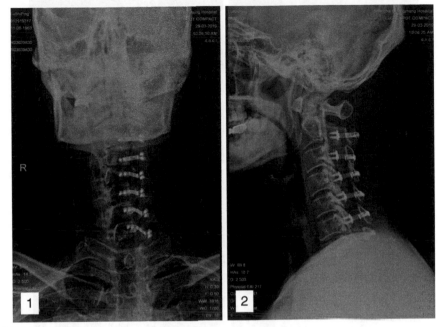

FIGURE 3.49.1

Preoperative X-ray of the cervical spine.
(1) Anteroposterior view.
(2) Lateral view.

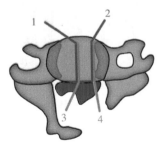

Reference of the sagittal planes

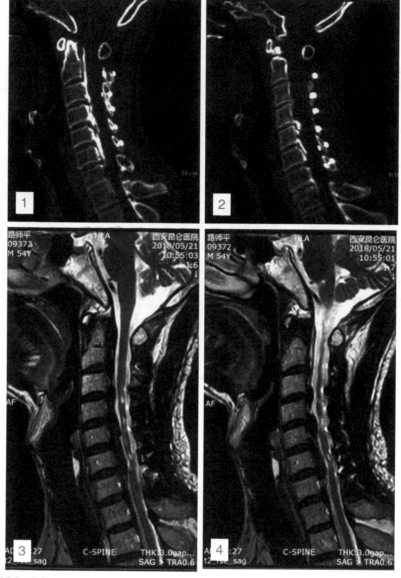

FIGURE 3.49.2

Preoperative sagittal images of the cervical spine and their reference on the axial diagram.

(1) Midsagittal CT.
(2) Sagittal CT of the left uncinate process.
(3) Midsagittal MRI.
(4) Sagittal MRI at the left uncinate process.

Preoperative sagittal CT image: A continuous-type OPLL from C2 to C7, with a double-layer sign at C4 to C6 (Fig. 3.49.2, panel 1 and 2).

Preoperative sagittal MR image: A hypointense band posterior to the vertebral bodies from C2 to C7; hyperintense dots at C3/4, C4/5, and posterior to C6 vertebra; ample amount of posterior CSF column, partial elimination of the anterior CSF column from C5 to C6/7, and "S"-shaped spinal cord (Fig. 3.49.2, panel 3 and 4).

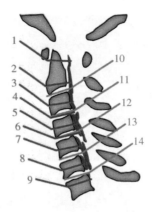

Reference of the axial planes

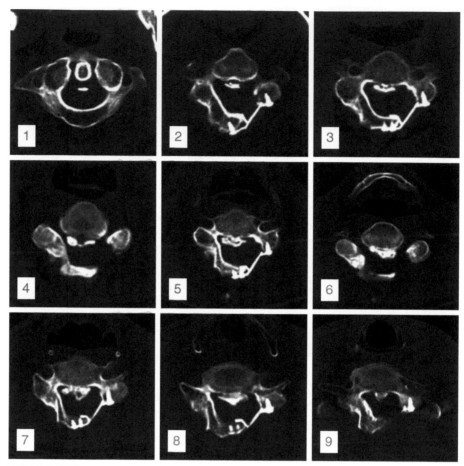

FIGURE 3.49.3

Preoperative axial images of the cervical spine and their reference on the sagittal diagram.
(1) Axial CT of C1.
(2) Axial CT of the inferior surface of C2.
(3) Axial CT of C3.
(4) Axial CT of C3/4.
(5) Axial CT of C4.
(6) Axial CT of C4/5.
(7) Axial CT of C5.
(8) Axial CT of C6.
(9) Axial CT of C7.
(10) Axial MRI of C2/3.
(11) Axial MRI of C3/4.
(12). Axial MRI of C4/5.
(13) Axial MRI of C5/6.
(14) Axial MRI of C6/7.

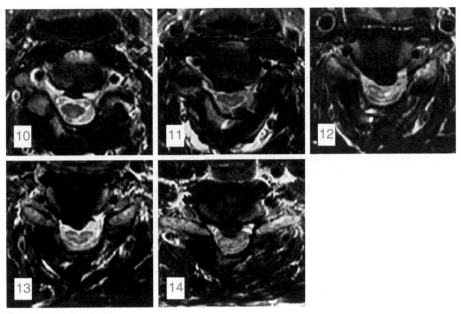

FIGURE 3.49.3 cont'd.

Preoperative axial CT images: The OPLL is more severe at C5 to C6, with a double-layer sign at C3 to C4/5. It measures:6.4 mm thick (anteroposterior) and 15.2 mm wide (mediolateral) at C3/4, 14.2 mm thick and 5.7 mm wide at C4, 6.9 mm thick and 16 mm wide at C4/5, 8.8 mm thick and 17.6 mm wide at C5, and 9.4 mm thick and 14.5 mm wide at C6 (Fig. 3.49.3, panel 1 to 9).

Preoperative axial MR images: Residual cord compression at C5/6 and C6/7, boomerang-shaped spinal cord due to anterior indentation, and partial effacement of CSF (Fig. 3.49.3, panel 10 to 14).

Highlights

This case features recurrent neural deficit following symptom resolution after a posterior single-door laminoplasty due to "hyperextension injury of the cervical spine." Imaging studies taken upon this presentation showed the size of the laminae's opening, the number of decompression levels, and the posterior shift of the spinal cord were appropriate. However, the spinal cord was still under stress, evidenced by the ventral ossification from C4 to C6 and partial obliteration of CSF. Also, the spinal cord was found rotated at the C5/6 level.

Surgical planning

A revision surgery via an anterior approach applies to this case, such as a three-level ACCF from C4 to C6.

The expanded spinal canal from the index posterior surgery was a favorable factor for an anterior procedure. Nevertheless, given the possible multilevel dural ossification, suggested by a double-layer sign from C4 to C6, a direct decompression may risk a dural tear or CSF leak.

The patient received ACAF for C4 to C6, and undercut decompression of the superior rim of the C7 vertebra via the C6/7 disc space.

With an expanded spinal canal from the index posterior surgery, VOC displacement distance in the ACAF technique should be smaller than the ossification thickness.

The amount of bone resection from the anterior vertebral bodies was benchmarked with the ossification thickness at C2 to C3. The OPLL thickness at the VOC levels was compared with the benchmark, whose difference became the bone thickness to be resected anteriorly (Fig. 3.49.4).

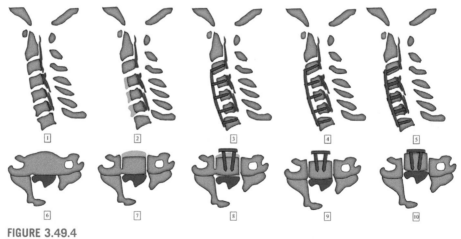

FIGURE 3.49.4

Illustration of the surgical plan on sagittal and axial planes.
(1, 6) Illustration of the OPLL on sagittal and axial views before surgery.
(2, 7) Resection performed to the anterior part of C4 to C6 vertebral bodies, a complete trough developed on the left vertebral bodies from C4 to C6 while a half one on the right side with the posterior bone yet to be dissected.
(3, 8) Plate and screws placed on vertebral bodies from C3 through C7.
(4, 9) The bottom of the right half-groove on C4 through C6 dissected.
(5, 10) Antedisplaced C4 to C6 vertebral bodies as screws were tightened.

Results

Postoperative function: JOA score was 8, Nurick score: 3, VAS: 3, and NDI: 24.

Cobb angle of 15.2° from C2 to C7 in a cervical spine with restored curvature (Fig. 3.49.5).

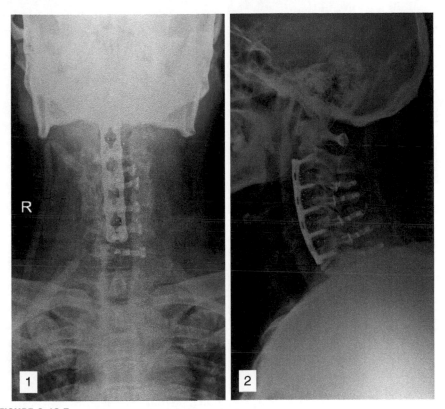

FIGURE 3.49.5

Postoperative cervical spine X-ray.
(1) Anteroposterior view.
(2) Lateral view.

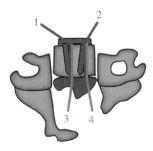

Reference of the sagittal planes

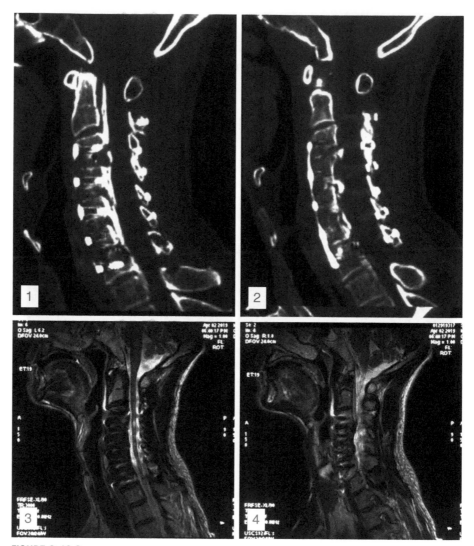

FIGURE 3.49.6

Postoperative sagittal views and their reference on the axial diagram.
(1) Left parasagittal CT.
(2) Right parasagittal CT.
(3) Left parasagittal MRI.
(4) Right parasagittal MRI.

Based on postoperative sagittal CT and MR image, antedisplaced VOC from C4 to C6 and widened spinal canal shown on postoperative midsagittal CT image (Fig. 3.49.6, panel 1 and 2). Spinal cord with restored curvature free of compression and surrounded by CSF (Fig. 3.49.6, panel 3 and 4).

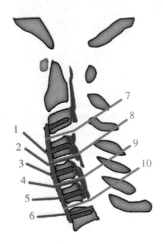

Reference of the axial planes

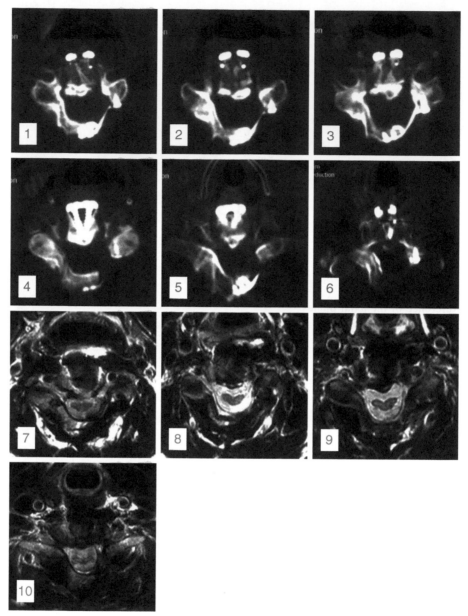

FIGURE 3.49.7

Postoperative axial cervical images and their reference on the sagittal diagram.

(1) Axial CT of C4.

(2) Axial CT of C4/5.

(3) Axial CT of C5.

(4) Axial CT of C5/6.

(5) Axial CT of C6.

(6) Axial CT of the superior surface of C7.

(7) Axial MRI of C3/4.

(8) Axial MRI of C4/5.

(9) Axial MRI of C5/6.

(10) Axial MRI of C6/7.

Based on postoperative axial CT images, the vertebral bodies from C4 to C6 have been dissected with parasagittal cuts on both sides 21.2 mm apart and ventrally displaced VOC by 4.7 mm (Fig. 3.49.7, panel 1 to 6). Based on axial MR images, the spinal cord has recovered to an oval and triangular shape (Fig. 3.49.7, panel 7 to 10).

Discussion

Why were C2 and C3 excluded from the antedisplacement complex?

The OPLL, in this case, spanned from C2 to the posterosuperior rim of the C7 vertebra. Locally at C2 to C3, the compression was focused at the inferior surface of the C3 vertebra, and an ample amount of CSF was still present behind C2 and the superior surface of the C3 vertebra. The prior surgery resolved cord compression at C2 to C3 and reduced the spinal cord to its natural shape. But cord deformation and rotation were still present from C4 to C6, which suggested residual compression.

The dissociation within the ossification at C3/4 was palpated with a nerve hook before dissection in case of insufficient advancement.

If this gap was unidentifiable or too narrow, the ossification could be debulked to widen the gap. As this gap may be reduced by the hyperextended surgical positioning, the access could be increased by partial resection of the C3 vertebra on the cephalad side and osteophyte removal.

Case 50: Ossification of posterior longitudinal ligament (OPLL) of cervical spine (At C3 to C6), history of cervical surgery, cervical kyphosis

Index terms

Antedisplacement of two vertebral bodies, local-type OPLL, narrow-based disease, cervical kyphosis, status postposterior cervical surgery, and thickness of ossification 6.1 mm.

History

Patient: A 59-year-old man.

Chief complaint: Weakness of the extremities for five years and status postposterior cervical surgery.

Physical exam: The patient was wheeled in. Physical exam was noted for the straightened cervical spine; limited range of cervical motion; an impaired sense of light touch, pinprick, and temperature on all the extremities, the trunk and the genital area; hypertonicity on all the extremities; muscular atrophy; and compromised fine movements. Muscle strength was tested at 3+/5 on the deltoid, biceps and triceps brachii, wrist flexion and extension, hand grips, iliopsoas, quadriceps femoris, biceps femoris, semitendinosus, semimembranosus, and anterior tibialis on both sides, triceps surae, dorsal and plantar flexion on both sides. Cremasteric reflex was indifferent. Brisk tendon reflexes were noted on bilateral biceps and triceps brachii, radiobrachialis, knees, and ankles.

Preoperative function: JOA score was 10, Nurick score: 3, VAS: 0, and NDI: 15.

Imaging studies

A kyphotic cervical spine with a Cobb angle of 3.8° from C2 through C7 and −2.1° from C2 to C5, and OPLL from C3 to C5 (Fig. 3.50.1).

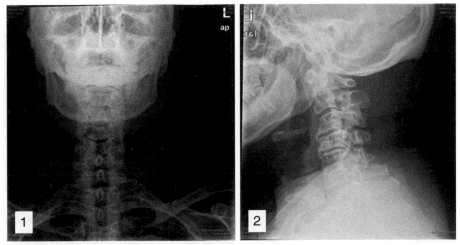

FIGURE 3.50.1

Preoperative X-ray of the cervical spine.
(1) Anteroposterior view.
(2) Lateral view.

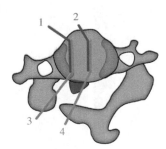

Reference of the sagittal planes

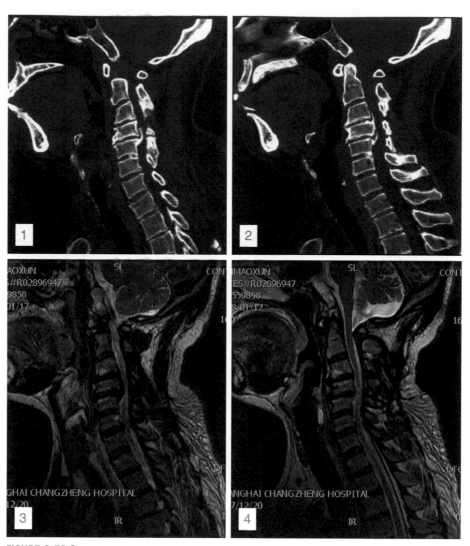

FIGURE 3.50.2

Preoperative sagittal images of the cervical spine and their reference on the axial diagram.
(1) Sagittal CT at the right uncinate process.
(2) Midsagittal CT.
(3) Sagittal MRI at the right uncinate process.
(4) Midsagittal MRI.

Postposterior cervical surgery and local-type OPLL from C3 to C5 shown on preoperative sagittal CT images (Fig. 3.50.2, panel 1 and 2).

A kyphotic spinal cord compressed and deformed at C3/4 to C4/5 with CSF obliteration shown on preoperative sagittal MR images (Fig. 3.50.2, panel 3 and 4).

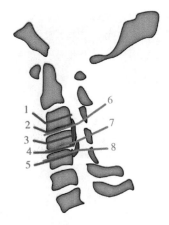

Reference of the axial planes

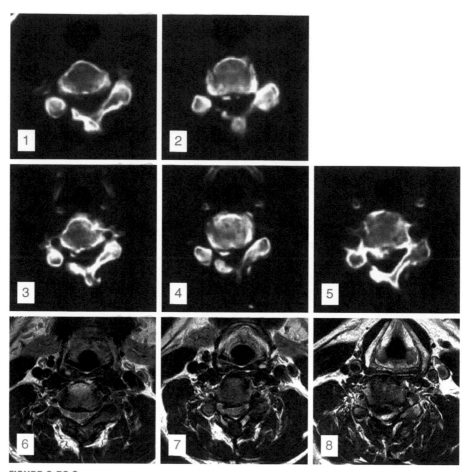

FIGURE 3.50.3

Preoperative axial images of the cervical spine and their reference on the sagittal diagram.
(1) Axial CT of C3.
(2) Axial CT of C3/4.
(3) Axial CT of C4.
(4) Axial CT of C4/5.
(5) Axial CT of C5.
(6) Axial MRI of C3/4.
(7) Axial MRI of C4/5.
(8) Axial MRI of C5.

Based on axial CT images, the OPLL is eccentric to the right and narrow-based, with a larger cross-section area at C3/4 and C4. The OPLL measures 2.1 mm thick (anteroposterior), 5.6 mm wide (mediolateral), and 21% in canal occupancy at C3; 2.6 mm thick, 10.6 mm wide, and 25% in canal occupancy at C3/4; 5.1 mm thick, 8.1 mm wide, and 43% in canal occupancy at C4; 5.4 mm thick, 12.7 mm wide, and 33% in canal occupancy at C4/5; and 6.1 mm thick, 14.7 mm wide, and 41% in canal occupancy at C5 (Fig. 3.50.3, panel 1 to 5).

Based on axial MR images, the spinal cord deformed into triangular and boomerang shape at C3/4 to C4/5; intramedullary signal hyperintensity suggesting myelopathy at C4/5, the level of maximum cord compression (Fig. 3.50.3, panel 6 to 8).

Highlights

This case features a short-segment OPLL from C3 to C5 in a locally kyphotic cervical spine. The patient presented with recurrent neural deficit sometime after a laminoplasty opened on the right side. Imaging studies from this presentation revealed inadequate expansion from the prior surgery, osteogenesis along the edge of the partial laminectomy, particularly at C5, and residual cord compression.

Surgical planning

Cervical kyphosis, short-segment OPLL, and status post right-based laminectomy lead to the option of ACCF for further decompression and curvature correction.

However, given the right paracentral component of the OPLL, the subtotal corpectomy of ACCF may lead to a residual lesion that is too risky and challenging to remove.

An ACAF with antedisplacement of C4 and C5 vertebral bodies and ossification resection at C3 through the disc space was planned for this case.

As the curvature correction provides extra decompression in a kyphotic cervical spine, the anterior resection shall measure thinner than the ossification thickness (Fig. 3.50.4).

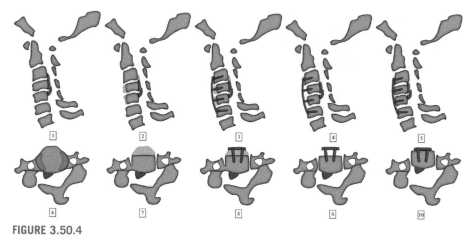

FIGURE 3.50.4

Illustration of the surgical plan on sagittal and axial planes.

(1, 6) Illustration of the OPLL on sagittal and axial views before surgery.

(2, 7) Resection of the anterior part of C4 to C5 vertebral bodies and the posteroinferior border of C3, a complete trough developed on the left vertebral bodies from C4 to C5 while a half one on the right side with the posterior bone yet to be dissected.

(3, 8) Plate and screws placed on vertebral bodies from C3 through C6.

(4, 9) The bottom of the right half-groove on C4 and C5 dissected.

(5, 10) Antedisplaced C4 and C5 vertebral bodies as screws were tightened.

Results

Postoperative function: JOA score was 14, Nurick score: 2, VAS: 0, and NDI: 10.

Lordotic cervical spine, Cobb angle of 12.9° from C2 to C7, and antedisplaced C4 to C5 vertebral bodies (Fig. 3.50.5).

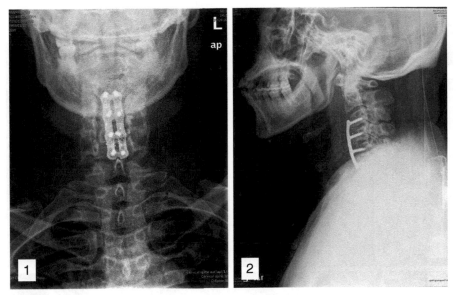

FIGURE 3.50.5

Postoperative cervical spine X-ray.
(1) Anteroposterior view.
(2) Lateral view.

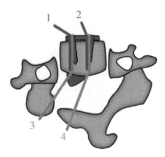

Reference of the sagittal planes

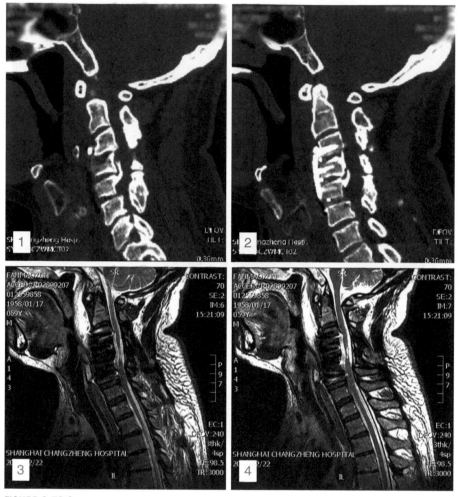

FIGURE 3.50.6

Postoperative sagittal views and their reference on the axial diagram.
(1) Sagittal CT at the right uncinate process.
(2) Midsagittal CT.
(3) Sagittal MRI at the right uncinate process.
(4) Midsagittal MRI.

Ventrally displaced VOC from C4 to C5, and ossification of the posteroinferior rim of C3 vertebra removed shown on postoperative sagittal CT images (Fig. 3.50.6, panel 1 and 2).

The spinal cord in restored curvature free of compression and surrounded by CSF, with residual intramedullary signal hyperintensity shown on postoperative sagittal MR images (Fig. 3.50.6, panel 3 and 4).

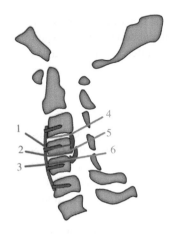

Reference of the axial planes

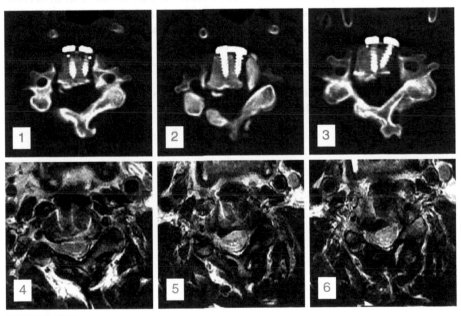

FIGURE 3.50.7

Postoperative axial cervical images and their reference on the sagittal diagram.
(1) Axial CT of C4.
(2) Axial CT of C4/5.
(3) Axial CT of C5.
(4) Axial MRI of C3/4.
(5) Axial MRI of C4/5.
(6) Axial MRI of the superior surface of C5.

Based on axial CT images, the vertebral bodies have been dissected with para-sagittal cuts on both sides 22.8 mm apart and antedisplaced by 4.6 mm, and the canal occupancy reduced to 20% (Fig. 3.50.7, panel 1 to 3).

Based on axial MR images, free of compression, the spinal cord has recovered to oval and triangular shape, surrounded by an ample amount of CSF, with residual dots of intramedullary signal hyperintensity at C4/5 and C5 (Fig. 3.50.7, panel 4 to 6).

Discussion

Is decompression achieved with antedisplacement of C4 alone?

The OPLL spanned from C3 to C5 with discontinuity, shown on preoperative imaging studies.

Specifically, the lesion involved less than half the height of C3 and C5 vertebral bodies, the component at C4 extended to C3, and that at the superior part of C5 extended cephalad to C4.

The idea of a three-level decompression achieved through antedisplacement of one vertebra does not work because there was a gap within the ossification at C4. A single-level antedisplacement could be considered with ossification dissection at C4/5 and undercutting for the lesion at C5, which is technically challenging.

Therefore, this case was decompressed via antedisplacement of C4 and C5 vertebral bodies and lesion resection posterior to C3 via the undercutting technique.

The instrumentation could have been done better as it ended up eccentric to the right. The right paracentral plate and the screws on the right side lead the VOC to deviate toward the right, leaving the screws on the left side of C4 and C5 vertebral bodies with a reduced purchase in the bone.

Case 51: Cervical canal stenosis, history of cervical surgery

Index terms

Antedisplacement of two vertebrae, circumscribed (localized) ossification of the posterior longitudinal ligament (OPLL), and status postanterior cervical surgery.

History

Patient: A 53-year-old man.

Chief complaint: Numbness of the extremities for one year and weakness of the extremities and gait instability for two months.

Physical exam: Physical exam was noted for gait disturbance, and muscle strength was tested at 4/5 on four extremities. Muscle tension of both lower limbs is increased, left triceps reflex is hyperreflexia, bilateral knee reflex is hyperreflexia, and bilateral Hoffmann sign is positive.

Preoperative function: Japanese Orthopedic Association (JOA) score was 10, Nurick score: 3, visual analog scale (VAS): 1, and neck disability index (NDI): 18.

Imaging studies

Status postsubtotal corpectomy of C6, osteophytes violating the spinal canal at the inferior rim of C5 and the superior rim of C7 (Fig. 3.51.1).

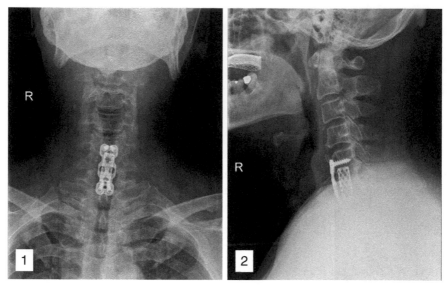

FIGURE 3.51.1

Preoperative X-ray of the cervical spine.
(1) Anteroposterior view.
(2) Lateral view.

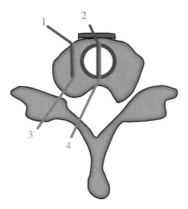

Reference of the sagittal planes

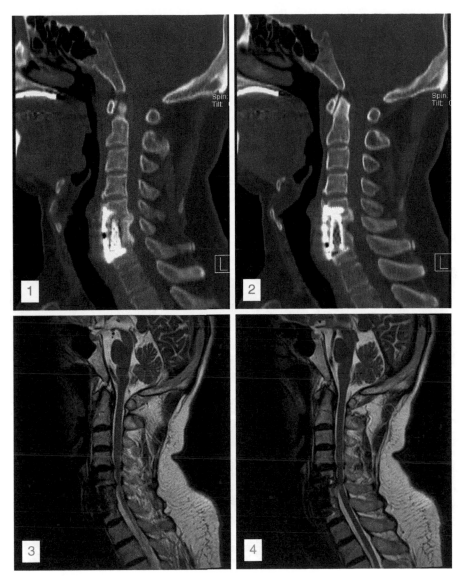

FIGURE 3.51.2

Preoperative sagittal images of the cervical spine and their reference on the axial diagram.

(1) Sagittal CT at the right uncinate process.

(2) Midsagittal CT.

(3) Sagittal MRI at the right uncinate process.

(4) Midsagittal MRI.

Preoperative sagittal computed tomography (CT) images: Status postanterior cervical corpectomy and fusion (ACCF) of C6 and osteophytes at the inferior rim of C5 and the superior rim of C7, with those at C5 being more protuberant (Fig. 3.51.2, panel 1 and 2).

Preoperative sagittal magnetic resonance (MR) images: The spinal cord compressed at C4/5 and C5/6, more severe at C5/6, and intramedullary signal hyperintensity suggesting myelopathy (Fig. 3.51.2, panel 3 and 4).

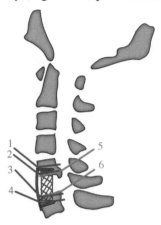

Reference of the axial planes

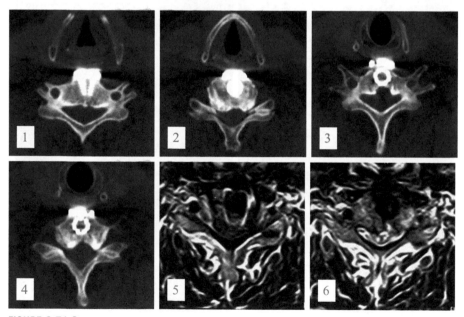

FIGURE 3.51.3

Preoperative axial images of the cervical spine and their reference on the sagittal diagram.
(1) Axial CT of C5.
(2) Axial CT of the inferior surface of C5.
(3) Axial CT of the superior surface of C7.
(4) Axial CT of the disc space above C7.
(5) Axial MRI of the interior surface of C5.
(6) Axial MRI of the superior surface of C7.

Osteophytes along the posterior rim of C5 vertebra in the neural exit foramen on both sides shown on axial CT images (Fig. 3.51.3, panel 1 to 4).

The spinal cord deformed into a triangular shape at C5 and C6, with an intramedullary snake-eyes sign at C6 shown on preoperative axial MR images (Fig. 3.51.3, panel 5 and 6).

Highlights

This case presented with recurrent neural deficit after ACCF surgery. The spinal cord was impinged at both ends of the mesh, more severe at C5 due to the indentation of its posterior rim. The spinal cord was also impinged at C4/5 due to disc herniation.

Surgical planning

Indirect decompression through the posterior approach in the revision surgery may cause incomplete cord decompression due to the poor cervical curvature.

Another option is hardware and bone removal through anterior surgery and reconstruction with a new mesh. Given the lateral-based impingement on both sides, after hardware removal, the lateral bone in the residual vertebra should be further resected for thorough decompression, which may risk excessive anterior shift of the spinal cord, nerve tethering, and palsy.

The patient received an anterior controllable antedisplacement fusion (ACAF) with antedisplacement of C5 and the mesh and intervertebral decompression of C4/5.

During the surgery, a transverse wedge was developed from the vertebra inferior to the mesh and C5 vertebra was resected from the front to the anterior surface of the mesh. The decompression was finished as the C5 displaced, and the wedge closed (Fig. 3.51.4).

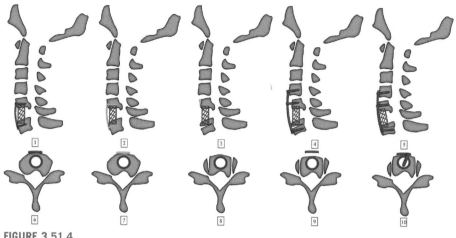

FIGURE 3.51.4

Illustration of the surgical plan on sagittal and axial planes.

(1, 6) Illustration of the OPLL on sagittal and axial views before surgery.

(2, 7) Removal of plate and screws, resection of the anterior part of the C5 vertebra, and wedge developed in the C7 vertebra.

(3, 8) A complete trough developed on the left vertebra while a half one on the right side with the posterior bone yet to be dissected.

(4, 9) The bottom of the right half-groove dissected.

(5, 10) Antedisplaced C5 vertebra and closed wedge in C7 as screws were tightened.

Results

Postoperative function: JOA score was 12, Nurick score: 3, VAS: 0, and NDI: 14.

Antedisplaced C5 vertebra and the mesh and instrumentation from C4 to C7 (Fig. 3.51.5).

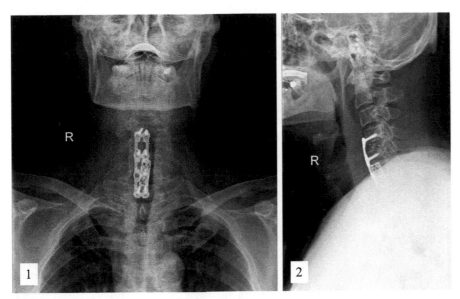

FIGURE 3.51.5

Postoperative cervical spine X-ray.
(1) Anteroposterior view.
(2) Lateral view.

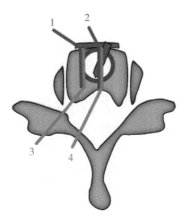

Reference of the sagittal planes

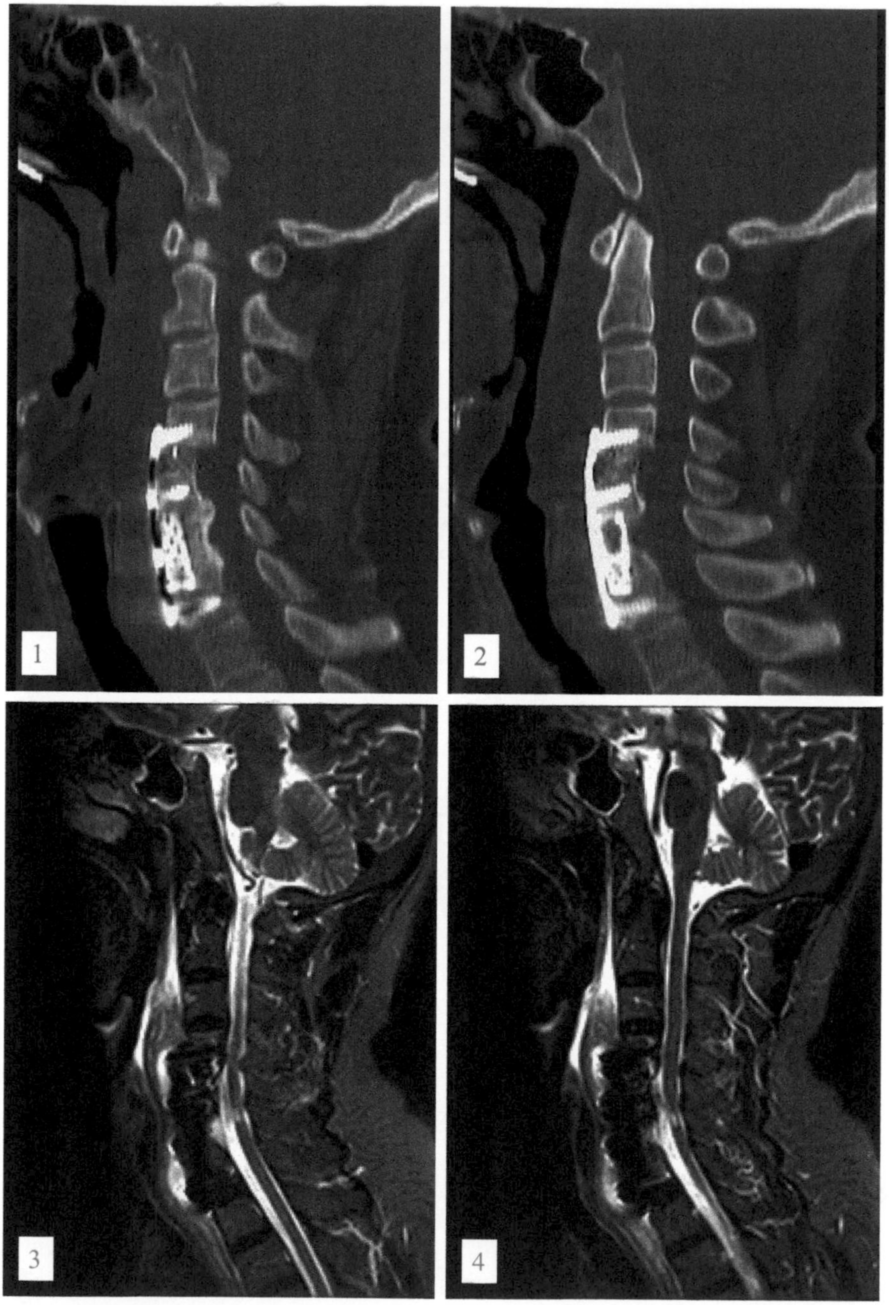

FIGURE 3.51.6

Postoperative sagittal views and their reference on the axial diagram.

(1) Axial CT of the inferior surface of C5.

(2) Axial CT of the superior surface of C7.

(3) Axial MRI of C5.

(4) Axial MRI of C6.

Based on sagittal CT images, ventrally displaced C5 and the mesh, expanded spinal canal, and well-engaged plate and mesh (Fig. 3.51.6, panel 1 and 2).

Based on sagittal MR images, the spinal cord free of compression and surrounded by CSF (Fig. 3.51.6, panel 3 and 4).

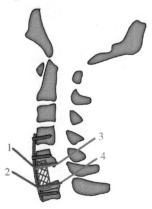

Reference of the axial planes

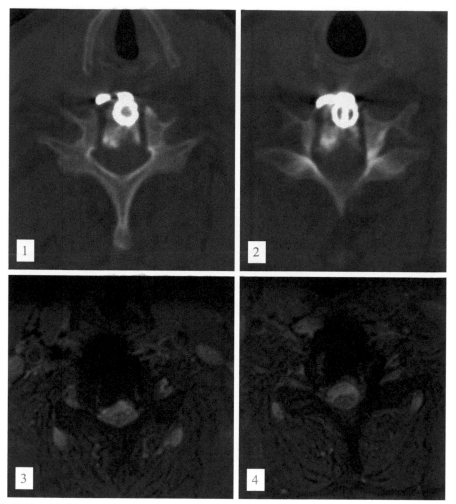

FIGURE 3.51.7

Postoperative axial cervical images and their reference on the sagittal diagram.
(1) Axial CT of the inferior surface of C5.
(2) Axial CT of the superior surface of C7.
(3) Axial MRI of the inferior surface of C5.
(4) Axial MRI of the superior surface of C7.

The vertebral bodies have been dissected with parasagittal cuts on both sides 20.7 mm apart and antedisplaced by 5.5 mm shown on postoperative axial CT images (Fig. 3.51.7, panel 1 and 2).

The spinal cord has recovered to oval shape with CSF filling shown on postoperative axial MR images (Fig. 3.51.7, panel 3 and 4).

Discussion

The antedisplacement complex was not from C5 to C7. What was the rationale?

The spinal cord had been under compression due to the residual lesion dorsal to the C5 vertebra after the index ACCF.

We gave up the thought of C5 to C7 antedisplacement, considering the relation between the plate and mesh. They were tightly engaged at the caudal end but well separated at the cephalad end.

This allowed minimal displacement at the caudal end of the construct unless the mesh was partly trimmed off. Otherwise, the mesh might contact the plate on the distal part prematurely and block the migration of the proximal mesh.

The proximal mesh was entitled to an adequate room for antedisplacement with strategies of bone resection of the anterior vertebra and plate contouring.

To adequately antedisplace C5 for a thorough decompression independent of the potential barrier from the distal end of the mesh, a wedge was developed below the distal end of the mesh at C7 with converging bone cuts toward the posterior cortex without going through it. As the screws were tightened, C5 was hoisted anteriorly, and the wedge in C7 closed, causing only microfracture of the posterior cortex of the C7 vertebra.

Case 52: Cervical canal stenosis, history of cervical surgery

Index terms

Antedisplacement of three vertebral bodies and status postanterior and posterior cervical surgeries.

History

Patient: A 54-year-old man.

Chief complaint: Status postcervical surgeries performed four years ago.

Physical exam: Physical exam was noted for gait disturbance; limited range of cervical motion; impaired sense on the genital and perianal area; an impaired sense of light touch, pinprick, and temperature distal to the shoulders and knees; tightness and numbness of the trunk below the intermammary line; hypertonicity on hands and lower extremities; and muscular atrophy of the left thigh. Muscle strength was tested at 4+/5 on bilateral deltoid, biceps and triceps brachii, wrist flexion and extension; 3/5 on hand grips; 4−/5 on bilateral iliopsoas and quadriceps femoris; 4+/5 on anterior tibialis, triceps surae, dorsal and plantar flexion on both sides. Brisk tendon reflexes were noted on knees and ankles.

Preoperative function: JOA score was 12, Nurick score: 3, VAS: 0, and NDI: 16.

Imaging studies

Status postsubtotal corpectomy of C5 vertebra and posterior decompression, instrumentation, grafting, and fusion from C4 to C7 (Fig. 3.52.1).

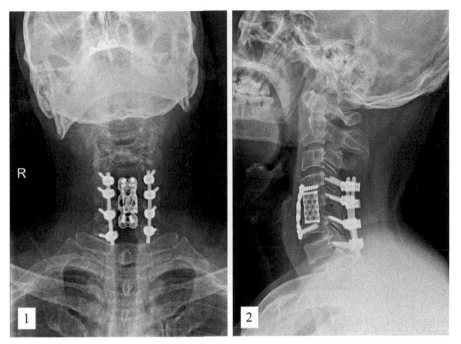

FIGURE 3.52.1

X-ray of the cervical spine prior to the revision surgery.
(1) Anteroposterior view.
(2) Lateral view.

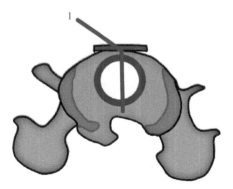

Reference of the sagittal plane

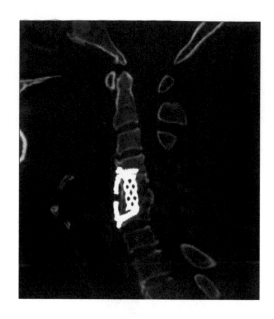

FIGURE 3.52.2

Preoperative sagittal image of the cervical spine and its reference on the axial diagram.
(1) Midsagittal CT.

Shown on preoperative sagittal CT images, status postsubtotal corpectomy of C5 vertebra, hill-shaped residual vertebra posterior to the mesh suggesting incomplete resection of the ossification, and devoid laminae and posterior elements from C4 to C7 (Fig. 3.52.2, panel 1).

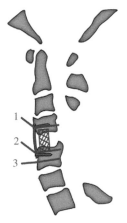

Reference of the axial planes

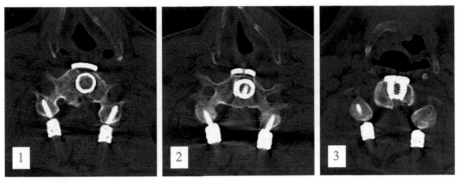

FIGURE 3.52.3

Axial images of the cervical spine before revision and their reference on the sagittal diagram.
(1) Axial CT of C4.
(2) Axial CT of the inferior surface of C6.
(3) Axial CT of the superior surface of C6.

Shown on preoperative axial CT images, the residual bone dorsal to C5 vertebra 5 mm thick and 8 mm wide violates the spinal canal (Fig. 3.52.3, panel 1 to 3).

Highlights

This patient had received C5 subtotal corpectomy for OPLL but experienced recurrent neural deficit, which was caused by residual OPLL dorsal to the residual C5 vertebra from the oblique bone cuts during the prior surgery. The second stage of the prior surgery was composed of a posterior laminectomy and instrumentation for curvature restoration and further decompression. However, the neurologic decompression was not thorough, as seen from imaging studies, and the spinal cord had not shifted back adequately.

Surgical planning

If treated with a conventional anterior procedure during the revision, the compression-related OPLL would be resected and the index mesh substituted with a longer one. Mesh removal was particularly risky in iatrogenic injuries and hardware-related complications since the mesh had been robustly fused with the residual vertebra.

During the consultation, the patient and his family declined surgeries that substitute the mesh.

The patient received ACAF with antedisplacement of C4 to C6, where the grooves were developed wider apart to maintain the index mesh. Decompression was achieved without hardware-related complications as the vertebral-OPLL complex (VOC) was ventrally displaced.

Sagittal grooves were developed off the anterior root of uncinate processes 21 mm apart. The mesh diameter was 14 mm.

The anterior part of the vertebrae was resected by the same thickness as the ossification, and the plate contoured to fit the preoperative cervical curvature. Care was taken not to overbend the plate (Fig. 3.52.4).

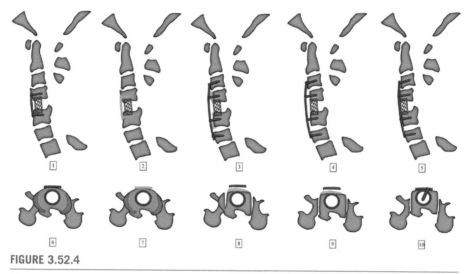

FIGURE 3.52.4

Illustration of the surgical plan on sagittal and axial planes.

(1, 6) Illustration of the OPLL on sagittal and axial views before surgery.

(2, 7) Screws removed, a left groove and a right half-groove with the posterior cortex still intact on C4, C5, and C6 developed.

(3, 8) Titanium plate and screws placed in vertebral bodies from C3 to C7.

(4, 9) Completion of the right groove on C4, C5, and C6.

(5, 10) Antedisplaced C4, C5, and C6 vertebral bodies as screws were tightened.

Results

Postoperative function: JOA score was 15, Nurick score: 1, VAS: 0, and NDI: 8 (Fig. 3.52.5).

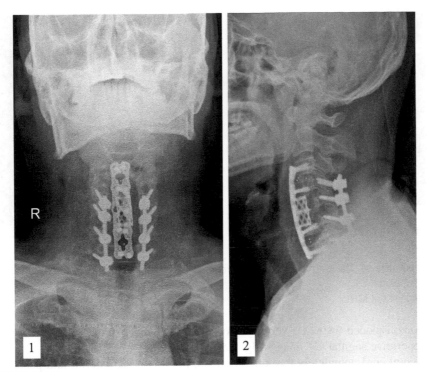

FIGURE 3.52.5

Postoperative cervical X-ray.
(1) Anteroposterior view.
(2) Lateral view.

Antedisplaced VOC from C4 to C6 with the titanium mesh and plate fit completely.

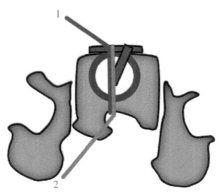

Reference of the sagittal plane

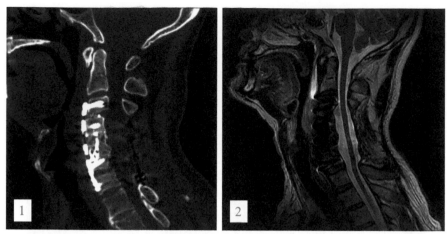

FIGURE 3.52.6

Postoperative sagittal images and their reference on the axial diagram.
(1) Midsagittal CT.
(2) Midsagittal MRI.

Antedisplaced C4 to C6 vertebral bodies and expanded spinal canal shown on postoperative sagittal CT image (Fig. 3.52.6, panel 1).

Spinal cord completely free of compression between the anterior and posterior columns of cerebrospinal fluid (CSF) shown on postoperative sagittal MR image (Fig. 3.52.6, panel 2).

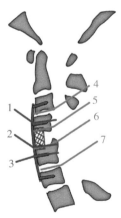

Reference of the axial planes

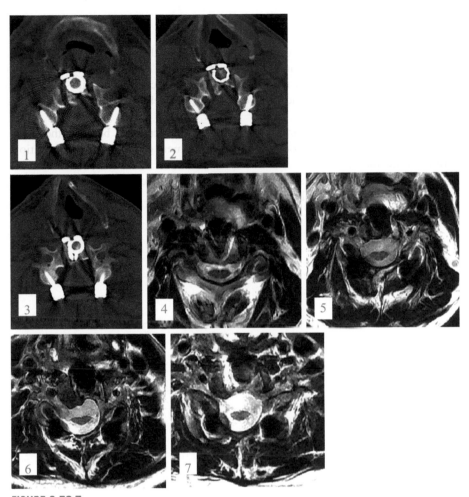

FIGURE 3.52.7

Postoperative axial cervical images and their reference on the sagittal diagram.

(1) Axial CT of C4.
(2) Axial CT of the superior surface of C6.
(3) Axial CT of the C6.
(4) Axial MRI of the C3/4.
(5) Axial MRI of the inferior surface of C4.
(6) Axial MRI of the superior surface of C6.
(7) Axial MRI of the C6/7.

Shown on postoperative axial CT image, the VOC has been antedisplaced by 3 mm with sagittal bone cuts 20 mm apart (Fig. 3.52.7, panel 1 to 3). The spinal cord resumes to an oval shape surrounded by CSF (Fig. 3.52.7, panel 4 to 7).

Discussion

The mesh may have restricted the anterior resection of the vertebra. Did it restrict vertebra displacement? How can this barrier be resolved?

The decision was made to resect the residual ossification posterior to the C5 vertebra through the antedisplacement of C4 to C6 vertebral bodies, based on pre-operative imaging studies.

This case was different from case 51 in that there were gaps between the mesh and the index plate. As such, room for antedisplacement came from bone resection anterior to the mesh.

Extra room for decompression was gained with a properly contoured plate that allowed space between the plate and the mesh.

Case 53: Ossification of posterior longitudinal ligament (OPLL) of cervical spine (At C2 to C5), history of cervical surgery

Index terms

Antedisplacement of three vertebral bodies, mixed-type OPLL, the thickness of ossification 7—9 mm, canal stenosis above 70%, shelter technique, status postposterior cervical surgery, cervical kyphosis, and K-line (−) OPLL.

History

Patient: A 75-year-old man.

Chief complaint: Worsen neurological deficit with quadriplegia for three years presented four years after cervical surgery.

Physical exam: The patient was wheeled in with paresthesia (tightness and numbness) of the trunk below the xiphoid, diminished cremasteric reflex, hypertonicity of the extremities, impaired tactile sensation of both hands, paresthesia of lower limbs, tendon hyperreflexia of all the extremities, and patellar and ankle clonus. Hoffmann and Babinski signs were present bilaterally.

Preoperative function: JOA score was 1, Nurick score: 5, VAS: 0, and NDI: 24.

Imaging studies

Kyphotic cervical spine, Cobb angle of −7.6° from C2 to C7, K-line (−) OPLL at C2—C6, and status postposterior cervical surgery (Fig. 3.53.1).

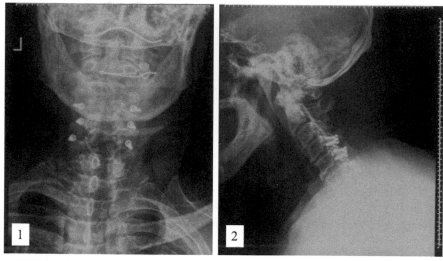

FIGURE 3.53.1

Preoperative X-ray of the cervical spine.
(1) Anteroposterior view.
(2) Lateral view.

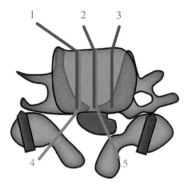

Reference of the sagittal plane

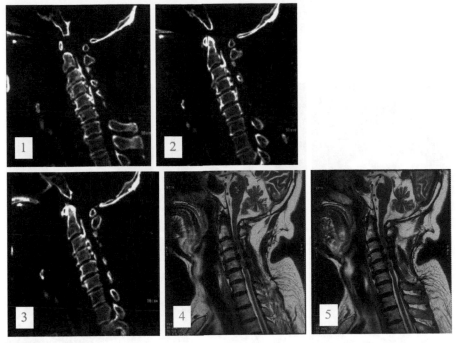

FIGURE 3.53.2

Preoperative sagittal images of the cervical spine and their reference on the axial diagram.

(1) Right parasagittal CT.

(2) Midsagittal CT.

(3) Left parasagittal CT.

(4) Right parasagittal MRI.

(5) Midsagittal MRI.

A flat, mixed-type OPLL from C2 to C5 and status postposterior surgery on C3 to C6 shown on preoperative sagittal CT images (Fig. 3.53.2, panel 1 to 3).

Status postposterior surgery of C3 to C6; secondary spinal canal stenosis; spinal cord impinged at C3/4, C4/5, and C5/6 due to anterior and posterior scar-based indentation, more severe from the posterior components; obliteration of the anterior and posterior CSF columns; intramedullary signal hyperintensity suggesting myelopathy, shown on preoperative sagittal MR images (Fig. 3.53.2, panel 4 and 5).

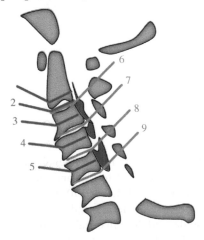

Reference of the axial planes

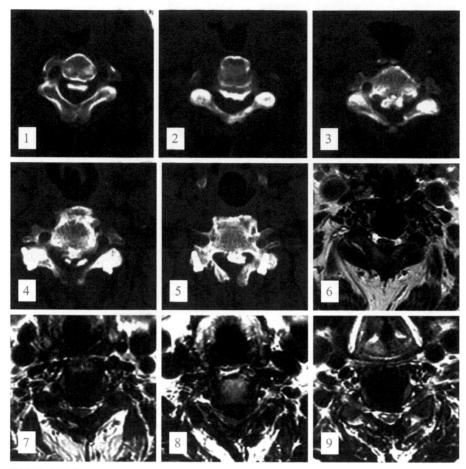

FIGURE 3.53.3

Preoperative axial images of the cervical spine and their reference on the sagittal diagram.
(1) Axial CT of the inferior surface of C2.
(2) Axial CT of C2/3.
(3) Axial CT of C3.
(4) Axial CT of C4.
(5) Axial CT of C5.
(6) Axial MRI of the C2/3.
(7) Axial MRI of the C3/4.
(8) Axial MRI of the C4/5.
(9) Axial MRI of the C5/6.

Based on preoperative axial CT image, devoid left lamina of C3, status postdouble-door laminoplasty from C4 to C6, and absence of fusion signs on the fenestrated right laminae of C4 and C5. The OPLL measures: 6.1 mm thick (anteroposterior), 11.8 mm wide (mediolateral), and 65.6% in canal occupancy at C3; 7.1 mm thick, 11.1 mm wide, and 76% in canal occupancy at C4; and 7.1 mm thick and 12.5 mm wide at C5 (Fig. 3.53.3, panel 1 to 5).

Based on preoperative axial MR image, the spinal cord impinged and deformed into a boomerang or triangle shape, with intramedullary snake-eyes sign at C5/6 (Fig. 3.53.3, panel 6 to 9).

Highlights

This case features segmental OPLL of C2 to C5, wide-based at C2/3, and double-layered at C3 and C4. After receiving a double-door laminoplasty with screws, the patient experienced symptom relief before recurrent myelopathy a few months later. Imaging studies upon presentation revealed moor cervical curvature, malunion of the right laminae, and collapsed opening of some levels, which suggested incomplete decompression.

Surgical planning

With the scars and adhesion from the previous surgery, a posterior procedure bore a high risk for dural tear and the spinal cord.

Therefore, an anterior decompression was preferred for decompression of C3 to C5. With dural ossification, suggested by preoperative imaging studies, the direct resection of the ossification may lead to dural tear and CSF leak. The use of a long cylindrical mesh is relevant to fusion failure and hardware-related complications.

An ACAF of C3 to C5 and a shelter technique for C2 decompression were planned for this patient. Also, kyphosis was to be corrected with a properly contoured plate.

The spinal canal had not been expanded despite the prior surgery that ended up in poor cervical curvature and scars. Thus, an anterior part of the vertebrae of the same thickness as the ossification was resected.

As the ossification extended high up the C2 level, its tip is frequently palpated for its relation to the bone resection on the posterior C2 vertebra to avoid residual compression (Fig. 3.53.4).

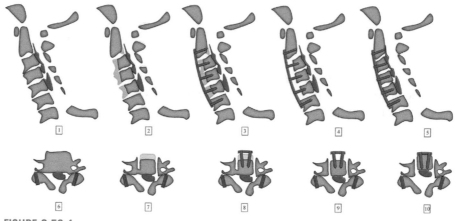

FIGURE 3.53.4

Illustration of the surgical plan on sagittal and axial planes.

(1, 6) Illustration of the OPLL on sagittal and axial views before surgery.

(2, 7) Resection of the anterior part of the vertebral bodies of C3 to C5; a left groove and a right half-groove with the posterior cortex still intact on C3 to C5.

(3, 8) Titanium plate and screws are inserted in vertebral bodies from C2 to C6.

(4, 9) Completion of the right groove on C3 to C5.

(5, 10) Antedisplaced C3 to C5 vertebral bodies as screws were tightened.

Results

Postoperative function: JOA score was 2, Nurick score: 4, VAS: 0, and NDI: 21.
    Cobb angle of 7° from C2 to C7 and restored cervical curvature (Fig. 3.53.5).

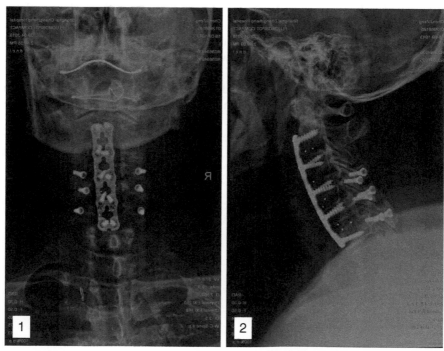

FIGURE 3.53.5

Postoperative cervical X-ray.

(1) Anteroposterior view.

(2) Lateral view.

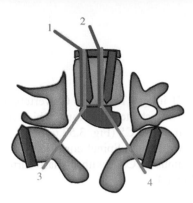

Reference of the sagittal plane

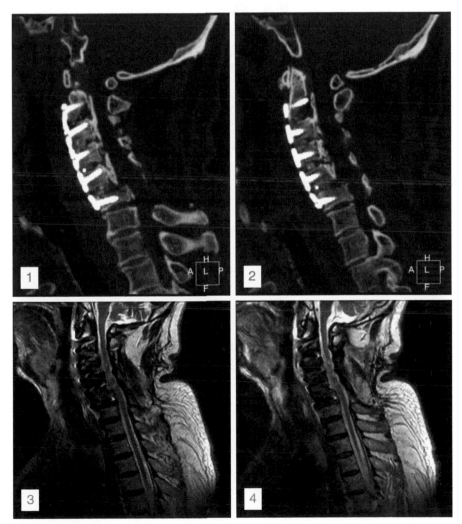

FIGURE 3.53.6

Postoperative sagittal images and their reference on the axial diagram.

(1) Sagittal CT at the right uncinate process.

(2) Midsagittal CT.

(3) Sagittal MRI at the right uncinate process.

(4) Midsagittal MRI.

Postoperative sagittal CT image: The C3 to C5 vertebral bodies have been ante-displaced and C2 undercut with shelter technique, which results in 5.8 mm antedisplacement of the VOC from C2 to C5 (Fig. 3.53.6, panel 1 to 2).

Postoperative sagittal MR image: Spinal cord free of compression between the anterior and posterior columns of CSF, with a sharp turn at C5/6 in the shape of "S" (Fig. 3.53.6, panel 3 and 4).

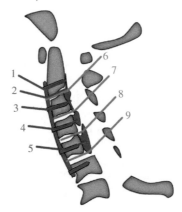

Reference of the axial planes

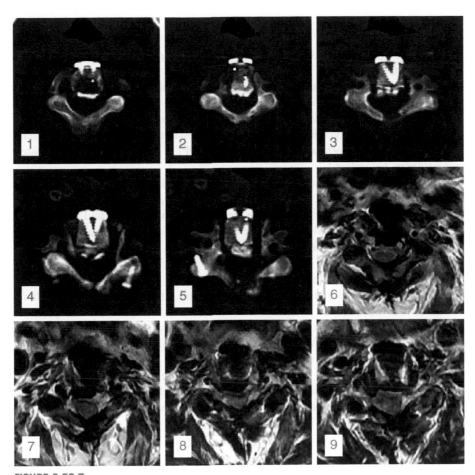

FIGURE 3.53.7

Postoperative axial cervical images and their reference on the sagittal diagram.

(1) Axial CT of the inferior surface of C2.
(2) Axial CT of C2/3.
(3) Axial CT of C3.
(4) Axial CT of C4.
(5) Axial CT of C5.
(6) Axial MRI of the C2/3.
(7) Axial MRI of the C3/4.
(8) Axial MRI of the C4/5.
(9) Axial MRI of the C5/6.

The antedisplacement has been achieved with sagittal bone cuts 22.0 mm apart shown on postoperative axial CT images (Fig. 3.53.7, panel 1 to 5).

The spinal cord free of compression resumes a triangular or oval shape and normal intramedullary signal intensity shown on postoperative axial MR images (Fig. 3.53.7, panel 6 to 9).

Discussion

What are the merits of ACAF for a revision surgery compared with the conventional anterior techniques?

Posterior fusion or nonfusion procedures, such as laminectomy and laminoplasty, have been validated strategies for multilevel OPLL but carry the risks of kyphosis development, C5 palsy, axial pain, and neurological deterioration. Anterior techniques also apply to revision with direct decompression. However, they may yield moderate results and noticeable complications in OPLL patients treated with posterior surgeries beforehand.

As an option in revision surgery, ACAF provides decompression to the spinal cord and the nerve roots at the same time. Specifically, the parasagittal bone cuts offer significant decompression to the nerve roots bilaterally, and the ventral displacement of VOC results in thorough decompression of the spinal cord. The decompression was amplified in this case as the lesion was converted to a K-line (+) one.

For the case presented here, the ventrally displaced VOC achieved decompression of the spinal cord and the bilateral nerve roots, in particular at C2/3 where the lesion was wide-based. The risks inherent to the ossified dura, including durotomy and CSF leak, were addressed since lesion removal was not involved in the ACAF technique. The ACAF lent extra benefit as the lesion had been converted from a K-line negative to a positive disease.

This surgery could have been performed better since there were residual osteophytes along the anterosuperior rim of C6. This resulted in the excessive displacement of C5 and a step along the posterior vertebral bodies between C5 and C6 that pushed the spinal cord into an "S" shape.

Case 54: Cervical canal stenosis, ossification of anterior longitudinal ligament, atlantoaxial instability

Index terms

Antedisplacement of three vertebral bodies, atlas subluxation, developmental stenosis of the spinal canal, bulky ossification of the anterior longitudinal ligament (OALL), and ACAF + posterior atlas reduction, decompression, grafting, and instrumentation.

History

Patient: A 65-year-old man.

Chief complaint: Numbness of both hands for four years with symptom aggravation, dysphagia, and gait disturbance for one year.

Physical exam: Physical exam was noted for gait instability and impaired fine movements. Muscle strength was tested at 4/5 on the deltoid, biceps and triceps brachii, wrist flexion and extension, hand grips, iliopsoas, quadriceps femoris, biceps femoris, semitendinosus, semimembranosus, and anterior tibialis on both sides, triceps surae, dorsal and plantar flexion on both sides. Brisk tendon reflexes were documented on bilateral biceps and triceps brachii, radiobrachialis, knees, and ankles, with positive ankle clonus. Hoffmann and Babinski signs were present bilaterally.

Preoperative function: JOA score was 10, Nurick score: 1, VAS: 0, and NDI: 20.

Imaging studies

Subluxed atlas; atlantodental interval (ADI) of 6.4 mm; space available for the cord (SAC) of 15.4 mm; spinal stenosis from C4 to C6; Pavlov ratio at 54%, 58%, and 66% at C4, C5, and C6, respectively; OALL from C2 through C6, and severe disc degeneration from C2/3 to C5/6 (Fig. 3.54.1).

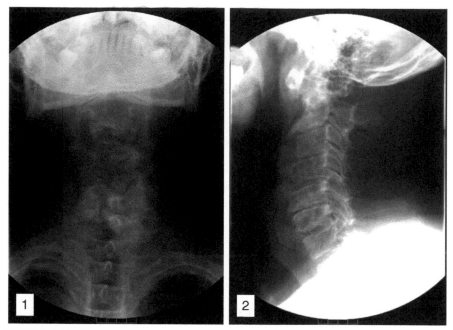

FIGURE 3.54.1

Preoperative X-ray of the cervical spine.
(1) Anteroposterior view.
(2) Lateral view.

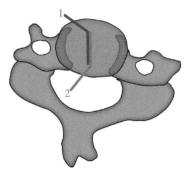

Reference of the sagittal plane

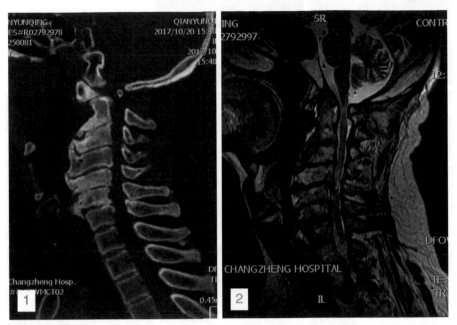

FIGURE 3.54.2

Preoperative sagittal images of the cervical spine and their reference on the axial diagram.
(1) Midsagittal CT.
(2) Right parasagittal MRI.

Subluxed atlas, OALL from C2 to C6 and fused, and severe disc degeneration from C2/3 to C5/6 shown on preoperative sagittal CT images (Fig. 3.54.2, panel 1).

Straightened spinal cord, subluxated atlas, pincer-pattern impingement of the spinal cord, spinal canal stenosis from C4 to C6, obliteration of the anterior and posterior CSF columns, and intramedullary signal hyperintensity at C4 and C5 suggesting myelopathy shown on preoperative sagittal MR images (Fig. 3.54.2, panel 2).

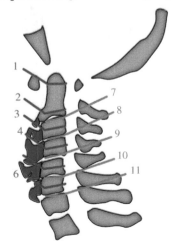

Reference of the axial planes

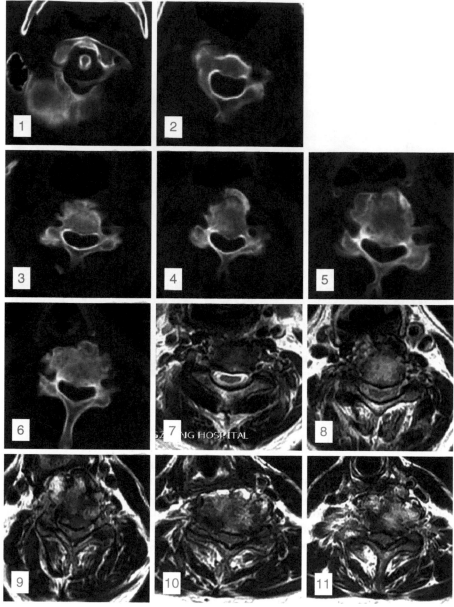

FIGURE 3.54.3

Preoperative axial images of the cervical spine and their reference on the sagittal diagram.

(1) Axial CT of C1.
(2) Axial CT of C2.
(3) Axial CT of C3.
(4) Axial CT of C4.
(5) Axial CT of C5.
(6) Axial CT of C6.
(7) Axial MRI of C2/3.
(8) Axial MRI of C3/4.
(9) Axial MRI of C4/5.
(10) Axial MRI of C5/6.
(11) Axial MRI of C6/7.

ADI of 5.4 mm, multilevel OALL measuring 12.9 mm thick (anteroposterior) and 45.7 mm in maximum width (mediolateral), and soft tissue in the neck pushed to the right shown on preoperative axial CT images (Fig. 3.54.3, panel 1 to 6).

A spinal cord significantly impinged from C4/5 to C5/6, appearing triangular and boomerang-shaped with intramedullary dotted signal hyperintensity shown on preoperative axial MR images (Fig. 3.54.3, panel 7 to 11).

Highlights

This case features atlas subluxation with developmental spinal canal stenosis from C4 to C6, bulky OALL that pushed the esophagus and trachea toward the right, according to imaging studies. The patient reported foreign body sensation during swallowing.

Surgical planning

The conventional strategy for atlas subluxation is a posterior reduction, decompression, instrumentation, and fusion.

In a posterior approach, spinal canal expansion surgery can be performed along side with the atlas reduction. However, these procedures require muscle elevation from the occiput to C7, which may leave the patient with sustained nuchal pain. In addition, a posterior surgery does not provide much relief for the spondylotic dysphagia.

A posterior atlas reduction, decompression, grafting, instrumentation, and fusion as well as ACAF for C4 to C6 vertebral bodies were performed on this patient.

During the surgery, the ossified anterior longitudinal ligament was skinned off to reveal the anterior cortex of the vertebral bodies and confirmed to be cleared with fluoroscopy.

Calculation of the distance of antedisplacement was based on the target of resumption of the spinal canal volume to the normal range and Pavlov ratio at 75% (Fig. 3.54.4).

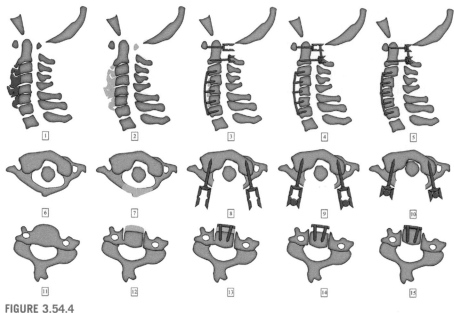

FIGURE 3.54.4

Illustration of the surgical plan on sagittal and axial planes.

(1, 6, 11) Illustration of the disease on sagittal and axial views before surgery.

(2, 7, 12) Resection performed to the anterior part of C4, C5, C6 vertebral bodies and posterior arch of atlas, a complete trough developed on the left vertebral bodies from C4 to C6 while a half one on the right side with the posterior bone yet to be dissected.

(3, 8, 9, 13) Titanium plate and screws placed in vertebral bodies from C3 to C7. Bilateral pedicle screws placed into C1–C2.

(4, 14) Completion of the right groove on C4, C5, and C6.

(5, 15) Antedisplaced C4, C5, and C6 vertebral bodies and C1 reset with screws were tightened.

Results

Postoperative function: JOA score was 12, Nurick score: 1, VAS: 1, and NDI: 10.

Reduced atlas, ADI of 3 mm, devoid posterior arch of the atlas, anterior instrumentation from C3 to C7, and antedisplaced C4 to C6 vertebral bodies (Fig. 3.54.5).

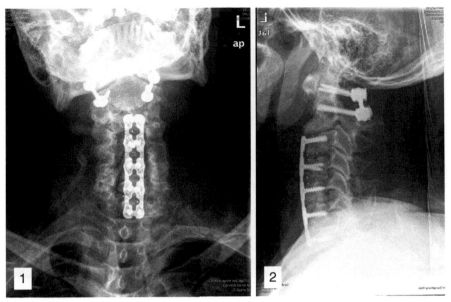

FIGURE 3.54.5

Postoperative cervical X-ray.
(1) Anteroposterior view.
(2) Lateral view.

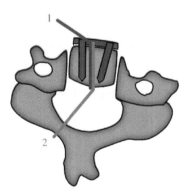

Reference of the sagittal plane

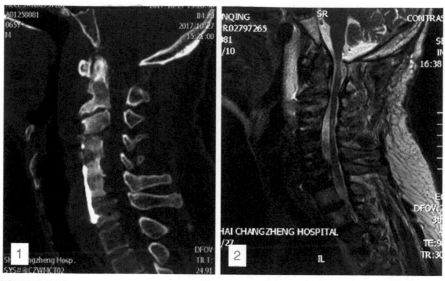

FIGURE 3.54.6

Postoperative sagittal images and their reference on the axial diagram.
(1) Midsagittal CT.
(2) Midsagittal MRI.

Adequately reset C1, devoid posterior arch of the atlas, antedisplaced C4 to C6 vertebral bodies, and expanded spinal canal shown on postoperative sagittal CT images (Fig. 3.54.6, panel 1).

Postoperative magnetic resonance imaging (MRI): Spinal cord free of compression and restored to lordosis, residual but diminished signal hyperintensity within the spinal cord, and residual deformation of the spinal cord due to indentation shown on postoperative sagittal MR images (Fig. 3.54.6, panel 2).

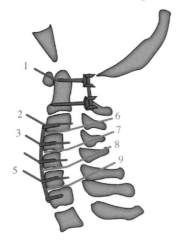

Reference of the axial planes

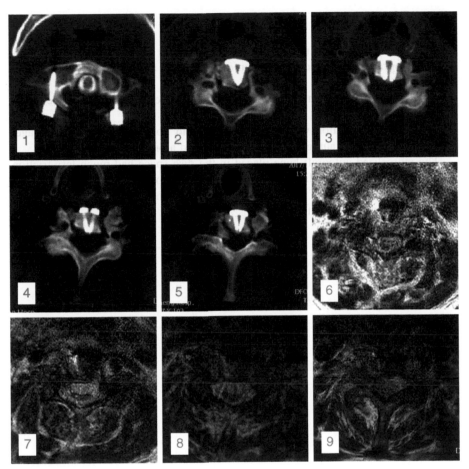

FIGURE 3.54.7

Postoperative axial cervical images and their reference on the sagittal diagram.
(1) Axial CT of C1.
(2) Axial CT of C3.
(3) Axial CT of C4.
(4) Axial CT of C5.
(5) Axial CT of C6.
(6) Axial MRI of C3/4.
(7) Axial MRI of C4/5.
(8) Axial MRI of C5/6.
(9) Axial MRI of C6/7.

Anterior tubercle of the atlas attached with the dens and vertebral bodies from C4 to C6 ventrally displaced by 5.7 mm with left-deviated bone cuts 22 mm apart. The left bone cuts at C5 and C6 have gone through the pedicles shown on postoperative sagittal CT images (Fig. 3.54.7, panel 1 to 5).

The spinal cord free of compression with an ample amount of CSF, though with residual deformation shown on postoperative sagittal MR images (Fig. 3.54.7, panel 6 to 9).

Discussion

Intervertebral cage was not used at C5/6. What were the considerations? Does morselized autograft bone placed within intervertebral space affect the antedisplacement process?

Severe disc degeneration affected every level of the cervical spine, most severe at C5/6 with collapsed space.

Even after preparation with a curette, C5/6 did not allow the smallest cage. Therefore, morselized autograft bones were applied alone in C5/6.

The morselized autograft bone placed in the disc space had much less friction than a cage during the antedisplacement process. Less compact than a cage, morselized bones bears the risk of anterior dislodgement during antedisplacement, which may block the displacement process.

Case 55: Cervical canal stenosis

Index terms

Antedisplacement of three vertebral bodies, cervical kyphosis, segmental ossification, and thickness of ossification 6.1 mm.

History

Patient: A 61-year-old man.

Chief complaint: Discomfort around the neck and shoulders for three years and numbness of the extremities for three months.

Physical exam: On physical exam, the patient demonstrated gait disturbance and mildly limited range of motion. Muscle strength was tested at 4+/5 on bilateral deltoids, biceps, and triceps brachii, wrist extension and flexion, and hand grips. Knee and ankle tendon hyperreflexia was noted on both sides.

Preoperative function: JOA score was 12, Nurick score: 3, VAS: 3, and NDI: 16.

Imaging studies

Kyphotic cervical spine with a Cobb angle of $-9.9°$, spinal canal stenosis, Pavlov ratio of 63%, 61%, 65%, and 74% from C3 to C6, respectively (Fig. 3.55.1).

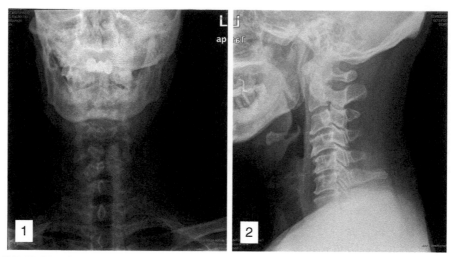

FIGURE 3.55.1

Preoperative X-ray of the cervical spine.
(1) Anteroposterior view.
(2) Lateral view.

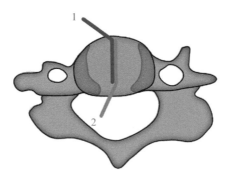

Reference of the sagittal plane

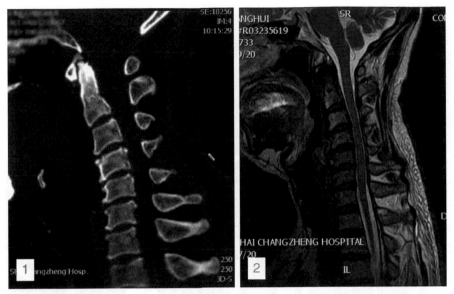

FIGURE 3.55.2

Preoperative sagittal images of the cervical spine and their reference on the axial diagram.
(1) Midsagittal CT.
(2) Midsagittal MRI.

Kyphotic cervical spine and increased anteroposterior of the vertebral bodies from C3 to C6 shown on preoperative sagittal CT image (Fig. 3.55.2, panel 1).

Kyphotic spinal cord, spinal canal stenosis from C4 to C6, obliteration of the anterior and posterior CSF columns, and spinal cord compression shown on preoperative sagittal MR image (Fig. 3.55.2, panel 2).

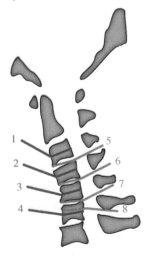

Reference of the axial planes

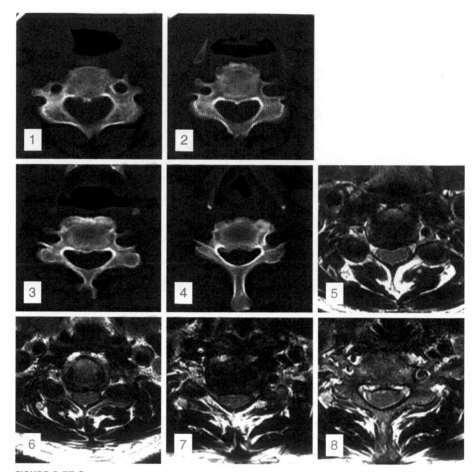

FIGURE 3.55.3

Preoperative axial images of the cervical spine and their reference on the sagittal diagram.

(1) Axial CT of C3.
(2) Axial CT of C4.
(3) Axial CT of C5.
(4) Axial CT of C6.
(5) Axial MRI of C3/4.
(6) Axial MRI of C4/5.
(7) Axial MRI of C5/6.
(8) Axial MRI of C6.

Developmental stenosis of the spinal canal shown on preoperative axial CT images (Fig. 3.55.3, panel 1 to 5).

CSF obliteration from C3/4 to C5/6 and triangular spinal cord due to indentation shown on preoperative axial MR images (Fig. 3.55.3, panel 6 to 9).

Highlights

This case features developmental stenosis of the spinal canal from C4 to C7 in a kyphotic cervical spine.

Surgical planning

Conventionally, long-segment spinal canal stenosis has been treated with indirect decompression through a posterior approach.

The poor cervical curvature may hamper the posterior shift of the spinal cord and lead to incomplete decompression, whereas the motion-preserving laminoplasty may aggravate the poor cervical curvature further down the road.

A conventional alternative is ACCF, which requires significant bone resection and the use of long instrumentation construct. As such, pseudoarthrosis and fusion-related complications, such as mesh subsidence, are likely to develop after surgery.

The patient received ACAF with antedisplacement of C4 to C6 vertebral bodies. Given the spinal canal component of this case, rather than OPLL alone, the anterior resection aimed for a Pavlov ratio above 75% (Fig. 3.55.4).

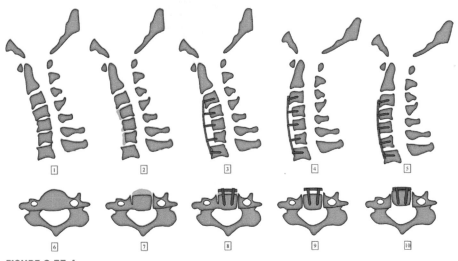

FIGURE 3.55.4

Illustration of the surgical plan on sagittal and axial planes.

(1, 6) Illustration of the disease on sagittal and axial views before surgery.

(2, 7) Resection performed to the anterior part of C4, C5, and C6 vertebral bodies, a complete trough developed on the left vertebral bodies from C4 to C6 while a half one on the right side with the posterior bone yet to be dissected.

(3, 8) Titanium plate and screws placed in vertebral bodies from C3 to C7.

(4, 9) Completion of the right groove on C4, C5, and C6.

(5, 10) Antedisplaced C4, C5, and C6 vertebral bodies as screws were tightened.

Results

Postoperative function: JOA score was 15, Nurick score: 2, VAS: 0, and NDI: 8.

Restored cervical curvature, a Cobb angle of 0.9° from C2 to C7 and 14.7° from C3 to C7, and antedisplaced C4 to C6 vertebral bodies (Fig. 3.55.5).

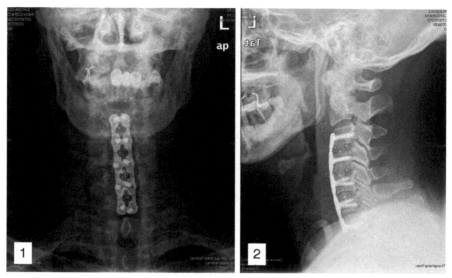

FIGURE 3.55.5

Postoperative cervical spine X-ray.
(1) Anteroposterior view.
(2) Lateral view.

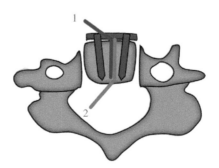

Reference of the sagittal plane

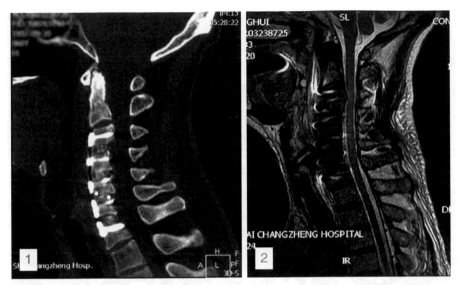

FIGURE 3.55.6

Postoperative sagittal views and their reference on the axial diagram.
(1) Midsagittal CT.
(2) Midsagittal MRI.

Shown on postoperative midsagittal CT image, the vertebral bodies from C4 to C6 have been ventrally displaced VOC by 4.3 mm and expanded spinal canal (Fig. 3.55.6, panel 1). Shown on postoperative midsagittal MR images, spinal cord with restored lordotic curvature free of compression and surrounded by CSF (Fig. 3.55.6, panel 2).

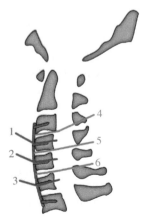

Reference of the axial planes

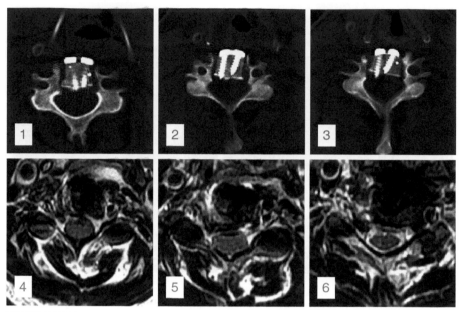

FIGURE 3.55.7

Postoperative axial cervical images and their reference on the sagittal diagram.
(1) Axial CT of C4.
(2) Axial CT of C5.
(3) Axial CT of C6.
(4) Axial MRI of C3/4.
(5) Axial MRI of C4/5.
(6) Axial MRI of C5/6.

Shown on postoperative axial CT images, the vertebral bodies have been dissected with parasagittal cuts on both sides 22 mm apart, and the left bone cut on C6 is deviated laterally and gone through the pedicle (Fig. 3.55.7, panel 1 to 3). Shown on postoperative axial MR images, the spinal cord has recovered to an oval shape surrounded by CSF (Fig. 3.55.7, panel 4 to 6).

Discussion

What are the values of ACAF for spinal canal stenosis compared with ACCF?

First, for multisegmental stenosis of the spinal canal, ACCF involves resection of much more bone volume, and thus it should be applied to a limited number of levels. In contrast, as more volume of the vertebra is preserved in ACAF, the risk of hardware-related complications is lower, fusion rate is higher in the longer-term, and it applies to extensive stenosis of the cervical spinal canal.

Second, the bone cuts developed in ACCF should not be lateral to the dura lest excessive anterior shift of the spinal cord and nerve root tethering, but medialized bone cuts that prevent the spinal cord's anterior shift may end up with incomplete decompression. As a procedure that allows bone cuts wider apart, ACAF addresses the anterior shift of the spinal cord with the reconstructed anterior wall of the spinal canal.

One thing that should have been done better was the bone resection on the right side of the C4 vertebra. It was excessively removed, and the screw on the right side ended up partially through the posterior vertebral wall. In this case with spinal canal stenosis but not OPLL, the proud screw tip may engage the dura and cause CSF leak and even spinal cord injury. Therefore, when performing ACAF for spinal canal stenosis, caution should be taken to resect the necessary volume of bone from the vertebral bodies and select screws of proper length.

Case 56: Cervical canal stenosis

Index terms

Antedisplacement of two vertebral bodies and spinal canal stenosis.

History

Patient: A 30-year-old man.

Chief complaint: Nuchal pain and numbness and weakness of the extremities for three months, and aggravation for two months.

Physical exam: Physical exam was noted for gait disturbance; straightened cervical spine; limited range of cervical motion; an impaired sense of light touch, pinprick, and temperature and hypertonicity of all the extremities; and compromised fine movements. Muscle strength was tested at 4/5 on the deltoid, biceps and triceps brachii, hand grips, dorsal and plantar flexion on both sides. Symmetric brisk tendon reflexes were noted on the biceps and triceps brachii, brachioradialis, knees, and ankles on both sides. Hoffmann and Babinski signs were positive bilaterally.

Preoperative function: JOA score was 11, Nurick score: 3, VAS: 1, and NDI: 14.

Imaging studies

Preserved cervical lordosis, Cobb angle of $21.2°$ from C2 to C7 and $-13.4°$ from C2 to C4 with intervertebral instability of C4/5, spinal canal stenosis of C4 and C5, and Pavlov ratio of 56% and 60% at C4 and C5, respectively (Fig. 3.56.1).

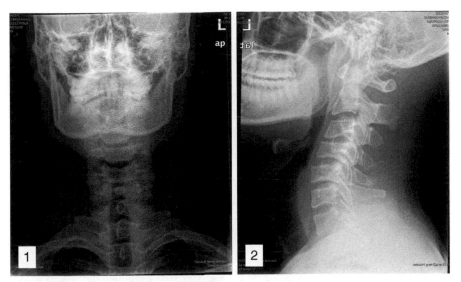

FIGURE 3.56.1

Preoperative X-ray of the cervical spine.

(1) Anteroposterior view.

(2) Lateral view.

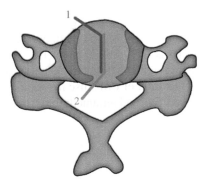

Reference of the sagittal plane

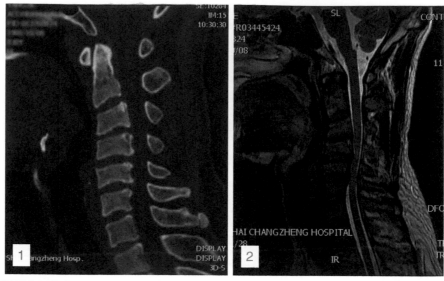

FIGURE 3.56.2

Preoperative sagittal images of the cervical spine and their reference on the axial diagram.
(1) Midsagittal CT.
(2) Midsagittal MRI.

Shown on preoperative midsagittal CT image, focal kyphosis from C2 to C5, increased anteroposterior dimension of the vertebral bodies from C3 to C5, OPLL, and spinal canal stenosis (Fig. 3.56.2, panel 1).

Shown on preoperative midsagittal MR image, kyphotic spinal cord, spinal canal stenosis from C4 to C5, obliteration of CSF, disc herniation at C4/5 to C5/6, hypertrophic ligamentum flavum at C5/6, and intramedullary signal hyperintensity at C4/5 (Fig. 3.56.2, panel 2).

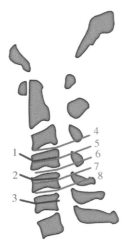

Reference of the axial planes

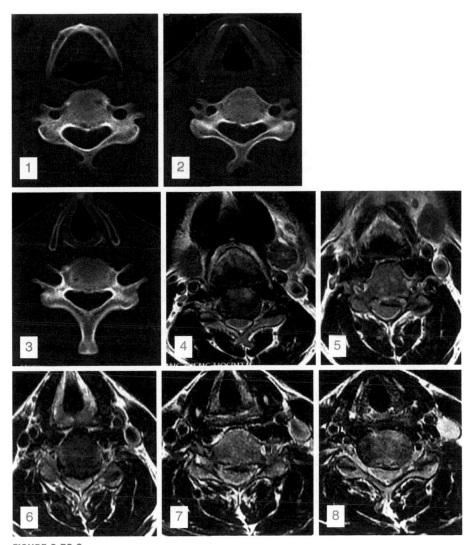

FIGURE 3.56.3

Preoperative axial images of the cervical spine and their reference on the sagittal diagram.
(1) Axial CT of C4.
(2) Axial CT of C5.
(3) Axial CT of C6.
(4) Axial MRI of C3/4.
(5) Axial MRI of C4.
(6) Axial MRI of C4/5.
(7) Axial MRI of C5.
(8) Axial MRI of C5/6.

Incipient OPLL and kidney-shaped spinal canal shown on preoperative axial CT images (Fig. 3.56.3, panel 1 to 3).

Spinal cord in the shape of a triangle or boomerang due to indentation from C3/4 to C5/6, total and partial CSF obliteration of the ventral and dorsal column, respectively, shown on preoperative axial MR images (Fig. 3.56.3, panel 4 to 8).

Highlights

This case features developmental spinal canal stenosis complicated with cervical kyphosis, C4/5 segmental instability, and C4 retrolisthesis.

Surgical planning

For short-segment spinal canal stenosis complicated with cervical kyphosis and segmental instability, a conventional strategy is ACCF that provides corpectomy, spinal canal expansion, segmental stabilization, and curvature correction.

ACAF serves as an alternative with antedisplacement of C4 to C5, preserved bone stock, and lower risk of fusion-related complications.

The anterior part of the vertebrae was resected by the thickness that restores the Pavlov ratio to above 75% (Fig. 3.56.4).

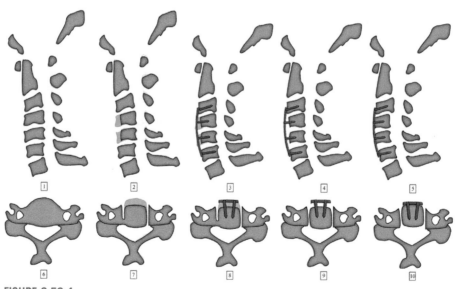

FIGURE 3.56.4

Illustration of the surgical plan on sagittal and axial planes.

(1, 6) Illustration of the disease on sagittal and axial views before surgery.

(2, 7) Resection of the anterior part of the vertebral bodies of C4 and C5, a left groove and a right half-groove with the posterior cortex still intact on C4 and C5.

(3, 8) Titanium plate and screws placed in vertebral bodies from C3 to C6.

(4, 9) Completion of the right groove on C4 and C5.

(5, 10) Antedisplaced C4 and C5 vertebral bodies as screws were tightened.

Results

Postoperative function: JOA score was 16, Nurick score: 1, VAS: 2, and NDI: 5.

Cobb angle of 9.9° from C2 to C7, instrumentation from C3 to C6 with 14 mm screws in C3 and C6, and 12 mm screws in C4 and C5, and antedisplaced C4 and C5 vertebral bodies (Fig. 3.56.5).

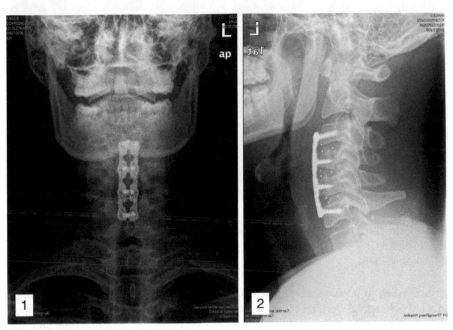

FIGURE 3.56.5

Postoperative cervical X-ray.
(1) Anteroposterior view.
(2) Lateral view.

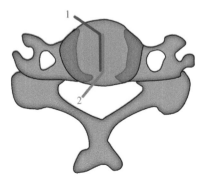

Reference of the sagittal plane

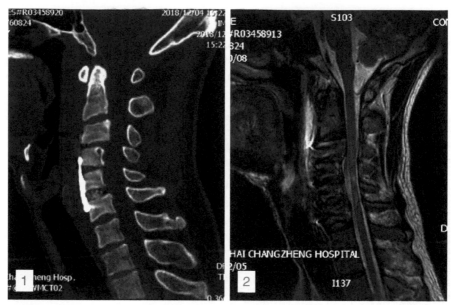

FIGURE 3.56.6

Postoperative sagittal images and their reference on the axial diagram.
(1) Midsagittal CT.
(2) Midsagittal MRI.

According to postoperative sagittal CT image, antedisplacement of the partially resected C4 and C5 vertebral bodies (Fig. 3.56.5, panel 1). According to postoperative sagittal MR image, straightened spinal cord free of compression and surrounded by CSF at C4 to C5, and residual intramedullary signal hyperintensity at C4/5 and C5/6 (Fig. 3.56.6, panel 2).

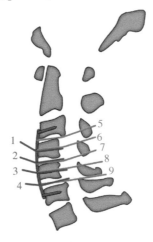

Reference of the axial planes

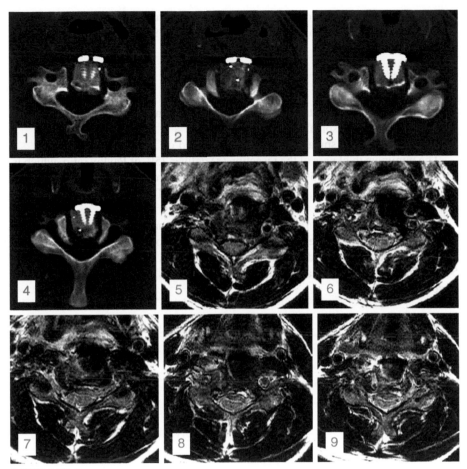

FIGURE 3.56.7

Postoperative axial cervical images and their reference on the sagittal diagram.

(1) Axial CT of C4.
(2) Axial CT of C4/5.
(3) Axial CT of C5.
(4) Axial CT of C5/6.
(5) Axial MRI of C3/4.
(6) Axial MRI of C4.
(7) Axial MRI of C4/5.
(8) Axial MRI of C5.
(9) Axial MRI of C5/6.

The vertebral bodies have been antedisplaced by 4.4 mm with parasagittal grooves on both sides 22.5 mm apart; the left cut on C4 is so lateralized that it violates the transverse foramen shown on postoperative axial CT images (Fig. 3.56.7, Figs. 1—4).

The spinal cord has recovered to an oval shape surrounded by CSF shown on postoperative axial MR images (Fig. 3.56.7, panel 5 to 9).

Discussion

How can we properly plan the thickness of the resection on the anterior part of the vertebra in cases with spinal canal stenosis?

This calculation in spinal canal stenosis is based on the target Pavlov ratio.

The minimum thickness of the resection (x) deliver 75% of Pavlov ratio, which is $(d\_sc + x)/(d\_vb + x) = 75\%$. D_sc represents the anteroposterior dimension of the spinal canal while d_vb, that of the vertebra. Thus, x is calculated as $(0.75*d\_vb-d\_sc)/1.75$.

In this patient, a Pavlov ratio above 75% through surgery would achieve spinal cord decompression. The level of maximum stenosis, or lowest Pavlov ratio, was used for calculation. Its' d_vb was 24.8 mm, d_sc 13.8 mm, and Pavlov ratio 54%. Aiming at 75%, at least 3 mm thick of bone was resected from the anterior vertebral bodies.

Case 57: Cervical developmental malformation, cervical canal stenosis

Index terms

Antedisplacement of one vertebra.

History

Patient: A 54-year-old woman.

Chief complaint: Numbness of hands and weakness of lower limbs for three months.

Physical exam: The patient had preserved gait stability. A physical exam was noted for a straightened cervical spine and a limited range of cervical motion. Muscle strength was tested at 4/5 on bilateral deltoid, biceps and triceps brachii, wrist flexion and extension, hand grips, iliopsoas, quadriceps femoris, biceps femoris, semitendinosus, semimembranosus, and anterior tibialis on both sides, and triceps surae; and 4-/5 on dorsal and plantar flexion on both sides.

Preoperative function: JOA score was 14, Nurick score: 1, VAS: 0, and NDI: 7.

Imaging studies

Straightened cervical spine, a Cobb angle of 6.6° from C2 to C7, Pavlov ratio of 53% at C4, dysplastic segmentation anomaly of C5 and C6 vertebral bodies, and arthrodesis (Fig. 3.57.1).

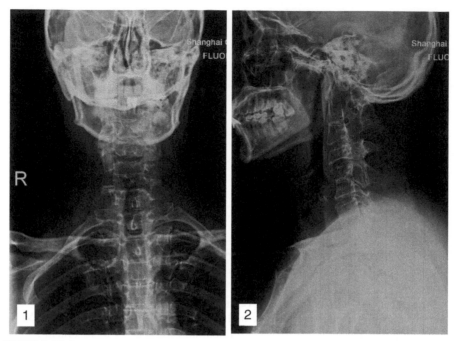

FIGURE 3.57.1

Preoperative X-ray of the cervical spine.
(1) Anteroposterior view.
(2) Lateral view.

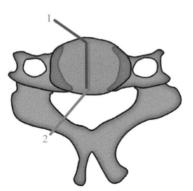

Reference of the sagittal plane

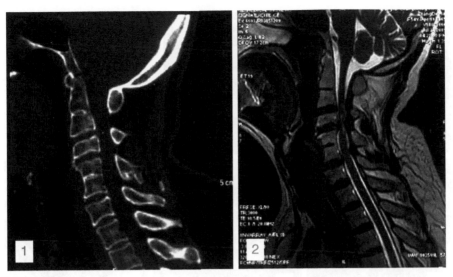

FIGURE 3.57.2

Preoperative sagittal images of the cervical spine and their reference on the axial
diagram
(1) Midsagittal CT.
(2) Midsagittal MRI.

Vertebra dysplasia that features atlantooccipital assimilation, and dysplastic segmentation anomaly involving the vertebral bodies and posterior elements among C1
to C3 and C5 to C6 shown on preoperative sagittal CT image (Fig. 3.57.2, panel 1).

Spinal cord compression at C3/4 to C4/5 and C6/7, disc protrusion at disc spaces,
hypertrophic ligamentum flavum, and intramedullary signal hyperintensity suggesting myelopathy shown on preoperative sagittal MR image (Fig. 3.57.2, panel 2).

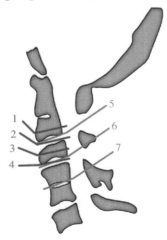

Reference of the axial planes

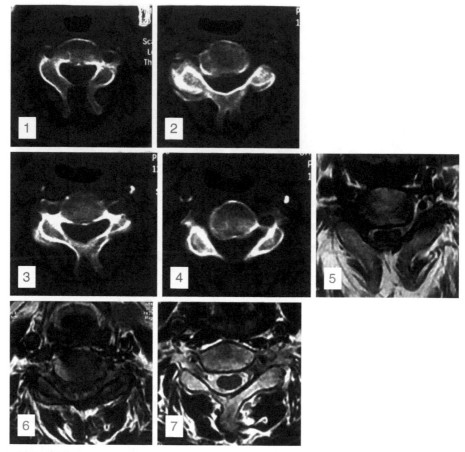

FIGURE 3.57.3

Preoperative axial images of the cervical spine and their reference on the sagittal diagram.
(1) Axial CT of C3.
(2) Axial CT of C3/4.
(3) Axial CT of C4.
(4) Axial CT of C4/5.
(5) Axial MRI of C3/4.
(6) Axial MRI of C4/5.
(7) Axial MRI of C5/6.

The spinal canal features kidney shape at C4 shown on preoperative axial CT images (Fig. 3.57.3, panel 1 to 4).

The spinal cord impinged and deformed into a boomerang shape, with an intramedullary snake-eyes sign at C4/5 shown on preoperative axial MR images (Fig. 3.57.3, panel 5 to 7).

Highlights

This case features dysplastic fusion of multiple cervical segments, spinal canal stenosis at C4, disc protrusion, and hypertrophy of ligamentum flavum.

Surgical planning

Single-level spinal canal stenosis is readily addressed with direct anterior decompression. An ACAF with antedisplacement of C4, the culprit level of stenosis, was planned for this patient.

Given the diffuse arthrodesis of the uncovertebral joints and impaired cervical curvature, the amount of bone resection on the anterior vertebra was calculated based on the Pavlov ratio (Fig. 3.57.4).

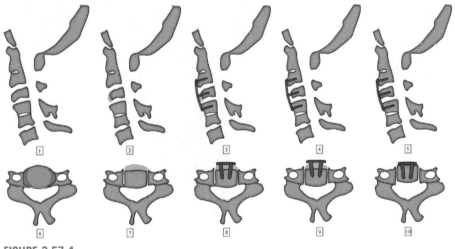

FIGURE 3.57.4

Illustration of the surgical plan on sagittal and axial planes.
(1, 6) Illustration of the disease on sagittal and axial views before surgery.
(2, 7) Resection of the anterior part of the vertebra of C4, a left groove, and a right half-groove with the posterior cortex still intact on C4.
(3, 8) Titanium plate and screws placed in vertebral bodies from C3 to C5.
(4, 9) Completion of the right groove on C4.
(5, 10) Antedisplaced C4 vertebra as screws were tightened.

Results

Postoperative function: JOA score was 15, Nurick score: 1, VAS: 0, and NDI: 85.

Minimally restored cervical curvature, Cobb angle of 8.7° from C2 to C7, and antedisplaced C4 vertebra (Fig. 3.57.5).

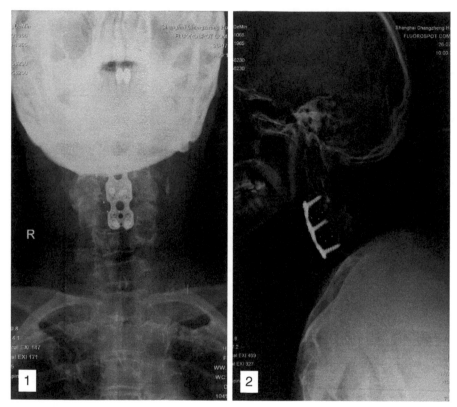

FIGURE 3.57.5

Postoperative cervical X-ray.
(1) Anteroposterior view.
(2) Lateral view.

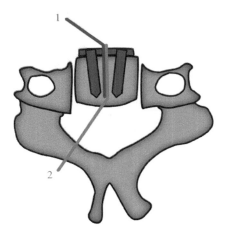

Reference of the sagittal plane

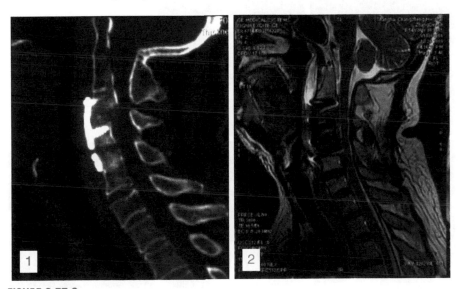

FIGURE 3.57.6

Postoperative sagittal images and their reference on the axial diagram.
(1) Midsagittal CT.
(2) Midsagittal MRI.

   Antedisplaced VOC from C4 and widened spinal canal shown on postoperative midsagittal CT image (Fig. 3.57.6, panel 1).

   Spinal cord free of compression between the anterior and posterior columns of CSF, and ill-defined intramedullary signal hyperintensity, suggesting improvement shown on postoperative midsagittal MR image (Fig. 3.57.6, panel 2).

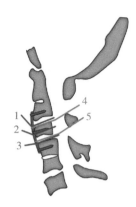

Reference of the axial planes

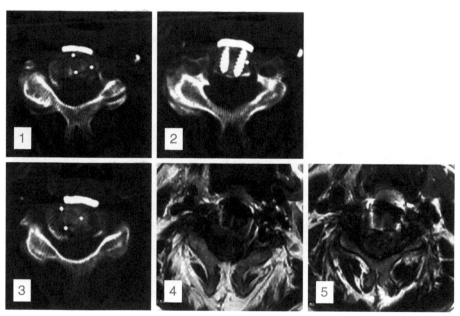

FIGURE 3.57.7

Postoperative axial cervical images and their reference on the sagittal diagram.
(1) Axial CT of C3/4.
(2) Axial CT of C4.
(3) Axial CT of the superior surface of C5.
(4) Axial MRI of C3/4.
(5) Axial MRI of C4/5.

Shown on postoperative axial CT images, the C4 vertebra has been antedisplaced by 3.3 mm with parasagittal bone cuts 20.5 mm on both sides (Fig. 3.57.7, panel 1 to 3). Shown on postoperative axial MR images, impingement from the hypertrophic ligamentum flavum has improved (Fig. 3.57.7, panel 4 and 5).

Discussion

Given the dysplastic cervical spine and osteoporosis, what were the pitfalls of this case when treated with ACAF?

Osteoporosis constitutes a major challenge for screw purchase, the fundamental mechanics for antedisplacement. The readers can refer to the previous cases for discussion of this topic. Described here are hemostasis strategy during bone resection.

Poor visualization was encountered due to the oozing bone surfaces when resecting bone and developing the parasagittal bone cuts.

Bone wax was applied as a sealant on the surface of the oozing cancellous bone. As the bone cut on one side was developed, it was filled with gauze and gel form chips, covered with a brain cotton pad, and pressed for hemostasis.

Upon wound closure, a drain was placed in front of the plate. Sixty hours after the surgery, the drain was removed, given less than 15 mL of light yellow fluid on a 12-hour basis.

Case 58: Ossification of posterior longitudinal ligament (OPLL) of thoracic spine (At T2/3 to T4/5)

Index terms

Antedisplacement of thoracic vertebral bodies.

History

Patient: A 54-year-old woman.

Chief complaint: Weakness of the lower limbs, tightness and numbness of the trunk, and bowel and bladder dysfunction for six months, with aggravation for two months.

Physical exam: Being wheeled in the clinic, the patient reported tightness and numbness of the trunk below the sternal angle. On physical exam, anal wink and sense of light touch, pinprick, and temperature were impaired on the lower limbs. Muscle strength was tested at 5/5 on the upper limbs and 3/5 on the lower limbs. Hyperreflexia was noted on the lower limbs. Babinski sign was positive on both sides.

Preoperative function: M-JOA was 4.

Imaging studies

Upper thoracic kyphosis of 17.4° and OPLL from T2 to T5 (Fig. 3.58.1).

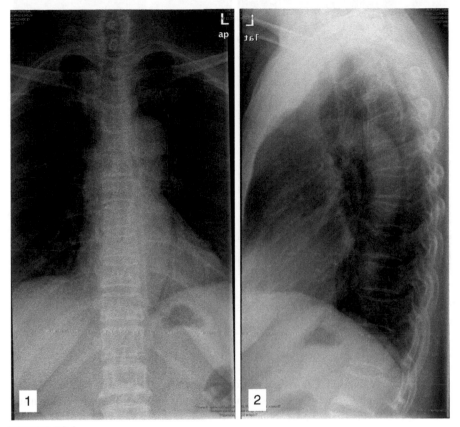

FIGURE 3.58.1

Preoperative X-ray of the thoracic spine.
(1) Anteroposterior view.
(2) Lateral view.

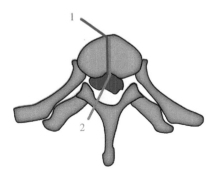

Reference of the sagittal plane

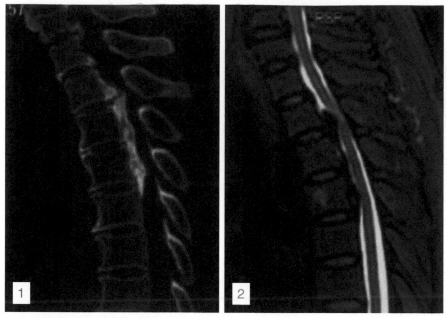

FIGURE 3.58.2

Preoperative sagittal images of the thoracic spine and their reference on the axial diagram.
(1) Midsagittal CT.
(2) Midsagittal MRI.

Preoperative sagittal CT image: A continuous-type OPLL from T2 to T5 that peaks at T2/3 and violates the spinal canal with; and breaks within the ossification at disc space levels (Fig. 3.58.2, panel 1).

Preoperative sagittal MR image: A hypointense, canal occupying, and cord compressing mass from T2 to T5 behind the vertebral bodies. The impingement is most severe at T2/3 and T4. Deformed spinal cord due to indentation, intramedullary signal hyperintensity at T2/3, and ectasia of the intramedullary central canal above the impinged levels (Fig. 3.58.2, panel 2).

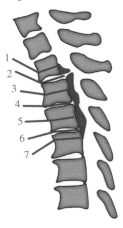

Reference of the axial planes

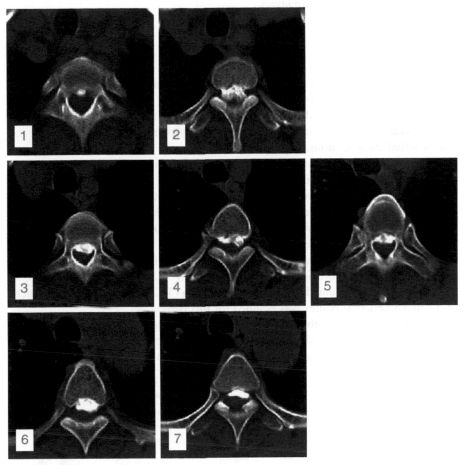

FIGURE 3.58.3

Preoperative axial images of the thoracic spine and their reference on the sagittal diagram.
(1) Axial CT of T2.
(2) Axial CT of T2/3.
(3) Axial CT of T3.
(4) Axial CT of T3/4.
(5) Axial CT of T4.
(6) Axial CT of T4/5.
(7) Axial CT of T5.

Based on preoperative axial CT images, the OPLL measures: 9.8 mm thick (anteroposterior), 17.6 mm wide (mediolateral), and 67.3% in canal occupancy at T2/3; 7.0 mm thick, 17.3 mm wide, and 58.3% in canal occupancy at T3/4; and 8.0 mm thick, 13.9 mm wide, and 57.2% in canal occupancy at T4/5 (Fig. 3.58.3, panel 1 to 7).

Highlights

This case features a continuous and bulky OPLL of the upper thoracic spine, which peaks and violates the spinal canal at T2/3 and T4/5. The spinal canal occupancy is above 60% at the most severe levels.

Surgical planning

This case features OPLL of the upper thoracic spine, namely T2 to T5, that peaks at multiple levels and spans T4.

The unique anatomy at the upper thoracic spine necessitates a sternal splitting or anterolateral approach, which is less practiced due to technical challenges and the risk of lethal complications.

Another option is posterior indirect decompression via laminectomy and kyphosis correction, allowing the posterior shift of the spinal cord away from the ventral indentation. However, the peak components of the OPLL may render a posterior-alone approach ineffective. To this end, a circumferential decompression can be added to the levels with residual compression due to the OPLL's peak.

Alternatively, an anterior decompression can be achieved via a posterior approach, an extremely challenging technique with an increased risk of durotomy and postoperative neurological deterioration.

A thoracic column antedisplacement and fusion (TCAF) with antedisplacement of T2 to T5 vertebral bodies was planned for this patient.

This case was among the first series of this technique where costotransversectomy was performed on both sides. Laminar plates were used on the levels of antedisplacement, and the posterior wall of the spinal canal was preserved (Fig. 3.58.4).

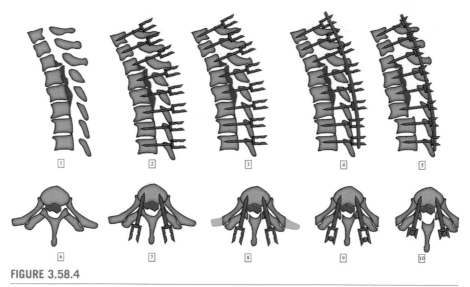

FIGURE 3.58.4

Illustration of the surgical plan on sagittal and axial planes.

(1, 6) Illustration of the OPLL on sagittal and axial views before surgery.

(2, 7) Pedicle screws were placed from C7 to T7 with the ones of T2 to T5 partially inserted.

(3, 8) Completed grooves were performed at both right and left base of lamina from T2 to T5 with bilateral ribs resected.

(4, 9) Implantation of prebent titanium rod, and fixed at C7, T1, T6 and T7.

(5, 10) Antedisplaced T2 to T5 vertebral bodies as tightening the nuts.

Results

Postoperative function: m-JOA was 8.

Thoracic kyphosis corrected to 15.4° (Fig. 3.58.5).

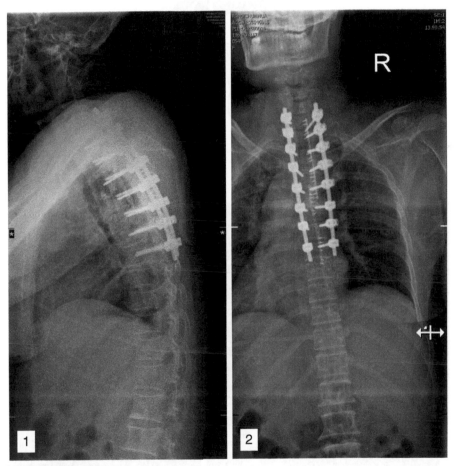

FIGURE 3.58.5

Postoperative thoracic X-ray.
(1) Anteroposterior view.
(2) Lateral view.

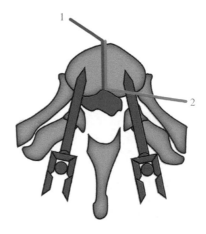

Reference of the sagittal plane

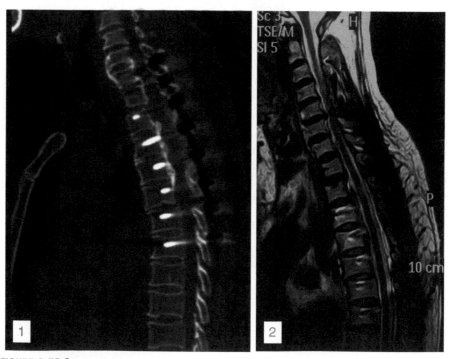

FIGURE 3.58.6

Postoperative sagittal images and their reference on the axial diagram.
(1) Midsagittal CT.
(2) Midsagittal MRI.

The VOC from T2 to T5 has been antedisplaced by 6.4 mm shown on postoperative sagittal CT image (Fig. 3.58.6, panel 1).

Spinal cord free of compression between the anterior and posterior columns of CSF, with the anterior indentation ventrally displaced shown on postoperative sagittal MR image (Fig. 3.58.6, panel 2).

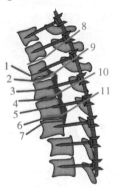

Reference of the axial planes

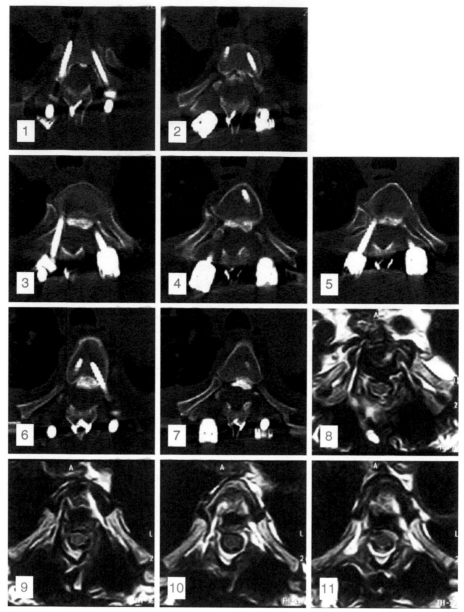

FIGURE 3.58.7

Postoperative axial thoracic images and their reference on the sagittal diagram.

(1) Axial CT of T2.

(2) Axial CT of T2/3.

(3) Axial CT of T3.

(4) Axial CT of T3/4.

(5) Axial CT of T4.

(6) Axial CT of T4/5.

(7) Axial CT of the superior surface of T5.

(8) Axial MRI of T1/2.

(9) Axial MRI of T2/3.

(10) Axial MRI of T3/4.

(11) Axial MRI of T4/5.

The canal stenosis at T2/3 reduced to 26.7% shown on postoperative axial CT images (Fig. 3.58.7, panel 1 to 7).

The morphology of spinal cord recovered and the CSF filling around shown on postoperative axial MR images (Fig. 3.58.7, penal 8 to 11).

Discussion

What are the values of antedisplacement of thoracic vertebrae compared with the conventional techniques?

The OPLL, in this case, spanned from T2 to T5 with a maximum thickness of 9.8 mm.

Given the bulky ossification and significant thoracic kyphosis, an indirect decompression may not yield an adequate posterior shift of the spinal cord. The residual symptomatology due to compression may necessitate a second surgery from the anterior.

Due to the involvement of the upper thoracic spine, the single-stage direct decompression via an anterior surgery is so challenging that the surgical team should involve the cardiothoracic service. In terms of surgical access, an anterior midline approach requires sternotomy and exposure of the vasculature, trachea, and esophagus in the mediastinum, whereas the posterolateral approach requires partial costectomy.

Another option is a direct or circumferential decompression via a posterior approach. However, the risks of durotomy and iatrogenic spinal cord injury are extremely high during bone retrieval since it would be a large bulk with multilevel diseases, let alone the potential need for nerve root resection.

The decompression effect is more deliverable with an antedisplacement procedure, which offers direct decompression via a posterior approach, than an indirect decompression.

What is more, the antedisplacement procedure is safer and more easily applicable than the conventional posterior decompression because it minimizes disruption to the spinal cord environment. Specifically, the antedisplacement procedure involves dissection of the laminae and posterior elements of the vertebrae and intervertebral preparation of both ends of the antedisplacement complex, rather than the extensive resection of the pedicles and the anterior vertebral bodies.

Case 59: Ossification of posterior longitudinal ligament (OPLL) of thoracic spine (At T6 to T9)

Index terms

Antedisplacement of thoracic vertebral bodies.

History

Patient: A 45-year-old woman.

Chief complaint: Numbness, pain, and weakness of the lower extremities for three months.

Physical exam: The patient walked into the clinic with crutches. Physical exam was noted for gait disturbance, an impaired superficial sensation of the trunk below the costal arch. Muscle strength was tested at 2/5 on lower limbs. Hyperreflexia and Babinski signs were documented on both lower limbs.

Preoperative function: M-JOA was 7.

Imaging studies

Thoracic kyphosis measured 18.5° from T4 to T10 (Fig. 3.59.1).

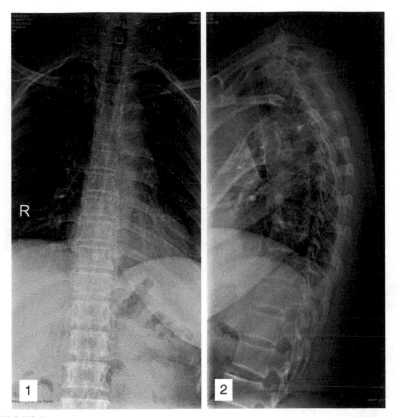

FIGURE 3.59.1

Preoperative X-ray of the thoracic spine.
(1) Anteroposterior view.
(2) Lateral view.

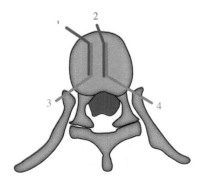

Reference of the sagittal plane

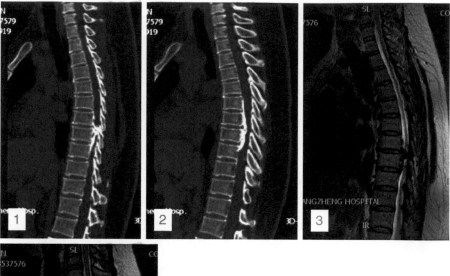

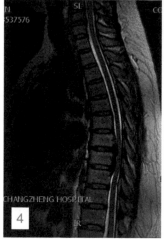

FIGURE 3.59.2

Preoperative sagittal images of the thoracic spine and their reference on the axial diagram.
(1) Right parasagittal CT.
(2) Midsagittal CT.
(3) Right parasagittal MRI.
(4) Midsagittal MRI.

A continuous OPLL from T6 to T9, most severe at T7/8 and T8 shown on preoperative sagittal CT images (Fig. 3.59.2, panel 1 and 2).

A hypointense mass from T7/8 to T8/9 anterior to the spinal cord violates the spinal canal and causes spinal cord indentation. The spinal cord is compressed at the disc levels with intramedullary signal hyperintensity suggesting myelopathy at T7/8 shown on preoperative sagittal MR images (Fig. 3.59.2, panel 3 and 4).

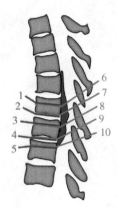

Reference of the axial planes

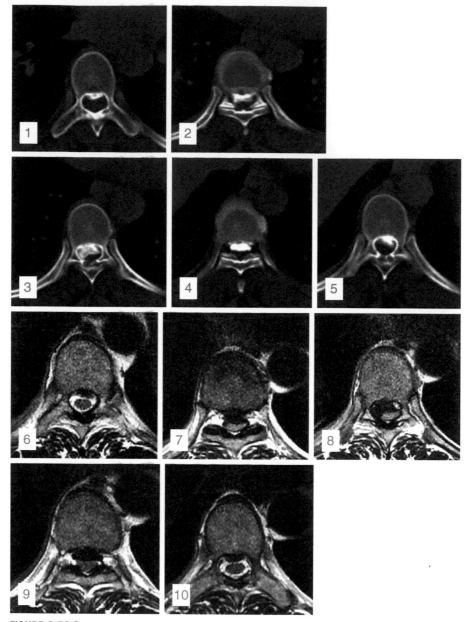

FIGURE 3.59.3

Preoperative axial images of the thoracic spine and their reference on the sagittal diagram.

(1) Axial CT of T7.
(2) Axial CT of T7/8.
(3) Axial CT of T8.
(4) Axial CT of the inferior surface of T8/9.
(5) Axial CT of T9.
(6) Axial MRI of T7.
(7) Axial MRI of T7/8.
(8) Axial MRI of T8.
(9) Axial MRI of T8/9.
(10) Axial MRI of T9.

Based on preoperative axial CT images, the OPLL measures: 10.1 mm thick (anteroposterior), 15 mm wide (mediolateral), and 86.3% in canal occupancy at T8 where it is midline-centered and more protuberant on the right; and 8.0 mm thick, 16.2 mm wide, and 68.4% in canal occupancy at T8/9 (Fig. 3.59.3, panel 1 to 5).

Based on preoperative axial MR images, preoperative MRI transverse position showed compression and deformation of spinal cord with axial rotation, and CSF disappeared.

Highlights

This case featured a long-segment OPLL from T6 to T9, which peaked at T7/8 to T8 and violated the spinal canal. The spinal cord had been severely compressed and deformed due to the anterior indentation with intramedullary signal hyperintensity. The patient presented with tightness and numbness of the trunk, which located the myelopathy at T10. She also reported impaired sensation and mobility of the lower limbs.

Surgical planning

Given the length of the ossification, a direct lesion removal bears the tremendous risk of neurological deterioration and morbidities.

Another conventional option is posterior laminectomy with circumferential decompression, which achieves indirect decompression and allows an adequate posterior shift of the spinal cord via laminectomy, compression via the upper and lower instrumented vertebrae, and dekyphosis.

For the protuberant component at T7/8, the result of decompression of the ventral spinal cord can be validated intraoperatively with ultrasound. Alternatively, this level can be addressed with a second-stage circumferential decompression.

This patient received an antedisplacement of the thoracic vertebral bodies. It is a safer technique that allows in situ decompression of the spinal cord via the ventral displacement of the ossification and obviates resection of the pedicles, ossification, or the vertebra (Fig. 3.59.4).

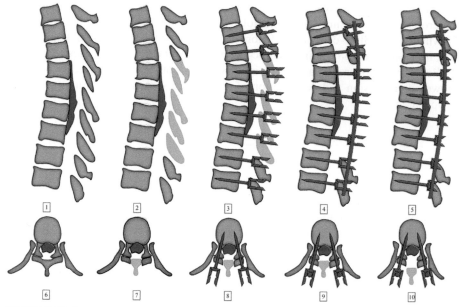

FIGURE 3.59.4

Illustration of the surgical plan on sagittal and axial planes.
(1, 6) Illustration of the thoracic spin on sagittal and axial views before surgery.
(2, 7) Total laminectomy was performed from T5 to T9.
(3, 8) Pedicle screws were placed from T4 to T11 with the ones of T6 to T9 partially inserted.
(4, 9) Implantation of prebent titanium rod, and fixed at C4, T5, T10 and 11.
(5, 10) Antedisplaced T6 to T9 VOC as tightening the nuts.

Results

Postoperatively function: M-JOA was 9.

Decreased thoracic kyphosis with Cobb angle measured 9.2° from T4 to T10 (Fig. 3.59.5).

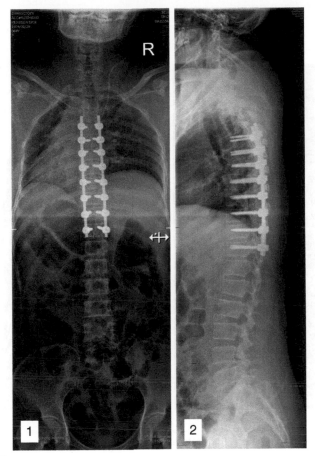

FIGURE 3.59.5

Postoperative X-ray of the thoracic spine.

(1) Anteroposterior view.

(2) Lateral view.

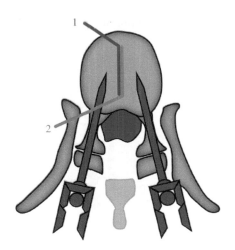

Reference of the sagittal plane

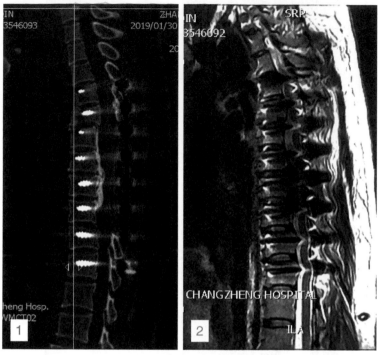

FIGURE 3.59.6

Postoperative sagittal views and their reference on the axial diagram.
(1) Midsagittal CT.
(2) Midsagittal MRI.

Postoperative sagittal CT, antedisplaced VOC from T6 to T9 by 6.7 mm (Fig. 3.59.6, panel 1).

Postoperative sagittal MRI, artifacts from the instrumentation, spinal cord free of ventral compression, and restored anterior and posterior CSF columns (Fig. 3.59.6, panel 2).

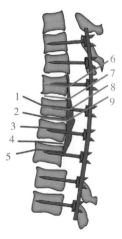

Reference of the axial planes

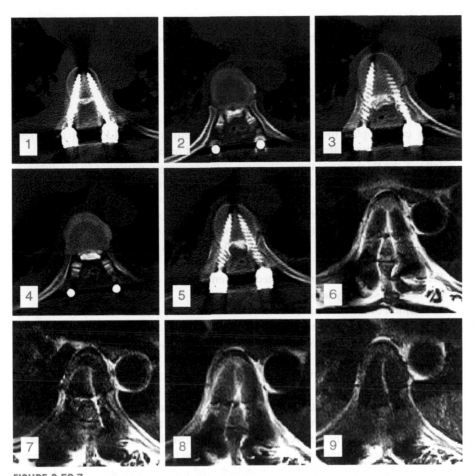

FIGURE 3.59.7

Postoperative axial thoracic images and their reference on the sagittal diagram.
(1) Axial CT of T7.
(2) Axial CT of T7/8.
(3) Axial CT of T8.
(4) Axial CT of T8/9.
(5) Axial CT of T9.
(6) Axial MRI of T6.
(7) Axial MRI of T6/7.
(8) Axial MRI of T7.
(9) Axial MRI of T7/8.

Postoperative CT cross section showed a small amount of pleural effusion, and the bilateral ribs of the operative segment were intact (Fig. 3.59.7, panel 1 to 5).

The transverse position of MRI showed the spinal cord decompressed with recovery of CSF around the cord, based on postoperative axial MR images (Fig. 3.59.7, panel 6 to 9).

Discussion

1. How can we plan the distance of antedisplacement in OPLL with a marked difference between the thinnest and the thickest levels?

   Indeed, the thickness of the ossification is the primary contributor to the distance of antedisplacement. In cases with heterogeneous thickness across the lesion, there are other parameters aside from lesion thickness alone.

   The challenge with lesions with a marked difference between the thinnest and the thickest levels is that antedisplacement based on the thickest part may result in excessive displacement, excessively shifted spinal cord, tethered neural axis, and nerve palsy.

   What is worse, the excessive antedisplacement may cause durotomy when the ossification severely adheres to the dura mater.

   In addition to the meticulous calculation before surgery, the neurophysiological monitoring guides the antedisplacement process. A change or obliteration of signal indicates excessive migration and no more attempt of antedisplacement should be made.

2. The ribs were not dissected in this case. Does this restrain the antedisplacement process?

   Postoperative imaging studies revealed that the antedisplacement was not hampered by the preserved ribs, reflecting the elastic recoil of the thoracic cage. Preserving the ribs helped reduce surgical risks, such as injuries of the pleura, intercostal nerves, and vasculature. Also, it prevents postoperative issues such as pleural irritation, pain at the dissection, and pseudoarthrosis.

Case 60: Ossification of ligamentum flavum of thoracic spine (at T2/3 to T5/6)

Index terms

Bridge crane technique.

History

Patient: A 54-year-old woman.

Chief complaint: Numbness and weakness of the lower limbs for three months.

Physical exam: Physical exam was noted for gait disturbance, tightness and numbness of the trunk below the intermammary line, hypertonicity on the lower extremities, and impaired superficial sensation of the lower limbs. Muscle strength was tested at 3/5 on both lower limbs. Brisk tendon reflexes and Babinski signs were noted on sides.

Preoperative function: M-JOA was 7.

Imaging studies

Upper thoracic kyphosis of 15.1° and ossification of the ligamentum flavum (OLF) from T2/3 to T4/5 (Fig. 3.60.1).

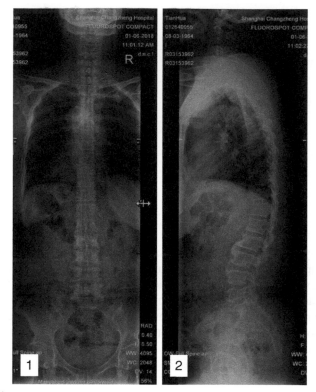

FIGURE 3.60.1

Preoperative X-ray of the thoracic spine.
(1) Anteroposterior view.
(2) Lateral view.

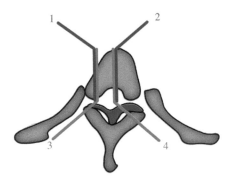

Reference of the sagittal plane

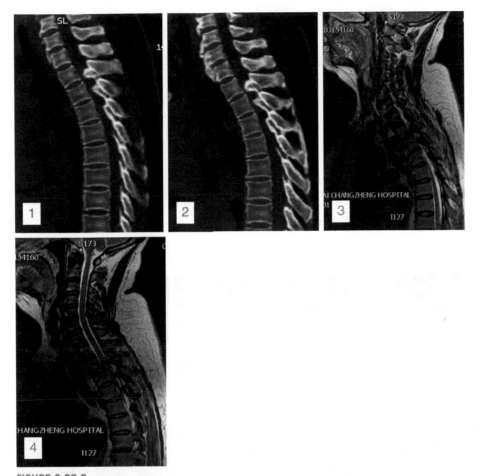

FIGURE 3.60.2

Preoperative sagittal images of the thoracic spine and their reference on the axial diagram.

(1) Right parasagittal CT.
(2) Midsagittal CT.
(3) Right parasagittal MRI.
(4) Midsagittal MRI.

OLF across multiple levels, more severe at T2/3 to T4/5 where it peaks and violates the spinal canal shown on preoperative sagittal CT images (Fig. 3.60.2, panel 1 and 2).

Hypointense masses along the posterior wall of the spinal canal between spinous processes from T2 to T6, which have violated the spinal canal and impinged upon the spinal cord shown on preoperative sagittal MR images (Fig. 3.60.2, panel 3 and 4).

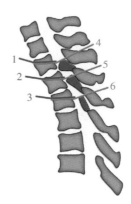

Reference of the axial planes

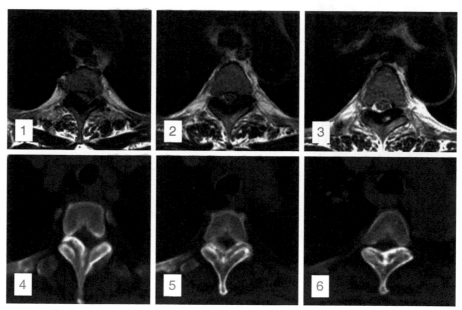

FIGURE 3.60.3

Preoperative axial images of the thoracic spine and their reference on the sagittal diagram.
(1) Axial CT of T2/3.
(2) Axial CT of T3/4.
(3) Axial CT of T4/5.
(4) Axial MRI of T2/3.
(5) Axial MRI of T3/4.
(6) Axial MRI of T4/5.

Shown on preoperative axial CT image, the OLF measures: 7.2 mm thick (anteroposterior) and 16.5 mm wide (mediolateral) at T2/3 where it is extended and eccentric to the right; 6.4 mm thick and 30.8 mm wide at T3/4; and 9.3 mm thick and 31.3 mm wide at T4/5. The lesion at T3/4 extends transversely posterior to T3 and into the spinal canal along the right pedicle of T4 (Fig. 3.60.3, panel 1 to 3).

Shown on preoperative axial MR image, severely impinged spinal cord with obliteration of the anterior and posterior CSF columns (Fig. 3.60.3, panel 4 to 6).

Highlights

This case features the fused or tuberous OLF from T2/3 to T5/6. This wide-based lesion extends anteriorly along the pedicles from C2/3 and C3/4.

Surgical planning

Conventionally, this case can be treated with total laminectomy that allows direct resection of the ossified ligamentum flavum.

Given the fused and tuberous components, the ossification has potentially adhered to the dura mater. If the conventional strategy is used, the ossification should be meticulously dissected from the dura mater lest durotomy and CSF leak.

The bridge crane technique with the hoisting of C2 to C4 laminae was planned for this patient. As the OLF extended beyond the bilateral pedicles at T2/3 and T3/4, parts of the pedicles were also resected to ensure adequate decompression (Fig. 3.60.4).

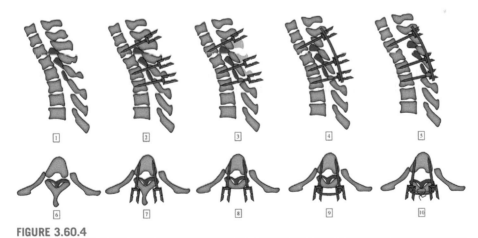

FIGURE 3.60.4

Illustration of the surgical plan on sagittal and axial planes.

(1, 6) Illustration of the OPLL on sagittal and axial views before surgery.

(2, 7) Pedicle screws inserted in T2 and from T4 to T5.

(3, 8) Spinous processes from T2 to T4 resected.

(4, 9) Rods and cross-links placed.

(5, 10) Hoisting of T2 to T4 laminae and fixed.

Results

Postoperative function: m-JOA of 9.

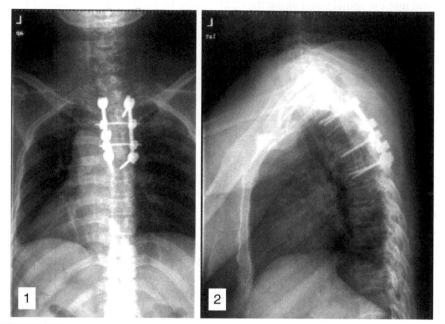

FIGURE 3.60.5

Postoperative thoracic X-ray.
(1) Anteroposterior view.
(2) Lateral view.

Upper thoracic kyphosis of 13.2°, the instrumentation on T2 and from T4 to T5, and hoisted T2 to T4 laminae (Fig. 3.60.5).

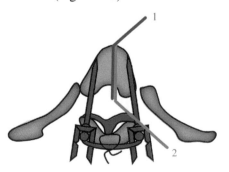

Reference of the sagittal plane

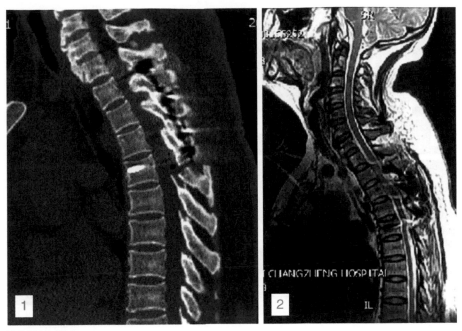

FIGURE 3.60.6

Postoperative sagittal Images and their reference on the axial diagram.
(1) Midsagittal CT.
(2) Midsagittal MRI.

Dorsally displaced T2 to T4 laminae and expanded spinal canal shown on postoperative sagittal CT image (Fig. 3.60.6, panel 1).

Expanded spinal canal from T2/3 to T5/6 and spinal cord surrounded by CSF shown on postoperative sagittal MR image (Fig. 3.60.6, panel 2).

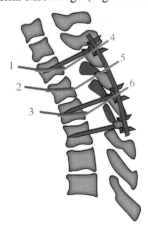

Reference of the axial planes

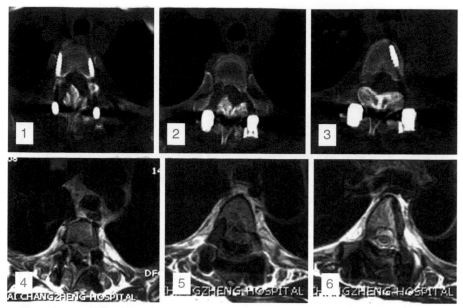

FIGURE 3.60.7

Postoperative axial thoracic images and their reference on the sagittal diagram.
(1) Axial CT of T2/3.
(2) Axial CT of T3/4.
(3) Axial CT of T4/5.
(4) Axial MRI of T2/3.
(5) Axial MRI of T3/4.
(6) Axial MRI of T4/5.

Based on postoperative axial CT images, the posterior element has been dissected at multiple levels at the junction between the lamina and the articular process; the dissected complex, made up of the ossification and laminae, has been displaced dorsally by 4.8 mm (Fig. 3.60.7, panel 1 to 3). Based on postoperative axial CT images, the spinal cord has resumed natural morphology surrounded by CSF (Fig. 3.60.7, panel 4 to 6).

Discussion

What are the values of the bridge crane technique in thoracic OLF compared with the conventional strategies?

Conventionally, thoracic OLF has been mostly managed with direct decompression from posterior. In cases as severe as this one, laminectomy is likely to cause dural tear and even aggravation of myelopathy.

Such risks are averted with the bridge crane technique where the laminae are dissected and immobilized to the posterior instrumentation. As such, the ossification is dorsally displaced without laminectomies. In other words, decompression is achieved without risk to dural tear and neurological deterioration.

In addition, due to the adhesion and ossification of the dura mater, the dorsal displacement of laminae expands the spinal canal in a fashion similar to setting up a tent. This helps avoid spinal cord compression due to postoperative hematoma.

How can we ensure the laminae and ligamentum flavum are sufficiently displaced?

The displacement of the dissected laminae hinges on the distance between the cross-links and the residual laminae.

First, the spinous processes are removed at the junction with the laminae to allow for adequate migration. During the displacement maneuver, a suture is threaded through the residual laminae and tied with a sliding knot on the cross-links. The displacement is achieved as the sutures are tightened and held with a clamp between tightenings. With fluoroscopy, sufficient displacement is confirmed, and knots are tied firmly.

Care should be taken to avoid the excessive displacement of the laminae. Otherwise, due to the adhesion and ossification of the dura mater, the spine may be subject to unfavorable stress on nerve roots or durotomy.

Case 61: Ossification of ligamentum flavum of thoracic spine (at T2/3 to T5/6)

Index terms

Bridge crane technique.

History

Patient: A 52-year-old man.

Chief complaint: Numbness and weakness of the lower limbs for two months.

Physical exam: The patient was wheeled in the clinic. Physical exam revealed an impaired sensation of the body below T8. Muscle strength was tested at 2/5 on the lower limbs. Hyperreflexia was noted on bilateral triceps and biceps brachii, brachioradialis, and lower extremities. Hoffmann and Babinski signs were positive bilaterally.

Preoperative function: m-JOA scored at 4.

Imaging studies

Upper thoracic kyphosis of 16.4° and OLF from T2 to T6 (Fig. 3.61.1).

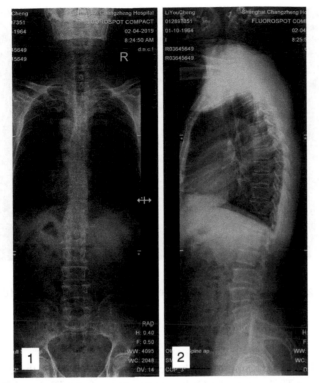

FIGURE 3.61.1

Full-length X-ray of the spine before surgery.
(1) Anteroposterior view.
(2) Lateral view.

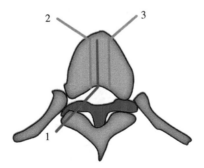

Reference of the sagittal plane

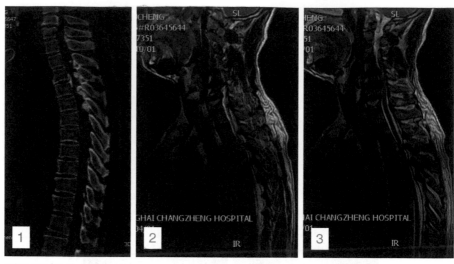

FIGURE 3.61.2

Preoperative sagittal images of the thoracic spine and their reference on the axial diagram.
(1) Midsagittal CT.
(2) Right parasagittal CT.
(3) Left parasagittal CT.

OPLL and OLF across multiple thoracic levels. Specifically, there is a circumscribed OPLL at T3/4, while the OLF is more severe from T2/3 to T5/6 shown on preoperative sagittal CT image (Fig. 3.61.2, panel 1).

Multiple hypointense masses in the spinal canal and spinal cord compressed at C4 to C6 and T2/3 to T5/6. The cervical compression is primarily from the anterior indentation, while the thoracic one, both anterior and posterior, with T3/4 being the most severe shown on preoperative sagittal MR images (Fig. 3.61.3, panel 2 and 3).

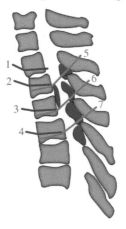

Reference of the axial planes

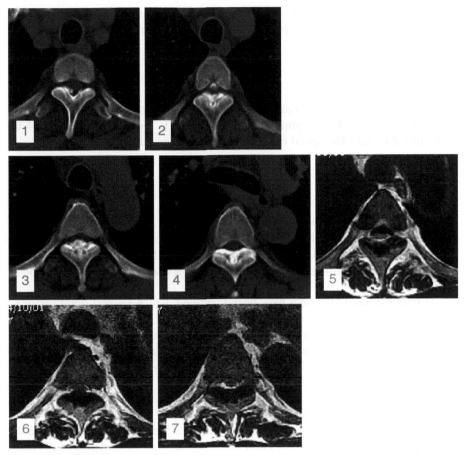

FIGURE 3.61.3

Preoperative axial images of the thoracic spine and their reference on the sagittal diagram.

(1) Axial CT of the inferior surface of T2.

(2) Axial CT of T3.

(3) Axial CT of T4.

(4) Axial CT of the inferior surface of T5.

(5) Axial MRI of the inferior surface of T3.

(6) Axial MRI of the inferior surface of T4.

(7) Axial MRI of the inferior surface of T5.

Based on axial CT images, the OLF is smaller and lateral on the right at T2/3, fused at T3/4, tuberous at T4/5, and fused at T5/6. The OLF measures 10.2 mm thick (anteroposterior) and 19.7 mm wide (mediolateral) at T3/4 in the spinal canal of 5.8 mm long anteroposteriorly; 13.5 mm thick and 19.7 mm wide at T4/5 in the spinal canal of 5.5 mm long; and 12.4 mm thick and 31.4 mm wide at T5/6 where the spinal canal is 8.0 mm long (Fig. 3.61.3, panel 1 to 4).

Based on axial MR images, severely impinged and deformed spinal cord with obliteration of the anterior and posterior CSF columns (Fig. 3.61.3, panel 5 to 7).

Highlights

This case features extensive ossification of ligaments composed of OPLL of T3/4 and OFL at T2/3 to T5/6. Spinal cord compression is most severe from T3/4 to T5/6 from the OLF. The spinal cord has been deformed due to indentation.

Surgical planning

Conventionally, a direct decompression via posterior approach is performed to remove the laminae and the ossified ligamentum flavum.

Since the OLF from T3/4 to T5/6 converge toward the midline and extend into the spinal canal, it is difficult to decompress the spinal canal via a double-door laminectomy.

As multiple fused OLF foci have been identified, which suggest dural ossification, the laminectomy bears a high risk for a dural tear.

A bridge crane procedure was planned for the patient to decompress the spinal cord via dorsal displacement of the laminae and the ossified ligamentum flavum. The decompression was achieved without resectioning the ossification, which reduced the risk of durotomy and CSF leak.

A tunnel was developed on both sides of the spinous process at its base or its junction with the lamina. The tunnels on both sides of the spinous process were conjoined by a towel clamp and threaded with a cable. Both limbs of the cable were brought and joined over the cross-link. The laminae were displaced dorsally as the joined cable limbs are twisted. Care was exercised to prevent overtightening the cable as this would cut through the vertebrae (Fig. 3.61.4).

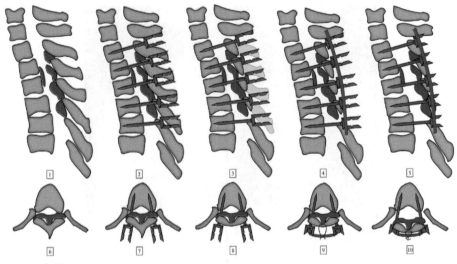

FIGURE 3.61.4

Illustration of the surgical plan on sagittal and axial planes.

(1, 6) Illustration of the OPLL on sagittal and axial views before surgery.

(2, 7) Screws inserted in T2 to T6 vertebral bodies.

(3. 8) T2 to T5 spinous processes resected.

(4, 9) Rods and cross-links installed with titanium cables threaded through the bases of the spinous processes.

(5, 10) The laminae-ossification complex from T2 to T6 dorsally displaced and fixed by titanium cables.

Results

Postoperative function: m-JOA was scored at 6.

Upper thoracic kyphosis of 11.2°, instrumentation from T2 to T5, devoid spinous processes, and hoisted laminae from T2 to T5 (Fig. 3.61.5).

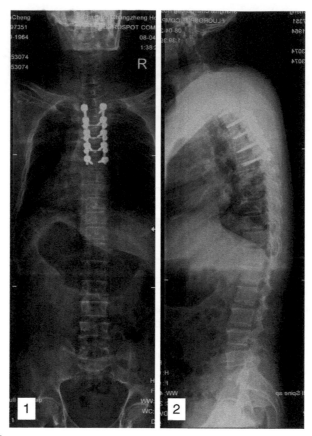

FIGURE 3.61.5

Postoperative thoracic X-ray.
(1) Anteroposterior view.
(2) Lateral view.

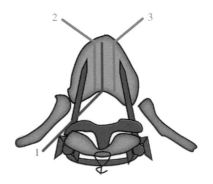

Reference of the sagittal plane

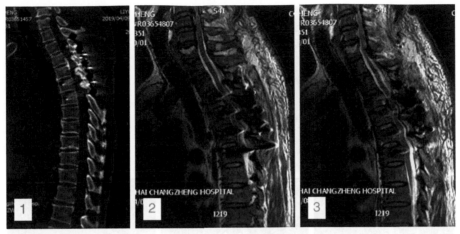

FIGURE 3.61.6

Postoperative sagittal images and their reference on the axial diagram.
(1) Midsagittal CT.
(2) Right parasagittal MRI.
(3) Left parasagittal MRI.

Postoperative CT: Ventrally displaced T2 to T5 laminae and expanded spinal canal shown on postoperative midsagittal CT image (Fig. 3.61.6, panel 1).

Expanded spinal canal from T2/3 to T5/6 and spinal cord surrounded by CSF shown on postoperative sagittal MR images (Fig. 3.61.6, panel 2).

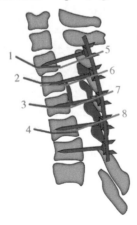

Reference of the axial planes

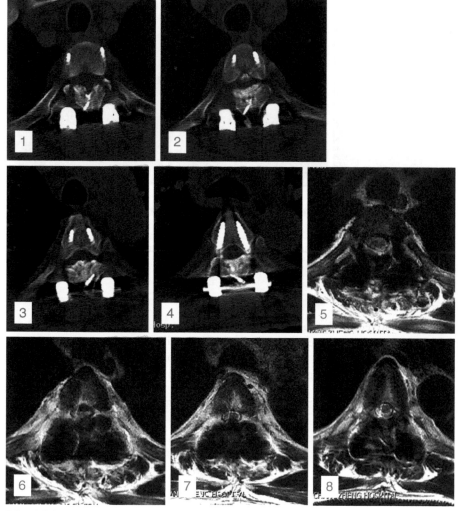

FIGURE 3.61.7

Postoperative axial thoracic images and their reference on the sagittal diagram.
(1) Axial CT of T2.
(2) Axial CT of T3.
(3) Axial CT of T4.
(4) Axial CT of T5.
(5) Axial MRI of T2.
(6) Axial MRI of T3.
(7) Axial MRI of T4.
(8) Axial MRI of T5.

Shown on postoperative axial CT images, the posterior element has been dissected at multiple levels at the junction between the lamina and the articular process; the dissected complex, made up of the 8.0 mm at T3/4, 8.8 mm at T4/5, and 10.9 mm at T5/6 (Fig. 3.61.7, panel 1 to 4). Shown on postoperative axial MR images, the spinal cord has resumed natural morphology surrounded by CSF (Fig. 3.61.7, panel 5 to 8).

Discussion

What are the values of titanium cable compared with suture for the dorsal displacement?

When thick absorbable sutures are used, the knot-tying process generates transverse or vertical micromotion of the VOC, which may still be attached to the dura. Such micromotion may exert stress on the spinal cord.

What is more, if the knots become loose or slipped, the construct is subject to inadequate or failed displacement.

In contrast, when titanium cables are used, they stabilize the construct as the cable ring is reduced, which constitutes a safer and more controllable displacement process that generates little micromotion.

Case 62: Ossification of posterior longitudinal ligament (OPLL) of cervical and thoracic spine (At C3 to C5 and T2/3 to T6/7)

Index terms

Combined surgeries of ACAF and TCAF.

History

Patient: A 54-year-old woman.

Chief complaint: Pain over the neck and the right shoulder for one month and weakness of the lower limbs for 20 days.

Physical exam: Physical exam was noted for gait disturbance, straightened cervical spine, and mildly limited range of cervical motion. Muscle strength was tested at 4/5 on the deltoid, biceps and triceps brachii, wrist flexion and extension, and hand grips on both sides; 4-/5 on bilateral iliopsoas, quadriceps femoris, biceps femoris, semitendinosus, semimembranosus, and anterior tibialis, triceps surae; and 4/5 on bilateral dorsal and plantar flexion. Brisk tendon reflexes were noted on the knees and ankles.

Preoperative function: JOA was measured at 15, Nurick score: 1, VAS: 0, and NDI: 6.

Imaging studies

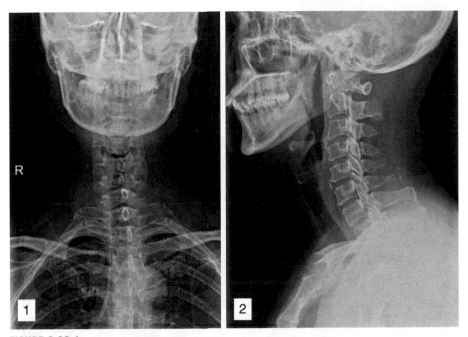

FIGURE 3.62.1

Preoperative X-ray of the cervical spine.
(1) Anteroposterior view.
(2) Lateral view.

Lordotic cervical spine, Cobb angle of 18.5° from C2 to C7, a dense band behind C2 to C6 vertebral bodies, and Pavlov ratio below 75% from C3 to C5 (Fig. 3.62.1).

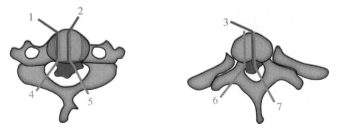

Reference of the sagittal plane of cervical and thoracic spine

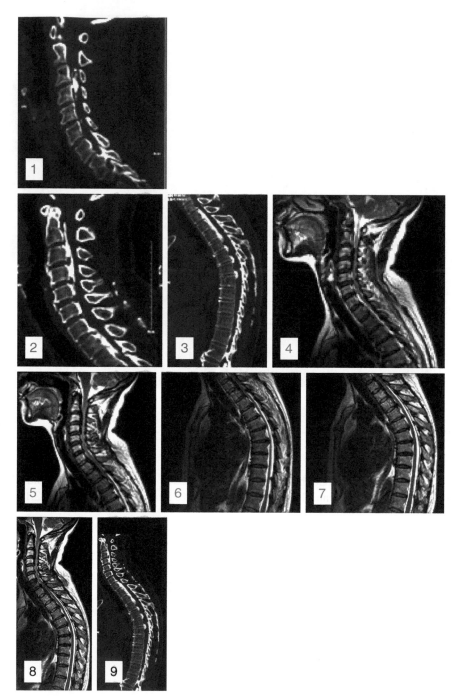

FIGURE 3.62.2

Preoperative sagittal images of the cervical and thoracic spine and their reference on the axial diagram.

(1) Parasagittal CT at the right uncinate processes.

Extensive ossification from C2 to T6 composed of OPLL of the cervical and thoracic spine. A mixed-type OPLL of C2 to C6 comprises a continuous-type component from C2 to C4 and a segmental one from C5 to C6. The lesions feature wide-based with double-layer sign noticed at multiple levels The thoracic OPLL is flat and continuous from C7/T1 to T4 whereas beak-typed from T4/5 to T6/7 shown on sagittal CT images (Fig. 3.62.2, panel 1 to 3,9).

Preoperative MRI: Hypointense masses posterior to the vertebral bodies, extensive cord compression, and straightened spinal cord curvature. The compression involves C2 to C6/7 and T1 to T3/4. Signal hyperintensity is present within the deformed spinal cord shown on sagittal MR images (Fig. 3.62.2, panel 4 to 7).

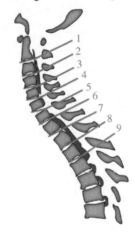

Reference of the axial planes

(2) Midsagittal CT of the neck.
(3) Midsagittal CT of the thorax.
(4) Parasagittal MRI at the right uncinate processes.
(5) Midsagittal MRI of the neck.
(6) Parasagittal MRI of the medial wall of the right pedicles.
(7) Midsagittal MRI.
(8) Midsagittal MRI of full-length spine.
(9) Midsagittal CT of full-length spine.

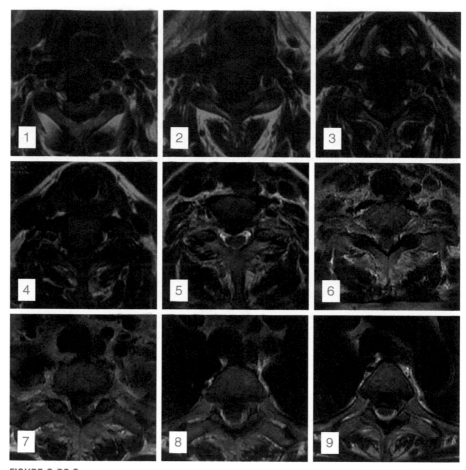

FIGURE 3.62.3

Preoperative axial images of the cervical spine and their reference on the sagittal diagram.

(1) Axial MRI of C2/3.

(2) Axial MRI of C3/4.

(3) Axial MRI of C4/5.

(4) Axial MRI of C5/6.

(5) Axial MRI of C6/7.

(6) Axial MRI of C7/T1.

(7) Axial MRI of T1/T2.

(8) Axial MRI of T2/T3.

(9) Axial MRI of T3/T4.

The cross-sectional position of preoperative MRI showed that the cervical spinal cord was compressed and deformed. The shape of the spinal cord was triangular or boomerang. The CSF band before and after the spinal cord disappeared. In the thoracic spinal cord, at the level of C7/T1 ～ T1, spinal cord was compressed anteriorly and posteriorly, and the CSF disappeared. At remaining levels, the cord was mainly compressed on the ventral side. The shape of the spinal cord features triangular, with the CSF band still appeared behind the spinal cord (Fig. 3.62.3, panel 1 to 9).

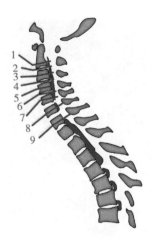

Reference of the axial planes of cervical spine

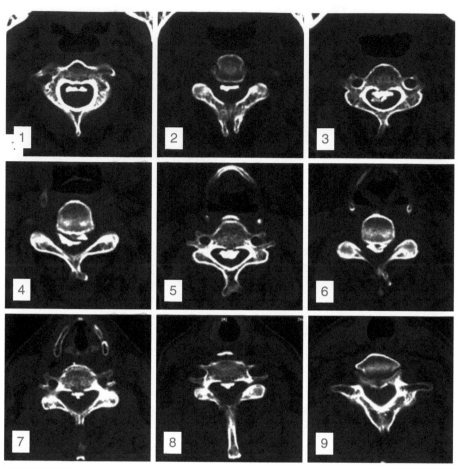

FIGURE 3.62.4

Preoperative cervical axial CT images and their reference on the sagittal profile.
(1) Axial CT of the inferior surface of C2.
(2) Axial CT of C2/3.
(3) Axial CT of C3.
(4) Axial CT of C3/4.
(5) Axial CT of C4.
(6) Axial CT of C4/5.
(7) Axial CT of C5.
(8) Axial CT of C6.
(9) Axial CT of C7.

As shown on axial CT images, the ossified mass from C2 to C5 measures: 4.1 mm thick (anteroposterior), 13.1 mm wide (mediolateral), and 39.3% in canal occupancy at C2; 7.0 mm thick, 13.7 mm wide, and 61.4% in canal occupancy at C3; 6.7 mm thick, 15.1 mm wide, and 56.3% in canal occupancy at C3/4 where the lesion is right paracentral; 4.7 mm thick, 11.9 mm wide, and 42.3% in canal occupancy at C4; and 5.8 mm thick, 7.8 mm wide, and 52.3% in canal occupancy at C5.

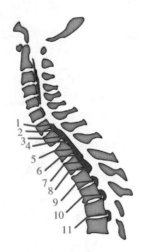

Reference of the axial planes of thoracic spine

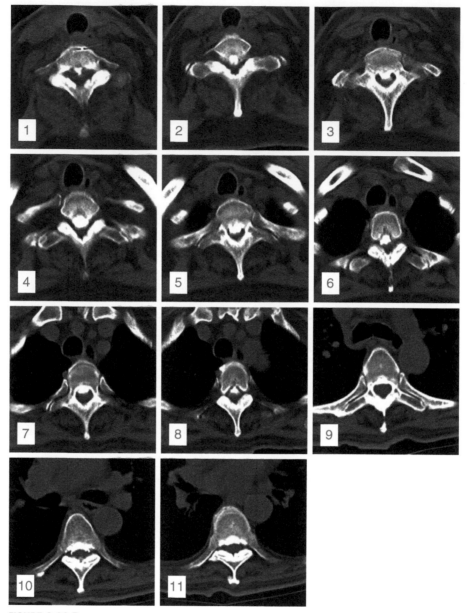

FIGURE 3.62.5

Preoperative thoracic axial CT images and their reference on the sagittal profile.
(1) Axial CT of C7.
(2) Axial CT of C7/T1.
(3) Axial CT of T1.
(4) Axial CT of T1/2.
(5) Axial CT of T2.
(6) Axial CT of T2/3.
(7) Axial CT of T3.
(8) Axial CT of T3/4.
(9) Axial CT of T4.
(10) Axial CT of T5/6.
(11) Axial CT of T6/7.

As shown on axial CT images of thoracic spine, the ossified mass measures 6.0 mm thick, 8.6 mm wide, and 47.6% in canal occupancy at C7; 5.8 mm thick, 10.8 mm wide, and 55.2% in canal occupancy at T1; 6.9 mm thick, 11.1 mm wide, and 49.3% in canal occupancy at T2; 4.8 mm thick, 14 mm wide, and 38.1% in canal occupancy at T3; and 6.1 mm thick, 15.6 mm wide, and 40.7% in canal occupancy at T4 (Fig. 3.62.4, panel 1 to 9; and Fig. 3.62.5, panel 1 to 11).

Highlights

This case features extensive flat-type OPLL that spans from the upper cervical spine to the mid-thoracic levels. As shown in preoperative MRI studies, the spinal cord compression is located at C2 to C6 and C7/T1 to T4 due to the OPLL. Hypointense masses are also present at other levels but have not generated cord compression or deformation. CSF still surrounds the spinal cord at these levels. Therefore, the surgery should involve C2 to C6 and C7/T1 to T4.

Surgical planning

In this case of K-line (+) OPLL that involves more than three levels, including the upper cervical spine, and double-layer sign, a direct decompression through anterior approach carries significant technical challenge and risk of complications such as neural or dural injury and hardware-associated morbidities. Conventionally, a posterior approach is better than an anterior one.

In addition, the thoracic component constitutes another challenge to direct anterior decompression, which often comes with increased morbidities. As such, the conventional indirect posterior decompression is favored over an anterior procedure. On top of these, the levels of incomplete decompression can be managed with circumferential decompression.

This patient received a three-level ACAF, from C3 to C5, and a TCAF from C7 to T4.

Though the OPLL extended to the C2 level, the impingement was relevant to C2/3. Therefore, the decompression involved interspace preparation and dissection of the lesion at C2/3 instead of resecting the ossification posterior to the C2 vertebra. Care should be taken to balance the need for successful antedisplacement of the thoracic levels and the increased stress on the bent point of the plate in case of rod breakage (Fig. 3.62.6).

In the first stage procedure, we prepared the C6/7 disc space, removed disc materials, dissected the OPLL, and placed a cage (Fig. 3.62.7).

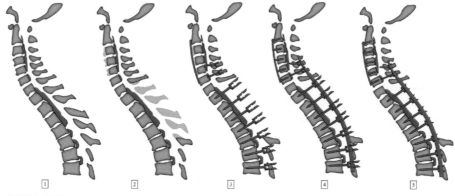

FIGURE 3.62.6

Illustration of the surgical plan on sagittal planes.

(1) Illustration of the OPLL on sagittal and axial views before surgery.

(2) Resection of the anterior part of the vertebral bodies of C3 to C5; the inferior surface of the C7 spinous process, T1 to T4 spinous processes, and the superior surface of T5 spinous process; a left groove and a right half-groove with the posterior cortex still intact on C3 to C5.

(3) Plate and the left screws inserted in vertebral bodies from C2 to C6, and pedicle screws placed on C5 to C6 and from T1 to T7.

(4) Completion of the right groove on C3 to C5, T1 to T4 laminae resected, and rods and cross-links placed.

(5) Antedisplaced C3 to C5 and C7 to T4 vertebral bodies as screws were tightened.

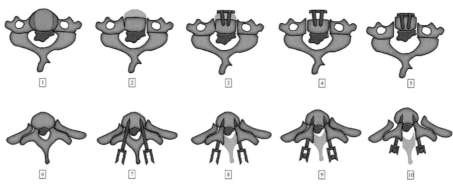

FIGURE 3.62.7

Illustration of the surgical plan on axial planes.

(1) The cervical OPLL on axial views before surgery.

(2) Resection of the anterior cortex of the vertebral bodies, a left groove and a right half-groove with the posterior cortex still intact.

(3) Plate and screws placed in the vertebral bodies.

(4) Completion of the right groove on the vertebral bodies.

(5) Antedisplaced VOC.

(6) The thoracic OPLL on axial views before surgery.

(7) Pedicle screws placed.

(8) Spinous process and the lamina resected with bone cuts on both sides.

(9) Rods and cross-links placed.

(10) Antedisplaced VOC as set screws are placed.

Results

Postoperative function: JOA score was 15, Nurick score: 1, VAS: 0, and NDI: 8.

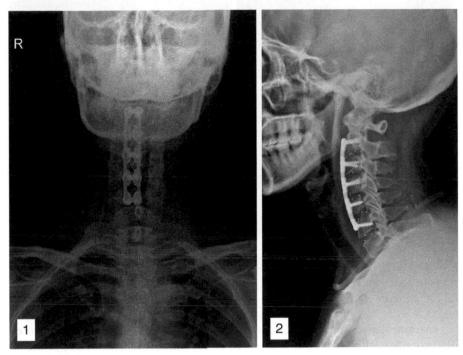

FIGURE 3.62.8

Postoperative cervical spine X-ray.
(1) Anteroposterior view.
(2) Lateral view.

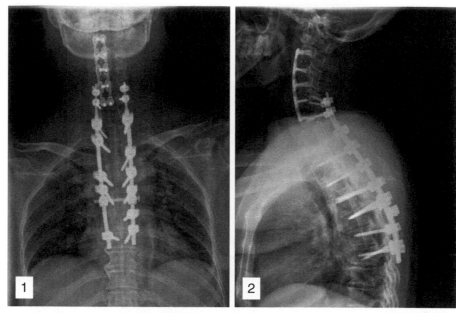

FIGURE 3.62.9

Postoperative thoracic spine X-ray.
(1) Anteroposterior view.
(2) Lateral view.

Instrumentation from C2 to C6, antedisplaced C3 to C5 vertebral bodies, posterior instrumentation from C5 to C6, and T1 to T7, and devoid laminae and posterior elements from T1 to T5. At the level of C6/7, a cage was only placed without internal fixation (Figs. 3.62.8 and 3.62.9).

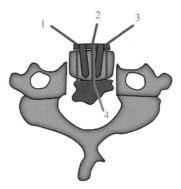

Reference of the sagittal plane

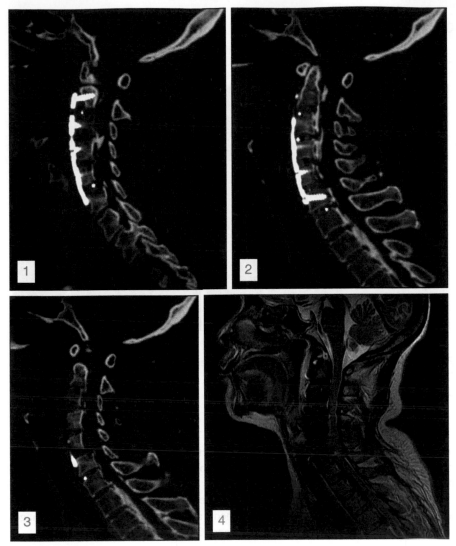

FIGURE 3.62.10

Postoperative sagittal cervical images and their reference on the axial diagram.

(1) Right parasagittal CT.

(2) Midsagittal CT.

(3) Left parasagittal CT.

(4) Midsagittal MRI.

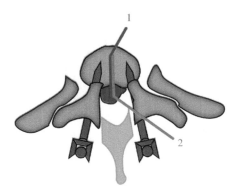

Reference of the sagittal plane

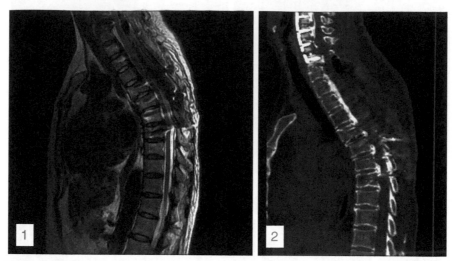

FIGURE 3.62.11

Postoperative sagittal thoracic images and their reference on the axial diagram.
(1) Midsagittal CT.
(2) Midsagittal MRI.

Antedisplaced VOCs of C3 to C5 and C7 to T4, expanded spinal canal, the proximal tip of OPLL left posterior to C2 and dissected at C2/3, and devoid spinous processes and laminae from C7 to T4, as shown on sagittal CT images (Fig. 3.62.10, panel 1 to 3, and Fig. 3.62.11, panel 1).

Spinal cord free of compression with restored cervical lordosis, and the anterior and posterior CSF columns have resumed, as shown on sagittal MR images (Fig. 3.62.10, panel 4; and Fig. 3.62.11, panel 2).

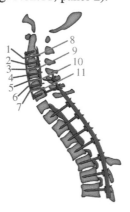

Reference of the axial planes

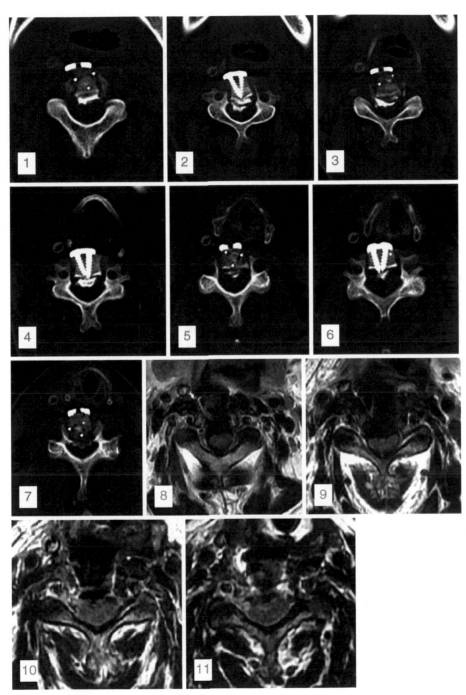

FIGURE 3.62.12

Postoperative axial cervical images and their reference on the sagittal diagram.
(1) Axial CT of C2/3.
(2) Axial CT of C3.

Details of the ACAF are shown on axial views. Parallel bone cuts are seen 18.6 mm apart on C3 and 21.2 mm apart on C4 to C5. The cervical VOC has been antedisplaced by 4.7 mm. The spinal canal stenosis has been reduced to 46.1% at C3, 24.1% at C4, and 0% at C5 (Fig. 3.62.12, panel 1 to 5, and Fig. 3.62.13, panel 1 to 11).The spinal cord has recovered to oval shape surrounded by CSF (Fig. 3.62.12, panel 1 to 7; and Fig. 3.62.13, panel 1 to 4).

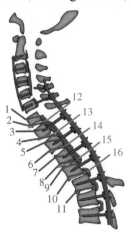

Reference of the axial planes

(3) Axial CT of C3/4.
(4) Axial CT of C4.
(5) Axial CT of C4/5.
(6) Axial CT of C5.
(7) Axial CT of C5/6.
(8) Axial MRI of C2/3.
(9) Axial MRI of C3/4.
(10) Axial MRI of C4/5.
(11) Axial MRI of C5/6.

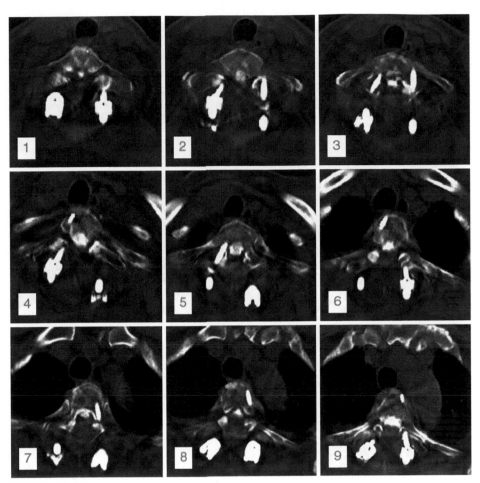

FIGURE 3.62.13

Postoperative axial thoracic images and their reference on the sagittal diagram.

(1) Axial CT of C7.

(2) Axial CT of C7/1.

(3) Axial CT of T1.

(4) Axial CT of T1/2.

(5) Axial CT of T2.

(6) Axial CT of T2/3.

(7) Axial CT of T3.

(8) Axial CT of the inferior surface of T3.

(9) Axial CT of the superior surface of T4.

(10) Axial CT of T4/5.

(11) Axial CT of T5/6.

(12) Axial MRI of C7/T1.

(13) Axial MRI of T1/2.

(14) Axial MRI of T2/3.

(15) Axial MRI of T3/4.

(16) Axial MRI of T4/5.

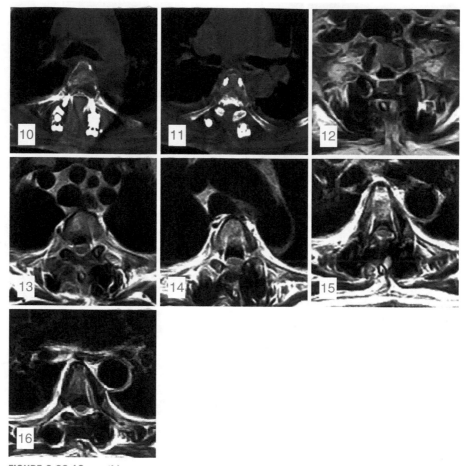

FIGURE 3.62.13 cont'd.

Shown on axial CT and MR image, the thoracic VOC has been antedisplaced by 5.7 mm and spinal cord resumes to oval shape with normal CSF around it.

Discussion

A cage was placed in C6/7 disc space in the first-stage procedure. Why was the segment excluded from the plate construct?

The C6/7 preparation primarily served the antedisplacement of C7 to T4. It was prepared during the first-stage procedure so that the second-stage procedure does not have to address it.

If C7 were immobilized with the plate during the first-stage surgery, the intended thoracal VOC antedisplace would fail.

The patient used a brace during the two-week interval between the two stages. The second-stage procedure should be performed soon after two weeks to prevent fusion or pseudoarthrosis of C6/7 as long as the patient could tolerate it. A sustained fusion at C6/7 was achieved with posterior screw and rod construct placed during the second-stage procedure.

Case 63: Ossification of posterior longitudinal ligament (OPLL) of cervical and spine (at C3 to C5) and ossification of ligamentum flavum (OLF) of thoracic Spine (at T2/3 to T6/7)

Index terms

Antedisplacement of three vertebral bodies, continuous OPLL, the thickness of ossification 5 to 7 mm, canal stenosis above 50% to 60%, ACAF + bridge crane technique, and oblique bone cuts.

History

Patient: A 58-year-old man.

Chief complaint: Numbness of all the extremities and gait disturbance for one year.

Physical exam: Physical exam was noted for gait disturbance and impaired superficial sensation of all the extremities with muscle strength of 4/5. Hoffmann and Babinski signs were present bilaterally.

Preoperative function: JOA score was 12, Nurick score: 3, VAS: 0, and NDI: 9.

Imaging studies

Cobb angle of 25.6° from C2 to C7 and a K-line (+) OPLL from C3 to C5, OLF at T3/4 to T6/7, and T1 to T3 vertebral bodies poorly appreciable due to superimposed structures (Fig. 3.63.1).

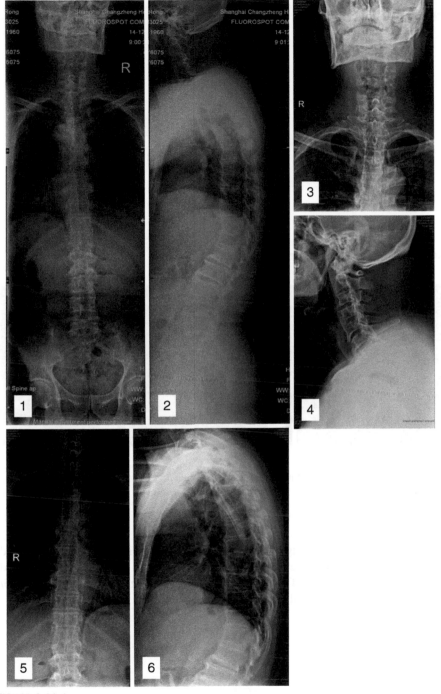

FIGURE 3.63.1

Preoperative X-ray of the spine.
(1) Full-length anteroposterior view.
(2) Full-length lateral view.
(3) Anteroposterior cervical view.
(4) Lateral cervical view.
(5) Anteroposterior thoracic view.
(6) Lateral thoracic view.

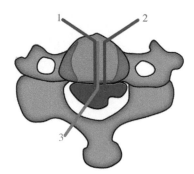

Reference of the sagittal plane

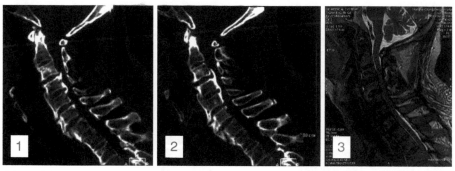

FIGURE 3.63.2

Preoperative sagittal images of the cervical spine and their reference on the axial diagram.

(1) Midsagittal CT.

(2) Left parasagittal CT.

(3) Midsagittal MRI.

Based on preoperative sagittal images, extensive ectopic ossification composed of a flat and continuous-type OPLL from C3 to C5, more protuberant at C3/4 and C4/5. Disc protrusion from C3/4 to C6/7, hypertrophic ligamentum flavum of C5/6 to C6/7, compressed spinal cord (Fig. 3.63.2, panel 1 to 3).

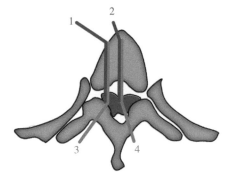

Reference of the sagittal plane

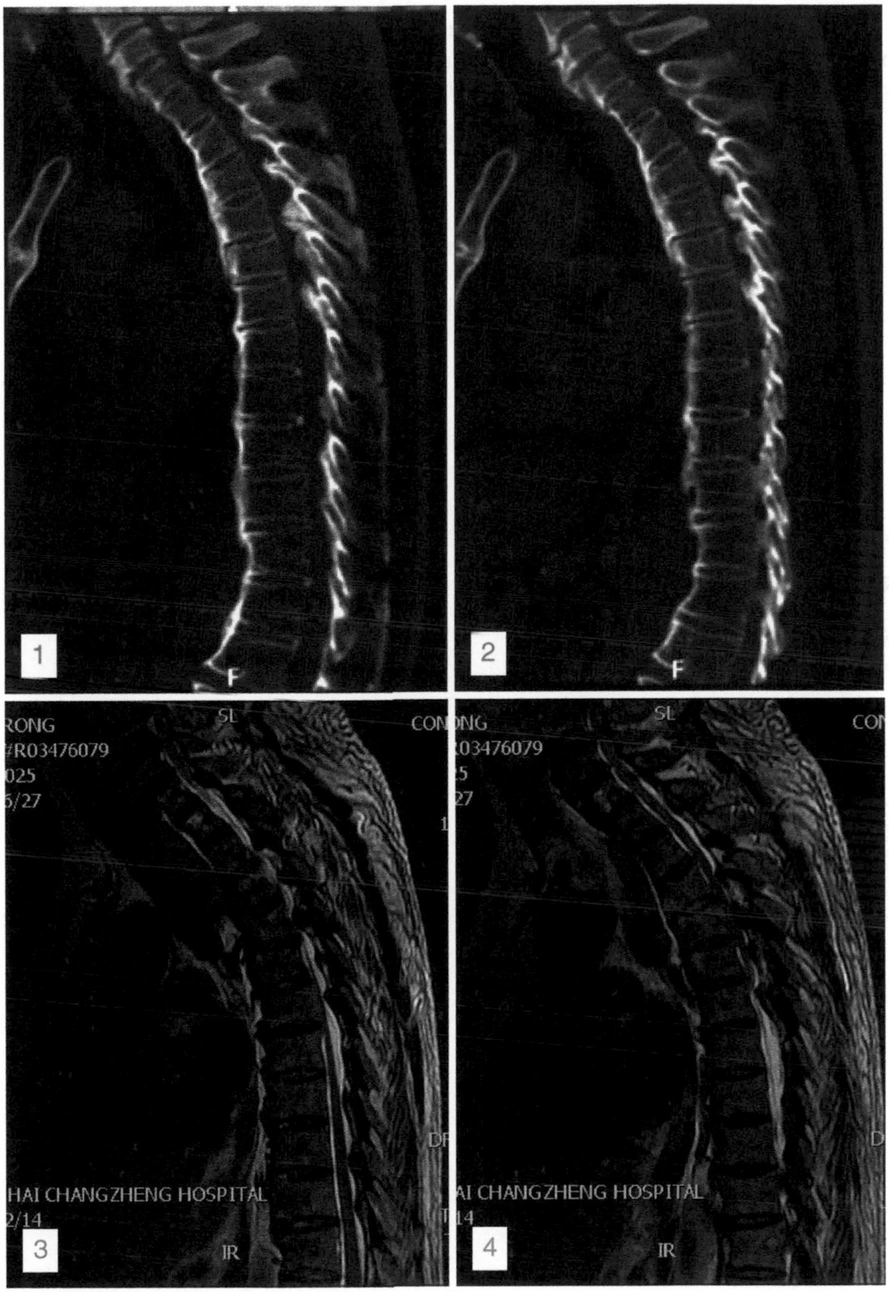

FIGURE 3.63.3

Preoperative sagittal images of the thoracic spine and their reference on the axial diagram.
(1) Right parasagittal CT.
(2) Midsagittal CT.
(3) Right parasagittal MRI.
(4) Midsagittal MRI.

OLF from T2/3 to T6/7. Obliterated anterior and posterior CSF columns, and hypertrophic and ossified ligamentum flavum from T2/3 to T6/7 protuberant into the spinal canal, most severe at T4/5 and T6/7 (Fig. 3.63.3, panel 1 to 4).

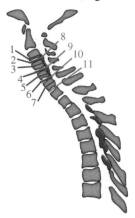

Reference of the axial planes of cervical spine

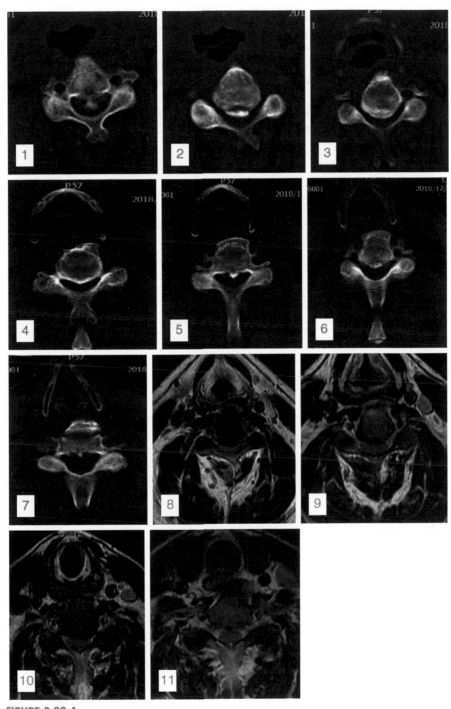

FIGURE 3.63.4

Preoperative axial images of the cervical spine and their reference on the sagittal diagram.

Preoperative axial CT: the cervical OPLL measures: 5.8 mm thick (anteroposterior), 12.2 mm wide (mediolateral), and 47.2% in canal occupancy at C3/4; 4.2 mm thick, 12.5 mm wide, and 42% in canal occupancy at C4; 5.8 mm thick, 19.7 mm wide, and 50% in canal occupancy at C4/5; 5.8 mm thick, 7.4 mm wide, and 50% in canal occupancy at C5; and 5.8 mm thick, 7.8 mm wide, and 52.3% in canal occupancy at C5.

Preoperative axial MRI: the spinal cord impinged and deformed into a boomerang or triangle shape from C3/5 to C5/6 (Fig. 3.63.4, panel 8 to 11).

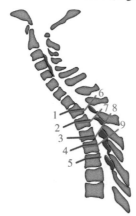

Reference of the axial planes

(1) Axial CT of the inferior surface of C3.
(2) Axial CT of C3/4.
(3) Axial CT of C4.
(4) Axial CT of C4/5.
(5) Axial CT of C5.
(6) Axial CT of C5/6.
(7) Axial CT of C6.
(8) Axial MRI of C3/4.
(9) Axial MRI of C4/5.
(10) Axial MRI of C5/6.
(11) Axial MRI of C6/7.

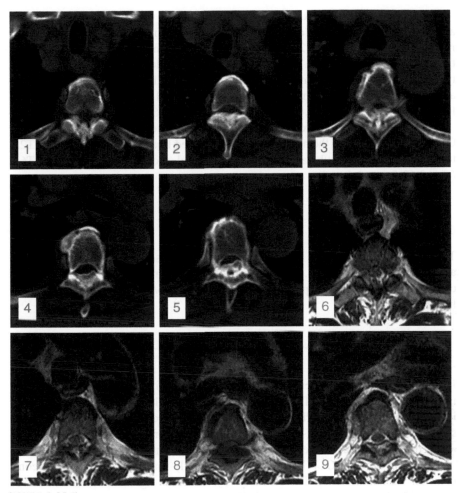

FIGURE 3.63.5

Preoperative axial images of the thoracic spine and their reference on the sagittal diagram.
(1) Axial CT of T2.
(2) Axial CT of the superior surface of T3.
(3) Axial CT of the inferior surface of T4.
(4) Axial CT of the superior surface of T5.
(5) Axial CT of the superior surface of T6.
(6) Axial MRI of T2.
(7) Axial MRI of T3.
(8) Axial MRI of T4/5.
(9) Axial MRI of the superior surface of T5.

Based on preoperative axial thoracic CT images, the OLF features enlarged type at T2/3 with 9 mm long (anteroposterior) spinal canal; tuberous type at T3/4 measuring 12.8 mm thick, 22.7 mm wide with 7.7 mm long spinal canal; fused type at T4/5 measuring 22.7 mm wide with 9.0 mm long spinal canal; tuberous type at T5/6 measuring 8.1 mm thick, 17.1 mm wide with 7.7 mm long spinal canal; and tuberous type at T6/7 measuring 11.3 mm thick, 15.0 mm wide with 6.0 mm long spinal canal (Fig. 3.63.4, panel 1 to 7; and Fig. 3.63.5, panel 1 to 5).

Based on preoperative axial thoracic MR images, the deformed spinal cord and CSF obliteration due to the hypertrophic and ossified ligamentum flavum from T2/3 to T6/7, which are protuberant into the spinal canal, most severe at T4/5 and T6/7 (Fig. 3.63.5, panel 6 to 9).

Highlights

This case features extensive ectopic ossification composed of OPLL from C3 to C5 and OLF from T2/3 to T6/7, complicated with developmental stenosis of the spinal canal from C4 to C6, disc protrusion from C5/6 to C6/7, and ligamentum flavum hypertrophy.

Surgical planning

In the case, cervical spinal canal stenosis and thoracic ligamentum flavum ossification were to be addressed. The cervical procedure would involve C3 to C6, which included the continuous OPLL from C3 to C5 and decompression of the stenosed spinal canal at C6. The long-segment and K-line (+) components necessitate an indirect decompression via the posterior approach conventionally.

The long-segment OLF has been conventionally managed with direct decompression via laminectomy. The centrally fused ossified ligamentum flavum leaves the double-door laminectomy too challenging and the single-door laminectomy too risky (Fig. 3.63.6).

An ACAF of C4 to C6 and undercutting technique for the C3 compression was planned for the cervical disease and a bridge crane technique for T2 to T6 VOC for the thoracic OLF (Fig. 3.63.7).

Results

Postoperative function: JOA score was 16, Nurick score: 0, VAS: 0, and NDI: 2.

Instrumentation from C3 to C7, antedisplaced C4 to C6 vertebral bodies, posterior instrumentation from T2 to T6, and dorsally displaced T3 to T6 laminae (Fig. 3.63.8, panel 1 to 4).

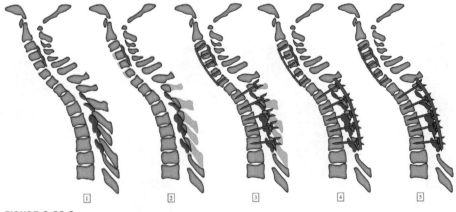

FIGURE 3.63.6

Illustration of the surgical plan on sagittal planes.

(1) Illustration of the diseases on sagittal views before surgery.

(2) Resection of the anterior part of the vertebral bodies of C4 to C6; a left groove and a right half-groove with the posterior cortex still intact on C4 to C6.

(3) Plate and left screws inserted on C4 to C6, and pedicle screws on T2 to T6.

(4) Completion of the right groove on C4 to C6, bilateral bone cuts along the laminae from T2 to T6, and rods and cross-links installed.

(5) VOC of C4 to C6 antedisplaced as screws are tightened and T2 to T6 laminae dorsally displaced via cables.

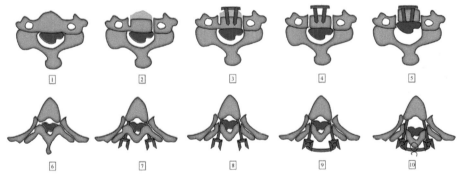

FIGURE 3.63.7

Illustration of the surgical plan on axial planes.

(1) The cervical disease on axial views before surgery.

(2) Resection of the anterior cortex of the vertebral bodies, a left groove and a right half-groove with the posterior cortex still intact.

(3) Plate and screws placed in the vertebral bodies.

(4) Completion of the right groove on the vertebral bodies.

(5) Antedisplaced VOC.

(6) The thoracic disease on axial views before surgery.

(7) Pedicle screws inserted and spinous processes resected.

(8) Bone cuts on both sides on the laminae.

(9) Rods and cross-links placed.

(10) VOC dorsally displaced via cables.

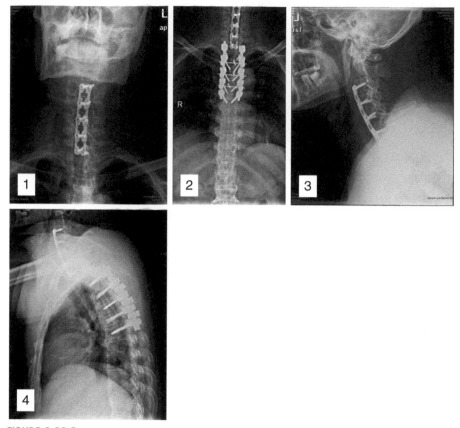

FIGURE 3.63.8

Postoperative X-ray.
(1) Cervical anteroposterior view.
(2) Thoracic anteroposterior view.
(3) Cervical lateral view.
(4) Thoracic lateral view.

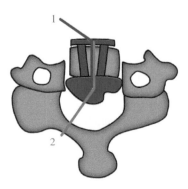

Reference of the sagittal plane

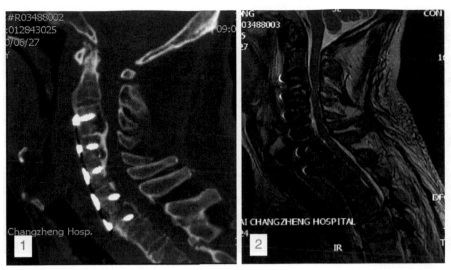

FIGURE 3.63.9

Postoperative sagittal cervical images and their reference on the axial diagram.
(1) Midsagittal CT.
(2) Midsagittal MRI.

Undercutting posterior part of the C3 vertebra, antedisplaced C4 to C6 vertebral bodies, and expanded spinal canal, as shown on postoperative sagittal cervical CT images (Fig. 3.63.9, panel 1).

Spinal cord free of compression between the anterior and posterior columns of CSF from C2 to C6 and from T2/3 to T5/6, and spinal cord with residual deformation due to indentation though surrounded by CSF at C/4, as shown on postoperative sagittal cervical MRI images (Fig. 3.63.9, panel 2).

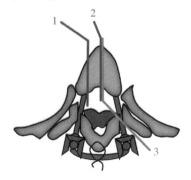

Reference of the sagittal plane

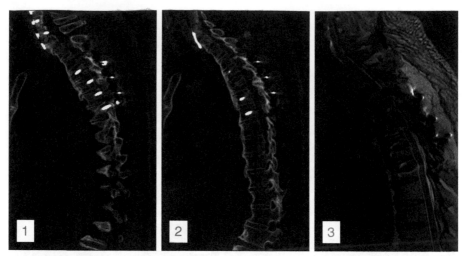

FIGURE 3.63.10

Postoperative thoracic sagittal images and their reference on the axial diagram.
(1) Right parasagittal CT.
(2) Midsagittal CT.
(3) Midsagittal MRI.

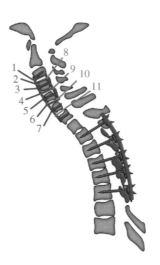

Reference of the axial planes

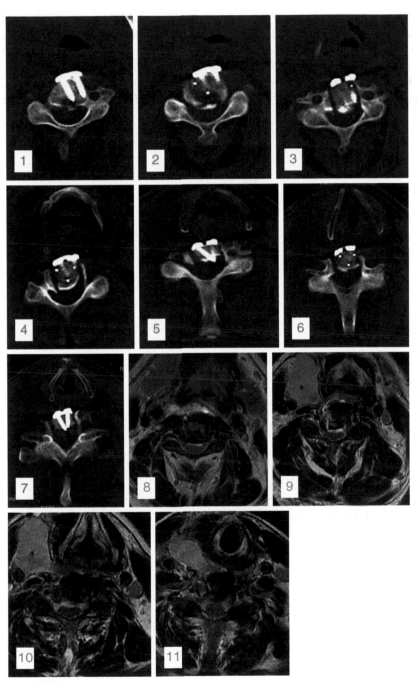

FIGURE 3.63.11

Postoperative axial cervical images and their reference on the sagittal diagram.

With sagittal bone cuts 17.7 mm apart, the C3/4 and C4 ossification have been antedisplaced by 2.8 mm, and spinal canal stenosis reduced to 38.5%; and the C4/5 to C6 complex has been antedisplaced by 5.3 mm, and stenosis is reduced to 0% (Fig. 3.63.11, panel 1 to 7).

The spinal cord resumes to triangular or oval shape surrounded by CSF (Fig. 3.63.10, panel 3 to 5; Fig. 3.63.11, panel 8 to 11; and Fig. 3.63.12, panel 6 to 10).

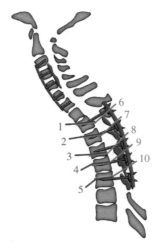

Reference of the axial planes

(1) Axial CT of the inferior surface of C3.
(2) Axial CT of C3/4.
(3) Axial CT of C4.
(4) Axial CT of C4/5.
(5) Axial CT of C5.
(6) Axial CT of C6/7.
(7) Axial CT of C7.
(8) Axial MRI of C3/4.
(9) Axial MRI of C4/5.
(10) Axial MRI of C5/6.
(11) Axial MRI of C6/7.

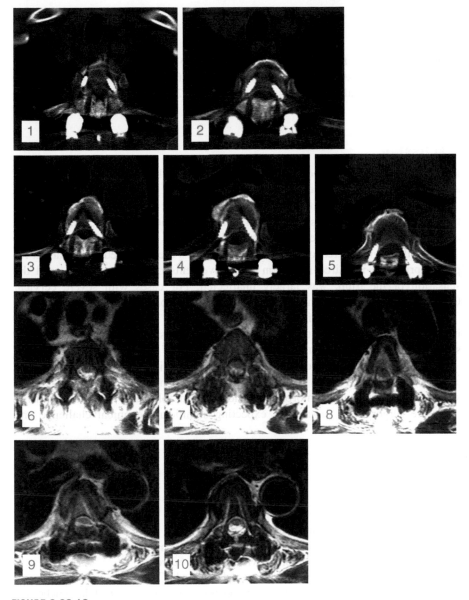

FIGURE 3.63.12

Postoperative axial thoracic images and their reference on the sagittal diagram.

(1) Axial CT of T2.
(2) Axial CT of T3.
(3) Axial CT of T4.
(4) Axial CT of the disc space of T5.
(5) Axial CT of T6.
(6) Axial MRI of T2.
(7) Axial MRI of T3.
(8) Axial MRI of T4.
(9) Axial MRI of T5.
(10) Axial MRI of T6.

With the laminae from T2/3 to T6/7 dorsally displaced by 5.4 mm, the spinal canal length (anteroposterior) has been restored to 12.0 mm at T2/3, 8.0 mm at T3/5, 10.0 mm at T4/5, and 11.2 mm at T5/6 (Fig. 3.63.12, panel 1 to 5).

Discussion

In treating cases with concomitant cervical and thoracic ligament ossifications, what are the rationales behind the decision on the surgical segments?

In extensive ectopic ossification of the ligaments that affect both the cervical and the thoracic spine, the bases for surgical planning are the levels affected, the extent of the surgery, and the patient's general health.

First, the segments responsible for the symptoms are identified. This patient reported primarily impaired sensation and movements of the extremities, and the sensation of the trunk was largely unaffected. For cases with severe cervical OPLL, a single-stage decompression for the cervical spine is preferable.

If the patient presents with significant tightness and numbness of the trunk and impaired sensation and function of the lower extremities, a single-stage decompression of the thoracic spine can provide symptom relief.

The decision on a single-stage cervical and thoracic procedure hinges on the extent of the surgical levels and the patient's general health. The surgery is often staged in patients with comorbidities and reduced tolerance, diseases requiring extensive surgery, and procedures expecting significant technical challenge and blood loss.

Addendum

Glossary

Anterior cervical discectomy and fusion (ACDF)
   asurgical procedure for the cervical spine that involves disc material resection and fusion of the adjacent vertebral bodies performed via an anterior approach.
Anterior cervical corpectomy decompression and fusion (ACCF)
   asurgical procedure for the cervical spine that involves a major resection of the vertebra and fusion of the adjacent vertebral bodies performed via an anterior approach.
Mixed decompression and fusion
   theuse of ACDF together with ACCF in managing cervical spondylosis.
Spinal cord decompression in situ
   thedecompression achieved via direct removal of compressors of any nature without subjecting the spinal cord to displacement.
Anterior controllable antedisplacement and fusion (ACAF)
   asurgical procedure for spinal cord decompression that involves ventral displacement of the cervical vertebral bodies and the ossified posterior longitudinal ligament as a whole.
Saint Venant's Principle

aload forces a change in the material's stressed state only in the regions close to the applied load.

Space available for the cord (SAC)

thespace in the spinal canal that readily accepts the occupation of the spinal cord.

Ossification of posterior longitudinal ligament (OPLL)

adisease entity where the patient presents with impaired sensation and movement of the extremities and autonomic dysfunction as the spinal cord and nerve roots have sustained impingement from the ossified posterior longitudinal ligament, primarily in the cervical spine.

Diffuse idiopathic skeletal hyperostosis (DISH)

anextensive thick bony hardening along the anterior vertebral bodies due to diffuse and conjoining osteophytes along the anterior and lateral side of vertebral bodies.

Vertebral-OPLL complex (VOC)

theintegration composed of the tightly attached posterior wall of the vertebra and the ossified posterior longitudinal ligament.

Expansive laminoplasty (ELP)

acategory of surgical procedure where the laminae are dissected and restabilized to enlarge the cross-section of the spinal canal.

Single open-door laminoplasty

atype of expansive laminoplasty where the lamina is dissected on one side, opened with the hinge developed on the other side and restabilized.

Bilateral open-door laminoplasty

atype of expansive laminoplasty where the spinous processes are split at midline, partially flipped open hinging on the bilaterally dissected lamina and restabilized.

Intervertebral cage

adevice that facilitates intervertebral fusion. For example, an Innesis cage.

Lamina

ossifiedligamentum flavum complex (LOC): the integration composed of the tightly attached lamina and the ossified ligamentum flavum.

Undercutting decompression

amechanism of decompression involved in the ACAF technique where decompression of the spinal cord at a given level is achieved by resecting the posterior part of the vertebra to accommodate the ossification of that level when it is advanced together with the vertebral-OPLL complex.

Bridge crane technique

asurgical procedure tailored to spinal cord decompression due to thoracic ossification of ligamentum flavum (OLF) where the laminae are dissected to allow the dorsal displacement of the laminae-OLF complex.

Wide-based OPLL (WBO)

onthe axial view of the vertebra divided into three parts by two parasagittal axes drawn along the uncinate processes, if the OPLL is present in the two lateral parts, it is deemed as a wide-based OPLL.

Narrow-based OPLL (NBO)

onthe axial view of the vertebra divided into three parts by two parasagittal axes drawn along the uncinate processes, if the OPLL is present only in the central part, it is deemed as a narrow-based OPLL.

Incomplete displacement

inthe ACAF procedure, the antedisplaced vertebra ending up > 1 mm away from the plate is defined as an incompletely antedisplaced vertebra. When this occurs to more than one level, the result is called incomplete displacement.

Virtual surgical planning

theparameters of the spine morphology and surgical instrument are entered in a surgical simulator, such as 3-matic software, where the surgeons have a sense of the resection and moves expected during the true surgery presented with modifiable transparency.

Shelter technique

aprocedure that involves the dissection of the ossification off the C2 vertebra and partial resection of the posterior part of C2 vertebra to accommodate the lesion of this level as the entire VOC is antedisplaced.

Appendix

Ossification characteristics

Range of ossified segments	Hoist below 3 vertebrae	Case2 Case3 Case4 Case5 Case6 Case10 Case12 Case14 Case22 Case26 Case27 Case28 Case29 Case30 Case36 Case37 Case38 Case39 Case40 Case41 Case45 Case50 Case51 Case56 Case57
	Hoist 3 vertebrae	Case1 Case7 Case8 Case9 Case11 Case23 Case24 Case25 Case32 Case33 Case35 Case42 Case43 Case44 Case46 Case47 Case48 Case49 Case52 Case53 Case54 Case55
	Hoist 4 vertebrae	Case13 Case15 Case20 Case21 Case31 Case34
	Hoist more than 4 vertebrae	Case16 Case17 Case18 Case19
Sagittal pattern of ossification	Focal ossification	Case3 Case5 Case6 Case10 Case39 Case50 Case51
	Segmental ossification	Case1 Case4 Case7 Case8 Case9 Case14 Case20 Case24 Case25 Case29 Case32 Case36 Case47
	Continuous ossification	Case2 Case12 Case18 Case23 Case26 Case27 Case28 Case30 Case35 Case37 Case40 Case41 Case45 Case49
	Mixed ossification	Case11 Case13 Case15 Case16 Case17 Case19 Case21 Case22 Case31 Case33 Case34 Case38 Case42 Case46 Case48 Case53
Cross-sectional characteristics of ossification	Wide base	Case2 Case7 Case8 Case9 Case11 Case12 Case13 Case16 Case17 Case18 Case19 Case20 Case21 Case22 Case25 Case26 Case27 Case28 Case29 Case31 Case33

949

Ossification thickness		Case34 Case37 Case38 Case40 Case41 Case45 Case46 Case48 Case49 Case53
	Ossification enters the intervertebral foramen	Case3 Case8 Case9 Case17 Case18 Case19 Case21 Case22 Case25 Case28 Case29 Case31 Case33 Case34 Case40 Case45 Case46 Case47 Case48 Case50
	Less than 5 mm	Case4 Case5 Case24 Case39
	5–7 mm	Case1 Case6 Case7 Case11 Case12 Case13 Case14 Case21 Case23 Case26 Case27 Case28 Case30 Case32 Case33 Case34 Case36 Case38 Case40 Case42 Case50
	7–9 mm	Case2 Case8 Case9 Case10 Case15 Case18 Case20 Case22 Case25 Case29 Case35 Case37 Case41 Case45 Case47 Case48 Case53
	More than 9 mm	Case3 Case16 Case17 Case19 Case31 Case46 Case49
The rate of spinal stenosis	Less than 50%	Case1 Case4 Case14 Case24 Case26 Case28 Case36 Case37 Case39
	50%–60%	Case2 Case5 Case6 Case7 Case13 Case27 Case30 Case32 Case33 Case35 Case38 Case40 Case41
	60%–70%	Case3 Case10 Case11 Case12 Case15 Case17 Case19 Case21 Case22 Case23 Case29 Case34 Case42
	More than 70%	Case8 Case9 Case16 Case18 Case20 Case25 Case31 Case51

Surgical technique

Shelter technique	Case2 Case16 Case17 Case18 Case19 Case20 Case 21 Case22 Case23 Case26 Case28 Case30 Case31 Case32 Case37 Case38 Case53
Stealth decompression technique	Case2 Case11 Case12 Case20 Case31 Case40 Case41 Case46 Case49
Bridge crane technique	Case60 Case61

Anterior hoisting of thoracic vertebrae technique	Case58 Case59
ACAF technique + ACDF technique	Case7 Case14 Case16 Case35
ACAF technique + anterior hoisting of thoracic vertebrae technique	Case62
ACAF technique + bridge crane technique	Case63
ACAF technique + atlantoaxial fusion technique	Case54

Medial history

History of deep injury	Case5 Case18 Case24 Case49
History of posterior surgery	Case45 Case46 Cases47 Case48 Case49 Case50 Case52 Case53
History of anterior surgery	Case43 Case44 Case51 Case52

Cervical curvature

Cervical kyphosis	Case8 Case11 Case12 Case17 Case18 Case22 Case25 Case34 Case35 Case43 Case45 Case50 Case53 Case55
K-line(-)	Case4 Case8 Case11 Cases15 Case16 Case17 Case18 Case19 Case22 Case23 Case25 Case31 Case32 Case33 Case34 Case37 Case45 Case53

Regrettable cases

Oblique slotting	Case9 Case15 Case17 Case18 Case20 Case21 Case31 Case45 Case52
Not enough lifting	Case6 Case11 Case 17 Case20 Case22 Case30 Case32 Case54
Residual ossification	Case8 Case14 Case17 Case19 Case37 Case53
Slotting width	Case17 Case37

Index

'*Note:* Page numbers followed by "f" indicate figures and "t" indicate tables.'

9780323880497